Clinical Surgery

Clinical Surgery

Alfred Cuschieri

MD ChM FRCS(Ed) FRCS FRCPS(Glas)
Head of Department
Department of Surgery
Ninewells Hospital and Medical School
Dundee

Thomas P.J. Hennessy

MD MCh FRCS FRCSI FACS
Regius Professor of Clinical Surgery
Department of Clinical Surgery
St James' Hospital, Dublin

Roger M. Greenhalgh

MA MD MChir FRCS
Dean and Professor of Surgery
Charing Cross and Westminster Medical School
London

David I. Rowley

BMedBiol MD FRCS
Professor of Orthopaedic Surgery
Department of Orthopaedic & Trauma Surgery
Caird Block, Royal Infirmary
Dundee

Pierce A. Grace

MCh FRCSI FRCS
Adjunct Professor of Surgical Science
University of Limerick
Limerick Regional General Hospital
Limerick

b

**Blackwell
Science**

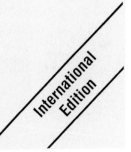

International
Edition

© 1996 by
Blackwell Science Ltd
Editorial Offices:
Osney Mead, Oxford OX2 0EL
25 John Street, London WC1N 2BL
23 Ainslie Place, Edinburgh EH3 6AJ
238 Main Street, Cambridge
  Massachusetts 02142, USA
54 University Street, Carlton
  Victoria 3053, Australia

Other Editorial Offices:
Arnette Blackwell SA
  224, Boulevard Saint Germain
  75007 Paris, France

Blackwell Wissenschafts-Verlag GmbH
  Kurfürstendamm 57
  10707 Berlin, Germany

  Zehetnergasse 6
  A-1140 Wien
  Austria

First published in 1996

Set by Expo Holdings Sdn Bhd, Malaysia
Printed and bound in Italy
by Rotolito Lombarda S.p.A., Milan

A catalogue record for this title
is available from the British Library

ISBN 0–632–03146–8 (BSL)
ISBN 0–86542–691–0 (IE)

Library of Congress
Cataloging-in-publication Data

Clinical surgery/
[edited by] Alfred Cuschieri ... [et al.].
        p.   cm.
  Includes bibliographical references
  and index.
  ISBN 0–632–03146–8
  1. Surgery. I. Cuschieri, A. (Alfred)
  [DNLM: 1. Surgery, Operative.
  WO 500 C641 1996]
617—dc20
DNLM/DLC
for Library of Congress   96–13646
                                        CIP

DISTRIBUTORS
Marston Book Services Ltd
PO Box 269
Abingdon
Oxford OX14 4YN
(*Orders*: Tel: 01235 465500
            Fax: 01235 465555)

USA
Blackwell Science, Inc.
238 Main Street
Cambridge, MA 02142
(*Orders*: Tel: 800 215–1000
            617 876–7000
            Fax: 617 492–5263)

Canada
Copp Clark, Ltd
2775 Matheson Blvd East
Mississauga, Ontario
Canada, L4W 4P7
(*Orders*: Tel: 800 263–4374
            905 238–6074)

Australia
Blackwell Science Pty Ltd
54 University Street
Carlton, Victoria 3053
(*Orders*: Tel: 03 9347 0300
            Fax: 03 9349 3016)

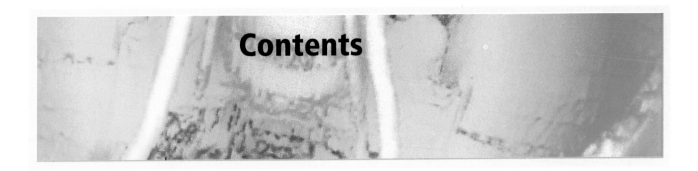

Contents

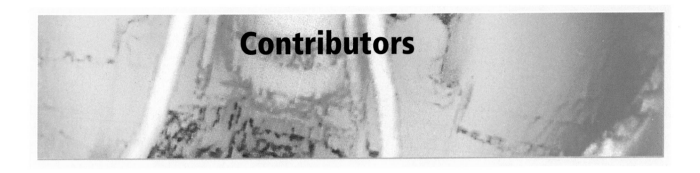

Contributors

T. Ahmad MA FRCS
Department of Plastic Surgery, St Johns Hospital, Howden, Livingston, West Lothian, Scotland

D. Bouchier-Hayes MCh FRCSI FRCS
Professor of Surgery, Royal College of Surgeons in Ireland, St Stevens Green, Dublin 2, Ireland

T. Creagh BSC MCh FRCSI
Consultant Surgeon Urologist, Kingston Hospital, Goldsworthy Road, Kingston Upon Thames, KT2 7QB

A. Cuschieri MD ChM FRCS(Ed) FRCS FRCPS(Glas)
Head of Department, Department of Surgery, Ninewells Hospital and Medical School, Dundee, DD1 9AY

J. M. Fitzpatrick MCh FRCSI
Professor of Surgery, University College Dublin, Mater Misericordiae Hospital, Surgical Professorial Unit, 47 Eccles Street, Dublin 7, Ireland

P. A. Grace MCh FRCSI FRCS
Adjunct Professor of Surgical Science, University of Limerick, Limerick Regional General Hospital Limerick, Ireland

R. M. Greenhalgh MA MD MChir FRCS
Dean and Professor of Surgery, Charing Cross and Westminster Medical School, Fulham Palace Road, London, W6 8RF

T. P. J. Hennessy MD MCh FRCS FRCSI FACS
Regius Professor of Clinical Surgery, Department of Clinical Surgery, St James' Hospital, Dublin 8, Ireland

P. Hornick BSC MB BChir FRCS
Department of Cardiothoracic Surgery, B Block 2nd Floor Surgical Directorate, Hammersmith Hospital, DuCane Road, London, W12 0HS

R. Illingworth MB BS FRCS
Consultant Neurosurgeon, Regional Neurosciences Department, Charing Cross Hospital, Fulham Palace Road, London, W6 8RF

P. Kinnear FRCS FRCOphth
Ophthalmic Surgeon, Charing Cross Hospital, Fulham Palace Road, London, W6 1RF

B. G. H. Lamberty MA FRCS
Consultant Plastic Surgeon, Department of Plastic & Reconstructive Surgery, Addenbrooke's Hospital, Hills Road, Cambridge, CB2 2QQ

T. J. K. Leonard MRCP FRCS FRCOphth
Consultant Ophthalmic Surgeon, 149 Harley Street, London, W1N 2DE

P. Richards MB BS FRCS
Consultant Paediatric Neurosurgeon, Radcliffe Infirmary, Woodstock Road, Oxford, OX2 6HE

D. I. Rowley BMed Biol MD FRCS
Professor of Orthopaedic Surgery, Department of Orthopaedic & Trauma Surgery, Caird Block, Royal Infirmary, Dundee, DD1 9ND

A. Sarazen, Jr MD
38 Powell Avenue, Newport Road Island, RI 02840, USA

K. Taylor MD MB ChB FRCS
Professor of Surgery, British Heart Foundation, Royal Postgraduate Medical School, Hammersmith Hospital, London, W12 0NN

J. A. Wilson FRCS MD
Professor of Otolaryngology, Department of Head and Neck Surgery, Freeman Hospital, High Heaton, Newcastle Upon Tyne, NE7 7DN

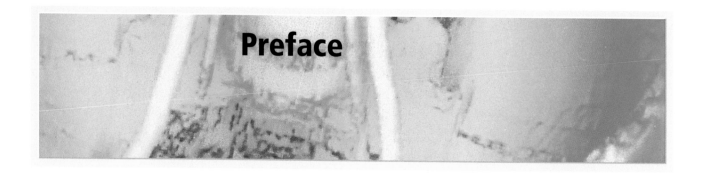

Preface

Why another undergraduate textbook? This is a valid question; its answer is linked to the significant changes in undergraduate medical education encompassing the 'Core plus Special Study Modules' system suggested by the Educational Committee of the General Medical Council some years back, and currently being implemented by all UK medical schools. The philosophy behind the new curriculum is designed to ensure core teaching and acquisition of practical cognitive and psychomotor skills in the clinical subjects by all the medical students. At the same time, Special Study Modules are included. These provide students with the opportunity for active, independent, albeit-tutor guided, studies on subjects of their choice which are relevant to the practice of medicine. Aside from ensuring knowledge of particular topics in some detail, the ability for independent learning, so essential to all good doctors throughout their career, is developed and enhanced by the participation of medical students in these special study modules.

Clinical Surgery has been written by a group of senior clinical academic surgeons with the requirements of the new undergraduate curriculum in mind. It covers all the relevant aspects of the subjects — clinical methods, management of acute surgical disorders and trauma, general and specialist surgery, perioperative care and rehabilitation. Throughout the book, particular emphasis has been laid on core material which we have defined as 'necessary for a proficient general practitioner'. This approach has been emphasized by the inclusion of *At A Glance* boxes which summarize the important features of all the common surgical disorders. These boxes not only highlight the core material, but should also facilitate rapid revision. Special attention has been paid to the layout of the book to enhance retention and recall of assimilated factual knowledge. A special four-colour text has been adopted for this purpose and the book is heavily illustrated with line drawings and clinical photographs. Our objectives in writing *Clinical Surgery* have been to ensure a well laid out account of the subject that medical undergraduates will find easy to read, understand and assimilate in a form that is attractive, concise and affordable.

The period of gestation of this book has been longer than initially envisaged, but we, as teachers, are very happy with the result and trust that *Clinical Surgery* will be well received and popular with medical undergraduates. We are grateful to the publishers, Blackwell Science, for the support given throughout and in particular, we are indebted to Dr Andrew Robinson who has been the main driving force, ensuring coordination and completion without significant delays, a task which may have seemed difficult at times but which he performed with tact and great patience.

Alfred Cuschieri
Thomas Hennessy
Roger Greenhalgh
David Rowley
Pierce Grace

Acknowledgements

The Editors would like to thank the following for their invaluable contributions to the development of this textbook. Every chapter was reviewed by a combination of medical students, junior doctors and surgeons, and illustrations have generously been donated from collections far and wide:

Joe Abrahams, Margaret Ambrose, G. J. Bates, Michael Benson, Crystal Blackmoore, Martin Blomley, Neil Borley, B. J. Britton, Claire Cousins, D. Cranston, John Dart, C. Entwhistle, Patricia Fitzgerald, Michael Greenall, Linda Hands, John Harrison, Suzanne Heazlewood, Anne Hennessy, Nuzhat Khanim, Kate Lankester, Peadar Keogh, Gearoid Lynch, who provided a significant number of illustrations, Matt McHugh, Ken Mealy, Prad Patel, Joseph Pflug, Andrew Robinson, Jonathan Rowley, Rebecca Salter, Peter Smith, Jo Stockwell, Robin Strachan, Bill Svennsen, P. J. Teddy, D. Wade, Tom Walsh, Steve Westaby, Professor Robin Williamson, and the students of St Mary's Hospital Medical School.

List of Abbreviations

AAA	abdominal aortic aneurysm
ABI	ankle/brachial index
ACE	angiotensin-converting enzyme
ACTH	adrenocorticotrophic hormone
ADH	antidiuretic hormone
AFP	α-fetoprotein
AIDS	acquired immune deficiency syndrome
ALT	alanine aminotransferase
AMI	acute mesenteric ischaemia
AMV	assisted mechanical ventilation
APACHE	acute physiology and chronic health evaluation
APS	acute physiological score
APTT	activated partial thromboplastin time
APUD	amine precursor uptake and decarboxylation
ARDS	adult respiratory distress syndrome
ARF	acute renal failure
ASD	atrial septal defect
AST	aspartate aminotransferase
ATN	acute tubular necrosis
AVM	arteriovenous malformations
AZT	azidothymidine
BCC	basal cell carcinoma
BCG	bacillus Calmette-Guérin
BPH	benign prostatic hypertrophy
CABG	coronary artery bypass graft
CCD	charge-coupled device
CDH	congenital dislocation of the hip
CI	cardiac input
CIS	carcinoma *in situ*
CISC	clean intermittent self-catheterization
CMF	cyclophosphamide, methotrexate and 5-fluorouracil
CO	cardiac output
COAD	chronic obstructive airways disease
CPAP	continuous positive airway pressure
CPK	creatine phosphokinase
CPR	cardiopulmonary resuscitation
CRP	C-reactive protein
CSF	cerebrospinal fluid
CT	computed tomography
CVA	cerebrovascular accident
CVP	central venous pressure
CXR	chest X-ray
DIC	disseminated intravascular coagulation
DIPJ	distal interphalangeal joint
DMSA	dimercaptosuccinic acid
DSA	digital subtraction arteriography
DTPA	diethylenetriaminepentaacetic acid
DU	duodenal ulcer
DVT	deep vein thrombosis
DXT	deep X-ray therapy
ECG	electrocardiogram
EDTA	ethylenediaminetetra-acetic acid
EEG	electroencephalography
EMG	electromyography
ENG	electronystagmography
ENT	ear, nose and throat
EPVF	extrapulmonary ventilatory failure
ER	oestrogen receptor
ERCP	endoscopic retrograde cholangiopancreatography
ESR	erythrocyte sedimentation rate
ESWL	extracorporeal shock-wave lithotripsy
FBC	full blood count
FDP	fibrin degradation product
FSH	follicle stimulating hormone
FVC	forced vital capacity
GCS	Glasgow coma scale
GFR	glomerular filtration rate
GH	growth hormone
GU	gastric ulcer
GvHD	graft versus host disease
HAFLOE	high air-flow oxygen enrichment
HAS	human albumin solution
HCG	human chorionic gonadotrophin
HDU	high-dependence unit
HES	hydroxyethyl starch
HIT	heparin-induced thrombocytopenia
HIV	human immunodeficiency virus
HLA	human leukocyte antigen
HRT	hormone replacement therapy
HvGR	host versus graft reaction
IAM	internal auditory meatus

ICA	internal carotid artery	PAP	pulmonary artery pressure
ICU	intensive care unit	PAWP	pulmonary artery wedge pressure
ICP	intracranial pressure	PCA	patient-controlled analgesia
IMV	intermittent mandatory ventilation	PCV	packed cell volume
INR	international normalized ratio	PCWP	pulmonary capillary wedge pressure
IPPV	intermittent positive-pressure ventilation	PE	Pulmonary embolus
ISS	injury severity score	PEEP	positive end expiratory pressure
IVC	inferior vena cava	PEFR	peak expiratory flow rate
IVU	intravenous urogram	PEG	percutaneous endoscopic gastrostomy
JVP	jugular venous pulse	PET	positron emission tomography
KUB	kidney, ureter, bladder	PND	paroxysmal nocturnal dyspnoea
LATS	long-acting thyroid-stimulating factor	PNET	primitive neuroectodermal tumour
LDH	lactic acid dehydrogenase	POAD	peripheral occlusive arterial disease
LH	luteinizing hormone	POP	plaster of Paris
LH-RH	luteinizing hormone-release hormone	PPL	postphlebitic limb
LIF	left illiac fossa	PSA	prostate-specific antigen
LLQ	left lower quadrant	PT	prothrombin time
LOS	lower oesophageal sphincter	PTC	percutaneous transhepatic cholangiography
LPS	lipopolysaccharide	PTFE	polytetrafluoroethylene
LUQ	left upper quadrant	PUJ	pelviureteric junction
LVEF	left ventricular ejection failure	PV	per vaginam
MALT	mucosa-associated lymphoid tissue	PVR	pulmonary vascular resistance
MAP	mean arterial pressure	PVR	pulse volume recordings
MCH	mean corpuscular haemoglobin	RA	rheumatoid arthritis
MCV	mean corpuscular volume	REM	rapid eye movement
MEN	multiple endocrine neoplasm	RLQ	right lower quadrant
MHC	major histocompatibility complex	RPLND	retroperitoneal lymph node dissection
MI	myocardial infarction	RTA	road traffic accident
MODS	multiple organ dysfunction syndrome	RUQ	right upper quadrant
MoTT	mycobacteria other than typical tubercle	RVH	renovascular hypertension
MPAP	mean pulmonary arterial pressure	SAH	subarachnoid haemorrhage
MRA	magnetic resonance angiography	SCC	squamous cell carcinoma
MRI	magnetic resonance imaging	SGOT	serum glutamic oxaloacetic transaminase
MRSA	methicillin-resistant *Staphylococcus aureus*	SIRS	systemic inflammatory response syndrome
MSH	melanocyte-stimulating hormone	SPECT	single-photon emission computed tomography
MSOF	multiple system organ failure		
MSU	mid-stream urine	SSEP	somatosensory evoked potential
NGU	non-gonococcal urethritis	STD	sexually transmitted disease
NORF	non-oliguric renal failure	SVC	superior vena cava
NPH	normal-pressure hydrocephalus	SVR	systemic vascular resistance
NSAID	non-steroidal anti-inflammatory drug	SVT	supraventricular tachycardia
NYHA	New York Heart Association	T_4	thyroxine
OGD	oesophagogastroduodenoscopy	TCC	transitional cell carcinoma

TENS	transcutaneous nerve stimulation	TTE	transthoracic echocardiography
TIA	transient ischaemic attacks	TURP	transurethral resection of the prostate
TIPS	transinternal jugular portosystemic shunt	TURT	transurethral resection of tumour
TLC	total lung capacity	U&E	urea and electrolytes
TNF	tumour necrosis factor	UTI	urinary tract infection
TOE	transoesophageal echocardiography	VMA	vanillylmandelic acid
t-PA	tissue plasminogen activator	VSD	ventricular septal defect
TPN	total parenteral nutrition	vWF	von Willebrand's disease
TRUS	transrectal ultrasound	WCC	white cell count
TSH	thyroid-stimulating hormone		

PART 1 Clinical Skills and Investigations

The trouble with doctors is not that they don't know enough but that they don't see enough.   Sir Dominic Corrigan (1802–80)

Introduction

The acquisition of clinical and psychomotor skills is fundamental to the safe practice of clinical medicine. These skills are acquired by talking to and examining patients in the wards and outpatient clinics. It requires an active commitment on the part of the medical student to master the techniques of history-taking, physical examination and other bedside clinical skills necessary for interpreting the nature of the patient's problems. The patient may have a number of problems for which he or she requires help and we should remember that we are dealing with a person and not (as one too often hears) 'the bowel tumour' or 'the black foot'! Proficiency comes with practice and, as cerebral recognition patterns are established and reinforced, the ability to make clinical diagnoses improves. The essentials of history-taking and physical examination are presented in Chapter 1.

A considerable amount of time and money — whether the patient's, the insurance company's or the tax-payer's (i.e. yours!) — is spent on investigations in medicine and there seems to be no end to the number of tests that can be ordered for a patient. In science there are two approaches to a problem: first, in the *inductive method* data are accumulated and then a theory is proposed based on the observations; second, in the *hypotheticodeductive method* a hypothesis is tested by appropriate well-designed experiments. Similar approaches can be adopted when planning a series of investigations for a patient. Either every investigation possible could be performed in the hope of finding something abnormal or a specific series of investigations could be requested to confirm or refute the initial clinical diagnosis. Clearly the latter approach should be adopted and only those investigations which are likely to provide further useful information for diagnosis or management should be ordered. In Chapter 2, a brief analysis of the types of investigations available is presented but the investigations performed in the assessment of specific pathologies are presented throughout the book in the relevant chapters.

1 History-Taking and Physical Examination

The most essential part of a student's instruction is obtained, not in the lecture room, but at the bedside. Nothing seen there is lost; the rhythms of disease are learned by frequent repetition; its unforeseen occurrences stamp themselves indelibly on the memory. Before the student is aware of what he has acquired he has learned the aspects and causes and probable issue of the diseases he has seen with his teacher and the proper mode of dealing with them, so far as his master knows. Oliver Wendell Holmes (1867)

Introduction

The mastery of clinical skills is different from knowing how the various clinical tasks are performed. It has several components:
- the ability to communicate freely and efficiently with patients;
- the ability reliably to detect abnormal physical signs, e.g. an enlarged liver, rebound tenderness;
- the ability to recognize acute and life-threatening situations; and
- the ability to confirm normality when present.

No amount of encyclopaedic knowledge gained from reading and lectures can ever impart clinical competence. The requirements for proficiency as a doctor are a core knowledge of the common medical and surgical disorders and full clinical competence. Rare and obscure illnesses will be encountered by every clinician from time to time. One needs only to be aware of these disorders since the competent doctor will recognize that the patient does not fit in any of the common disease patterns and seek advice or expert opinion.

Clinical presentation

Patients may present in two ways:
- *electively*: with chronic symptoms of variable duration; or
- *acutely*: with life-threatening disorders.

Table 1.1 Management of the elective patient.

Establish the diagnosis and confirm it, whenever necessary, by the appropriate investigations
Decide on the nature of the treatment required — surgical or medical
Impart this information to the patient and carry out the treatment if the patient consents to this

The pathways in management of the two are quite different.

In the elective (cold) situation, the surgeon proceeds as shown in Table 1.1.

If surgical treatment is required, the patient is usually put on the waiting list or is given a date for the operation at the time of the outpatient interview. A priority system based on disease severity is adopted in deciding which patients are operated on soon after the diagnosis is confirmed. Thus a patient with cancer takes precedence over a patient with an uncomplicated inguinal hernia. Cancer patients undergo a process of staging by appropriate investigations based on the TNM (tumour, regional nodes, distant metastases) system before the appropriate treatment is selected. This staging process influences management in several ways. In some patients, the disease is found to be inoperable, when non-surgical treatment (chemotherapy, radiotherapy) may be employed. In others, the disease, though operable, is advanced and adjuvant therapy (endocrine, chemotherapy, radiotherapy) before or after surgery is needed in addition

3

Table 1.2 Management of the acutely ill patient.

Prompt diagnosis and assessment of the condition

Resuscitation (**A**irway, **B**reathing, **C**irculation; Chapters 3 and 4)

Decision on treatment: emergency surgical intervention or conservative management with close clinical observation

Table 1.4 Approach to history-taking.

Establish a rapport with the patient: introduce yourself, shake hands

Initiate the process by asking the patient to tell you what made him or her seek medical advice

Listen without interruption to the patient as he or she relates the history of the presenting complaint(s). During this process make a mental note of the key symptoms

Wait for the answer before asking another question

Obtain further details on specific symptoms, including duration, nature of severity and associations by specific questions

Briefly review the systems by key questions

Obtain details of the past medical history, including drug medication, surgical conditions, operations and exposure to general anaesthesia. Past medical incidents are important because they may relate to the patient's current illness and may also influence management

Obtain details of social history and habits, including alcohol consumption and smoking

Obtain a brief family history

to surgical extirpation of the primary tumour. Staging (clinical and pathological) is also the best overall guide to prognosis in the individual patient.

Acute patients are admitted as emergencies with life-threatening disorders or trauma. The pathway of management in these patients is shown in Table 1.2. Frequently, resuscitation and diagnosis go hand in hand in the seriously ill or injured patient.

Prompt and efficient resuscitation of seriously ill patients, which necessitates an understanding of the underlying pathophysiological mechanisms (Chapters 3–7) is crucial to the survival of these patients. Not all acute conditions need surgical intervention and some are managed conservatively in the first instance with recourse to surgery if progress is not made or the clinical condition deteriorates. The relief of acute pain by appropriate analgesia (Chapter 31) is a very important part of the clinical management of acutely ill patients, whether they need emergency surgery or not.

In the management of trauma victims the priorities in order of precedence are shown in Table 1.3.

The history

Much has been written and said about the technique of history-taking. For most individuals this is an acquired attribute. Basic to successful history-taking is the ability to establish a rapport with the patient, allowing him or her to relate the story (history) of the illness. In essence, history-taking is the art of conversation and requires a fine balance between the ability to listen and interject with relevant

questions to clarify points and obtain details as the history unfolds (Table 1.4).

In this process there are dos and don'ts. The only way in which a student can confirm that he or she has obtained an accurate history is to summarize the history to the patient for confirmation. This provides a valid check of the accuracy of the history-taking process and is highly recommended until full proficiency in history-taking is obtained. The wrong information can be obtained if the technique is poor and the patient is confused by the interviewer. In this respect one should avoid the mistakes outlined in Table 1.5.

Symptoms

Patients can present with specific or non-specific symptoms or a combination of both. Specific symptoms are those which relate to disease in specific organs, e.g. difficulty with swallowing (dysphagia), indicating disorders of deglutition or organic narrowing of the oesophagus. Each system has

Table 1.3 Priorities in the management of the acutely injured patient.

A	**A**irway
B	**B**reathing
C	**C**ardiovascular system
D	Neurological **D**efects
E	**E**xposure to detect all injuries

Table 1.5 Don'ts of history-taking.

Do not interrupt the patient
Do not use medical terminology
Do not ask ambiguous or irrelevant questions
Do not use leading questions in the first instance
Do not be abrupt or impatient

Table 1.6 Specific symptoms.

Nervous system: headache, nausea and vomiting, visual disturbances, motor defects (paralysis), incoordination, sensory loss and disturbances (paraesthesiae), altered levels of consciousness

Respiratory system: cough, espectoration, breathlessness, wheezing, chest pain, diminished exercise tolerance

Cardiovascular system: loss of consciousness (syncope), breathlessness, diminished exercise tolerance, retrosternal chest pain, intermittent pain in limbs on walking (intermittent claudication), rest pain in the limbs, gangrene (necrosis of tissue)

Hepatobiliary – pancreatic system: nausea and vomiting, pain, jaundice, itching, bleeding tendency, weight gain due to water retention, weight loss

Gastrointestinal system: loss of appetite (anorexia), nausea and vomiting, difficulty in swallowing, indigestion, abdominal pain, altered bowel habit (diarrhoea and/or constipation), blood in vomit (haematemesis), passage of slime and fresh or altered blood in the faeces

Genitourinary system: loin pain, fever, suprapubic pain, frequency, painful micturition (dysuria), micturition at night (nocturia), poor stream, dribbling and incontinence, blood in urine (haematuria), enlarged or tender testis

Table 1.7 Diagnostic clinical information on pain.

Site
Radiation
Severity
Nature
Duration
Relieving factors
Aggravating factors
Associations

its own specific symptoms, although there is considerable overlap (Table 1.6).

Patients vary considerably in their clinical presentation. Although a few present with all the characteristic symptoms of a specific illness (classical presentation — full-house), in the majority of patients the history is not typical and the clinician has to decipher the situation. The ability to identify specific symptoms is one of the reasons for the increasing diagnostic efficiency that comes with clinical experience. Non-specific symptoms do not immediately give a clue to the diagnosis or site of the disease. In this situation, a tentative diagnosis is made on the history as a whole. In this group of patients more reliance is placed on investigations in establishing the diagnosis.

Common important symptoms in general surgery

Pain

Pain is the most common and important symptom in surgical practice. (It used to be said with some truth that pain and blood were the only two events that brought patients quickly to the doctor.) Pain is universal and can be caused by benign or malignant disorders and elective or acute conditions. It is the symptom that is least commonly overlooked by patients, although the threshold for pain varies considerably from one patient to another. The information required to establish the clinical significance of pain is shown in Table 1.7.

The most reliable way to obtain precise information on the location of pain is to ask the patient to point to the exact site of the pain and where it radiates. Pain may be localized or diffuse and can be referred. Localized pain is either musculoskeletal in origin or is indicative of disease, trauma or inflammation in the affected region. Pain may be referred to the corresponding sensory dermatome. This is exemplified by shoulder tip pain due to a subphrenic abscess causing irritation of the ipsilateral phrenic nerve.

Types of pain

• *Colicky pain* is indicative of an obstructed hollow organ. It is griping in nature and fluctuates, with peaks of intensity followed by partial or complete relief before a further bout occurs. Colicky pain is always severe and makes the patient restless. The patient rolls about in agony, unable to find a comfortable position. It is usually accompanied by nausea and vomiting.

• *Somatic pain*, i.e. the severe pain due to inflammation of the parietal peritoneum from localized or general peritonitis, is aggravated by movement and the patient lies still and breathes shallowly to diminish the abdominal wall excursion with respiration (e.g. perforated peptic ulcer) or assumes a position which releases tension on the abdominal musculature, i.e. draws the knees up — a posture often observed in patients with acute pancreatitis. The pain of acute peritonitis is also aggravated by coughing.

• *Burning pain* signifies mucosal injury/inflammation and is typified by heartburn of reflux oesophagitis, the burning indigestion encountered in patients with peptic ulceration (Chapter 13) and dysuria which accompanies inflammation of the urinary bladder (cystitis; Chapter 20).

• *Intermittent claudication* is the term used to signify cramp-like pain in the muscles of the lower limbs (usually calf, but may involve the thighs and gluteal regions) which develops with walking and subsides with rest, after which the patient can resume walking before the pain comes on again. It is caused by peripheral occlusive vascular disease (atherosclerosis) with a resultant defective blood supply leading to the accumulation of metabolites, such as lactic acid, with exertion. The claudication distance — the distance the patient can walk before the onset of the muscle cramps — reflects the severity of the peripheral vascular disease (Chapter 18).

• *Rest pain* is a much more serious type of vascular pain. The patient experiences pain in the affected limb at rest. The pain is severe, constant and interrupts sleep. Some relief is obtained by dangling the affected limb over the edge of the bed. Rest pain denotes threatened viability of the limb and requires urgent vascular treatment to prevent the development of gangrene (Chapter 18).

• *Root pain* is caused by irritation of the spinal dorsal roots and can be caused by compression (vertebral collapse) or direct malignant involvement. The pain radiates from the back around the body, usually on either side, in the distribution of the respective dermatomes. It is often accompanied by both sensory (paraesthesiae) and motor changes (muscle weakness/paralysis). Pain due to inflammation, partial injury or neoplastic involvement of nerves or nerve roots is known as *neuralgia*. It is always severe, often intractable and requires special measures which may include neurosurgical intervention (Chapter 22).

Indigestion

Indigestion or *dyspepsia* are loosely defined words which refer to epigastric discomfort or pain occurring either during fasting or during or after meals and indicate disease within the upper digestive and biliary tract. The practical problem encountered with these symptoms relates to the frequency with which normal individuals experience indigestion. One study has shown that 70% of people living in the UK experience episodes of indigestion and heartburn from time to time and reports from other western countries indicate a similar prevalence. The key issue in clinical practice is what constitutes abnormal indigestion. This is difficult to define and for this reason diagnosis of serious conditions, such as gastric cancer, is often delayed as the general practitioner usually prescribes medication designed to produce symptomatic relief. Meantime the tumour progresses and is often incurable by the time the diagnosis is made. Thus in most western countries 90% of all gastric cancers are advanced at the time of presentation. There are certain practical considerations in relation to dyspepsia which must never be overlooked and which require investigation by endoscopy rather than empirical symptomatic treatment (Table 1.8).

Dysphagia

Dysphagia signifies inability to swallow and may be caused by motility disorders or organic disease which encroaches

Table 1.8 Indications for upper gastrointestinal endoscopy.

Frequent or persistent indigestion irrespective of age
Indigestion accompanied by other gastrointestinal symptoms
Indigestion occurring for the first time in a patient above the age of 40 years

on the lumen of the oesophagus such as stricture or neoplasm (Chapter 13). This symptom always warrants urgent investigation by flexible endoscopy and a barium swallow. The difficulty in swallowing may be experienced in relation to liquids and solids. In some patients with inflammatory mucosal disease, the dysphagia is accompanied by pain. This symptom complex is known as *odynophagia*. Dysphagia due to organic disease is progressive and eventually, without treatment, the patient may be unable to swallow saliva due to complete occlusion of the oesophageal lumen. Dysphagia caused by motility disorders such as achalasia (Chapter 13) may be intermittent. High dysphagia due to bulbar palsy or cricopharyngeal spasm is accompanied by spluttering and choking as the bolus, unable to negotiate the upper oesophageal sphincter, spills over into the larynx.

In the presence of significant oesophageal occlusion, dysphagia is accompanied by *regurgitation* which is passive and effortless, as opposed to vomiting. In patients with dysphagia, spillage of retained food debris in the dilated oesophagus across the cricopharyngeus into the larynx may occur in the supine position during sleep, leading to aspiration and pneumonitis. This accounts for the chronic productive cough and fever encountered in patients with long-standing dysphagia.

Anorexia and weight loss

Anorexia refers to loss of appetite. This may be due to an abnormal psychiatric state, e.g. anorexia nervosa, but in surgical patients loss of appetite is usually caused by malignant neoplasms, usually of the upper digestive tract and pancreas. Anorexia must be distinguished from fear of eating because of precipitation of symptoms or inability to eat consequent on a disordered swallowing mechanism from any cause. Anorexia is invariably accompanied by weight loss due to diminished protein-calorie intake. However, there are other causes of weight loss. Some malignant tumours are accompanied by the development of a catabolic state such that the weight loss is out of proportion to the reduced dietary intake — *cachexia*.

Some patients lose weight because they are unable to assimilate the ingested food. This may be the result of impaired digestion of the foodstuffs (e.g. diminished pancreatic enzymes in chronic pancreatitis), reduced bile salt pool from any cause (malabsorption of fats), bacterial overgrowth, intrinsic disease of the small-bowel mucosa (coeliac disease, brush-border enzyme deficiencies), disorders affecting the small bowel (Crohn's disease) or extensive resection of the small intestine (short gut syndrome).

Vomiting

Vomiting is an active process and involves violent contractions of the abdominal musculature forcibly to expel in a retrograde fashion the gastric contents. During vomiting the lower oesophageal sphincter and the cricopharyngeus are reflexly opened and the glottis is closed. In surgical practice, vomiting may have a cerebral cause such as raised intracranial pressure by a space-occupying lesion. More commonly, however, it is the result of acute intra-abdominal disease or obstruction of hollow organs. Thus, nausea and vomiting may be a feature of such diverse conditions as acute appendicitis, acute gastritis (drug- or alcohol-induced), exacerbation of peptic ulceration, acute pancreatitis, renal and biliary colic. Vomiting is a predominant feature of an obstructed stomach (pyloric stenosis).

The nature of the vomit is important. In obstructions proximal to the pylorus, the vomit does not contain bile. Vomiting of blood (*haematemesis*) is encountered in bleeding lesions of the lower oesophagus, stomach and duodenum. The blood may be fresh or dark and 'coffee-ground' in appearance due to digestion by the hydrochloric acid and pepsin in the stomach. In pyloric stenosis, the vomit often contains portions of food which the patient had ingested several hours, sometimes days, beforehand. In some of these patients, the vomiting may be self-induced in an effort to relieve the upper abdominal discomfort caused by a distended stomach.

Vomiting in the unconscious state (e.g. head injury, alcoholic stupor and during recovery from general anaesthesia) is particularly dangerous in view of the distinct possibility of inhalation of the vomit into the tracheobronchial tree with severe pulmonary damage and the development of the adult respiratory distress syndrome (ARDS; Chapter 19). Vomiting is a major clinical presentation of acute small-bowel obstruction (Chapter 13) where it is accompanied by variable abdominal distension and constipation.

Altered bowel habit

Strictly speaking, this term is applied to patients with previous regular bowel habits, who suddenly develop constipation, diarrhoea or diarrhoea alternating with constipation. This is a feature of some but not all patients who develop a colonic neoplasm in the left colon or upper rectum. The difficulty lies in establishing what was normal for the patient beforehand. Undoubtedly, in western countries due to a diminished dietary intake of fibre, constipation and low bulk stools are very common, as are disorders of colonic transit (diverticular disease, slow transit constipation). There is also a tendency towards constipation with increasing age.

In patients with rectal or lower sigmoid carcinoma, the constipation may also be accompanied by a feeling of incomplete evacuation after defecation. This is often referred to as *tenesmus*. Other symptomatic accompaniments in these patients include the passage of mucus and rectal bleeding which is mixed with the motion.

Bloody diarrhoea is a feature of colonic inflammatory bowel disease and infective colitis. Diarrhoea may also signify the presence of colonic motility disorders exemplified by the irritable bowel syndrome. This common obscure condition can also present with constipation.

Foul-smelling diarrhoea which floats and is difficult to flush away is encountered in malabsorption. Because the faeces contains a large amount of fat, the term *steatorrhoea* is often used in this condition. Passage of foul-smelling tar-like liquid or solid motion (*melaena*) indicates a proximal source of bleeding in the gastrointestinal tract.

Physical examination

General principles

Physical examination must be thorough and efficient without being overdone and exhausting to the patient. Whichever system or anatomical region is examined, the process relies on four skills: *inspection, palpation, percussion* and *auscultation*, and is designed to elicit the appropriate clinical signs. Whereas the examination of the various systems is crucial to the management of patients with medical disorders, in surgical practice physical examination is more commonly focused on anatomical regions: head and neck, ear, nose and throat, breasts, abdomen and limbs, although assessment of the important systems such as the respiratory, cardiovascular and renal systems is often necessary. Certain vital signs such as temperature, blood pressure, pulse rate and pulse volume and respiratory rate are performed routinely in all but minor cases.

Inspection

Inspection requires a trained eye actively to detect abnormalities. It consists of a detailed and systematic scrutiny of the anatomical region. Inspection entails close observation of abnormal movements of the parietes and body contour as well as surface abnormalities (scars, surface lesions, lumps, bulges) and complexion of the skin, lips, conjunctival membranes and sclera. Good lighting is essential, particularly for the detection of abnormal discoloration (pallor, cyanosis, jaundice).

Palpation

Palpation relies on the tactile sense organs in the fingers to outline surface irregularities, tension of the abdominal walls, lumps and enlarged organs. The exercise should be carried out by a relaxed warm hand and should be conducted gently and in an orderly fashion. In general, the more you press, the less you feel, and worse still, the patient is hurt.

Percussion

Percussion is very useful for establishing the consistency of a swelling or organ. Thus a solid lump or organ is *dull* to percussion. A fluid-containing cyst or body cavity (peritoneal, thoracic) is *stony dull* to percussion. For the same reason a distended urinary bladder is detected as a localized dull swelling in the suprapubic region. By contrast, air-containing organs (normal ventilated lung, air-containing hollow abdominal viscera) are *resonant* on percussion (much like a drum). When using percussion to outline the size or margins of an organ, one should *percuss from the resonant to the dull area*. The point where the note changes marks the margin of the organ.

Auscultation

Auscultation with the stethoscope requires considerable experience to recognize the normal from the abnormal, and is used to examine the lungs (normal and adventitial breath sounds), heart sounds and murmurs, abdominal bowel sounds and bruits over stenotic or dilated segments (aneurysms) of arteries.

Examination of an ulcer

An ulcer is defined as an *area of discontinuity of the surface epithelium* and may occur internally (mucosal) or externally, when it involves the skin and subcutaneous tissues. Ulceration has a varied aetiology and ulcers may be benign or malignant in nature. In establishing the nature of an ulcer, certain characteristics are important. These include the site of the ulcer, the floor, its base and the edges (Fig. 1.1). The history is also important and often provides useful diagnostic clues. The duration of the ulcer, history of trauma and the presence or absence of pain are all relevant.

The *floor of an ulcer* is made up of fibrovascular granulation tissue. If this consists of healthy pink granulations, the ulcer has an excellent chance of healing. By contrast, healing is compromised if the floor is covered by grey slough and pale granulation tissue. Neuropathic or trophic ulcers are examples of the latter situation. They are found on pressure areas of the feet in patients with absent or diminished sensation due to peripheral neuropathy from any cause (often diabetes). They are deep penetrating ulcers, often containing slough and poor granulation tissue. They are characteristically painless because of the anaesthesia, which is indeed involved in their aetiology, since they are attributable in part to repeated unrecognized trauma.

Ischaemic ulcers have virtually no granulation tissue and may expose underlying structures such as tendons, muscles and periosteum. They usually require limb revascular-

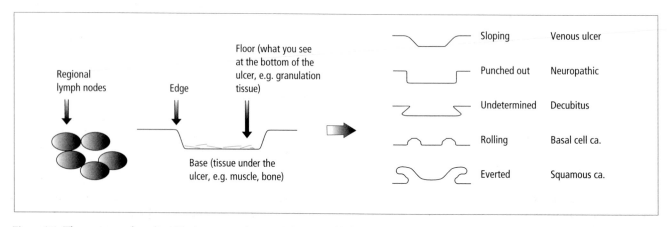

Figure 1.1 The anatomy of an ulcer. The important characteristics to establish with any ulcer are the site, size, shape, floor, base, edge, discharge, surrounding skin and regional lymph nodes.

ization (by arterial surgery to restore blood flow to the limb) and sometimes skin grafting.

The *base of an ulcer* refers to the state of the tissues underneath and around the floor of the ulcer. If there is inflammatory involvement, the surrounding tissues feel indurated and the ulcer appears fixed and is tender. Fixation and induration may be the result of neoplastic infiltration of the deeper tissues if the ulcer is malignant. In this instance, the fixation is not accompanied by tenderness.

The *edge of an ulcer* is often indicative of the nature of the lesion.

• *Sloping blue edges* indicate advancing epithelium (over the red granulation tissue) and signify healing. Blue healing edges are often encountered in venous (gravitational) ulcers.

• *Punched-out* ulcers with sharp edges used to be characteristic of syphilis in the preantibiotic days. These have virtually disappeared from clinical practice nowadays and a more typical example of a punched-out ulcer is the neuropathic ulcer due to peripheral neuropathy, most commonly encountered in diabetic patients.

• *Undermined edges* are typical of decubitus ulcers (pressure sores) and tuberculous ulcers which, though rare in the West, are still common in underprivileged countries. Decubitus ulcers are the result of poor medical and nursing care of patients who are confined to bed for prolonged periods as a result of illness or operation. They are caused by compression necrosis of the skin and subcutaneous tissues over pressure points: heels, sacral region, scapular region. Decubitus ulcers are largely preventable by ensuring clean soft bedding and frequent turning of these immobile patients.

• *Rolled* or *everted edges* are seen when central ulceration is accompanied by growth at the edges and are characteristic of malignant ulcers such as basal cell carcinoma (see Fig. 17.12) and squamous cell carcinoma of the skin (see Fig. 17.13). Eversion of the edges is more prominent in squamous carcinomas than in basal cell lesions, where the edges are gently rolled and the floor is often encrusted.

The *site of an ulcer* may be a clue to the diagnosis. Examples of this include the predilection of basal cell lesions for the upper third of the face and forehead, occurrence of venous ulcers around the medial malleolus, frequency of ischaemic ulcers on the anterior aspect of the shin and dorsum of the foot, location of trophic ulcers on the sole of the forefoot (especially underneath the ball of the big toe) and common occurrence of decubitus ulcers in the sacral region.

Whilst some ulcers are dry, a *discharge* is a common feature and may be thin and serosanguineous or thick and purulent if the ulcer is infected. If a discharge is present, a swab should be taken for culture and sensitivity testing. The *regional lymph nodes* are often enlarged due to infection but the lymphadenopathy may be due to metastatic spread in the case of squamous cell carcinomas. If the nature of an ulcer remains in doubt after clinical examination, a biopsy with histological examination is essential. The biopsy taken is a wedge which includes a portion of the floor, the edge of the ulcer and adjacent normal skin.

Examination of a lump or swelling

A lump may be visible on inspection or may not be detected until palpation is carried out. The lump may be discrete and localized or be diffuse, when it is more properly designated as a swelling. The important features which provide diagnostic information are site, anatomical plane, relationship to adjacent structures, temperature, tenderness, consistency, mobility, fluctuation, pulsatility (expansile, transmitted) and state of regional lymph nodes. In addition, specific lumps have additional characteristics which can be demonstrated by appropriate clinical tests.

Position, location, shape and size

The first feature that should be noted is the position of the lump and its relationship to adjacent anatomical structures, the plane of location (subcutaneous, intramuscular, intra-abdominal, etc.). A lump which is superficial to a muscular compartment, e.g. situated in the subcutaneous plane, is rendered more prominent when the patient is made to contract the relevant muscles. By contrast, this manoeuvre makes a lump become less distinct both on inspection and palpation if the lesion lies within or beneath a muscular compartment. In subcutaneous swellings, it is often possible to 'pinch' the skin over the summit of the lesion. This cannot be achieved with intracutaneous lumps such as sebaceous cysts. During this stage of the examination, a note is also made of the shape and size (in two diameters) of the lump. Size is important in planning surgical excision and in the assessment of the effect of non-surgical therapy for inflammatory and neoplastic lesions.

Inflammatory characteristics

Palpation of a lump should be carried out gently and, initially, the temperature of the lesion and the presence of any tenderness noted. Surface discoloration (erythema, bruising, etc.) should also be noted.

An inflammatory swelling will be tender, hot, erythematous, indurated and oedematous. It is important to note, however, that some rapidly growing malignant neoplasms may exhibit an inflammatory appearance which is virtually indistinguishable from that caused by infective conditions. This is encountered most commonly in the breast, where differentiation between a breast abscess and inflammatory cancer may be difficult.

Mobility

The mobility of a lump is tested in two planes at right angles to each other. For lumps that are situated over a muscle compartment, contraction of the muscle group is important before the mobility is assessed since a lesion may be infiltrating the muscles and still appear to be mobile if the muscle is not contracted. Mobility does not designate a lump as being benign. Indeed, many benign lumps exhibit limited mobility because of attachment of anatomical structure (e.g. ganglion because of its attachment to tendons and joint capsule, goitre as the thyroid is tethered to the trachea, etc.). The majority of neoplastic lesions are mobile in the early stages and become fixed only when they infiltrate surrounding tissues.

Consistency, dullness and resonance

The feel or consistency of a lump is probably its most important clinical feature. It may be solid and hard (when the possibility of neoplasia arises), tense, soft, cystic, or pulsatile (vascular origin). Most enlarged lymph nodes feel rubbery. Solid and fluid-containing lumps are dull on percussion. Some swellings contain gas or gas-filled viscera when they are resonant.

A superficial fluid-containing cavity or collection is *fluctuant*. The test for fluctuation is simple and is illustrated in Fig. 1.2. Fluctuation is very useful for the detection of non-inflamed localized collections of fluid and blood. Generally speaking, cystic lumps and swellings are soft, although a tense cyst may feel hard. The benign tumour of fat (*lipoma*) which often presents as a subcutaneous lump also fluctuates on testing.

A fluid thrill may be present in some cystic swellings. This may be elicited by tapping at one side of the swelling and detecting the transmitted percussion wave with the examining fingers placed on the opposite side of the swelling.

Transillumination

Transillumination involves shining a light through a swelling to detect whether the swelling transmits light brilliantly or not (Fig. 1.3). Transillumination is a function of the optical density of the component elements of the swelling. Thus, a cyst containing clear fluid (e.g. hydrocele, cystic hygroma) transilluminates brilliantly; one containing opalescent fluid (spermatocele) less so. Fat (lipoma) and

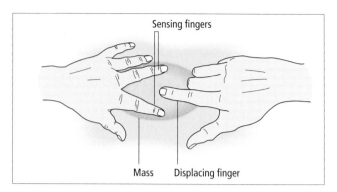

Figure 1.2 Test for fluctuation. The index and middle finger of the left hand are placed in a V-shaped configuration on the mass and the index finger of the right hand is used to depress the summit of the mass repeatedly. If fluid is present, the pressure waves created are felt by the sensing left fingers. The test is applied twice, with the second attempt being at right angles to the first. Obviously inflamed and tender masses (e.g. abscesses) should not be subjected to fluctuation as this causes considerable pain.

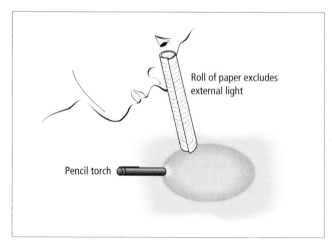

Figure 1.3 Test for transillumination of a swelling. Transillumination is elicited by a pencil torch light and a hollow cylinder (made of rolled paper) placed on opposite sides of the swelling. If the swelling contains clear fluid the light will be transmitted through the fluid and will be seen by the observer looking down the paper cylinder. The cylinder is used to exclude other light from the test region.

subcutaneous tissues also transilluminate to a varying extent.

Vascular swellings

A swelling arising from an artery is usually the result of localized dilatation (aneurysm) and demonstrates expansile pulsation. The most common example encountered in clinical practice is abdominal aortic aneurysm, which must be palpated gently because of the risk of rupture. In

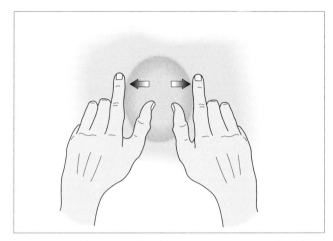

Figure 1.4 To elicit expansile pulsation (i.e. an aneurysm) the index fingers are placed one on either side of the swelling. Separation of the two index fingers occurs synchronously with each systolic impulse.

superficial aneurysms, a vascular thrill caused by the turbulent flow in the aneurysm is felt on palpation. Some non-vascular (solid or cystic) lesions which are apposed to large arteries transmit arterial pulsations. The differentiation between expansile and transmitted pulsations is important and requires bi-digital palpation with each index finger placed on either side of the swelling. If the lump is intrinsically pulsatile, the index fingers are separated with each systolic impulse (Fig. 1.4).

Dilated (varicose) veins are obvious on inspection, especially with the patient standing up. When the proximal part of the long saphenous vein is dilated (due to incompetence at the saphenofemoral junction), it forms a uniform bulge in the immediate subinguinal region and is known as a *saphena varix*. This swelling also exhibits a fluid thrill which is elicited by tapping the vein below the swelling and feeling the impulse with the fingers of the other hand placed over the varix.

Hernial swellings

The characteristic features of hernial swellings (inguinal, paraumbilical and incisional) are increased prominence with a rise in intra-abdominal pressure (cough, contraction of abdominal musculature, erect posture) and an impulse, visible and palpable, when the patient coughs. There is one important exception to these observations — a femoral hernia usually presents as a subinguinal lump which does not have a cough impulse and does not change in size with change in posture.

Examination of specific anatomical areas

Examination of the head and neck

General aspects and inspection

Examination of the head and neck begins with inspection. Lesions, abnormalities of bone structure and soft tissues of the face are obvious but lesions in the scalp are often not apparent on inspection except in bald males. Anatomically, the neck is divided into two triangles on either side of the midline (Fig. 1.5). Most abnormalities of the neck are visible as swellings. Size and location should be noted and confirmed later by palpation. Lumps attached to the trachea, e.g. thyroid swellings, move upwards (with the trachea) on swallowing. Central lumps attached to the hyoid bone such as thyroglossal cysts move upwards with both swallowing and protrusion of the tongue. The most common lump in the neck is due to cervical lymphadenopathy, which may be inflammatory but is often neoplastic (secondary carcinoma or lymphoma). The anatomical disposition of the cervical lymph nodes is shown in Fig. 1.6.

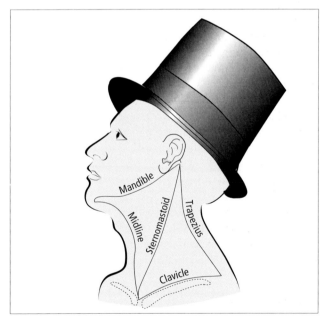

Figure 1.5 Anterior and posterior triangles of the neck. The boundaries of the anterior triangle are the midline, the anterior border of the sternomastoid muscle and the lower border of the mandible. The margins of the posterior triangle are the trapezius, the posterior border of the sternomastoid and the upper border of the clavicle. To determine whether an abnormality is in the anterior or posterior triangle, the sternomastoid muscle should be rendered tense by asking the patient to depress the chin against resistance.

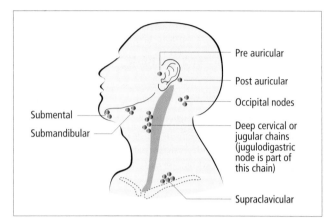

Figure 1.6 The anatomical disposition of the cervical lymph nodes.

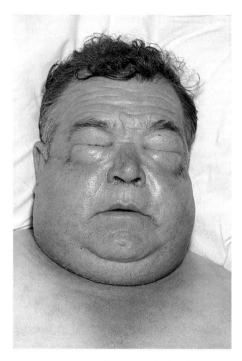

Figure 1.7 Severe surgical emphysema of the head and neck. This patient was crushed in a lift shaft.

An important feature of inspection of the head and neck relates to the venous drainage. Abnormal engorgement of the external jugular vein may be indicative of cardiac failure or circulatory overload. In patients with obstruction of the superior vena cava, usually caused by malignant lymphadenopathy in the superior mediastinum (primary or secondary), there is gross engorgement of the head and neck with prominent superficial veins, a congested suffused appearance and evidence of collateral pathways over the anterior chest wall.

Surgical emphysema most commonly appears in the head and neck region as soft crepitant diffuse swelling. It is caused by escape of air from lacerations or perforation of the tracheobronchial tree or the oesophagus. The extravasated air tends to occupy and cause swelling of regions with lax tissue planes such as the supraclavicular and periorbital regions. When marked, the resultant swelling leads to virtual occlusion of the eyelids (Fig. 1.7).

Palpation

Systematic palpation of the scalp is essential to detect lesions in this region. Parting of the hair over a lump which is identified by palpation enables closer inspection of the lesion. Scalp lesions superficial to the galea aponeurotica move with the scalp when the patient contracts the occipitofrontalis muscle. Lesions deep to this structure or those invading it and the subjacent pericranium are fixed.

Palpation of the anterior triangles of the neck is carried out from the front, whereas palpation of the posterior triangles is best conducted from behind the patient. The entire regions are covered and if an anterior lump is felt, the patient should be asked to swallow and any resulting displacement noted. The consistency of the lump is determined and fluctuation elicited if the swelling appears to be soft and

cystic. Transillumination of a large cystic swelling in infants and children, if positive, confirms the condition of cystic hygroma (Fig. 1.8; see Chapter 18). Palpation of the neck must cover the lymph node groups, especially the deep cervical and the supraclavicular regions. The left supraclavicular region is a common site for metastatic nodal disease from visceral cancer (oesophagus, stomach and pancreas). The carotid vessels must also be palpated for thrills, associated swellings and any aneurysmal dilatation.

Percussion

Percussion is seldom employed in the examination of the head and neck. It may provide useful information in swellings occupying or extending below the suprasternal notch, when percussion over the manubrium may elicit dullness, indicating probable retrosternal extension of the lump. This is most often encountered with swellings of the thyroid gland. It is, however, an imprecise clinical test and is unreliable, especially in patients with chronic obstructive airways disease and emphysema.

Auscultation

Auscultation is used if the swelling appears to be vascular and this is most commonly applicable to patients with toxic en-

Cervical lymphadenopathy

Enlargement of the cervical lymph nodes may be due to infection or neoplastic infiltration. The latter may consist of secondary deposits from a primary tumour elsewhere in the body or be primary in nature, i.e. lymphoma.

Infective conditions may be viral or bacterial, acute or chronic. Examples include tonsillitis, infectious mononucleosis, acquired immune deficiency syndrome (AIDS), scalp infestations, cat-scratch fever, etc. Pyogenic infections (usually staphylococcal in nature) may form large painful abscesses which require drainage. Cervical cellulitis due to streptococcal infection is fortunately rare nowadays. As the infection is confined by the deep cervical fascia, airway obstruction from pressure and laryngeal oedema can occur in these patients.

Although rare in western countries, *tuberculosis* of the cervical lymph nodes (*Mycobacterium tuberculosis*) is common in underprivileged countries and is encountered in the West in immigrant populations. Tuberculous cervical lymphadenopathy results in a collar-stud abscess (Fig. 1.9). In western countries infection is more commonly caused by atypical myobacteria, also known as MOTT (mycobacteria other than typical tubercle). These infections are nowadays most often encountered in patients suffering from AIDS.

Lymphomas

The neck forms one of the commonest sites for lymphoma which is a primary tumour of lymph nodes and is classified into two broad categories — Hodgkin's and non-Hodgkin's lymphoma — each category being subdivided into various types depending on the cell of origin of the tumour (T or B cell) and the degree of differentiation. When it arises in the neck, the tumour forms painless non-tender swellings. The enlarged lymph nodes are discrete, firm and rubbery and may be located in either the anterior or posterior triangles. When enlarged nodes are discovered in the neck, a systematic palpation of other lymph node sites (axillary, inguinal) and palpation of the abdomen for enlarged liver and spleen are essential to determine whether the disease appears to be localized to one region or has disseminated. The patient may or may not have systemic symptoms such as malaise, intermittent fever and weight loss. The staging of lymphomas, necessary for outlining the treatment regimen, necessitates the performance of special investigations including radiology of the chest, computed tomographic (CT) scanning, isotope bone scan and bone marrow biopsy. Within each stage, the absence or presence of systemic symptoms is designated by the letters A and B respectively.

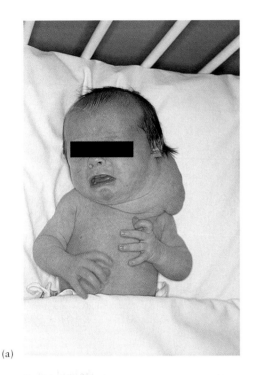

(a)

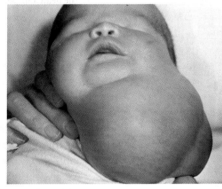

(b)

Figure 1.8 (a, b) Large cystic hygromas both present at birth. Cystic hygromas are large disfiguring lymphangiomas which are treated by surgical excision.

largement of the thyroid gland (Chapter 15). A systolic bruit is often present in patients with primary hyperthyroidism. Auscultation of the carotid vessels should be performed routinely in patients above the age of 50 years and is mandatory in patients with a history of fleeting blindness (*amaurosis fugax*) or recoverable attacks of muscle weakness or loss of consciousness. These symptoms are indicative of 'minor strokes' which are referred to as transient ischaemic attacks (TIAs) and are caused by emboli from atheromatous narrowing of the carotid vessels at the bifurcation into external and internal carotid branches. In these patients a carotid bruit is often heard on auscultation (Chapter 18).

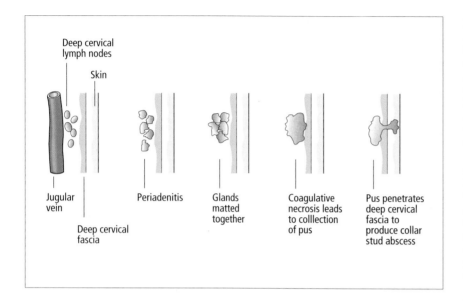

Deep cervical
lymph nodes

Skin

Jugular
vein

Deep cervical
fascia

Periadenitis

Glands
matted
together

Coagulative
necrosis leads
to colllection
of pus

Pus penetrates
deep cervical
fascia to
produce collar
stud abscess

Figure 1.9 The evolution of a collar-stud abscess. Initially, tuberculous lymph nodes are firm and discrete but as caseation (coagulative necrosis) progresses, the inflammatory process induces a marked periadenitis and the enlarged nodes become matted together. Eventually, the necrotic glands are converted into a collection of pus which burrows through the investing layer of the deep cervical fascia to form a superficial (subcutaneous) extension. This is referred to as a collar-stud abscess in view of the two localized collections superficial and deep to the investing layer of the deep cervical fascia Although often tender, the superficial component of a collar-stud abscess is not accompanied by inflammatory changes of the overlying skin (as obtains with ordinary pyogenic abscesses). For this reason, it is often described as a cold abscess. Untreated, it 'points' and eventually erodes through the skin, forming single or multiple discharging sinuses.

Metastatic cervical lymphadenopathy

Overall, metastatic deposits in one or more cervical lymph nodes constitute the most common cause of a lump in the neck. The common sites of primary tumour which may present in this way are squamous cell carcinomas of the pharynx and larynx, oral cavity (tongue, buccal mucosa), thyroid, bronchial tumours, breast cancer and cancer of the upper digestive system (oesophagus, stomach, pancreas). The deposits may occur anywhere in the neck but the commonest sites are the deep cervical and the supraclavicular, especially on the left side. Metastatic nodes are always hard in consistency and soon become fixed to surrounding tissues and matted together, although in early disease the enlarged nodes may be mobile on palpation. There is an important sequence of investigations whenever enlarged lymph nodes thought to be caused by secondary deposits are found in the neck with no other apparent abnormality on complete physical examination. This is outlined in Table 1.9.

It is very important that this protocol is followed before the lump is submitted to biopsy, since if the primary tumour is in the head and neck (usually squamous in nature), cervi-

cal block dissection of the enlarged lymph nodes is required together with excision of the primary. The success of this treatment is jeopardized if a preliminary excision biopsy of the involved nodes has been carried out.

Thyroid swellings

Thyroid swellings are designated by the general term *goitre* and move on swallowing. Enlargement of the thyroid gland may be unilateral or diffuse and bilateral. If a discrete lesion is located in the isthmus of the gland, it presents as a midline swelling; otherwise the majority of unilateral swellings are lateral or anterolateral. They are commonly solid but may be cystic. Diffuse multinodular enlargement is common — nodular goitre — and is associated with iodine deficiency. In some disorders such as primary hyperthyroidism the thyroid is uniformly enlarged with a smooth surface. A discrete solitary nodule in an otherwise normal thyroid should always arise suspicion of malignancy (papillary or follicular neoplasm) and must be accompanied by a systematic palpation of the neck to exclude or confirm associated lymphadenopathy (Chapter 15). However, the anaplastic cancers which are encountered in older patients present as diffuse infiltrative enlargement of the thyroid gland (Fig. 1.10). Because of the fixation to surrounding tissue, the mass does not move with swallowing and may be accompanied by features indicative of tracheal compression (dyspnoea and stridor) and involvement of the recurrent laryngeal nerve (hoarseness).

The position of the trachea should be checked in all patients with thyroid enlargement and with large swellings the

Table 1.9 Management of enlarged cervical lymph node suspected of metastic tumour.

Examination of other lymph node regions
Full ear, nose and throat examination
Chest X-ray
Full blood count

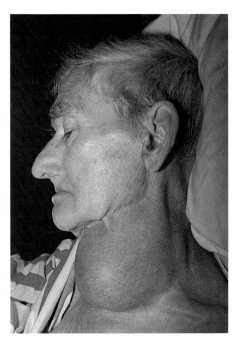

Figure 1.10 Large malignant goitre in an elderly man.

inferior part of the mass is palpated carefully to determine the lower margin. If this cannot be felt, a retrosternal prolongation is likely. A large benign goitre with a retrosternal extension can give rise to pressure symptoms such as engorgement of the head and neck veins and stridor. These are accentuated when the patient elevates both upper arms above the head. Clinical assessment of the thyroid status (euthyroid, hyper- or hypothyroid) is an integral part of the examination of a patient with thyroid enlargement (Chapter 15).

Enlargement of the salivary glands

There are four major salivary glands: two parotid and two submandibular. The *parotid gland* has been likened to 'a lump of bread dough poured over an egg whisk', the dough representing the glandular tissue and the egg whisk the branches of the facial nerve. The gland occupies and extends over the hollow between the masseter muscle anteriorly and the sternomastoid posteriorly (see Fig. 16.2). It is covered with a dense parotid fascia deep to which are attached the parotid lymph nodes.

The *submandibular gland* overlies the mylohyoid muscle under the ramus of the mandible. The posterior part of the gland bends around the posterior border of the mylohyoid and then gives rise to the submandibular duct which runs on the floor of the mouth to open at the frenulum of the tongue. The lingual nerve, the submaxillary ganglion and the hypoglossal nerve are situated close to the deeper part of the gland (see Fig. 16.1).

In practice, enlargement affects the parotid gland most commonly, followed by the submandibular gland. Although swellings of the salivary glands may be due to viral infections (e.g. mumps parotitis), in surgical practice the enlargement is most commonly caused by calculous disease blocking the ductal drainage system (submandibular more commonly than parotid) or by tumours (predominantly mixed parotid tumours). Enlargements of the submandibular gland appear as swellings in the submandibular triangle. By contrast, parotid swellings occur within a large inverted triangular area with boundaries extending from the tragus of the ear to the anterior border of the mandibular ramus and the gap between the mastoid process and the angle of the mandible inferiorly. Swellings caused by infection and stones obstructing the salivary duct are painful and tender, whereas tumours are painless and non-tender (see Chapter 16).

Face, oral cavity and scalp

Inspection forms an important part of the examination. The facial expression of the patient describes the mood of the patient and with practice, the physician can rapidly establish anxiety, depression, introversion and mania. Inspection of the skin and mucosal surfaces, conjunctivae and buccal mucosae identifies pallor (anaemia), central cyanosis (deoxygenation of the blood and polycythaemia) and abnormal pigmentation. The yellowish discoloration in jaundiced patients is obvious on inspection but minor grades of icterus are identified by examination of the sclera in a good light. Other features of hepatic disease include muscle wasting, bruising, spider naevi which are found in the territory of the superior vena cava and yellowish-white periocular fatty deposits (xanthelasma) encountered in certain hyperlipidaemic states.

The mucosal lining of the lips and buccal mucosa may exhibit areas of pigmentation in certain disorders. The most common ulcers of the lips are viral lesions (herpes simplex) which often accompany debility and infections of the upper respiratory tract and occur as painful lesions at the angle of the mouth. Malignant ulcers of the lip are squamous cell lesions which present as painless persistent ulcers usually on the lower lip (Fig. 1.11a). Spread is to the submental and submandibular lymph node groups in the first instance. Basal cell (rodent ulcers) carcinomas are much more frequent and occur in elderly patients predominantly in the upper third of the face and scalp above the maxillary line (Fig. 1.11b and c). The other common malignant tumour encountered in the face and scalp is malignant melanoma (Fig. 1.12), of which there

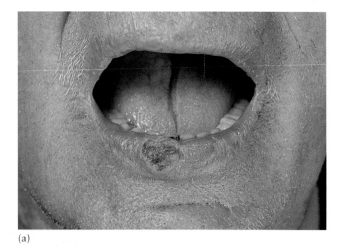

(a)

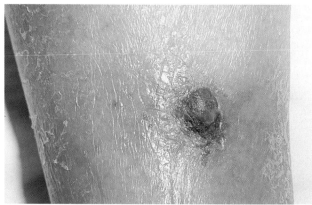

Figure 1.12 Malignant melanoma on the leg of a 'sun worshipper'.

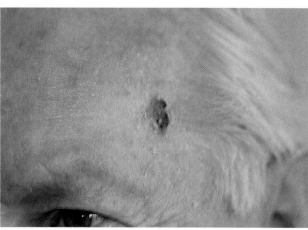

(b)

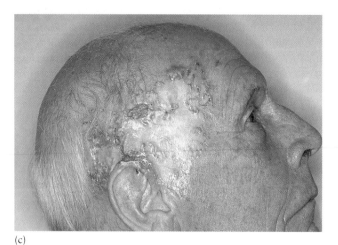

(c)

Figure 1.11 (a) Squamous carcinoma on the lower lip of an inveterate pipe smoker. (b) Early basal cell carcinoma on the forehead. At this stage treatment is straightforward and the prognosis is excellent. (c) A neglected basal cell carcinoma on the side of the head involving the ear and a large area of the scalp. Treatment is now extremely difficult and it may not be possible to remove the lesion completely.

are various types. Malignant melanomas occur as pigmented lesions over a wide age range and are prevalent in fair-skinned individuals who are exposed to sunshine (see Chapter 17).

The buccal cavity is examined for gingival hypertrophy (often drug-induced), inflammation (gingivitis) and tumours of the gums, and lesions (ulcers, thickenings and fissures) of the tongue and buccal mucosa. Oral and mucocutaneous candidiasis (infestation by *Candida albicans*) is encountered in debilitated individuals and may complicate antibiotic therapy. The infection causes a very sore mouth and throat and may extend to the oesophagus. The affected mucosa is red and covered with white adherent patches. The pharynx can be inspected directly or indirectly with a laryngeal mirror and light source. Ulcers of the tongue should always be viewed with suspicion. Whist some are traumatic (caused by a jagged tooth or ill-fitting dentures) or aphthous in nature, a significant percentage prove to be malignant. As approximately one-third of cancers of the tongue occur on the undersurface or on the lateral edge of the posterior third of the tongue, examination should include elevation of the organ for inspection of the inferior surface and protrusion forwards and laterally (to either side), whilst the appropriate angle of the mouth is retracted to enable adequate inspection or the posterior part of the lateral borders.

The commonest swelling of the scalp is a sebaceous cyst which is a retention cyst of a hair follicle. Sebaceous cysts are often multiple (Fig. 1.13). They are round in shape and are always attached to the skin. Their contents are cheesy in nature and on palpation they are firm and non-fluctuant. Sometimes, a punctum can be identified in the centre of the lesion. They become painful and swollen if infected, when they discharge pus and then resolve, although recurrence of the swelling is frequent.

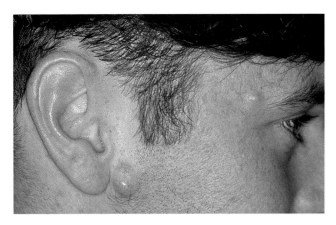

Figure 1.13 Sebaceous cysts are often multiple.

Examination of the breasts

The common breast complaints in females are discovery of a lump (benign or malignant), pain (mastalgia) and nipple discharge. In males, the commonest ailment is unilateral or bilateral hypertrophy (gynaecomastia), which may be idiopathic (postpubertal), drug-induced or secondary to certain disorders, e.g. liver disease.

Undoubtedly the most important presentation is a *palpable lump*, in view of the frequency of breast carcinoma which now affects 1 : 12 females in Western countries. *Breast pain* is a very common complaint and may either be diffuse and cyclical with pain and tenderness before and during menstrual periods (cyclical pronounced mastalgia) or localized to a specific area with or without a palpable lesion at this site (trigger-point mastalgia). *Nipple discharge* may occur alone or in association with other symptoms (e.g. lump or pain). The nature and colour of the discharge vary but when blood-stained, nipple discharge signifies the presence of a duct papilloma or carcinoma. The examination of the breasts should always include palpation of the neck and both axillae for lymph node enlargement.

Inspection

This necessitates removal of clothing to the waist and therefore requires privacy and the presence of a nurse. Inspection is carried out in two postures:
• Initially the breasts are inspected with the patient sitting up straight and the arms by the side facing the doctor. At this stage one is assessing size, contour of breast mounds, surface abnormalities and the state and direction of the nipples. A certain amount of disparity in breast size is quite common and normal, but the nipples should point in the same direction. Inversion of the nipples is frequently en-

countered and may be normal, due to benign disease (usually bilateral retraction) or an underlying cancer (unilateral retraction).

The skin over a breast abscess is red, shiny and oedematous. However, a similar appearance is encountered in patients with inflammatory breast cancer (mastitis carcinosa). The thickening of the skin in these patients is due to oedema secondary to cutaneous lymphatic permeation, the pitted appearance simulating orange skin — hence the term *peau d'orange*.
• The patient is then asked to lift her upper arms above her head. This manoeuvre normally results in uplifting of the breasts with diminished protrusion of the nipples but the surface contour of the breast mounds should remain smooth and convex. Dimpling or localized depression or obvious inversion of the nipple is indicative of an underlying malignant mass which is causing tethering of the superficial tissues.

Palpation

Palpation of the breast

The unaffected breast is palpated first. The patient must be comfortable in the sitting or semirecumbent position with her elbows resting on the couch and the arms on her flanks. Palpation of the breast is carried out with the flat of the hand gently compressing the breast tissue against the chest wall (Fig. 1.14). It starts in the areolar region and covers, in a systematic manner, the entire breast, including the axillary tail. If a lump is found, its position is noted but the general palpation is continued to determine whether any other lumps are present. Normal breast tissue feels soft and smooth. In many adult females, the breasts have a nodular, lumpy consistency and the distinction between normal and abnormal may be

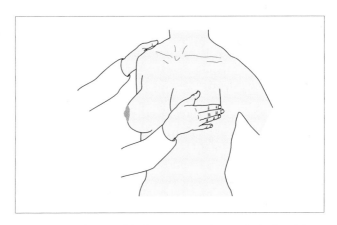

Figure 1.14 Palpation of the breast is carried out with the flat of the hand gently compressing the breast tissue against the chest wall.

difficult and requires considerable experience. Pathological diffuse thickening may be localized or generalized.

Palpation of an identified breast lump

If a lump is identified during the general palpation, the following information is essential: tenderness, position, size, consistency, margins, mobility and involvement of adjacent structures and tissues. A breast abscess is exquisitely tender. Tenderness is also encountered in mammary duct ectasia, Mondor's disease (thrombophlebitis of the subcutaneous breast veins) and in traumatic fat necrosis of the breast.

In terms of precise location of a lump, the breast is divided into the areolar region and four quadrants: upper inner, upper outer, lower outer, lower inner (see Fig. 14.1). The size of the lump is best measured by callipers in two directions. Size is one of the variables used in the staging of cancer of the breast. *Breast cancer* feels firm to hard, is not tender and has indistinct margins. By contrast, benign lesions (fibroadenomas, breast cysts) are firm, smooth and always mobile. *Fibroadenoma* is very mobile and tends to slip away from the examining finger and, for this reason, has been described as 'a breast mouse'. The mobility of a lump is tested both in relation to the overlying skin and to the underlying pectoralis major fascia and muscle. Tethering or fixation of the lump to the underlying pectoral muscles is determined after the patient is asked to contract the ipsilateral pectoralis major muscle by pressing on her hips with her hand. Involvement of the superficial breast tissue varies from tethering such that the skin and subadjacent breast parenchyma cannot be rolled over the mass to actual involvement with puckering of the skin, ulceration and fungation.

Palpation of the axillae

Examination of the breasts is incomplete without careful palpation of both axillae and neck for palpable lymph nodes which could represent metastatic disease.

Palpation of the axilla is carried out from in front of the patient who is either in the semirecumbent or sitting position. The patient's upper arm is supported on the examiner's arm during the palpation (Fig. 1.15), which must be carried out in an orderly fashion, starting at the apex of the axillae followed by the medial (chest) wall, anterior wall (pectoral muscles) and posterior wall (over the subscapularis muscle). If palpable lymph nodes are present, their number and mobility or otherwise are noted (see Chapter 14).

Abdominal examination

An abdominal examination consists of several parts — examination of the abdomen, examination of the inguinal

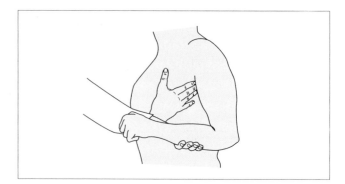

Figure 1.15 Palpation of the axilla is carried out from in front of the patient who is either in the semirecumbent or sitting position. The patient's upper arm is supported on the examiner's arm during the palpation.

region, examination of the scrotum and testes and a rectal examination.

Examination of the abdomen

Good examination of the abdomen entails certain requirements such as a well-lit room to detect skin colour changes and warm environment to prevent shivering, which results in contractions of the abdominal wall and thereby interferes with palpation of the abdomen. If the patient is in a multibed unit, curtains are drawn around the bed for privacy during the examination.

The patient is examined supine with one pillow beneath the head and a sheet or blanket which covers the pubic region and the lower limbs. Patients with an acute abdomen are often more comfortable with the legs drawn up as this relieves tension on the anterior abdominal musculature. No attempt must be made to straighten their lower limbs as this will exacerbate the pain and limit the scope of the examination. Right-handed individuals should examine patients from the right side of the bed and left-handed individuals from the other side. Ideally, the patient's abdomen should be at the level of the examiner's elbow. This is achieved either by elevating the bed to the right level or bending to the right level.

Surface anatomy of the abdomen

The various quadrants described in anatomical textbooks are not practical because of considerable overlap. A better subdivision for clinical purposes is shown in Fig. 13.1 which has the following components: four quadrants (right and left upper quadrants and right and left iliac fossae), epigastric, periumbilical (or central), suprapubic and two flank (or loin) regions.

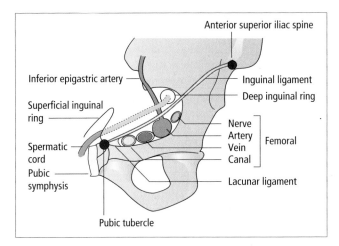

Figure 1.16 The anatomy of the inguinal canal. The *midpoint of the inguinal ligament* between the anterior superior iliac spine and the pubic tubercle marks the site of the internal or deep inguinal ring, whereas the *midinguinal point* between the anterior superior iliac spine and the pubic symphysis locates the superficial femoral artery as it emerges below the inguinal ligament. The important structures below the inguinal ligament, from the lateral to medial aspect, are the femoral nerve, femoral artery, femoral vein and the femoral ring which is bordered medially by the lacunar ligament and laterally by the femoral vein.

The important cutaneous landmarks on the anterior aspect are the costal margins, xiphoid process, umbilicus, anterior iliac spine, pubic tubercle, symphysis pubis and the inguinal ligament (Fig. 1.16). The useful cutaneous landmarks on the posterior aspect are the tip of the 11th rib (the 12th rib is not usually palpable), the ridge of the paraspinal muscles (erector spinae), the vertebral spinous processes and the iliac crest.

Inspection of the abdomen

Inspection should cover the following:
- contour of the abdomen;
- surface markings and abnormalities; and
- hernial defects.

Movement and contour In normal individuals, the anterior abdominal wall moves passively with respiration (expands with inspiration and recedes with expiration). This movement is abolished or considerably reduced in patients with an acute abdomen where the abdominal muscular walls are in spasm.

The contour of both the anterolateral abdominal wall and the flank provides useful information both in the elective and emergency situations. In normal individuals in the supine position, the abdomen is flat, although it may be scaphoid in thin people and the contour of the flank is flat in males and concave in females. Bulging of the flanks and abdominal distension are encountered in obesity ascites, pregnancy and intestinal obstruction.

Surface markings or abnormalities These include previous operation scars (normal, keloid, pitted due to previous infection), skin lesions, scratch marks (in jaundice), striae (previous pregnancy or obesity), bruising or staining of the skin of the abdomen (e.g. flank in acute pancreatitis — Turner's sign; periumbilical staining due to haemoperitoneum — Cullen's sign), obvious swellings, dilated abdominal wall veins (obstruction or compression of the inferior vena cava), previously constructed ostomies (colostomy, ileostomy), abnormal pulsations (abdominal aortic aneurysm).

Hernial defects Herniation may occur through natural orifices such as the inguinal or femoral canal (Chapter 13) or through weaknesses in the anterior abdominal wall such as besides the umbilical cicatrix (paraumbilical hernia) or through a poorly healed surgical wound (incisional hernia). When noticed during inspection with the patient in the supine position, an unobstructed hernia appears as a momentary bulge when the intra-abdominal pressure is raised either by asking the patient to cough or tense the abdominal muscles. In some patients atrophy of the recti abdominis muscles together with their separation from each other results in a central abdominal bulging defect. This is most commonly seen in multiparous females but is also encountered in males and is referred to as divarication of the recti or ventral hernia. An irreducible hernia (one that is stuck in the parietes) or an obstructed hernia appears as a constant bulge which is there all the time and cannot be reduced either by the patient or the doctor.

The demonstration of an incisional or ventral hernia is best achieved simply by asking the patient to lift his or her head (without support from the upper arms) from the pillow. This raises the abdominal pressure and produces a distinctive bulge. The same effect can be achieved by asking the patient to lift his or her lower limbs off the bed Fig. 13.54.

Abdominal palpation

Palpation is the most important aspect of the physical examination of the abdomen. Various techniques are used: light palpation, deep palpation, palpation of specific organs (liver and spleen), bimanual palpation (kidneys and retroperitoneum) and palpation of a fluid thrill.
- *General principles*: Aside from ensuring that the patient is in a comfortable supine position, palpation must be carried out gently with warm hands and in a systematic

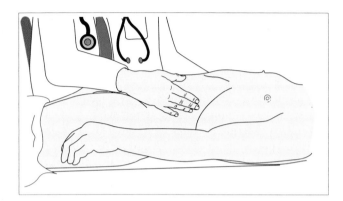

Figure 1.17 Light palpation of the abdomen is best performed by a doctor in the sitting or kneeling position so that the examiner's arm is comfortable and level with the anterior abdominal wall. Palpation should proceed in an orderly fashion around the quadrants of the abdomen, always starting diametrically opposite the area of interest (e.g. if the patient has right iliac fossa pain, start in the left upper quadrant). Note that the patient is exposed from the nipple line to the mid-thigh.

fashion from quadrant to quadrant. Long finger nails, by digging into the patient's skin, impair the ability to conduct the examination. A common mistake enacted by the inexperienced is to hurry the palpation (flitting palpation). The hand should not be transferred to another region until the doctor has registered whether the area concerned feels normal or not. Light palpation (Fig. 1.17) is conducted before deep palpation. In general, the more one presses the abdominal wall, the less one feels for two reasons. In the first instance, the tactile sensation is diminished with constant sustained pressure. Secondly, clumsy deep palpation hurts the patient and induces spasm of the abdominal muscular walls. The technique used varies with the state of the abdomen: acute or non-acute.

• *Palpation of the acute abdomen*: These patients are acutely ill, usually in considerable pain and some may be in shock from dehydration/hypovolaemia (Chapter 4). The primary concern is therefore resuscitation and relief of pain by intravenous opiates. Both these measures must precede palpation of the abdomen. Opiates should be administered via the intravenous route, especially in shocked patients, since the peripheral shutdown greatly reduces the uptake of the drug by the circulation when this is administered by the intramuscular route. Relief of pain is not only kind and humane, but also facilitates the conduct of the examination by increasing patient comfort and allaying anxiety. The belief that analgesia may mask physical signs is completely unfounded.

The abdominal palpation of patients with an acute abdomen must be conducted with the utmost gentleness

and is primarily designed to establish the presence of reflex spasm of the abdominal muscles (guarding and rigidity) and the presence, extent and location of abdominal tenderness. In the presence of peritoneal irritation due to infection or escape of gastrointestinal contents (e.g. perforated peptic ulcer), both the visceral and the parietal peritoneum become inflamed (peritonitis). The localized pain and tenderness and the resulting spasm of the overlying abdominal muscles are due to stimulation of the somatic nerves supplying the abdominal parietes. When the abdominal wall is depressed by palpation, the pain is enhanced over the inflamed area. Moreover, the pain is intensified further as the pressure from the fingers is released. This is known as rebound tenderness. The test, although valuable, must be elicited with the minimum of suffering possible. In the vast majority of patients, simple coughing will induce pain in the affected region and this is equivalent to eliciting rebound tenderness by light palpation. In others, gentle percussion on the examiner's left fingers (placed on the abdominal wall) by the right hand can elicit the sign. In any event, deep palpation must never be practised in these patients.

The extent of spasm of the abdominal musculature varies from increased tension of the abdominal wall (guarding) to board-like rigidity. To some extent, the degree of rigidity depends on the state of the individual patient's musculature. Thus, elderly patients with atrophic muscles may not exhibit significant rigidity despite an established generalized peritonitis, but they will always experience tenderness with rebound during the examination. By contrast, the abdomen of a previously fit athletic male patient with a perforated ulcer will be board-like in most instances. Physical signs, including guarding and rebound tenderness, may be abrogated by drugs (especially steroids), old age and immunosuppression from any cause. Thus, a high index of suspicion must be kept in these groups of patients.

• *Palpation of the non-acute abdomen*: Light palpation is used in the first instance and suffices for most patients. The technique entails using a slightly cupped hand which is warm and relaxed (almost dead weight) with the terminal phalanges gently depressing the anterior abdominal. The sensitivity and ability to feel lumps and normal organs increase with practice and experience, for which there is no substitute. Deep palpation is necessary in obese individuals and patients with well-developed abdominal musculature. The best technique (Fig. 1.18) entails the use of both hands: the left on the abdominal wall (as the sensing hand) is overlapped and depressed by the right hand. Again, as little force as is necessary is applied. Some clinicians perform deep palpation using one hand. Palpation of the abdomen in the non-acute situation is designed to detect the presence of tenderness, the enlargement of organs (liver, spleen and kidneys) and the presence of any intra-abdominal masses.

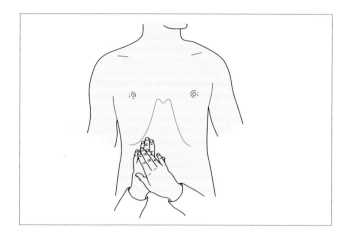

Figure 1.18 Technique of deep palpation using two hands.

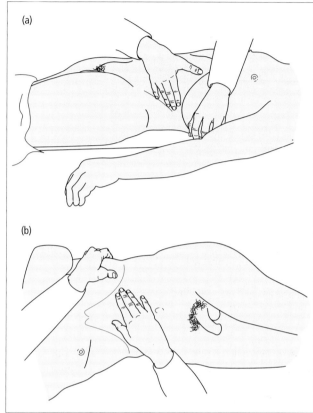

Figure 1.19 (a) Palpation of the spleen requires elevation of the left lower ribcage and flank as the abdomen is palpated with the right hand starting in the right iliac fossa. (b) When uncertainty remains as to whether a spleen is palpable, the patient should be positioned in the right semiprone position, as this results in anterior displacement of the organ.

- *Palpation of specific organs.*
  (a) *Liver and gallbladder.* The lower edge of the liver is just palpable in most normal individuals with the tips of the fingers pointing upwards, starting in the right lower quadrant and moving up towards the right costal margin. Normally, a distinct smooth edge is felt which moves and becomes more prominent with inspiration. The substance of the liver lies underneath the thoracic cage and its upper margin is therefore impalpable; however, its position can be identified by percussion (see below). When the liver enlarges as a result of disease, the anterior superior surface becomes palpable as a firm mass extending from the right hypochondrium to the epigastric region. Normally, the gallbladder is not palpable. When enlarged, as happens in patients with cancer of the head of the pancreas (Chapter 13), it is felt as a round smooth swelling which moves with respiration in the right hypochondrium along the mid clavicular line.
  (b) *The spleen.* This has to be enlarged to one-and-a-half to twice its normal size (splenomegaly) before it can be felt. As the spleen enlarges medially and inferiorly, it projects for a varying distance below the left costal margin towards the right lower quadrant. Palpation of the spleen requires elevation of the left lower ribcage and flank as the abdomen is palpated with the right hand starting in the right iliac fossa (Fig. 1.19a). When uncertainty remains as to whether a spleen is palpable or not, the patient should be positioned in the right semiprone position as this results in anterior displacement of the organ (Fig. 1.19b). Palpation of the spleen should be carried out during inspiration as the diaphragm pushes the organ downwards, rendering it more accessible to the tips of the fingers. In some enlarged spleens a distinct notch is palpable along the anterior margin, but this is by no means universal.

  (c) *The kidneys.* The kidneys are examined by the technique of bimanual palpation shown in Fig. 1.20. For the right kidney, the left hand is placed beneath the right flank and the right, anteriorly. The left hand is used to lift the retroperitoneal contents and thereby trap the mass or kidney between the two hands. The kidneys are not palpable in health, although in thin patients the lower poles may be felt occasionally. On the right side, an enlarged kidney has to be differentiated from a mass in the hepatic flexure or enlarged liver. On the left, the differentiation is between an enlarged spleen and mass in the descending colon.
- *Palpation of intra-abdominal masses.* Distinction between intra-abdominal masses and swellings within the abdominal wall is achieved by asking the patient to contract the abdominal muscles. This accentuates intramural masses and renders intra-abdominal swellings less distinct or impalpable. The most important clue to the nature of a swelling within the abdomen is the site (Table 1.10).

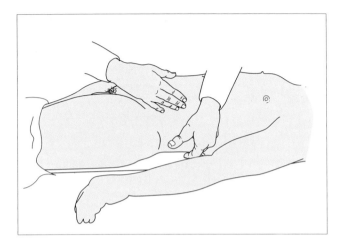

Figure 1.20 The kidneys are examined by the technique of bimanual palpation. The technique for examining the left kidney is shown here.

Table 1.10 Palpable abdominal masses.

Mass in RUQ: cancer of the hepatic flexure, enlarged gallbladder, enlarged right kidney

Mass in RUQ extending to the epigastrium: hepatomegaly

Mass in the epigastric region: liver, gastric cancer, abdominal aortic aneursym

Mass in LUQ: splenomegaly, cancer of the descending colon, swelling in tail of pancreas, enlarged left kidney

Mass in the periumbilical region: paraumbilical hernia, cancer of the transverse colon, tumour deposit from visceral neoplasm (Sister Mary Joseph's nodule)

Mass in LLQ: constipation (faecal scybala), cancer of the descending colon

Mass in the suprapubic region: distended urinary bladder, pregnancy, ovarian cyst

Mass in RLQ: appendiceal disease, cancer of the ascending colon, Crohn's disease of the terminal ileum

Mass in the inguinal region: hernia, enlarged lymph node (imflammatory, lymphoma, secondary tumour deposit), saphena varix, aneurysm

RUQ, Right upper quadrant; LUQ, left upper quadrant; LLQ, left lower quadrant; RLQ, right lower quadrant.

Other important features include presence of tenderness over the mass (denotes an inflammatory component), mobility with palpation, movement with respiration and consistency.

Percussion of the abdomen

Percussion is best regarded as an adjunct to palpation. It is used to determine the presence of tenderness, to estimate the size of an enlarged organ or mass, and to distinguish gaseous distension of hollow organs from an excessive amount of fluid in the peritoneal cavity (ascites), both of which cause generalized abdominal distension. The technique consists of gentle tapping with the right fingers (and a relaxed right wrist) on the index and middle finger of the left hand placed on the area to be percussed. A resonant note is obtained over a hollow organ which is distended with air (dilated stomach, colon, etc.) whereas a dull note is elicited over a solid organ (e.g. liver) or mass and fluid-filled cavities (e.g. distended urinary bladder, intra-abdominal cyst, ascites).

• *Percussion of the liver:* The objective of the exercise is to determine the size of the liver. The upper margin is defined first. This is normally situated at the level of the sixth rib in the mid clavicular line, but may be displaced downwards in patients with obstructive airways disease (emphysema) and in asthenic patients whose liver is loosely attached and ptotic. To determine the upper margin of the liver, percussion is started on the right anterior chest wall at the fourth intercostal space. A resonant note (due to aerated lung parenchyma) is obtained initially. This changes to relative dullness as the upper margin of the liver (still overlapped by lung) is reached. A few centimetres further down the percussion note becomes dull and remains so until the lower margin of the liver is reached. The normal anterior span of the liver varies with body size and ranges from 11 to 15 cm in males and 9 to 13 cm in females.

Auscultation of the abdomen

Auscultation of the abdomen is performed with the diaphragm end-piece of the stethoscope. It is used to listen for bowel sounds, bruits and venous hums and succussion splashes. An adequate technique is required to avoid spurious sounds caused by movement of the stethoscope over the abdominal wall, particularly in hairy individuals. During auscultation the diaphragm must be held absolutely still.

• *Bowel sounds:* The normal bowel sounds are difficult to describe and indeed exhibit a wide range of frequency, intensity and pitch. They are caused by peristaltic activity. In mechanical intestinal obstruction (Chapter 13), they become hyperactive due to the enhanced peristaltic activity proximal to the obstruction and can be heard as loud rushes which are coincident with episodes of colicky abdominal pain. Absent bowel sounds (during a 2-min period of auscultation) indicate loss of peristaltic activity and are encountered in adynamic ileus from any cause. In some of these patients, particularly those with hugely distended small intestine, tinkling sounds are heard. These result from the passive movement of fluid contents inside the cavernous intestinal loops.

- *Bruits*: Most bruits are heard in the midline between the xiphoid process and the umbilicus. These are caused by aneurysms (aorta, splenic artery) or stenosis (renal artery). A soft hum may be heard over the liver in portal hypertension and large vascular hepatic tumours, including hepatomas. A friction rub may be audible over the splenic region along the lower part of the left costal margin in patients with a splenic infarct or perisplenitis.
- *Succussion splash*: The stomach becomes distended with fluid (ingested liquid, saliva and gastric juice) when the pylorus is obstructed by tumour or cicatricial stenosis. The distended stomach gives rise to a dull fullness in the epigastrium. A splashing sound — succussion splash — heard (by the diaphragm of the stethoscope placed medial to the left costal margin) when the patient is shaken from side to side by the lower ribcage is pathognomonic of this condition. The test must, however, be carried out after a 4-h fast.

Examination of the abdomen for ascites

Ascites, which is the pathological accumulation of an excessive amount of fluid in the peritoneal cavity, causes abdominal distension which is dull to percussion. Similar findings on physical examination may be caused by large cysts which usually arise from the pelvis and are ovarian in origin, although some large cysts arise in the small-bowel mesentery. As distinct from large cysts, ascites is always accompanied by bulging of the flanks and the patients often have an everted umbilicus due to the formation of an umbilical hernia. Both specific palpation and percussion techniques are used to identify large cysts and differentiate one from the other.

The technique of *palpation of fluid thrill* which establishes the presence of fluid is illustrated in Fig. 1.21. The presence of ascites can only be established clinically by the detection of *shifting dullness* (Fig. 1.22).

Examination of inguinal region

The inguinal region is a site of common pathology — hernia formation, lymph node enlargement, etc. The important

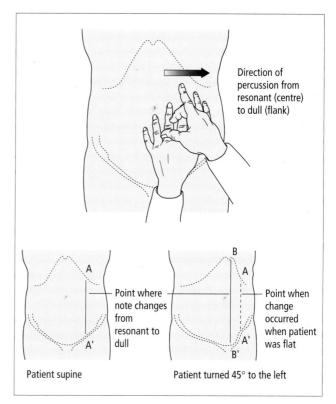

Figure 1.22 Tests for shifting dullness. In the *supine–lateral position test*, the abdomen is percussed from the umbilicus laterally in either direction and the line where resonance is replaced by dullness (A–A') is marked on either side. The patient is then rolled 45° on to one side and the abdomen percussed again, when (as a result of the fluid displacement by gravity) the level of dullness is seen to have shifted closer to the umbilicus on the dependent side (B–B'). This test is always positive when the ascites is accompanied by distension of the abdomen but may be negative or equivocal if the amount of fluid is less than 1500 ml. When doubt persists, the *knee–elbow–supine test*, which is more sensitive, is performed. The patient is first asked to assume the prone position for several seconds and then to elevate the trunk off the bed by assuming the knee–elbow position. Percussion reveals dullness around the central region of the abdomen, extending to the flanks. The lateral borders of the dullness are marked on either side. The patient is then turned to the supine position when the previous dull region becomes resonant.

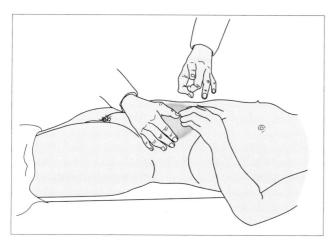

Figure 1.21 Technique of palpation of a fluid thrill. The right hand is placed flat on one side of the distended region and the swelling is tapped by the fingers of the left hand. This action produces sets of waves in the fluid (much like the ripples in a pool) which are felt by the right hand. The fluid thrill is accentuated if an assistant (or the patient) compresses the swelling with the edge of one hand.

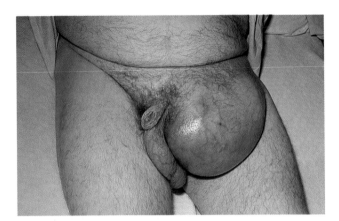

Figure 1.23 Massive metastatic inguinal lymph node deposits.

anatomical landmarks are described in Fig. 1.16. Inguinal lymph nodes are disposed both along the inguinal ligament (oblique) and vertically along the femoral vessels. They drain the lower abdominal wall, the genitalia, perineal region and the lower limbs (Fig. 1.23).

Inguinal herniae arise above the inguinal ligament and emerge through the external ring medial to the public tubercle. By contrast, a femoral hernia exits through the femoral canal below the inguinal ligament and lateral to the public tubercle. Inguinal herniae are anatomically classified into direct (weakness through the posterior wall made up of the transversalis fascia and conjoint tendon) and indirect, where the hernia enters the inguinal canal through the internal ring and courses down obliquely through the canal before it exits through the external ring. As it enlarges, an indirect inguinal hernia descends into the scrotum (inguinoscrotal hernia), which a direct hernia never does.

The examination for suspected hernia commences with inspection of the patient in the standing position, when a bulge may seen. This will become more prominent if the patient coughs. The hand is then placed over the lump and the patient is asked to cough again, when a cough impulse is felt. This establishes the diagnosis. It is important that both inguinal regions are examined for cough impulse as inguinal herniae are often bilateral. The patient is then put in the supine position. If the hernia disappears spontaneously in this position, it is likely to be of the direct variety. Otherwise an attempt is made to reduce the hernia. If this is unsuccessful, the hernia is labelled as irreducible. This stage is accompanied by a significant increase in the risk of obstruction and strangulation (Chapter 13).

A femoral hernia is usually not reducible and may not transmit a cough impulse. It forms a tense globular subcutaneous swelling below the inguinal ligament and lateral to the pubic tubercle and is sometimes difficult to differentiate from an enlarged lymph node (Fig. 13.54).

Examination of the scrotum and external genitalia

In surgical practice this is usually confined to examination of the male genitalia, since females with disorders of this region are managed by gynaecologists. The examination is best performed with the patient in the supine position. Phimosis (narrowing of the preputial orifice such that the prepuce cannot be retracted over the glans) is common in uncircumcised males and often causes infection (balanitis) and meatal stricture. The majority of penile tumours are confined to the glans penis and this region should always be inspected in patients with a history of blood-stained discharge.

Initially one should establish that the patient has two palpable testes. If only one testis is palpable, palpation of the groin may reveal an ectopic testis (usually in infants and children). The impalpable testis may of course be in the inguinal canal or the abdominal cavity (undescended testis).

Scrotal swellings may originate from disease of the testis and epididymis and their coverings or result from a swelling (an indirect inguinal hernia) which descends to and in time occupies the scrotum. Thus the first objective with any scrotal swellings is to determine whether one can get above the scrotal swelling by approximating the tips of the two hands above the upper limit of the swelling (Fig. 1.24). If the examiner is unable to establish this, the swelling is inguinoscrotal and caused by a large indirect inguinal hernia.

The common swellings encountered in the scrotum are: hydrocele, inflammation of the testis and epididymis (epididymo-orchitis), and tumours of the testis (seminomas and teratomas). *Torsion of the testis* presents acutely with a very painful tender swelling and may be very difficult to distinguish from epididymo-orchitis.

A *hydrocele* is a collection of fluid in the tunica vaginalis and therefore surrounds the testis which thus becomes difficult to palpate. The swelling caused by a hydrocele is smooth and uniform, fluctuates and is brilliantly transilluminable. *Cysts of the epididymis* (multiloculated epididymal cyst, spermatocele) are not surrounded by fluid and for this reason are felt as swellings above and behind the testis, which is also easily palpable in this situation. Because of the septation, multiloculated epididymal cysts have a characteristic 'Chinese lantern' appearance on transillumination. *Testicular tumours* form heavy painless swellings of the testis and may be surrounded by a lax secondary hydrocele which does not, however, obscure their presence. When suspected, palpation of testicular tumours should be gentle to minimize the risk of dissemination of these malignant

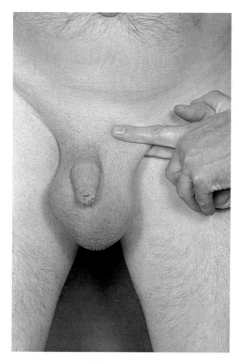

Figure 1.24 'Can I get above it?' The first objective with any scrotal swelling is to determine whether one can get above it by approximating the tips of the two hands above the upper limit of the swelling.

tumours. As the lymphatic spread from these tumours goes straight to the para-aortic lymph nodes, palpation of the abdomen for masses on either side of the umbilicus should be conducted.

Rectal examination

An abdominal examination is incomplete without a rectal examination. For this purpose, the patient is most commonly positioned in the left lateral decubitus position, although some prefer the knee–chest position.

Inspection

The examination starts with inspection of the perineum for external skin tags, perianal inflammation, sinuses, fissures, induration medial to the ischial tuberosity (base of the ischiorectal fossa).

Digital examination

Digital examination of the rectum is performed both in the elective situation and in patients with an acute abdomen. The actual rectal examination is carried out with a lubri-cated gloved hand. The tip of the index finger is placed inside the anal canal and directed initially towards the umbilicus before turning posteriorly towards the sacral concavity.

Deep rectal tenderness is encountered in acute appendicitis, salpingitis and in patients with peritonitis. A ballooned empty rectum may be found in patients with small-bowel obstruction. Alternatively, in patients with large-bowel obstruction due to severe constipation, a mass of impacted faeces is encountered.

In the elective situation, the rectal walls (anterior, lateral and posterior) are first felt for mucosal lesions (polypoidal growths, ulcers, etc.). The prostate gland is examined through the anterior wall. Normally, it should be possible to move the rectal wall over the prostate gland. The median sulcus between the two lobes of the prostate gland is also palpable. In benign disease, the prostate may be enlarged or fibrotic, whereas in cancer of the prostate, the gland feels craggy with loss of the normal outline and infiltration of the anterior rectal wall. No other structure should be palpable through the rectal walls. Ovaries and tubes are felt laterally only when enlarged and pathological. Tumour deposits in the pelvic peritoneum may be felt as a hard shelf anteriorly. When the digital examination is complete, the glove is inspected for the presence of blood and a haemoccult test is performed before being discarded.

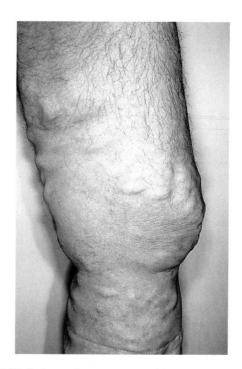

Figure 1.25 Varicose veins.

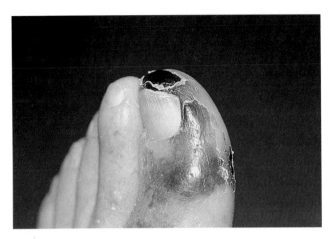

Figure 1.26 Gangrene of great toe in an elderly patient with peripheral vascular disease who presented with rest pain.

Examination of the limbs

Aside from tumours (skin, soft tissues and bone), the limbs are examined for disorders of the locomotor system (Chapters 10, 11, 22), the peripheral nervous system (Chapter 11) and the vascular system (Chapter 18). Detailed descriptions of the clinical examination of the limb are given in these chapters. Common conditions include varicose veins (Fig. 1.25) and peripheral vascular disease due to acute or chronic vascular insufficiency (Fig. 1.26). Lymphoedema which is caused by primary (Fig. 1.27) or secondary dis-

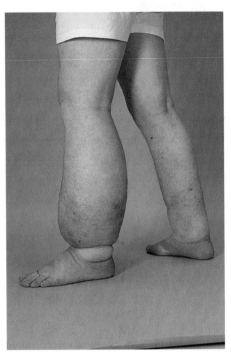

Figure 1.27 Primary lymphoedema of the legs in a 28-year-old man.

orders of the lymphatics (e.g. after radical surgery or radiotherapy) is less frequent. Peripheral nerve injury is a relatively common complication of trauma and produces characteristic clinical signs which are discussed in detail in Chapter 11.

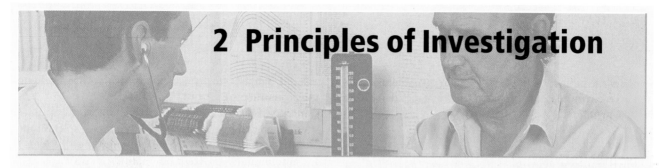

2 Principles of Investigation

Modern doctors regrettably prefer to look at the results on a piece of computer paper than to listen to the credible, consistent and reasoned observations of their patients who after all live with their bodies. If the blood tests are all normal the symptoms must be generated from a disturbed psyche. (John Dwyer, 1993)

Introduction

Throughout this book reference is made to the investigations which are carried out in patients suspected of having various surgical disorders. Although specific investigations provide valuable information, their indiscriminate use constitutes bad practice; not only is it wasteful of resources but it may also put patients and staff at risk (e.g. contrast media may induce anaphylaxis). The risk to the patient correlates with the degree of invasiveness of the procedure and a spectrum of risk exists. This ranges from no risk, when the examination is entirely non-invasive and has no harmful side-effects (e.g. ultrasonography), to considerable risk with invasive procedures (e.g. arterial puncture during arteriography may result in serious complications). In addition, there are risks to the staff (e.g. handling contaminated blood exposes staff to the risk of disease transmission, such as hepatitis and acquired immune deficiency syndrome (AIDS); X-ray staff have to be vigilant against radiation exposure).

Investigations may be classified into a number of large groups (Table 2.1). A key investigation is one that confirms or excludes a strongly suspected diagnosis and is always necessary, e.g. gastroscopy in a patient with a history suggestive of upper gastrointestinal bleeding. By contrast, routine or baseline haematological and biochemical tests are performed before surgery to establish normality or to obtain baselines. However, the ordering of baseline investigations, though widespread in hospital practice, is wasteful of resources and is gradually being replaced by selective testing based on the clinical findings. One study found abnormalities on routine testing in only 0.4% of asympto-

Table 2.1 Investigations commonly used in the assessment of patients.

Blood investigations	*Endoscopy*
Haematology	
Biochemistry	*Function tests*
Blood gas analysis	Pulmonary function
Immunology	Oesophageal motility
	Urodynamics
Microbiology	Anorectal manometry
	Nerve conduction studies
Imaging	
X-rays	*Vascular*
Barium studies	ECG
Gastrografin	Holter monitoring
Cholecystography and	Echocardiography
cholangiography	Duplex scanning
Intravenous urography, cystography	Plethysmography
Arteriography	Ankle/brachial index measurement
Venography	
Myelography	
Ultrasound	
CT and MRI	
Nuclear medicine studies	

CT, Computed tomography; MRI, magnetic resonance imaging; ECG, electrocardiogram.

matic patients undergoing surgery. Thus, asymptomatic healthy patients may have surgery *without any investigations* while specific tests should be ordered on the basis of the clinical preoperative evaluation (including urinalysis). For example, urea and electrolytes are indicated when there is evidence of water and electrolyte depletion, renal disease, in elderly patients or in patients taking diuretics. A preoperative chest X-ray is indicated only in patients with cardiorespiratory disease or symptoms, in the elderly, in smokers, in patients with possible pulmonary metastases and in recent immigrants from countries where tuberculosis is still endemic.

Blood investigations

Haematology

The standard investigation performed to assess the status of the elements in blood is the full blood count. The information derived from this investigation is given in Box 2.1.

• The *haemoglobin* is reduced in anaemia and elevated in dehydration and polycythaemia. Most 'surgical' anaemias are due to chronic blood loss, e.g. oesophagitis, carcinoma of the caecum, and will have a microcytic (mean corpuscular volume (MCV) <80 fl), hypochromic (mean corpuscular haemoglobin (MCH) <25 pg) picture. However, a macrocytic picture (MCV >96 fl) may be seen in anaemias following gastrectomy (due to loss of intrinsic factor) or in patients with ileal disease (e.g. Crohn's disease) or after ileal resection. Polycythaemia may be primary (haemoglobin >18 g/dl) with elevation of haematocrit (>0.55), white cell count (WCC >12 × 10^9/l) and platelets (>650 × 10^9/l), or secondary, due to hypoxia or increased erythropoietin production in renal disease.

• The *WCC* is often measured in surgical patients. A raised WCC is commonly due to the presence of excessive numbers of neutrophils (*neutrophilia/leukocytosis*) as a result of acute bacterial infections, haemorrhage or tissue necrosis. Rarely, an infection is so severe that white cell production is decreased leading to a reduced WCC (*neutropenia/leukopenia*). Raised lymphocyte counts should alert one to the possibility of viral infections or leukaemias, while reduced lymphocyte levels are seen with AIDS, radiation and chemotherapy.

• Increased platelet numbers (*thrombocytosis*) are seen after haemorrhage and especially after splenectomy. *Thrombocytopenia* (low platelet count) may be due to an autoimmune process (idiopathic thrombocytopenic purpura), hypersplenism secondary to splenomegaly, and drug reactions (e.g. heparin-induced thrombocytopenia).

• Occasionally, patients are seen who have a combination of anaemia, leukopenia and thrombocytopenia. This is referred to as *pancytopenia*. This may be drug-induced or result from marrow destruction (e.g. by tumour infiltration) and is diagnosed by bone marrow examination.

• *Tests for clotting.* Bleeding is arrested by vessel constriction, the development of a platelet plug and activation of the clotting cascade (see Chapter 18). The three investigations routinely used to assess clotting are the *platelet count* (deficiencies cause purpura), the *prothrombin time* (PT) and the *activated partial thromboplastin time* (APTT).

(a) The PT measures the extrinsic pathway and factors VII, X and V. It is prolonged in vitamin K deficiency and is used to monitor anticoagulation with warfarin. The normal PT is 12–15 s. The results of the PT in patients is now expressed as the INR (international normalized ratio), which is derived by dividing the patient's PT by an international reference standard (e.g. if a patient's PT is 30 s and the standard is 12 s then the INR is 30/12 = 2.5).

(b) The APTT measures deficiencies of factors V, VII–XI and XII (the intrinsic pathway) and is used to monitor anticoagulation with heparin. The APTT is prolonged in haemophiliacs.

Disseminated intravascular coagulation (DIC)

If extensive intravascular clotting occurs (e.g. in sepsis), the coagulation factors are consumed and the PT and APTT are prolonged. The vast amounts of fibrin formed in the coagulation process are broken down into *fibrin degradation products* (FDP), the levels of which are elevated in the serum and urine.

Blood grouping and cross-matching for transfusion are frequently required in surgical patients. Transfusion of blood may be hazardous and should not be undertaken lightly. This subject is discussed fully in Chapter 29.

Biochemistry

Measurement of various biochemical parameters is frequently performed in surgical patients. The main biochemical tests performed and the normal range of values are listed in Box 2.2. Similarly, blood gases are fre-

Full blood count, normal values		
Haemoglobin	Male	12.5–16.5 × 10^9/litre
	Female	11.5–15.5 × 10^9/litre
Packed cell volume (PCV)	Male	0.42–0.53
(Haematocrit)	Female	0.39–0.45
Red cell count	Male	4.4–6.5 × 10^{12}/litre
	Female	3.9–5.6 × 10^{12}/litre
Mean corpuscular volume (MCV)		80–96 fl
Mean corpuscular haemoglobin (MCH)		27–31 pg
White cell count (WCC)		4–10 × 10^9/litre
Platelet count		150–400 × 10^9/litre

Box 2.1

Normal serum biochemistry values

Sodium	135–146 mmol/litre
Potassium	3.5–5.0 mmol/litre
Urea	2.5–6.7 mmol/litre
Creatinine	60–120 μmol/litre
Glucose	4.0–7.0 mmol/litre
Calcium	2.2–2.6 mmol/litre
Phosphate	0.8–1.4 mmol/litre
Bicarbonate	22–30 mmol/litre
Uric acid	0.18–0.42 mmol/litre
Total protein	62–80 g/litre
Albumin	34–48 g/litre
Bilirubin	<17 μmol/litre
Osmolality	280–296 mosm/litre

Enzymes

Alkaline phosphatase	25–120 U/litre
Aspartate aminotransferase (AST)	10–40 U/litre
Alanine aminotransferase (ALT)	5–30 U/litre
Lactate dehydrogenase (LDH)	40–125 U/litre
Creatine phosphokinase (CPK)	24–195 U/litre

Box 2.2

Antibodies identified in autoimmune diseases

Disease	Antibodies produced
Graves' disease	Thyroglobin
Hashimoto's thyroiditis	Thyroid microsomal antigen
Pernicious anaemia	Gastric parietal cell
Addison's disease	Adrenal
Diabetes mellitus	Pancreatic islet cell
Connective tissue disease	Antinuclear (ANA)
Biliary cirrhosis	Mitochondrial
Chronic active hepatitis	Smooth muscle
Coeliac disease	Reticulin
Crohn's disease	
Rheumatoid arthritis	Anti-IgG antibody

Box 2.3

quently measured to assess the acid–base balance of surgical patients. Disorders of acid–base are closely allied to electrolyte disorders and both are discussed fully in Chapter 6.

Immunological tests

Antibodies

Antibodies are generated in response to extrinsic antigens (e.g. microorganisms, environmental allergens) or intrinsic antigens (autoantibodies). Measurement of serum auto-antibody levels is often required in surgical patients. These tests are usually requested as an autoantibody screen (Box 2.3).

Acute-phase proteins

The levels of a number of plasma proteins increase rapidly in response to infection or tissue injury. These include α_1-*antitrypsin*, *fibrinogen* and *C-reactive protein* (CRP). CRP is frequently measured in surgical patients and is useful in the diagnosis of bacterial infections when its level rises.

Microbiology

In patients with a suspected bacterial infection cultures should be obtained before starting antibiotic therapy. If the source of infection is suspected then the appropriate culture should be obtained (e.g. wound exudate in an infected wound). If the source is unclear urine, blood and sputum cultures should be obtained and central lines removed and cultured.

Urinalysis should be performed on all patients coming to hospital. This is a quick dipstix test which will identify the presence of glucose, blood and protein in the urine (Fig. 2.1). The presence of glucose should alert one to the possibility of diabetes and a blood sugar should be performed to confirm or refute the presence of diabetes. If haematuria is present on urinalysis, formal microscopy of the urine should be performed. The presence of nitrates or protein is an indication for urine culture. Samples for urine culture are obtained as midstream specimens (see Chapter 20).

Blood cultures should be obtained in all patients with suspected infection in whom the source is not obvious and in all patients with rigors. A blood culture is obtained by vein puncture following sterilization of the skin with alcohol. Ten millilitres of blood is withdrawn into a syringe. The blood is then decanted from the syringe into two sterile culture bottles, one for aerobic culture and one for anaerobic culture. A new needle is placed on the syringe and the top of the bottle is swabbed with alcohol prior to decanting the blood sample. Formal blood culture requires that three sets be taken from different sites around the body.

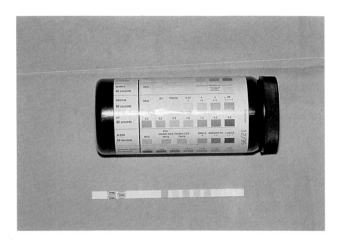

Figure 2.1 Dipstix test used for urinalysis.

Imaging

X-rays — a device which enables us to see how the bones in the back room are doing.   (Don Quinn)

Details of the various imaging techniques used to investigate specific systems are given in the relevant chapters. Only the principles underlying the specific imaging techniques are given here.

Radiography

• *Introduction.* X-rays were discovered by Wilhelm Roentgen in 1895 and were almost immediately applied to medicine (Box 2.4). X-rays are generated by passing an electric current through a vacuum tube. The quality and quantity of X-rays produced are determined by the electrical potential (kilovoltage: kV) applied to the tube and the electrical energy (measured in milliampere-seconds: mAs) passed through it. The X-rays produced diverge uniformly from the tube so that the area covered is directly proportional to the square of the distance travelled.

• *Plain film radiography.* When an X-ray beam passes through tissues it is differentially attenuated by the various structures present. The absorption of X-rays by tissues depends on the atomic number of the principal substance of which the tissue is composed. Thus, bone (containing calcium and other radiopaque salts) absorbs considerably more X-rays than surrounding tissues (e.g. muscle or lung tissue). This variable absorption produces a shadow on an X-ray plate which reflects tissue composition and structure (Fig. 2.2) and it is this phenomenon that forms the basis of plain film radiography.

Roentgen discovers X-rays

Wilhelm Roentgen (1845–1923) was professor of physics at Wurzburg. He was interested in phosphorescence of metallic salts exposed to light. In November 1895 he performed an experiment which involved passing an electrical current through a vacuum tube. While the current was passing through the tube he noticed that a screen 2 metres away gave off a greenish glow and on further investigation found that the screen had been painted with barium platinocyanide, a phosphorescent substance. He deduced that something given off by the tube was affecting the screen. He did some more experiments and found that the invisible (X) rays coming from the tube could pass through solid materials, e.g. wood. He also observed that when the rays were passed through his hand an image of the bones of his hand appeared on a photographic plate. He presented his findings to the Wurzburg Medical Society in December 1885. His discovery, surprisingly, was almost immediately taken up by the medical profession and Roentgen received the Nobel prize for physics in 1901.

Box 2.4 Roentgen discovers X-rays.

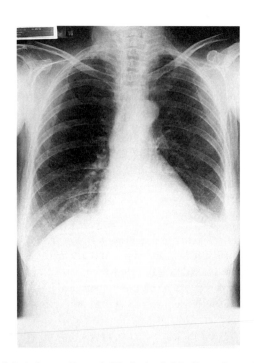

Figure 2.2 A chest radiograph. The basis of plain film radiography is that differential absorption of X-rays by tissues produces a shadow on a sensitized plate. The resulting image is called a radiograph (not an X-ray!).

• *Contrast media* are substances which are introduced into the body to enhance the differences in absorption and thereby delineate a particular tissue. Contrast material may have either a high atomic number and provide positive contrast (e.g. barium sulphate, organic iodine compounds) or a

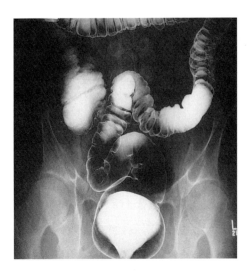

Figure 2.3 Double-contrast barium enema. Both barium (positive contrast) and air (negative contrast) are passed into the colon per-rectum to enhance the quality of the image obtained.

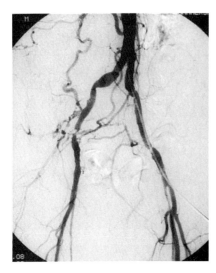

Figure 2.4 Digital subtraction fluorography. Digital subtraction angiogram of the aorta and iliac arteries in a patient with peripheral vascular disease. Note the catheter in the left iliac artery and the stenosis in the right iliac artery.

low atomic number and provide a negative contrast (e.g. gases such as air). In some situations both positive and negative contrast materials are used together, e.g. in a double-contrast barium enema both barium sulphate and air are used to outline the colon (Fig. 2.3).

• Subtraction techniques are now widely used to obtain enhanced images with lower concentrations of parenterally administered contrast media. In the subtraction technique a positive-image radiograph is obtained first. Contrast material is then injected and a second identical negative image is obtained. The two images are then superimposed; the positive and negative images common to both radiographs cancel out, leaving only the negative image of the injected contrast material. The modern technique is called *digital subtraction fluorography*. The analogue images are converted to digital signals and held in a computer memory. The computer mixes, subtracts and manipulates the images to give the optimum detail. The image is reconverted to analogue form and displayed on a screen (Fig. 2.4).

• *Tomography* is a technique whereby a structure in a preselected plane, e.g. a kidney, is highlighted radiographically by causing blurring of the images from the tissues anterior and posterior to the preselected plane. The simplest way to achieve this effect is by moving the tube and film in opposite directions while the patient remains stationary so that only the images of the preselected plane remain sharp. Tomography has been superseded by computed tomography (CT) and is seldom used now (Fig. 2.5).

• *CT* is a technqiue that uses tomography to produce cross-sectional images of the body. A large number of images

taken in different directions by a CT scanner (Fig. 2.6a) are fed into a digital computer which constructs the cross-sectional image. The system is very sensitive, so that small

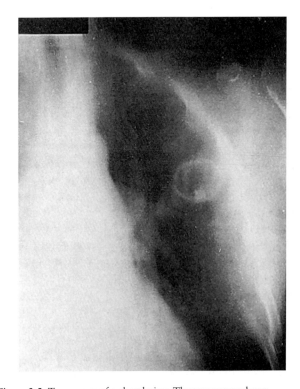

Figure 2.5 Tomogram of a chest lesion. The tomogram shows cavitation and calcification due to active pulmonary tuberculosis.

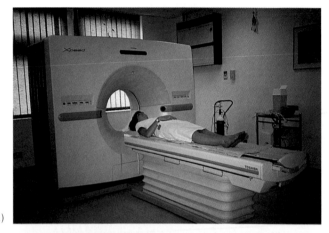

(a)

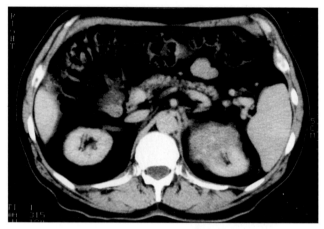

(b)

(c)

Figure 2.6 (a) A CT scanner. As the patient passes through the scanner several images in different directions are accumulated and a computer constructs a cross-sectional image. (b) A CT scan of the abdomen. The image is viewed from 'below'. In this case a tumour of the left kidney can be seen. (c) 3D CT scan of the upper abdomen showing the aorta, both kidneys and the spleen.

differences in tissue density can be recognized and a very detailed two-dimensional picture constructed (Fig. 2.6b). It is possible to construct three-dimensional CT images of structures (3D CT) so that complex anatomy can be interpreted with ease (Fig. 2.6c). In conventional CT scanning 'slices' of the body are obtained at 1 cm intervals by a camera which rotates around the patient at each 1 cm level. A newer, faster technique, known as helical or spiral CT scanning, produces a continuous image as the camera spirals around the patient.

• *Xeroradiography* is exactly the same as conventional radiography but the image is projected on to a selenium plate and appears as a positive rather than a negative image. It was mainly used for mammography but has now been displaced by conventional soft-tissue mammograms.

Ultrasonography

Ultrasonography is a diagnostic technique that uses high-frequency sound waves to generate an image. Ultrasound is generated in pulses from a special transducer disc when a voltage is placed across it. The interfaces of different body tissues reflect the sound waves as echoes. The echoes are returned to the transducer disc and converted into electrical impulses which can be converted into images. The images can be displayed in various different ways.

• A-mode or amplitude-modulated scan.
• M-mode or motion scan.
• B-mode or brightness-modulated scan.
• Real-time or two-dimensional scan.

Most diagnostic scanning now uses B-mode or real-time scanning. M-mode scanning is used (with pulsed Doppler and real-time scanning) in *echocardiography*.

The *Doppler effect* is the change in frequency of a sound due to the relative movement of the source of the sound and the observer. Simple Doppler probes (Fig. 2.7) can be used to detect arterial or venous blood flow, while pulsed Doppler probes, which emit short bursts or pulses of ultrasound, are very useful in cardiology for the detection of shunts and in the assessment of valvular heart disease. Pulsed Doppler is also combined with real-time scanning in *Duplex scanners* (Fig. 2.8) which are used to assess flow and anatomy in peripheral vessels, especially the carotid.

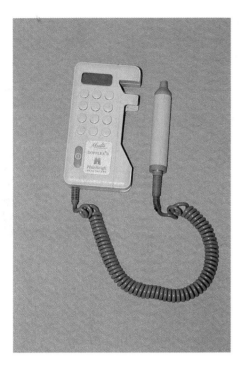

Figure 2.7 Doppler probe.

Radionuclide imaging (scintigraphy)

Radionuclide imaging is a technique which uses a special radiation detector (γ-camera) to depict the distribution of an administered isotope within an organ or the whole body (Fig. 2.9). Radionuclide imaging is mainly used to measure function but it can also demonstrate anatomy. Several radionuclide tests are now available, but all conform to the principle that an injected, inhaled or ingested pharmaceutical compound labelled with a suitable radionuclide is concentrated in the organ under review and the emitted radiation is detected by the γ-camera. Areas of increased or decreased activity are thus easily detected.

Technetium 99m (^{99m}Tc) is an ideal radionuclide as it emits only γ radiation, has a single energy peak, is readily available, has a half-life of 6 h and is suitable for many investigations (e.g. brain, thyroid, bone, kidney, adrenal glands). Other isotopes used are krypton (^{81m}Kr) for ventilation studies, iodine 131 (^{131}I) for thyroid studies and Gallium 67 (^{67}Ga), which is used to locate abscesses and tumours.

Patients are sometimes concerned that they are being given a radioactive material. The radiation dose is usually less than an equivalent radiological investigation but as the isotope is excreted by the body, tissues other than the tissue under examination are exposed to some radiation. Radionuclide examinations should be avoided in lactating

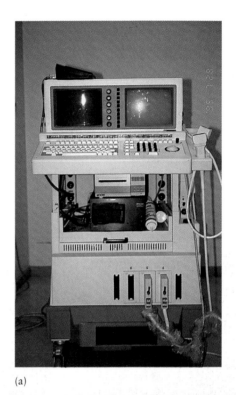

(a)

(b)

Figure 2.8 (a) Duplex scanner. (b) Colour duplex scan of blood vessels. Arterial blood flowing in one direction appears red/orange in colour while venous blood flowing in the opposite direction appears blue.

mothers as the radionuclide will be excreted into the breast milk.

Magnetic resonance imaging

Magnetic resonance imaging (MRI) is a diagnostic technique based on the fact that an externally applied magnetic field causes protons in tissues to align in the direction

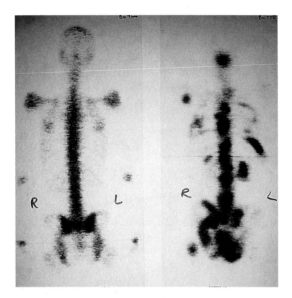

Figure 2.9 Radionuclide scan. Isotope bone scans. The image on the left is normal while the image on the right shows multiple 'hot' spots indicating metastatic disease.

of the magnetic field. By applying a second smaller magnetic field (in the form of a radiofrequency (RF) pulse) perpendicular to the main magnetic field, the alignment of the protons is changed. When the RF pulse is stopped the protons return to equilibrium and in so doing they produce another RF signal. This signal is the *magnetic resonance* (MR) signal which is amplified and transformed by computer into images.

The process whereby the protons give off energy is called *relaxation*. This process is characterized by two time constants: T_1 refers to the time for the protons to return to their original state of equilibrium; T_2 refers to the time for the protons to become out of phase with each other. Different tissues have different relaxation times and this gives rise to

image contrast. It is possible to optimize contrast by enhancing either T_1 or T_2 images. This is referred to as weighting, e.g. T_1-weighted images are used to demonstrate neural tissues (Fig. 2.10).

Magnetic resonance angiography (MRA) is a technique which has been developed over the last few years to provide angiographic data without the need for catheter insertion. MRA images are acquired by exploiting the differences between stationary tissues that have been saturated with RF pulses and unsaturated blood which flows into the saturated area from outside the excited section. Two slightly different techniques, called time of flight (TOF) and phase contrast (PC), are used to acquire the images. MRA is especially useful in assessing patients with suspected neurological dissease (Fig. 2.11).

MRI has brought with it its own hazards. Patients (or staff) with pacemakers should not go near an MR scanner. There have been horror stories of scissors and scalpels flying into the centre of MR scanners and injuring patients. Credit cards should also be kept at a safe distance. It would be rather embarrassing if you could not pay your hospital bill because your credit card was 'cleaned' while you were having your MR scan!

Endoscopy

Doctors have been trying to peer inside their patients' bodies for centuries (open your mouth, please!) but only in the last 150 years have instruments been developed which allow them to achieve this aim with any degree of precision (e.g. the first electrically lighted cystoscope was developed by Max Nitze in 1877, but fully flexible endoscopes for gastroscopy were not available until the late 1960s). Today several types of scope are available, not only for examining

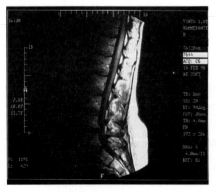

(a)

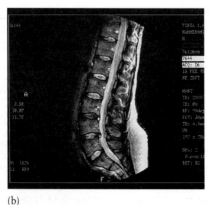

(b)

Figure 2.10 Magnetic resonance scan. (a) T_1-weighted image, (b) T_2-weighted image.

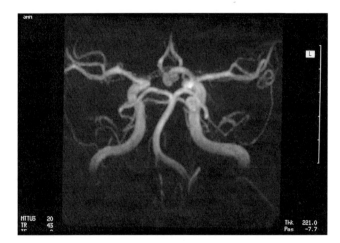

Figure 2.11 Magnetic resonance angiography demonstrating the circle of Willis.

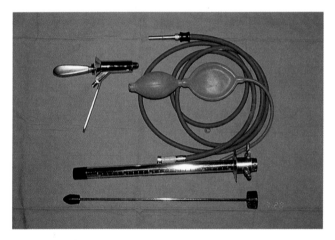

Figure 2.12 Proctoscope, and rigid sigmoidoscope.

the inside of the body but also for facilitating endoscopic surgical operations.

Rigid scopes

Scopes are of two kinds — rigid and flexible. Rigid scopes are simply straight tubes through which light is passed from an external source into the part of the body under examination. The simplest are proctoscopes (used to illuminate the anal canal) and rigid sigmoidoscopes (for the rectum and sigmoid colon; Fig. 2.12). Rigid bronchoscopes and oesophagoscopes are rarely used now but occasionally a rigid scope is employed to examine the mediastinum (mediastinoscope). Rigid cystoscopy is used regularly and a rigid scope with a resecting wire and irrigating channels (resectoscope) is used to perform transurethral pro-

statectomy or resection of bladder tumours. The scopes used for laparoscopy and arthroscopy are also rigid.

Flexible scopes

Flexible endoscopes are complex pieces of equipment consisting of:
- a head with controls and an eyepiece;
- a flexible shaft with a manoeuvrable tip; and
- an external light source.

The head is connected to the light source via a connecting flexible shaft which also contains tubes supplying air insufflation, suction and irrigation to the scope. The light from a high-intensity light source is transmitted down the scope via fibreoptic light bundles. This light illuminates the body cavity being inspected. The image generated is transmitted back up the scope via fibreoptics to the eyepiece or, more recently, via a charge-coupled device (CCD) chip to a television monitor. This is known as videoendoscopy (Fig. 2.13).

Flexible endoscopes are used to examine the bronchial tree (bronchoscopy), the upper gastrointestinal tract (oesophagogastroduodenoscopy: OGD; Fig. 2.14), the biliary and pancreatic ducts (endoscopic retrograde cholangiopancreatography: ERCP), the sigmoid colon (flexible sigmoidoscopy), the entire colon (colonoscopy), the urethra and bladder (flexible cystoscopy) and the lumina of blood vessels (angioscopy). Most flexible scopes also have working channels incorporated into them which facilitate the passage of a variety of instruments:
- biopsy forceps for obtaining specimens for histology;
- brushes for obtaining specimens for cytology;
- flexible needles for injection of sclerosants or drugs (e.g. adrenaline) to stop bleeding from varices or ulcers;

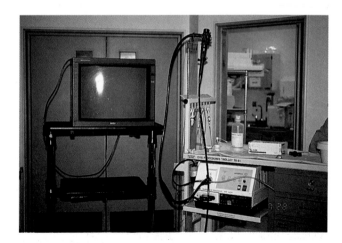

Figure 2.13 Videoendoscopy set-up.

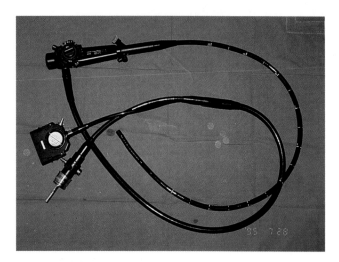

Figure 2.14 Gastroscope.

• heater probes and laser fibres to stop bleeding from ulcers;
• snares for removing polyps;
• graspers for removing foreign bodies;
• papillotome for dividing the papilla of Vater; and
• wire baskets to remove stones, e.g. from the biliary tract.

Most gastrointestinal endoscopy is now performed in purpose-designed endoscopy units. Formal written consent should be obtained prior to endoscopy. Patients have to starve before upper gastrointestinal endoscopy and a bowel preparation will be required before colonoscopy. Pharyngeal anaesthesia is given to patients before OGD or ERCP and most patients require sedation (midazolam and diazepam are the commonly administered sedatives). Patients having colonoscopy also require sedation, usually with a benzodiazepine and an opiate. Sedated patients should be monitored with ECG, frequent blood pressure estimation and pulse oximetry. The antagonists to benzodiazepines (adnexate) and opiates (naloxone) should be immediately available when performing endoscopy. Specific endoscopic investigations will be discussed in the relevant chapters throughout the book.

Measurement of function

Many investigations are undertaken to measure how well a system is functioning or to detect abnormalities in the function of an organ or structure. Clearly, some blood investigations (e.g. creatinine clearance for assessment of renal function, thyroid function tests) and many imaging techniques (DTPA scanning) achieve this aim. However, specific investigations have been developed to assess function in most of the body's major systems. These are discussed in the relevant chapters but are listed briefly in Table 2.2.

Table 2.2 Investigations commonly used to assess physiological function.

RESPIRATORY SYSTEM	GASTROINTESTINAL TRACT
Pulmonary function tests	*Tests of oesophageal function*
The peak expiratory flow rate (PEFR)	Oesophageal manometry
Spirometry	pH studies
Blood gas analysis	
	Tests of gastric function
CARDIOVASCULAR SYSTEM	Pentagastrin test
Tests of heart function	*Tests of anorectal function*
Echocardiography	Electromyography (EMG)
Electrocardiography	Anorectal manometry
Resting ECG	GENITOURINARY TRACT
Exercise ECG	*Urodynamics*
Holter monitoring	Uroflowmetry
	Cystometry
Investigations of peripheral	Urethral pressure profilometry
vascular disease	
Doppler velocimetry	NERVOUS SYSTEM
Ankle pressure measurement	
Ankle/brachial index	*Tests of CNS function*
Segmental pressure measurement	Electroencephalography (EEG)
Waveform analysis	Somatosensory evoked potential
Exercise response	(SSEP)
Plethysmography	
Pulse volume recording	*Tests of peripheral nerve function*
Digital plethysmography	Nerve conduction studies
Duplex colour ultrasonography	Electromyography (EMG)

ECG, Electrocardiogram; CNS, central nervous system.

PART 2 The Management of Acute Surgical Illness and Trauma

Introduction

Patients can become acutely ill from:
- acute malfunction or failure of specific organs;
- acute loss of circulating blood volume; and
- severe sepsis or major trauma.

Often the initial insult leads to a cascade of adverse consequences such that several pathophysiological factors account collectively for the acute illness which threatens the life of the patient. Thus, for example, in a patient with severe necrotizing pancreatitis, in addition to severe sepsis, the circulation is compromised and oxygenation is impaired.

In life-threatening situations (traumatic or otherwise), there are two important considerations which directly affect survival:

- early recognition of the disease and its severity; and
- prompt resuscitation.

The importance of these two factors is exemplified by the mortality following road traffic accidents in the UK where it has been documented that some 30% of deaths which occur within a few hours of the injury are preventable and are the result of inadequate resuscitation at the scene of the accident and delay in transport to the appropriate trauma centre (Fig. 1). The vast majority of these deaths are caused by correctable hypoxia and inadequate blood volume replacement. Efficient, early and adequate resuscitation prevents secondary complications, e.g. renal failure due to prolonged hypotension, brain damage from anoxia.

All seriously ill patients require management in *intensive care units* (ICUs) because of the need for life support systems and extensive, invasive monitoring (see Chapter 18). Others, though ill, have a stable cardiovascular system and adequate respiratory gas exchange but require careful

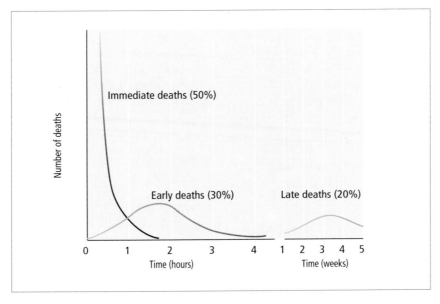

Figure 1 Death following trauma has a trimodal distribution. The first peak corresponds to people who die immediately or very soon after injury (*immediate deaths*). Fifty per cent of post-trauma deaths are immediate. The cause of death is usually a brain or brainstem laceration, spinal cord injury, heart or great vessel injury. Little can be done to save these people after the event, although preventive measures (e.g. ban on drink-driving, use of helmets and safety belts, gun control) could dramatically reduce the numbers injured. The second peak is people who die within the first few hours of injury (*early deaths*). These people die from blood loss secondary to internal haemorrhage and are potentially salvageable if effective treatment is instituted during the 'golden hour' after injury. The third peak occurs at 3–4 weeks and death is from infection or systemic inflammatory response syndrome (SIRS; *late deaths*), discussed fully in Chapter 7.

monitoring and may need support for acute renal failure by haemodialysis or haemofiltration. These patients are nursed in *high-dependency units* (HDUs). The decision on which type of facility is needed for an individual patient is taken jointly by the surgeon and the anaesthetist after the surgical treatment has been completed.

Assessment of outcome in seriously ill patients

Methods

• For the majority of patients, assessment of risk is based largely on clinical assessment. This is a judgement based on history and clinical examination (with bedside testing) of the clinical, physiological and nutritional state of the patient. If carried out by an experienced clinician, this overall assessment is probably as reliable as any complex scoring system.

• Usually, the clinical assessment is supplemented by taking into consideration the influence of individual factors (variables) which are known to have a documented adverse effect on outcome, e.g. old age, respiratory disease, cardiac disease, renal impairment, etc. This type of additional assessment of risk is known as *univariate* as the individual risk factors are considered one at a time.

• By contrast, *multivariate* (multifactorial) assessment provides a cumulative score made up of the collective contributions of various data (clinical and laboratory) which reflect the overall severity of illness and the likely outcome. Some of these systems are *disease-related*:

(a) the *Ranson and Imrie's criteria* for grading the severity of patients with acute pancreatitis;

(b) the *Glasgow Coma Scale* for head injuries;
(c) the *Pugh modification of Child's classification* of liver disease;
(d) the *multifactorial index of cardiac risk*;
(e) the *Revised Trauma Score*; and
(f) the *Injury Severity Score (ISS)*.

Others are designed to provide an *overall estimate of survival* in the acutely ill. The most comprehensive of such multivariate assessments is the *APACHE II (Acute Physiology and Chronic Health Evaluation)* system which is used to evaluate outcome of patients requiring intensive care treatment. It measures the severity of the acute disease by quantifying the degree of abnormality of multiple physiological variables. The APACHE system gives a score which is the sum total of:

• A: acute physiological score (APS);
• B: age points; and
• C: chronic health points.

The maximum possible score with the APACHE II system is 71. In practice, no patient has ever exceeded 55 and scores in excess of 35 are associated with a mortality exceeding 85%.

The assessment of outcome is an important consideration in patients requiring treatment in an ICU. Intensive care is extremely expensive and the cost–benefit ratio of therapy has to be considered. All are agreed that intensive care is inappropriate when the patient is not salvageable, i.e. the probability of survival is negligible. Within any hospital environment, the facilities for intensive care treatment are limited. If a selective policy is not adopted, the available resources become readily exhausted and salvageable patients who become acutely ill and require intensive care support may be denied this treatment.

A) **Acute Surgical Illness**

3 Hypoxic States and Airway Obstruction

An opening must be attempted in the trunk of the trachea, into which a tube of reed or cane should be put; you will then blow into this, so that the lung may rise again…the lung will swell to the full extent of the thoracic cavity and the heart become strong. (Andreas Vesalius, 1555)

Introduction

The general term for lack of oxygen is *hypoxia* and the specific term for lack of oxygen in the arterial blood is *hypoxaemia*. Hypoxia may be acute or chronic. Acute hypoxia is immediately life-threatening if left uncorrected for more than a few minutes. Acute hypoxia causes cardiac arrest and severe cerebral impairment, leading to brain death or gross permanent mental disability should the patient survive. Thus, acute hypoxia is seldom seen in isolation and usually requires cardiopulmonary resuscitation. Chronic hypoxia is seen in chronic obstructive or restrictive lung disease (see also Chapter 19). The causes of hypoxia are listed in Table 3.1.

Acute hypoxia

Impaired level of consciousness

Impaired level of consciousness from any cause (e.g. head injury, sedation, cerebrovascular accident) can be accompanied by depression of the respiratory centre (diminished ventilatory drive). Loss of consciousness is also accompanied by loss of the protective gag and cough reflexes such that aspiration of foreign material into the broncho-pulmonary tree is likely. In addition, the tongue musculature is relaxed and the neck muscles fail to lift the base of the tongue from the posterior pharyngeal wall. If the patient's head is in the flexed or mid-position, acute

Table 3.1 Causes of hypoxia.

Hypoxic hypoxia
Decreased Po_2 in inspired air (high altitude)

Hypoventilation
　Depression of respiratory centre (head injuries, opiates, cerebrovascular accident)
　Shallow respirations due to pain (after chest or upper abdominal surgery, pleurisy)
　Airway obstruction (foreign body, aspiration)
　Increased airway resistance (asthma, emphysema)
　Large pneumothorax (trauma, rupture of emphysematous bulla)

Alveolar/capillary diffusion block
　Decreased alveolar membrane area (pneumonia, pulmonary congestion)
　Fibrosis of alveolar or pulmonary capillary walls (pulmonary fibrosis)

Abnormal ventilation/ perfusion ratio
　Perfusion of unventilated alveoli (atelectasis)
　Ventilation of underperfused alveoli (pulmonary embolism)
　Shunting of venous blood into arterial circulation (cyanotic congenital heart disease)

Anaemic hypoxia
Anaemias (hypoxia is worse on exercise)
Carbon monoxide (CO) poisoning (CO binds to haemoglobin producing carboxyhaemoglobin which cannot release oxygen)

Stagnant hypoxia
During shock, slow circulation to the tissues produces hypoxia and damage (e.g. renal failure)

Histotoxic hypoxia
Inhibition of the cytochrome oxidase enzyme system in the tissues (cyanide poisoning)

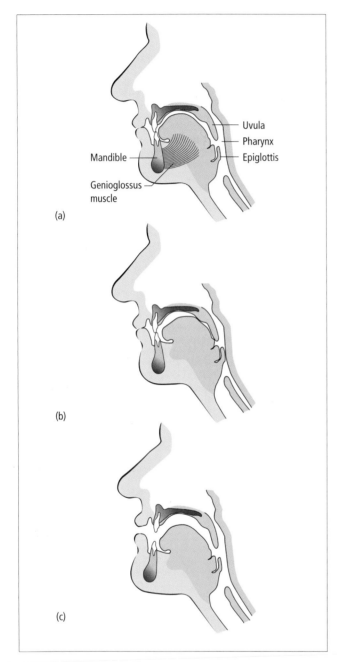

Mandible

Uvula
Pharynx
Epiglottis

Genioglossus
muscle

(a)

(b)

(c)

Figure 3.1 Upper-airway obstruction. (a) The tongue is normally lifted forwards in the mouth by the action of the genioglossi muscles which are attached to the inner surface of the symphysis of the mandible. (b) If the patient is unconscious or has a fracture of the mandible the tongue may fall back into the pharynx and cause airway obstruction. Flexion of the head causes more narrowing of the pharynx, exacerbating the situation. (c) The triple-airway manoeuvre is used to correct the resulting airway obstruction: the neck is extended, the mandible is displaced forwards and the mouth opened.

obstruction of the upper airway supervenes. Hypopharyngeal obstruction by this mechanism is the commonest cause of hypoxia encountered in clinical practice. This type of upper-airway obstruction is commonly seen after head injuries with loss of consciousness (Fig. 3.1).

Facial fractures

Occlusion of the laryngeal orifice by the prolapsed tongue is particularly prone to occur in patients with fractures of the body of the mandible. The upper airway may also be compromised directly by fractures of the middle third of the face, when the maxillae are driven backwards over the laryngeal orifice.

Aspiration

Aspiration of blood, vomit or gastric juice will result in severe laryngospasm in the stuporous or lightly comatose patient. In addition, and irrespective of the degree of coma, it causes lower-airway obstruction by a combination of bronchospasm, excessive bronchial secretions and mucosal oedema. If the aspirated fluid is irritant (e.g. gastric juice), it often progresses to pulmonary oedema and adult respiratory distress syndrome (ARDS; see Fig. 19.21).

Extrinsic upper-airway compression

Thyroid disease

Extrinsic compression of the upper airway in patients with thyroid disease may occur in several ways. *Bleeding inside a thyroid nodule* may result in rapid enlargement with compression of the trachea, especially if it occurs in a retrosternal thyroid, as the rigid boundary of the thoracic inlet cannot accommodate the sudden increase in volume. Tracheal compression is also encountered in advanced *thyroid cancer*, especially of the anaplastic variety, in the late stages of *Reidel's thyroiditis* (due to fibrous contracture) and after *thyroidectomy* due to postoperative bleeding with clot compression underneath the strap muscles. If, as rarely happens nowadays, *both recurrent laryngeal nerves* are damaged during thyroid surgery, severe asphyxia is encountered when the endotracheal tube is removed as the paralysed vocal cords become opposed in the midline occluding the laryngeal orifice.

Malignancy

Extrinsic compression from secondary tumour deposits or lymphomas in the mediastinum is usually part of the *superior vena cava compression syndrome*. In addition to the respiratory difficulties, there is marked congestion of the upper half of the body. When due to lymphomas, rapid relief is obtained by appropriate urgent therapy with chemotherapy and radiotherapy. Endovascular stents are also used to relieve superior vena cava compression syndrome.

Other important causes

The other important causes of acute hypoxia are:
- imbalance between alveolar ventilation and perfusion (i.e. there is a mismatch of blood and airflow to the lungs, e.g. atelectasis and pulmonary embolism);
- right-to-left shunting (blood returns to the left heart without being oxygenated);
- impairment of gaseous diffusion due to thickening of the alveolar–capillary interface between blood and inspired air;
- defective extrapulmonary ventilation due to diminished central (cerebral) ventilatory drive or disease/trauma limiting effective chest wall and diaphragmatic movement; and
- important medical disorders accompanied by hypoxaemia are heart failure, severe lobar pneumonia and status asthmaticus.

Clinical features of hypoxia

Symptoms

- If the patient is unconscious the only reliable clinical manifestations of hypoxia are *central cyanosis, abnormal respiration* (rapid, slow, apnoea, gasping) and *hypotension.* Complete airway obstruction leads to asphyxia and cardiac arrest within 5–10 min. Incomplete airway obstruction in the unconscious patient is noisy (rattling, stridor).
- The conscious hypoxic patient is *cyanosed, anxious, restless, sweating* and often *confused.* Accessory muscles of respiration are recruited with indrawing of the supraclavicular spaces. *Stridor* is an inspiratory whooping sound which indicates partial obstruction of the trachea (intrinsic or extrinsic).

Apnoea (defined as cessation of breathing in the expiratory position) is the most serious clinical situation and demands immediate active intervention (see below).

Physical examination

1 First examine the patient and ensure that there is no obstruction to the airway.
2 Then determine the presence or absence of pulse (femoral or carotid). If the patient is apnoeic and there is no pulse,

full cardiopulmonary resuscitation (CPR) should be instituted immediately (see below).
3 If spontaneous respiration is present, the essential physical examination consists of examination of the respiratory system (see Chapter 19). Briefly, this should include:
   (a) *inspection of the chest wall* (for injuries, expansion and paradoxical movement, i.e. chest wall moves in with inspiration and out with expiration);
   (b) *auscultation of both lung fields:* for air entry to both lungs, abnormal breath sounds (crepitations, bronchial breathing); and
   (c) *percussion:* if air entry is absent, this will determine whether the affected hemithorax is hyperresonant (air in pleural cavity), dull (pneumonic consolidation) or stony dull (fluid).

Investigations

The important immediate investigations are the taking of a femoral arterial blood sample for *blood gas analysis.* With respiratory failure the blood gases will indicate respiratory acidosis, but if there has been significant anoxia to the tissues, e.g. if there has been a cardiac arrest, there will also be a metabolic acidosis due to accumulation of lactic acid (see Chapter 6).

A *portable chest radiograph* should also be obtained. It is imperative that the hypoxic patient is never sent to the radiological department for the chest X-ray. Other investigations such as a portable electrocardiogram (ECG) are needed in the event of cardiac arrest.

Principles of treatment of the hypoxic patient

The principles underlying basic life support in the immediate management of the acutely hypoxic patient are:
A Airway control;
B Breathing support;
C Circulatory support; and
D Determine the cause.
   Once the critical situation has been controlled, the underlying cause must be treated.

Airway control

The first measure is to correct hypopharyngeal obstruction. This is achieved by the triple-airway manoeuvre:
1 extension of the neck;
2 forwards displacement of the mandible;
3 opening the mouth (Fig. 3.1c).

Next, any secretions or fluid (vomit, blood) in the mouth or pharynx are removed by suction, intraoral foreign bodies including dentures are removed and a nasopharyngeal or oropharyngeal airway is inserted (Fig. 3.2) if the patient is unconscious. If the upper airway is blocked, a laryngoscopic examination is performed to clear the pharynx

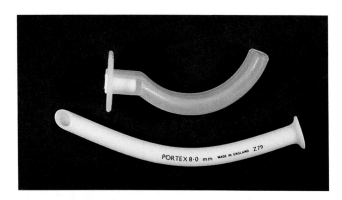

Figure 3.2 Oropharyngeal and nasopharyngeal airways.

and rapidly assess the situation. Then an endotracheal tube is passed or, if this fails, a cricothyrotomy or mini-tracheostomy is performed (Fig. 3.3). Usually senior staff are available for this contingency.

The *Heimlich manoeuvre* is a first-aid procedure used to try and relieve upper-airway obstruction classically caused by inhalation of a bolus of food, the so-called café coronary syndrome. Standing behind the patient, place your arms around the patient's upper abdomen and, clasping your hands together, firmly force upwards under the ribs. In this way the air in the chest is compressed and, with luck, the foreign body will be expelled from the upper airway.

Breathing support

Mouth-to-mouth breathing support

Expired air contains 16–18% oxygen and, when delivered adequately to the apnoeic patient via mouth-to-mouth or mouth-to-nose ventilation, achieves an arterial P_{O_2} of 10 kPa or 75 mmHg (normal: 13.3 kPa or 100 mmHg) if

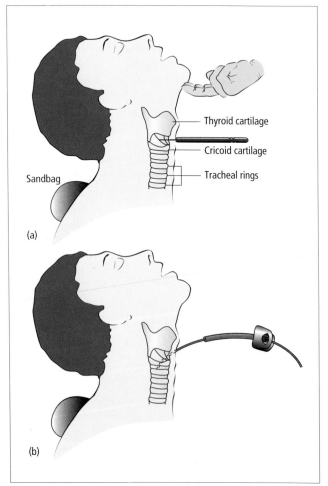

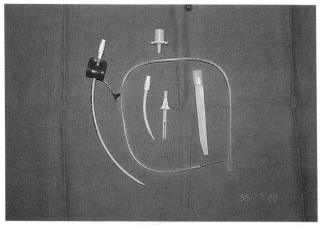

Figure 3.3 Minitracheostomy. (a) The head is extended and a small sandbag is placed between the shoulder blades. The cricothyroid membrane is identified between the thyroid and cricoid cartilages. The overlying skin and cricothyroid membrane are infiltrated with local anaesthetic and a few drops of anaesthetic are flushed into the trachea. A transverse stab incision is made through the skin and subcutaneous tissue and the cricothyroid membrane is punctured. (b) An introducer is then passed through the wound into the trachea and over this the minitracheostomy tube (internal diameter 4 mm) is passed. The introducer is removed and the minitracheostomy tube is secured. A minitracheostomy allows for very effective aspiration of sputum in postoperative patients and may obviate the need for intubation and ventilation. (c) The equipment required to perform a minitracheostomy.

the patient's lungs are normal. Mouth-to-mouth breathing is commenced immediately until oxygen delivery systems can be brought to the scene. The practical sequence is to tilt the patient's head backwards and inflate the lung by mouth-to-mouth ventilation. If this meets with an obstruction, the patient's mouth is closed and mouth-to-nose ventilation is tried. After an airway has been introduced one can change to mouth-to-airway ventilation.

Self-refilling bag-valve unit (Fig. 3.4)

This requires experience for efficient use with a mask in the non-intubated patient, but is particularly effective for maintaining oxygenation after the patient has been intubated. It permits ventilation during both spontaneous and artificial ventilation. The unit consists of a self-refilling bag with an inlet valve to which an oxygen cylinder is attached and has a non-rebreathing valve at the mask or endotracheal tube.

Circulatory support

Circulatory support involves *external cardiac massage* for cardiac arrest and the setting-up of adequate intravenous

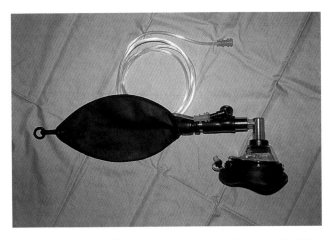

Figure 3.4 The self-refilling bag-valve unit. It consists of a self-refilling bag with an inlet valve to which an oxygen cylinder is attached and has a non-rebreathing valve at the mask or endotracheal tube.

lines for volume replacement and drug administration. For external cardiac massage the patient is placed supine on a hard surface. The aim is to compress the heart between the sternum and the spine, thereby forcing blood from the heart

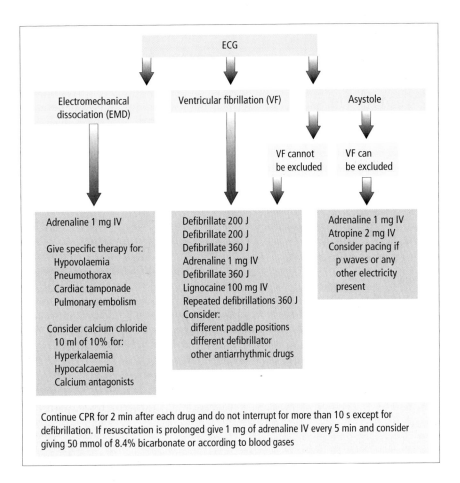

Figure 3.5 Algorithm for drug therapy and the use of defibrillation during cardiopulmonary resuscitation (CPR).

and producing a circulation. It is important to feel the femoral or carotid pulse during CPR to ensure that an adequate circulation is being produced. External cardiac massage is performed by placing the heel of one hand with the other hand on top, over the lower half of the sternum. With the arms extended the sternum is pressed down and then released at a rate of about 60 times per minute. Excessive force should be avoided as there is a risk of fracturing ribs during CPR. External cardiac massage must be coordinated with ventilation, with one respiration being given for every five compressions. CPR must not be interrupted for more than 10 s. An alogrithm for the use of drugs and defibrillation during CPR is given in Fig. 3.5.

Correction of underlying abnormality

Having resuscitated the patient, the specific condition which led to the hypoxic arrest must be treated, e.g. correction of maxillary fractures, pharmacological treatment of heart failure or asthma, antibiotics for pneumonia, etc. If the apnoea is thought to result from opioid-induced depression of the respiratory centre, *naloxone hydrochloride* is administered intravenously. In patients who aspirate gastrointestinal contents, acid damage to the lung with the development of ARDS is likely (see Chapter 19). These patients are given antibiotics and vigorous physiotherapy. If ARDS develops the patient will require ventilation.

Oxygen therapy

Oxygen is often administered by mask to patients who are hypoxic but breathing spontaneously. A number of different types of mask are available:
• Oxygen is usually administered by a mask of the type which does not deliver a constant known percentage of oxygen to the patient. This is due to the variable dilution of the oxygen in the mask by the inspired air. Examples of these masks are the *Mary Catteral* (MC) and the *Hudson* mask. They administer oxygen to the patient in a concentration varying from 35 to 60%. This is fine because, unless there is additional lung pathology, 35% oxygen is adequate for ensuring normal arterial oxygen tension and oxygen toxicity is unlikely if less than 60% of oxygen is administered.
• When more accurate oxygen administration is needed, a high-airflow oxygen enrichment (HAFLOE) mask such as the *Ventimask* (Fig. 3.6) is used. Several models are available which are capable of administering oxygen in defined concentrations ranging from 24 to 60%.
• Accurate masks delivering low inspired oxygen concentrations are essential for patients with *chronic lung disease*

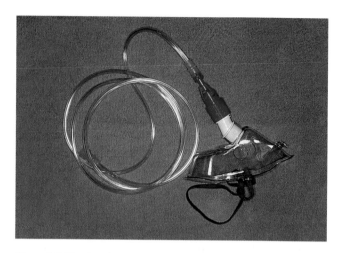

Figure 3.6 Ventimask.

who have lost the normal ventilatory control and depend on moderate hypoxaemia to stimulate the respiratory centre. Such patients require enough oxygen to avoid serious hypoxaemia but not so much that the arterial oxygen tension reaches the normal range, as this would result in apnoea from loss of the respiratory drive.
• When longer oxygen therapy is needed, *humidification* is necessary, especially in patients with sputum retention or mouth-breathers. Otherwise the tracheal secretions become inspissated by the cold, dry inspired air–oxygen mixture. In addition, ciliary activity is lost. This further exacerbates the retention of bronchial secretions. Humidification is best achieved by blower humidifiers of the heated water or ultrasonic type.
• When oxygen is administered in very high concentrations, *oxygen toxicity* may occur. In practice this is only seen in ventilated patients breathing >60% oxygen for more than 24 h. The manifestations of oxygen toxicity are lung damage, blindness from retrolental fibroplasia (seen in premature babies) and epilepsy.

Mechanical ventilation

Mechanical ventilation is indicated in patients with acute respiratory failure. The common clinical reasons for ventilation are given in Table 3.2.

Intermittent positive-pressure ventilation (IPPV)

When patients are put on a ventilator they are given IPPV. This requires endotracheal intubation with connection to a mechanical respirator, usually in an intensive care or high-dependency unit. IPPV ensures normal gas exchange and

Table 3.2 Clinical indications for mechanical ventilation.

Cardiopulmonary resuscitation
Hypoventilation, e.g. respiratory depression, muscle relaxants
Hypoxaemia, e.g. ARDS, chest trauma, asthma
Shock, e.g. septic shock
Postoperatively, e.g. after major surgery, in obese patients
Cerebral oedema, e.g. following head injury

ARDS, Adult respiratory distress syndrome.

abolishes the work (respiratory muscular activity) of breathing. This often results in reduced oxygen consumption and better arterial oxygenation with a reduced demand on the heart to maintain a high output. By varying the respiratory rate, tidal volume and the inspired oxygen concentration the optimum ventilation for a patient can be achieved. However, there are also a number of specific ventilator programmes that can be employed, depending on what one wants to achieve, e.g. increase PaO_2, wean the patient from the ventilator, etc. The commonly used programmes are:

• *Intermittent mandatory ventilation* (IMV) allows the patient to take spontaneous breaths during ventilation. The ventilator, however, is programmed to deliver a certain number of mandatory breaths per minute. This technique is used when weaning the patient from the ventilator. As the patient increases the number of spontaneous breaths taken, the number of mandatory ventilator breaths is reduced.

• *Assisted mechanical ventilation* (AMV) is a technique whereby any attempt by the patient to take a breath triggers the ventilator to deliver a tidal volume. For obvious reasons, the ventilator will deliver predetermined breaths if there is no attempt at spontaneous breathing by the patient!

• *Positive end expiratory pressure* (PEEP) is a system that applies positive pressure to the respiratory tree throughout the respiratory cycle. Such pressure prevents alveolar and small-airway collapse in expiration, thus maximizing the amount of alveolar membrane available for gas exchange. PEEP is indicated when adequate concentrations of inspired oxygen (i.e. 60%) fail to maintain satisfactory oxygenation. The usual PEEP applied ranges from 5 to 15 cmH$_2$O. This technique must be used with care as it results in increased intrathoracic pressure, decreased cardiac output and an increased risk of barotrauma.

• *Continuous positive airway pressure* (CPAP) may be applied to the airway of *spontaneously breathing* patients. CPAP applied to the endotracheal tube is used as part of the weaning process but it may also be applied via a well-fitting facemask if the patient is not intubated.

If it is anticipated that mechanical ventilation will be required for a prolonged period, e.g. more than 2–3 weeks, then consideration should be given to replacing the endotracheal tube (which may damage the vocal cords) with a tracheostomy (see Chapter 24).

Pulse oximetry

Pulse oximetry is a method of continuous measurement of oxygen saturation. A small device placed on a digit uses transillumination and plethysmography to obtain repeated measurements of light absorption during the cardiac cycle, from which the pulse rate and the arterial oxygen saturation can be determined and displayed on a screen (Fig. 3.7). Pulse oximetry is very useful in detecting hypoxic episodes during intubation and extubation, during the recovery period following surgery, especially in elderly and obese patients prone to hypoxaemia, and during gastrointestinal endoscopy. However, movement, peripheral vasoconstriction and the presence of carboxyhaemoglobin can produce inaccurate readings.

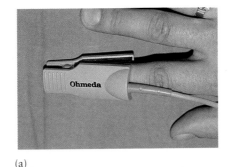

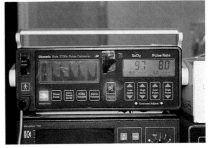

Figure 3.7 Pulse oximeter. (a) A small device placed on a digit detects blood flow by transillumination and plethysmography. (b) The oxygen saturation and pulse rate are displayed continuously on a small screen.

(a)   (b)

Hypoxia at a glance

DEFINITIONS

Hypoxia is defined as lack of oxygen generally. *Hypoxaemia* is lack of oxygen in arterial blood. *Apnoea* means cessation of breathing in expiration

COMMON CAUSES

- Impaired level of consciousness
- Facial fractures
- Aspiration of blood or vomit
- Upper-airway obstruction from thyroid disease or cervical malignancy
- Ventilation–perfusion mismatch (e.g. pulmonary embolism, pneumothorax)
- Right-to-left pulmonary shunt

CLINICAL FEATURES

In the unconscious patient
- Central cyanosis
- Abnormal respirations
- Hypotension

In the conscious patient
- Central cyanosis
- Anxiety and restlessness
- Confusion
- Stridor
- Apnoea

INVESTIGATIONS

Arterial blood gases
- Respiratory acidosis
- Metabolic acidosis later

Chest radiograph/ECG
- Portable

MANAGEMENT

- **A**irway control (triple-airway manoeuvre, suction secretions, clear oropharynx, endotracheal intubation/cricothyrotomy/minitracheostomy)
- **B**reathing support (mouth-to-mouth or mouth-to-airway ventilation, self-refilling bag unit)
- **C**irculatory support (external cardiac massage coordinated with ventilation, good intravenous line, do not fracture the ribs!)
- **D**etermine and treat the cause

4 Haemorrhage, Hypovolaemia and Shock

The patient in shock has the appearance of being seriously ill. (Norman E. Freeman MD, 1940)

Introduction

Shock may be defined as acute circulatory failure with inadequate or inappropriate perfusion resulting in generalized cellular hypoxia. Thus, inadequate tissue perfusion for whatever reason causes cellular hypoxia, thereby precipitating a number of intracellular reactions, culminating in a metabolic acidosis. The latter, by altering vascular permeability, creates a vicious circle through which there are increasing plasma losses from the circulation with reducing cardiac output and further acidosis, so that the state of shock becomes irreversible.

Classification of shock

Hypovolaemic shock

Hypovolaemic shock may be due to haemorrhage, loss of plasma or loss of extracellular fluid.
- *Haemorrhage* may occur following injury, e.g. ruptured spleen, multiple fractures, etc., gastrointestional disease, e.g. haematemesis from gastric or duodenal ulcer, or in vascular disease, e.g. ruptured aortic aneurysm.
- *Plasma losses* may follow severe burns when significant volumes of plasma and blood may be lost from the surface of the burn.
- *Extracellular fluid* is lost in large quantities in patients with vomiting or diarrhoea or those who have intestinal fistulae.

Cardiogenic shock

- Cardiogenic shock is most commonly seen after *myocardial infarction* when cardiac output is seriously reduced due to failure of the central pump mechanism.

- *Ventricular arrhythmias*, by rendering pump action ineffective, may also give rise to cardiogenic shock.
- A further cause may be the interruption of flow brought about by *massive pulmonary embolus*.
- Another cause of secondary cardiogenic shock is *cardiac tamponade*, usually caused by direct penetrating injuries to the myocardium. The subsequent haemorrhage into the pericardial sac prevents adequate filling of the ventricles during diastole and precipitates cardiogenic shock.

Septic shock

Septic shock may arise as a consequence of Gram-positive or Gram-negative infection — more usually the latter — in the urinary, biliary or gastrointestinal tracts. Shock results from the action of bacterial endotoxins and exotoxins on the cardiovascular system. The presence of vasoactive kinins gives rise to greatly increased capillary permeability and peripheral vasodilatation. Large quantities of fluid leak out of the circulation and the increased vascular capacity causes a relative hypovolaemia. A myocardial-depressant factor may be released from hypoxic cells; this restricts cardiac output. The common bacteria involved are *Escherichia coli*, *Proteus*, *Pseudomonas* and *Bacteroides*. Fungal infections are increasingly seen in patients on broad-spectrum antibiotics and in patients who are immunologically suppressed.

Anaphylaxis

Anaphylactic shock occurs when a hypersensitive patient is exposed to an antigen to which he or she has previously been sensitized. The binding of antigen and antibody releases histamine and other vasoactive substances which cause vasodilatation and increased capillary permeability. Bronchoconstriction also occurs; this interferes with

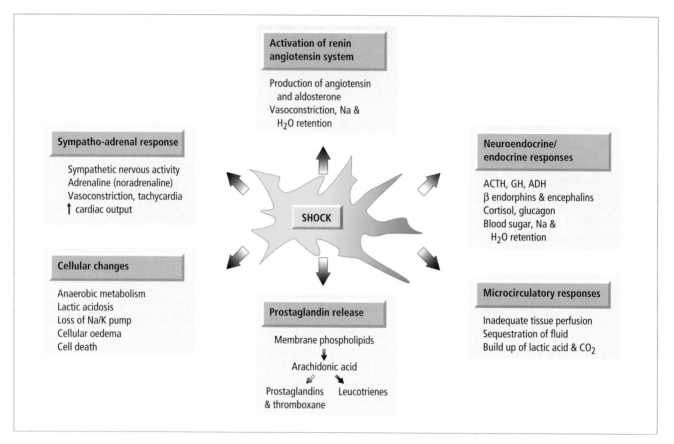

Figure 4.1 Shock, regardless of cause, initiates a series of pathophysiological changes aimed at protecting the organism and preserving its vital functions.

oxygenation. Common causes of anaphylactic shock are drugs such as penicillin and radiological contrast media.

The pathophysiological changes which occur in shock are summarized in Fig. 4.1.

Clinical features

The clinical features of shock are summarized in Table 4.1.

Patients in *hypovolaemic* or *cardiogenic shock* are pale, cold and sweating. The pulse is fast and weak. The blood pressure is low and there is oliguria. These clinical manifestations are due to the intense sympathetic and adrenal activity with release of catecholamines (Fig. 4.1). The tachycardia attempts to compensate for the low cardiac output and the peripheral vasoconstriction attempts to redistribute the intravascular volume. The change in the intracellular metabolism from aerobic respiration via the Kreb's cycle to the lactic acid production of anaerobic metabolism produces a metabolic acidosis which provokes

Table 4.1 The clinical features of shock. All patients will experience hypotension, tachycardia, dyspnoea, oliguria and restlessness to some degree.

	Hypovolaemic	Cardiogenic	Septic	Anaphylactic
Skin colour	Pale	Pale	Flushed	Urticarial rash
Sweating	Present	Present	Absent	Absent
Temperature	Cold	Cold	Warm	Warm
Capillary refill	Slow	Slow	Rapid	Normal or rapid
Mental status	Restless	Quiet	Drowsy	Variable

a compensatory hyperventilation. Oliguria is due to the reduction in renal blood flow.

In the early stages of *septic shock* the patient may present a different picture with warm flushed skin and bounding pulse. This is due to endotoxin-induced vasodilatation which is unresponsive to catecholamines and the reduced peripheral resistance is accompanied by an increased cardiac output. This phase is temporary, however, and soon reverts to the low-output state with increased peripheral resistance.

End-phase

The failing circulation is unable to provide the major organs with an adequate supply of oxygen and progressive cerebral hypoxia is manifested by agitation and restlessness, followed by confusion and coma. Diminished coronary blood flow leads to progressive heart failure, which may be aggravated by myocardial depressant factor and hypoxia. The fall in renal blood flow diminishes the glomerular filtration rate and induces oliguria, leading to acute tubular necrosis (see Chapter 5).

Assessment and treatment of shock

Patients in shock require invasive monitoring and vigorous treatment, which is usually performed in the accident and emergency department, the operating theatre or the intensive care unit (and sometimes in all three places!). Details of the type of monitoring performed on ill patients in intensive care units are given in Chapter 18. However, a summary of the assessment of the shocked patient is given here. Usually, assessment and treatment are performed concurrently.

Assessment of shock

• Clinical assessment includes *pulse rate*, *blood pressure*, respiratory rate and *temperature*. A rapid clinical examination may provide some clues to the underlying cause, whether it be haemorrhage, anaphylaxis, sepsis or cardiac insufficiency.
• An electrocardiogram (ECG) will provide evidence of cardiac status and may be helpful in identifying pulmonary embolus also. However, the classical ECG findings (S-wave in lead I and Q-waves and inverted T-waves in lead III: S1QT3) are found in only 10–20% of patients with pulmonary embolus (see Chapter 18).
• Venous blood samples are used for measuring *haemoglobin* level, *haematocrit*, *urea and electrolytes* and *cardiac enzymes*.
• *Grouping* and *cross-matching* are done if haemorrhage is the underlying problem.
• If sepsis is suspected, a blood sample is taken for aerobic and anerobic *blood culture*.
• *Urine output* should be documented hourly after insertion of a urinary catheter.
• *Central venous pressure* (CVP) is used to monitor the circulation blood volume.

Changes in blood volume, however, may be absolute or relative, depending on whether the patient is suffering from haemorrhage, fluid loss, sepsis or anaphylaxis. CVP may also reflect intrinsic myocardial disease in right ventricular failure or, more commonly, the pulmonary hypertension induced by left ventricular failure. Its interpretation, therefore, may be difficult and misleading and must be carried out in conjunction with other evidence.
• *Pulmonary artery wedge pressure* (PAWP) is an accurate reflection of left ventricular function and can be used to monitor cardiac output and pulmonary oedema.
• *Blood gas analysis* and arterial pH provide important information on arterial oxygen tension and partial pressure of carbon dioxide. Patients in shock usually have a metabolic acidosis due to accumulation of lactic acid, the main product of anaerobic metabolism (see Chapter 6).

Treatment of shock

The aim of treatment is to:
• resuscitate the patient and improve tissue perfusion and the delivery of oxygen to the cells to maintain aerobic respiration;
• deal with the cause of the shock, e.g. stop bleeding, treat infection, etc.; and
• prevent and treat complications of shock.

Resuscitation

• Ensure that the airway is clear, that breathing is spontaneous and adequate, and that the patient has a circulation (ABC; see Chapter 3).
• Provision of *100%* oxygen via a facemask (see Chapter 3) is immediately helpful.
• In *hypovolaemic shock* restoration of circulating volume must be carried out as quickly as possible. *Crystalloid solutions* (e.g. Ringer's lactate solution) are ideal in situations where water and sodium loss is predominant and will also serve as initial treatment in haemorrhagic shock. *Colloid solutions*, e.g. dextran, hydroxyethyl starch (HES), gelatins (Haemaccel), however, remain longer in the circulation and draw extracellular fluid into the circulation by osmotic pressure. The administration of intravenous crystalloid or colloid should be monitored by CVP observations and urine output.
• *Blood transfusion*: Blood, plasma or plasma substitutes should be given as indicated as soon as they become available, e.g. blood for haemorrhagic shock, plasma for burns. However, a number of problems may arise when large quantities of blood are given (Table 4.2; see also Chapter 29).
• In *cardiogenic shock*, the aim of treatment is to improve cardiac output without increasing excessively the workload on the heart, which might further compromise the coronary

Table 4.2 Problems which may be encountered when transfusing large amounts of blood.

Coagulation deficiency
Blood stored for more than 24 h contains no platelets and is deficient in clotting factors V, VIII and XI. If more than 10 units of blood are required, fresh frozen plasma and platelet concentrates should be given to correct these deficiencies

Citrate toxicity
Citrate toxicity may also develop, giving rise to muscle tremors and ECG changes related to hypocalcaemia. Administration of 10% calcium gluconate is necessary to correct the calcium level

Microemboli
Microemboli, consisting of aggregates of platelets, white cells and fibrin, develop in stored blood and may help precipitate failure unless filtered out with filters of pore size 40 μm

Hypothermia
In order to avoid the risk of hypothermia, blood stored at 4°C should be warmed before transfusion

Reduced 2,3 DPG
The reduction of 2,3 DPG in stored blood enhances the affinity of haemoglobin for oxygen, thus reducing its ability to release it to the tissues. This is a temporary phenomenon, lasting about 48 h

ECG, Electrocardiogram; 2,3 DPG, 2,3-diphosphoglycerate.

Table 4.3 Management of common arrhythmias seen after myocardial infarction.

Arrhythmia	Treatment
Supraventricular tachycardia (SVT)	Carotid massage Adenosine DC cardioversion
Atrial flutter or fibrillation	Digoxin Verapamil Amiodarone DC cardioversion
Complete heart block	Atropine Cardiac pacing
Ventricular arrhythmias	Lignocaine infusion Bretylate
Ventricular tachycardia	CPR DC cardioversion

DC, Direct current; CPR, cardiopulmonary resuscitation.

circulation. Patients should have *complete bedrest* and be *monitored in a coronary care unit. Pain relief* should be achieved with diamorphine or morphine. If the patient has had a myocardial infarction, *thrombolytic therapy* in the form of streptokinase or recombinant tissue plasminogen activator (rTPA) should be administered as well as aspirin. If the patient is in *heart failure*, diuretics (e.g. frusemide 40 mg), nitrates, angiotensin-converting enzyme (ACE) inhibitors, cardiac glycosides and dopexamine may be indicated. *Arrhythmias* must be avoided and controlled (Table 4.3).

• *Septicaemic shock* is commonly seen in surgical practice. The source of infection may arise *de novo* from a perforated viscus or may be due to postoperative complications, e.g. abscess, leaking anastomosis, etc. Treatment is aimed at *controlling infection* and *improving the hypovolaemic state* caused by endotoxin-induced peripheral vasodilatation. The latter is improved by the administration of colloid solutions, the volume of which is monitored by CVP and urine output. *Blood cultures* should always be carried out before antibiotic administration so that the sensitivity of the responsible organisms may be determined. In the interim a combination of penicillin, aminoglycoside and metronidazole should be effective against the most common organisms. The use of inotropes is often indicated in severely ill septic patients to maintain cardiac output and preserve vital functions. The most frequently used inotropes are listed in Table 4.4. These drugs are very potent, however, and should only be used in an intensive care setting and in conjunction with the treatment of abnormal-

Table 4.4 Inotropic agents frequently used in patients with shock.

Dopamine		
Low-dose	Peripheral resistance falls secondary to dilatation of splanchnic and renal vasculature. Renal and hepatic blood flow increase. Renal-protective effect	
High-dose	Causes noradrenaline release, leading to vasoconstriction and loss of renal-protective effect	
Dobutamine	Reduces systemic resistance and improves cardiac performance Possibly has better inotropic effect than dopamine	
Dopexamine	β_2-Adrenergic agonist and dopamine receptor agonist	Increased heart rate Increased cardiac index Increased cardiac output Decreased peripheral resistance No vasoconstriction
Adrenaline		
Low-dose	β_2-Adrenergic agonist effects	
High-dose	α-Adrenergic agonist effects	Vasoconstriction Decreased renal blood flow Peripheral gangrene
Noradrenaline	α-Adrenergic agonist effects	

ities which may impair cardiac performance, e.g. hypoxia, acidosis, hypocalcaemia. Intravenous hydrocortisone has been advocated in the treatment of septic shock but its use is controversial.

• *Anaphylactic shock* may be precipitated as a response to an antigen to which the individual has been previously sensitized. The release of histamine and other vasoactive amines causes widespread vasodilatation with increased capillary permeability. Bronchoconstriction is also a prominent feature which further exacerbates the tissue anoxia. The common causes of anaphylactic shock in hospital practice are the administration of radiological contrast media and intravenous drugs, e.g. penicillin. While most insect bites produce no more than a mild local hypersensitivity, wasp and bee stings may produce full-blown anaphylactic shock with circulatory collapse in some people. Treatment consists of:

(a) *intravenous fluids* to compensate for the relative hypovolaemia produced by widespread capillary vasodilatation;

(b) *subcutaneous administration of adrenaline* to improve cardiac output and induce vasoconstriction;

(c) *antihistamines* to block the histamine receptors; and

(d) *hydrocortisone* to prevent the release of histamine from the mast cells.

Specific treatment such as penicillinase is used if the anaphylactic reaction is due to penicillin.

Complications of shock

Apart from the profound effects on the cardiovascular system, shock may precipitate acute respiratory failure, acute renal failure, disseminated intravascular coagulation (DIC) or, more rarely, hepatic failure. Severely ill patients may develop the systemic inflammatory response syndrome (SIRS), which often results in multiple system organ failure (MSOF; this is also known as multiple organ dysfunction syndrome: MODS) and, ultimately, death (see Chapter 7).

Disseminated intravascular coagulation

DIC is a major complication of septic shock. In this condition the various factors involved in the clotting mechanism are activated and widespread intravascular clotting takes place, with consequent depletion of clotting factors, including platelets. Profuse spontaneous haemorrhage is then paradoxically produced and bleeding from operation sites may be uncontrollable. If the condition is suspected, diagnosis is confirmed by the high level of fibrin degeneration products (FDPs) present in the serum. Intravenous

heparin is administered to control the coagulation and the normal clotting factors are restored by giving fresh frozen plasma and platelets.

Stress ulceration

Severe haemorrhage may occur from multiple gastric erosions in critically ill patients. The erosions are secondary to mucosal ischaemia which is caused by hypotension or the effects of endotoxin. Alteration in mucosal permeability allows a back-diffusion of H^+ which stimulates excess acid secretion. Administration of antacids to raise the gastric pH to 7 may be of help; H_2-receptor antagonists have also been used, although their efficiency remains unproven. The elevation of the pH, however, may allow bacterial colonization of the stomach from the oropharynx where gram-negative colonization is common in seriously ill patients. To avoid bacterial overgrowth, which is encouraged by raising the pH, cytoprotection with sucralfate has been used as an alternative.

Acute respiratory failure

Severe respiratory problems may develop after successful resuscitation of the shocked patient. The so-called shock lung syndrome may be associated with a variety of abnormalities including sepsis, fat embolism, massive blood transfusion, oxygen toxicity and DIC. The varied aetiology has prompted the term adult respiratory distress syndrome (ARDS) to cover all these conditions. Increasing evidence implicates activated white cells (e.g. by endotoxin via the complement system in the case of Gram-negative septicaemia) as the mediators of ARDS. The activated white blood cells release free radicals and hydrolytic enzymes that damage the endothelium of the lung capillaries. The result is that the lungs become very oedematous; fibrin and microaggregates collect in the interstitial spaces around the alveoli and capillaries, thus reducing efficient gas exchange (see also Chapter 19).

Clinically, respiration becomes more rapid, the PaO_2 falls significantly, even when the patient is breathing high concentrations of oxygen and the increased respiration lowers the PCO_2, producing a respiratory alkalosis. Chest radiographs may change from normal to complete 'white-out' over a 24-h period. Treatment is mainly supportive and aimed at preserving adequate PaO_2. Intermittent positive-pressure ventilation is necessary if the oxygen tension falls below PaO_2 8 kPa. If intermittent positive-pressure ventilation fails to maintain adequate oxygenation, positive end-expiratory pressure at a pressure of between 5 and 15 cmH$_2$O is used (see Chapter 3). Other measures to reduce oedema such as maintaining plasma osmotic pressure by gastrointestinal or intravenous feeding and the administration of intravenous albumin and the judicious use of diuretics are important. Steroids and antibiotics are of doubtful value.

Acute renal failure

The commonest cause of acute renal failure in the surgical patient is a fall in the glomerular filtration rate (GFR) as a consequence of hypovolaemic shock. This is clinically manifest as oliguria with a daily urine output of between 400 and 700 ml, i.e. less than 20 ml/h.

When oliguria becomes established, fluid intake must be severely restricted and electrolyte concentrations carefully monitored. The blood urea will rise rapidly and the serum K+ tends to rise to dangerous levels, which can cause cardiac arrhythmias or cardiac arrest. A severe metabolic acidosis develops (see Chapter 6).

Fluid administration is restricted to 400 ml/day plus known losses. A rising K+ may be controlled by giving intravenous glucose and insulin, calcium gluconate or ion exchange resins. Sodium bicarbonate is used to control the metabolic acidosis. In most cases of acute renal failure some form of dialysis is necessary during the acute tubular necrosis phase. Peritoneal dialysis has the advantage of being a simple technique but haemodialysis is more efficient. At the end of the oliguric phase, assuming that acute tubular necrosis rather than acute cortical necrosis is the problem, the diuretic phase commences, during which large quantities of unconcentrated urine are passed and very high losses of Na+ and K+ may occur which need careful management (see also Chapter 5).

Shock at a glance

DEFINITIONS

Shock is defined as acute circulatory failure with inadequate or inappropriate tissue perfusion resulting in generalized cellular hypoxia

COMMON CAUSES

Hypovolaemic
- Blood loss (ruptured abdominal aortic aneurysm, upper gastrointestinal bleed, multiple fractures, etc.)
- Plasma loss (burns, pancreatitis)
- Extracellular fluid losses (vomiting, diarrhoea, intestinal fistula)

Cardiogenic
- Myocardial infarction
- Ventricular arrhythmias
- Pulmonary embolus
- Cardiac tamponade

Septic
- Gram-negative or, less often, Gram-positive infections

Anaphylactic
- Release of vasoactive substances when a sensitized individual is exposed to the appropriate antigen

CLINICAL FEATURES

Hypovolaemic and cardiogenic
- Pallor, coldness, sweating and restlessness
- Tachycardia, weak pulse, low blood pressure and oliguria

Septic
- Initially warm flushed skin and bounding pulse
- Later confusion and low output picture

INVESTIGATIONS AND ASSESSMENT

- Monitor pulse, blood pressure, temperature, respiratory rate and urinary output
- Establish good intravenous access and set up CVP line (possibly Swan–Ganz catheter as well)
- ECG and cardiac enzymes
- Hb, Hct, U&E, creatinine
- Group and cross-match blood
- Obtain blood cultures
- Arterial blood gases

MANAGEMENT

- Resuscitate the patient:
  Hypovolaemic (ABC, give 100% oxygen, restore circulating volume with crystalloids, colloids or blood depending on the cause)
  Cardiogenic (bedrest, adequate analgesia, thrombolytic therapy and aspirin if MI, treat heart failure and arrhythmias)
  Septic (give fluids to restore circulating volume, treat infection with antibiotics ± surgery; inotropes are frequently required)
  Anaphylaxis (intravenous fluids, adrenaline, antihistamines, hydrocortisone)
- Deal with the cause of the shock (stop the bleeding, drain the abscess, remove the source of the anaphylactic antigen, etc.)

COMPLICATIONS

- ARDS
- ARF   } SIRS
- DIC   } MODS
- Hepatic failure
- Stress ulceration

U&E, urea and electrolytes; MI, myocardial infarction; ARF, acute renal failure.

Acute hepatic failure

Rarely, severe shock may bring about acute hepatic failure. Encephalopathy, jaundice and coagulation disorders may supervene with progressive coma and respiratory failure. Treatment is mainly supportive and the mortality is very high. Hepatic failure is discussed fully in Chapter 13.

Prognosis

The prognosis of patients with two or more system failures is poor. Each organ failure carries a mortality of about 30%. However, these mortality rates are additive, so that patients with three or more system failures have mortality rates of 90–95%.

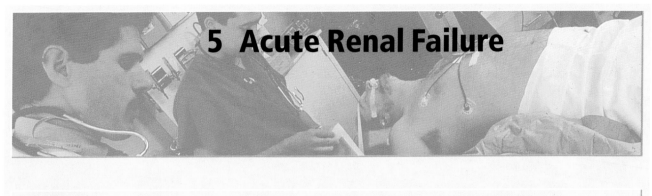

5 Acute Renal Failure

Introduction

Acute renal failure classically presents with sudden anuria (no urine) or oliguria (<400 ml/day) associated with a steep rise in serum urea and creatinine levels. However, non-oliguric renal failure (NORF) may also occur and is recognized by a persistently rising serum creatinine level in the presence of normal output of urine. The prognosis following oliguric renal failure is worse than NORF and this condition is frequently seen in, and contributes to, the mortality of patients in intensive care units.

Classification of renal failure

Renal failure may be classified into three groups (Fig. 5.1) — prerenal, intrinsic and postrenal. The commonest cause of a lowered urinary output in a surgical patient is inadequate intravenous fluid administration. Thus, prerenal oliguria and acute tubular necrosis (ATN) are the types of renal failure usually encountered following surgery; postrenal failure, which results from obstruction to urinary flow, is seen in urology patients (see Chapter 20). Medical causes of intrinsic renal failure are acute glomerulonephritis, severe pyelonephritis, malignant hypertension and end-stage chronic renal disease, e.g. secondary to diabetes mellitus.

Pathophysiology of acute renal failure

Acute renal failure may occur as a consequence of shock. The reduction in circulating blood volume, whether absolute or relative, which occurs produces a significant decrease in renal blood flow which may fall to one-third of its normal level. The glomerular filtration rate is correspondingly reduced and the patient becomes oliguric, producing only 400–700 ml of urine per 24 h or less than 20 ml/h.

When oligaemic states cause a reduction in renal blood flow, additional changes take place. There is a diversion of blood from the renal cortex and this exacerbates the situation by causing a further reduction in glomerular filtration rate. If the impairment in renal blood flow is of brief duration and blood volume is rapidly restored, the condition is reversible and normal urine output is resumed, although sometimes there is a lapse of some hours before this takes place. A more prolonged ischaemic period causes ATN with oliguria persisting for 1–3 or 4 weeks, followed by a period of diuresis when 4–5 litres of dilute urine are passed per day. More profound ischaemia gives rise to cortical necrosis, an irreversible condition requiring renal dialysis and eventually renal transplant.

Once acute renal failure becomes established, serious water and electrolyte disturbances occur.

- During the *oliguric phase* water retention with a relatively low Na^+ may precipitate cardiac failure, accompanied by pulmonary and systemic oedema. The degree of dyspnoea may be sufficiently severe to warrant ventilatory support. Inability to excrete K^+ leads to dangerously high plasma levels, which may give rise to arrhythmias and, if uncontrolled, to cardiac arrest. Retention of H^+ ions precipitates a metabolic acidosis. At first, hyperventilation and respiratory alkalosis compensate for this but this mechanism eventually fails and the pH of the blood falls rapidly. This phase may be exacerbated by respiratory failure and a developing lactic acidosis. Both the blood urea and serum creatinine levels progressively increase and calcium levels may fall.

- Careful monitoring and replacement of fluid and electrolytes are also required during the *diuretic phase.*

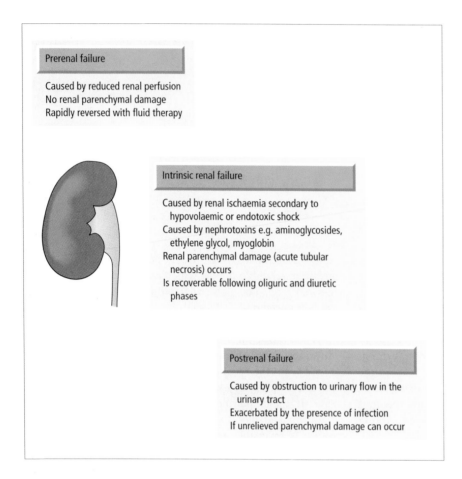

Prerenal failure

Caused by reduced renal perfusion
No renal parenchymal damage
Rapidly reversed with fluid therapy

Intrinsic renal failure

Caused by renal ischaemia secondary to
    hypovolaemic or endotoxic shock
Caused by nephrotoxins e.g. aminoglycosides,
    ethylene glycol, myoglobin
Renal parenchymal damage (acute tubular
    necrosis) occurs
Is recoverable following oliguric and diuretic
    phases

Postrenal failure

Caused by obstruction to urinary flow in the
    urinary tract
Exacerbated by the presence of infection
If unrelieved parenchymal damage can occur

Figure 5.1 Classification of renal failure.

Clinical features

• *Dyspnoea* is a frequent problem and in some patients respiratory failure may require intermittent positive-pressure ventilation (IPPV; Chapter 4). The respiratory problems are due to fluid retention with fluid overload giving rise to pulmonary as well as systemic oedema. *Metabolic acidosis* (see Chapter 6) and pulmonary infection may contribute further to the respiratory difficulties.

• *Hypertension* may also be a consequence of fluid overload and retention of K+ may give rise to *arrhythmias*.

• Gastrointestinal symptoms range from *nausea* and *vomiting* from water intoxication, to *hiccups* and *diarrhoea* which frequently accompany uraemia. Stress ulceration and gastric erosions are common with acute renal failure following shock and *gastrointestinal haemorrhage* may be severe.

• Cerebral oedema and toxic metabolites cause *confusion*, *drowsiness* and eventually *coma*.

• A progressive *anaemia* may develop and *coagulation defects* may occur. Disseminated intravascular coagulation is a not uncommon development.

• Finally, there is a generalized impairment of the immune system, increasing the risk of serious *infection*, which is probably the commonest cause of death in acute renal failure. The indiscriminate use of antibiotics exacerbates this risk by promoting the development of resistant strains of pathogenic bacteria.

Management of acute renal failure

Prevention

Acute renal failure may be prevented by careful attention to preoperative fluid balance, proper monitoring of the patient peroperatively and avoidance of hypotension and sepsis.

• Patients at risk of developing renal failure, e.g. patients with obstructive jaundice, should have an intravenous infusion established the night before surgery so that they are well-hydrated. Remember that they will be starved prior to surgery and will not be allowed oral fluids for about 12 h (but often longer) before surgery.

• Patients undergoing major surgery should have a urinary catheter, central venous line and arterial line placed and urinary output and haemodynamics measured regularly throughout the operation and postoperatively and appropriate action taken.

• Some drugs may help to avoid renal failure in certain situations. *Dopamine*, which at low doses (<5 μg/kg per min) induces vasodilation and increased renal perfusion, is frequently given to at-risk patients in an attempt to preserve renal function. *Mannitol*, an osmotic diuretic, may also protect renal function in some patients, such as those with obstructive jaundice or those at risk of rhabdomyolysis (e.g. following arterial embolectomy).

• Patients receiving known nephrotoxic drugs should have their renal function monitored regularly and in the case of aminoglycosides plasma concentrations should be measured 1 h after intramuscular or intravenous administration and just prior to the administration of the next dose. This ensures that excessive and subtherapeutic doses are avoided. For gentamicin the peak level should not exceed 10 mg/l, while the trough level should be less than 2 mg/l.

Treatment

• As already mentioned, prompt restoration of circulating volume of renal blood flow can prevent the occurrence of ATN. Once ATN is established, however, the first priority is the maintenance of fluid and electrolyte balance.

• Water intake must be restricted to 400 ml/day, in addition to whatever may be lost from other sources.

• Administration of Na^+ is limited to the amount lost in urine or through the gut, which should be measured so that replacement can be exact.

• The intake of K^+ is restricted and a rise of K^+ in the serum to dangerous levels should be controlled by intravenous glucose and insulin (e.g. 100 ml of 50% dextrose with 20 units of soluble insulin) and ion exchange resins (calcium resonium) given orally or rectally.

• It is often necessary to provide the patient's nutritional requirements intravenously as the patient is too ill for oral feeding and enteral feeding by tube may provoke diarrhoea. However, where possible enteral feeding should be used. A high caloric intake in a small fluid volume is needed and, since protein must be severely restricted, the calories are supplied as 50% dextrose via a central venous catheter.

• A metabolic acidosis is likely to develop and may require administration of sodium bicarbonate.

• Since many of these patients are suffering from infection, antibiotic therapy is frequently necessary. The aminoglycosides are nephrotoxic and the use of drugs such as gentamicin must be given in lower dosage and its use carefully monitored by checking plasma levels regularly.

• The definitive treatment of established ATN is renal dialysis. This may be accomplished either by the simple technique of peritoneal dialysis or by the more complicated but more efficient method of haemodialysis.

Dialysis

Peritoneal dialysis

Peritoneal dialysis requires an intact abdominal wall and peritoneal lining. A catheter is placed into the peritoneal cavity and dialysis is achieved by infusing and draining dialysis fluid from the peritoneal cavity. It relies for its effect on an osmotic gradient, allowing fluid and ions to be exchanged across the peritoneal membrane. The solutions used are either isotonic or hypertonic. The latter is of value when large volumes of fluid have to be taken out of the circulation rapidly. Like most concentrated fluids, it is very irritant and should only be used for short periods. The volume of fluid used in peritoneal dialysis averages around 2 l/h and the flow in and out should be continuous. Frequent postural change may be necessary for adequate drainage and the procedure may be painful. Severe pain may be controlled by including lignocaine in the dialysing solution.

Ultrafiltration

The accumulation of fluid following the onset of ATN may lead to cardiac failure, pulmonary oedema and water intoxication. Ultrafiltration/haemofiltration may be used if volume regulation is all that is required. Heparinized blood via an arterial line is circulated through a haemofiltration cartridge. The patient's blood pressure provides the necessary gradient for removal of plasma fluid (Fig. 5.2).

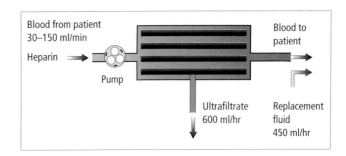

Figure 5.2 Haemofiltration circuit. In a haemofiltration circuit blood passes across a filtration membrane. Ultrafiltration rates of *600 ml/h* are usual, removing toxins and fluid with a clearance of 10 ml/h. Many patients in the intensive therapy unit with acute renal failure are managed with continuous venovenous haemofiltration which requires the use of a pump.

Haemodialysis

In haemodialysis, exchange of fluid and electrolytes is effected across a cellophane membrane using a pressure gradient to provide filtration. The membrane is distributed over a large surface area by means of plates or coils to achieve adequate filtration. Haemodialysis is a more complicated invasive procedure requiring arteriovenous access and expensive and sophisticated equipment, the use of which demands familiarity and practice (Fig. 5.3).

Prognosis

ATN usually lasts for 1–3 weeks. If oliguria continues for a few more weeks, acute cortical necrosis should be suspected and renal biopsy performed. If a diagnosis of cortical necrosis is confirmed, the patient must be transferred to a chronic renal dialysis programme and be considered for renal transplantation.

At the end of the oliguric phase in ATN the diuretic phase begins and may last a further 3 or 4 weeks, during which the patient passes large volumes of dilute urine with large losses of sodium and potassium. The management and control of water and electrolytes during this period must be as rigorous as in the oliguric phase.

The mortality in acute renal failure may be as high as 50%, with infection leading to multiple organ failure as the most common cause of death.

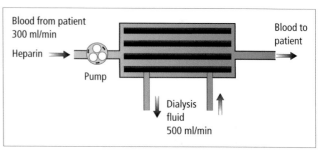

(a)

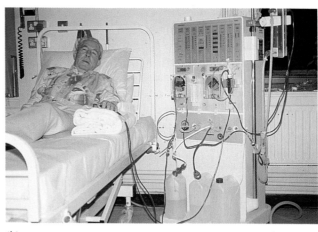

(b)

Figure 5.3 (a) Haemodialysis circuit. In a haemodialysis circuit blood and dialysis fluid circulate in a countercurrent fashion separated by a semipermeable membrane. Blood flow rates of *100–300 ml/min* are usual and patients undergo haemodialysis for 3–5 h three times per week. Creatinine clearances are 100–150 ml/min during dialysis or 5–10 ml/min when calculated for a week. (b) Patient undergoing haemodialysis.

Acute renal failure at a glance

DEFINITION

Acute renal failure is a sudden deterioration in renal function such that neither kidney is capable of excreting body waste products (e.g. urea, creatinine, potassium) which accumulate in the blood. It is fatal unless treated. *Anuria* means that no urine is passed in a day. *Oliguria* means that 400 ml/day is passed

COMMON CAUSES

Prerenal failure
- Shock causing reduced renal perfusion

Intrinsic renal failure
- Shock causing renal ischaemia (*acute tubular necrosis*)
- Nephrotoxins (aminoglycosides, myoglobin)
- Acute glomerulonephritis
- Severe pyelonephritis
- Hypertension and diabetes mellitus

Postrenal failure
- Urinary tract obstruction, e.g. prostatic hypertrophy

CLINICAL FEATURES

- Dyspnoea, confusion, drowsiness, coma
- Hypertension, arrhythmias
- Nausea, vomiting, hiccups, diarrhoea, gastrointestinal haemorrhage
- Anaemia and coagulation defects

U&E, Urea and electrolytes; ECG, electrocardiogram; CXR, chest X-ray.

INVESTIGATIONS

- U&E (especially K+) and creatinine estimations
- ECG/CXR
- Arterial blood gases (metabolic acidosis)

MANAGEMENT

Prevention
- Keep at-risk patients (e.g. patients with obstructive jaundice) well-hydrated pre- and peroperatively
- Protect renal function in selective patients with drugs such as *dopamine* and *mannitol*
- Monitor renal function regularly in patients on nephrotoxic drugs (e.g. gentamicin)

Treatment
- Maintain fluid and electrolyte balance

Water intake	400 ml/day + measured losses
Sodium intake	Limited to replace loss only
Potassium intake	Nil (frequently dextrose and insulin and/or ion exchange resins are required to control hyperkalaemia)
Diet	High-calorie, low-protein in a small volume of fluid
Acidosis	Sodium bicarbonate

- Treat any infection
- Dialysis   Peritoneal
                    Ultrafiltration

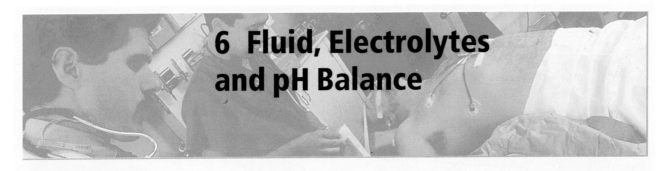

6 Fluid, Electrolytes and pH Balance

Water water everywhere
And all the boards did shrink;
Water water everywhere
Nor any drop to drink.   (Samuel Taylor Coleridge 1772–1834)

Introduction

Biochemical disorders of fluid and electrolyte balance and pH disturbances are often encountered in acutely ill patients and those with chronic renal, respiratory and liver disease. To a large extent, fluid and electrolyte disturbances and pH changes are interactive — pathological changes in one result in abnormal deviations in the other. Thus, contractions of the extracellular fluid compartment (e.g. shock) lead to acidosis and primary acid–base disturbances are often accompanied by significant volume changes.

Fluid and electrolyte balance

Body composition

Water constitutes 67–79% of the lean tissue mass. The exact amount depends on the body fat, as adipose tissue has a low water content. The various fluid compartments of the body are shown in Fig. 6.1.

The intracellular compartment is the largest fluid compartment with a volume of 25–30 litres. The extracellular compartment is made up of the plasma or intravascular compartment (4 l) and the interstitial space (10–12 l). Normally, there is a continuous bidirectional movement of water between the plasma and the interstitial fluid across the capillary bed. This is governed by the hydrostatic pres-

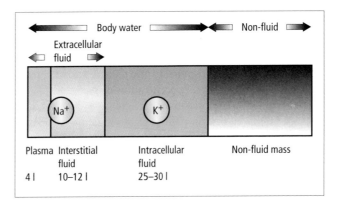

Figure 6.1 Body fluid compartments. The main extracellular cation is Na+ and the main intracellular cation is K+. The concentrations of these cations are maintained by the Na+/K+ pump. There is a daily net gain of fluid by the interstitial space. This is returned to the vascular compartment by the lymphatic system.

sure at the arteriolar end of the capillary, and the oncotic pressure of the plasma at the venular extremity. The exchange of fluid across the capillary membrane is, of course, essential for the supply of nutrients and oxygen to the tissues and the elimination of waste products of metabolism.

The osmolality (total particle concentration) is the same in all the fluid compartments and is normally 280–295 mosmol/kg water. By contrast, the electrolyte composition of the intracellular compartment is very

Table 6.1 Electrolyte composition of plasma and intracellular fluid (mmol/l).

Constituent	Symbol	Plasma*	Intracellular
Cations			
Sodium	Na$^+$	142	10
Potassium	K$^+$	4	150
Calcium	Ca^{2+}	2.5	2
Magnesium	Mg^{2+}	1.5	20
Anions			
Chloride	Cl$^-$	103	10
Bicarbonate	HCO$_3^-$	27	10
Sulphate	SO$_4^{2-}$	1.5	70
Phosphate	PO$_4^{2-}$	1	45

* Interstitial fluid has similar composition.

500 ml 0.9% NaCl + 20 mmol KCl 500 ml 0.5% Dextrose	8 hours
500 ml 0.5% Dextrose + 20 mmol KCl 500 ml 0.5% Dextrose	8 hours
500 ml 0.5% Dextrose + 20 mmol KCl 500 ml 0.5% Dextrose	8 hours

Box 6.1 This is a typical intravenous regime for uncomplicated cases requiring intravenous fluid replacement therapy. This regime provides 3000 ml of water, 77 ml of NaCl and 60 mmol of KCl. Each litre of fluid should be infused over 8 h.

different from that of the plasma and interstitial fluid (Table 6.1).

The main *cation* (a positively charged atom which is attracted to a negative electrode — cathode) in the plasma is Na$^+$ and the accompanying *anions* (negatively charged atoms that are attracted to a positive electrode — anode) are Cl$^-$ and HCO$_3^-$. In the normal state, the plasma electrolytes account for the large part of its osmolality and there is a good correlation between the plasma concentration of Na$^+$ and plasma osmolality, i.e. a high plasma Na$^+$ signifies hyperosmolality and vice versa. In certain pathological states, the osmolality may also be pathologically elevated by the accumulation of large amounts of organic solutes, e.g. excess urea in renal failure and excess glucose in uncontrolled diabetes mellitus.

Normal requirements

The normal daily requirements for fluids and electrolytes are shown in Table 6.2.

There is of course a significant individual variation and any excesses are excreted by the kidneys provided renal

Table 6.2 Daily requirements of water and electrolytes.

	per kg body weight	Total for average male adult
Water	35 ml	2500 ml
Sodium	1 mmol	70 mmol
Potassium	1 mmol	70 mmol
Chloride	1 mmol	70 mmol
Phosphate	0.2 mmol	14 mmol
Calcium	0.1 mmol	7 mmol
Magnesium	0.1 mmol	7 mmol

function is normal. A typical intravenous fluid regime for a patient for 24 h is given in Box 6.1, this regime provides 3000 ml of water, 77 mmol of NaCl and 60 mmol of KCl. Each litre of fluid should be infused over 8 h.

Water

The body incurs certain daily obligatory losses of water: in expired air, faeces, urine and insensible skin loss. The minimal or obligatory volume of urine necessary for the excretion of the daily solute load is 500 ml. This represents the absolute limit of the concentrating power of the kidney and the normal urine output is much higher, averaging 1500–2000 ml. Only a very small amount of water (250 ml) is actually produced by the body each day as a result of metabolic activity. Thus the daily losses have to be replaced by the daily intake.

Water intake is controlled by the sensation of thirst which is dependent on stimuli from the cerebral cortex and the limbic system. Satiation of thirst is influenced by stimuli from gastric stretch receptors and from receptors in the oropharynx which respond to moistening. The control of water excretion by the kidneys is regulated by *antidiuretic hormone* (ADH), the release of which is controlled by osmoreceptors in the hypothalamus and pressure receptors in the heart and great vessels. ADH alters the permeability of the distal convoluted and collecting tubules so that more water than solute is reabsorbed. The water reabsorbed in excess of the solute load is referred to as *free water*.

High-pressure stretch receptors are located both extra- and intrarenally. The extrarenal group stimulates the release of *renin* through the sympathetic system. The intrarenal pressure receptors are located in the juxtaglomerular complex which contains renin-secreting cells. Other components of the juxtaglomerular complex (macula densa) are capable of monitoring the Na+ load in the distal tubular fluid and thereby induce the release of renin. The latter converts *angiotensinogen* to *angiotensin I*. A plasma-converting enzyme subsequently hydrolyses angiotensin I to the octapeptide *angiotensin II*. This induces the release of *aldosterone* from the adrenal cortex, a potent mineralo-corticoid which causes increased renal tubular reabsorption of Na+ and water. Aldosterone secretion can also be directly stimulated by a decreased plasma Na+ or an increased plasma K+. The control of Na+ balance is also dependent on the release of a *natriuretic hormone*, which leads to the increased excretion of this cation by the proximal tubules of the kidney.

Fluid and electrolyte disturbances

In surgical practice deficiency states are more common than disturbances characterized by excess water or salt. The important disorders are excess water, water deple-tion, sodium deficiency, iso-osmolar sodium excess, potassium excess and deficiency, and raised or low serum calcium.

Water

Water intoxication

This condition is rare and is caused by the administration of excessive amounts of 5% dextrose, especially in the pres-ence of impaired renal function. Occasionally, it is associ-ated with excessive secretion of ADH. There is an expansion of both the intracellular and extracellular fluid compartments, a low serum sodium and widespread oedema. Irritability, drowsiness, convulsions and coma may occur. Treatment is by water restriction and sometimes administration of hypertonic saline.

Water depletion

Inadequate intake of water leads to dehydration and raised plasma Na+ (*hypernatraemia*) with a rise in the osmolality of the body fluids. Despite increased reabsorption of water by the kidney, there is contraction of both the extracellular and intracellular fluid compartments. Clinically there is thirst, drowsiness and coma. Treatment consists of slow intravenous replacement with hypotonic saline solution. Rapid intravenous infusion with 5% dextrose is contra-indicated as it will cause water intoxication with coma and convulsions.

Sodium

Hypernatraemia

Hypernatraemia may be due to excessive administration of sodium (usually iatrogenic from infusing excessive amounts of sodium in intravenous fluids) or dehydration from decreased fluid intake or water loss. The osmotic pressure of the extracellular fluid rises and the clinical picture is similar to that of water depletion (see above). Rarely, hypernatraemia is caused by primary hyperaldosteronism (Conn's syndrome; Chapter 15). If the serum sodium rises above 160 mmol/l, hypernatraemic encephalopathy may occur. Treatment of hypernatraemia is by slow intravenous replacement with hypotonic saline solution.

Sodium deficiency

Deficiency of Na+ (*hyponatraemia*) is the commonest acute biochemical disturbance encountered in surgical practice. The common causes of hyponatraemia (i.e. serum sodium <130 mmol/l) are listed below.

Sodium losses

• Sodium-rich losses from the gastrointestinal tract, e.g. vomiting, diarrhoea, intestinal obstruction, etc.
• Renal sodium loss, e.g. in Addison's disease (Chapter 15).
• Diuretic use, particularly those that promote sodium diuresis (naturesis), e.g. frusemide and the thiazide diuretics.

Water retention

• Prolonged infusion of dextrose 5% alone.
• Transurethal resection of the prostate (TURP) syndrome (Chapter 20).
• Cardiac failure and cirrhosis of the liver.
• Inappropriate ADH secretion (Fig. 6.2).

In its most usual mild form, hyponatraemia is asymp-tomatic. When plasma sodium falls below 120 mmol/l patients become confused. There is severe contraction of the extracellular fluid compartment with a hypovolaemia, poor venous filling, oliguria, dry skin with loss of turgor and sunken eyeballs. If the levels go below 110 mmol/l con-vulsions and coma may ensue. Therapy for hyponatraemia is directed at the underlying cause. Sodium losses can be replaced by increasing sodium intake without increasing daily fluid intake (e.g. giving normal saline continuously); water retention should be treated by fluid restriction.

Inappropriate ADH secretion	

Neurological
  Head injury
  Cerebral metastases
Pulmonary
  Oat cell carcinoma of lung
  Bronchial carcinoid
  Tuberculosis
  Lung abscess
  Pneumonia
Miscellaneous
  Prostatic cancer
  Pancreatic cancer
  Lymphomas
	ADH, antidiuretic hormone (vasopressin).
	It is a hormone normally secreted from the posterior lobe of the pituitary gland

Figure 6.2 Excess antidiuretic hormone increases renal tubular water reabsorption independently of sodium. Thus, water is retained, causing dilutional hyponatraemia. The urinary osmolality will be high while the serum osmolality is low.

Potassium

Hyperkalaemia

An elevated serum potassium (*hyperkalaemia*) is encountered in acidotic, hypoxic and ischaemic states. In these conditions potassium is released from cells. However, the most common cause of hyperkalaemia is potassium retention due to renal failure. Clinically hyperkalaemia is associated with diarrhoea, colicky abdominal pain and peaked T-waves on the electrocardiogram (ECG; Fig. 6.3). Irrespective of cause, a serum K⁺ level above 6 mmol/l may precipitate a cardiac arrest (usually ventricular fibrillation). The treatment of hyperkalaemia entails correction of the underlying cause, together with measures designed to reduce the level of the plasma K^+. These include:

- administration of intravenous *calcium gluconate* or *sodium bicarbonate* or *insulin* and *glucose*; the latter two act by promoting the movement of K^+ into the cells;
- the cation exchange resin, *calcium resonium*, administered by mouth or as an enema is also effective in removing excess body potassium; and
- severe hyperkalaemia associated with renal failure is an indication for *dialysis*.

Hypokalaemia

A low serum potassium (*hypokalaemia*) is encountered in pyloric stenosis, high jejunal obstructions, liver failure and diarrhoea from any cause. Rarely, hypokalaemia is caused by primary hyperaldosteronism (Conn's syndrome). Clinically, hypokalaemia is characterized by lethargy, muscle weakness, adynamic ileus and life-threatening ventricular dysrhythmias which may progress to cardiac arrest in asystole. The ECG shows a prolonged P-R interval, T-wave inversion and classical U-waves. Hypokalaemia is always accompanied by a *metabolic alkalosis* (see below). This is due to the increased reabsorption of HCO_3^- and excretion of H^+ from the proximal tubules of the kidney. The correction of hypokalaemia has to be done gradually. If hypokalaemia is severe, intravenous KCl in a concentration of *not more than 40 mmol/l* may be administered. Such therapy should be monitored by ECG as severe cardiac dysrhythmias may be encountered and require temporary interruption of the infusion.

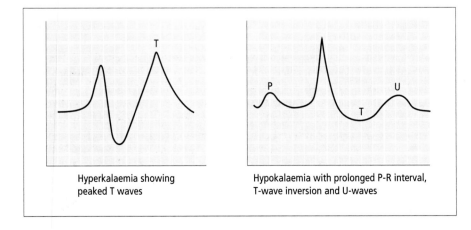

Hyperkalaemia showing peaked T waves

Hypokalaemia with prolonged P-R interval, T-wave inversion and U-waves

Figure 6.3 Typical electrocardiogram changes associated with hyper- and hypokalaemia.

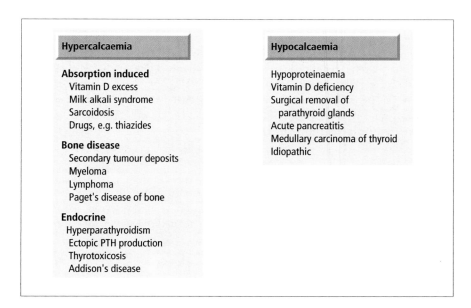

Hypercalcaemia	Hypocalcaemia
Absorption induced	Hypoproteinaemia
Vitamin D excess	Vitamin D deficiency
Milk alkali syndrome	Surgical removal of
Sarcoidosis	parathyroid glands
Drugs, e.g. thiazides	Acute pancreatitis
Bone disease	Medullary carcinoma of thyroid
Secondary tumour deposits	Idiopathic
Myeloma	
Lymphoma	
Paget's disease of bone	
Endocrine	
Hyperparathyroidism	
Ectopic PTH production	
Thyrotoxicosis	
Addison's disease	

Box 6.2 The common causes of hyper- and hypocalcaemia.

Calcium

Calcium metabolism is discussed fully in Chapter 15. However, the main causes of hyper- and hypocalcaemia are summarized in Box 6.2.

The normal total calcium range is 2.2–2.6 mmol/l. Calcium is usually bound to albumin and the levels of both calcium and albumin should be measured together. (To correct for low serum albumin, 0.025 should be added to the serum calcium for every 1 g/l that the albumin is lower than 40 g/l.)

Hypercalcaemia

Hypercalcaemia is usually asymptomatic below a serum level of 3.5 mmol/l. Above that level clinical features include muscle weakness, lassitude, drowsiness and hyperreflexia. Anxiety and mania may develop with coma as a terminal event. Polyuria and polydipsia indicate impaired renal concentration. Nausea, vomiting, constipation and peptic ulceration may also occur. Treatment is directed at dealing with the underlying cause but rapid reduction of serum calcium levels can be achieved by hydration with saline, calciuresis with diuretics (frusemide), steroids and specific drugs, e.g. mithramycin, calcitonin, ethylenediaminetetraacetic acid (EDTA) and biphosphonates.

Hypocalcaemia

Hypocalcaemia (serum calcium <2 mmol/l) results in a dramatic clinical picture characterized by *tetany*. In its mildest form, there may be paraesthesiae and muscle cramps. The full-blown picture is characterized by hyperexcitability of the nervous system, most commonly expressed as carpopedal spasm. This consists of severe tonic contractions of the muscles of the hand; the fingers are bunched together and flexed at the metacarpophalangeal joints and the wrist is acutely flexed (*main d'accoucheur*). Similarly, the toes are flexed and the ankle joint acutely plantar flexed. Latent tetany may be demonstrated by *Chvostek's sign* (tapping over the facial nerve inducing twitching of the facial muscles) and *Trousseau's sign* (carpal spasm induced by inflating a sphygmomanometer cuff above systolic pressure). Acute hypocalcaemia is treated by slow intravenous infusion of calcium gluconate (10% solution; see also Chapter 15).

Acid–base balance

The pH is a representation (the negative logarithm) of the hydrogen ion (H^+) concentration in the body fluids. Maintenance of a blood pH between 7.37 and 7.42 is essential for normal metabolic activity. As the latter results in the generation of acids (e.g. lactic acid), particularly during physical exertion, efficient compensatory mechanisms are invoked to prevent any significant deviations in the pH. These compensatory mechanisms include those listed below.
• *Buffer systems*: intracellular buffers are proteins and phosphates while blood buffers are bicarbonate and haemoglobin.

• *The lungs*: overall regulation of pH consists of immediate buffering of acid metabolites followed by pulmonary excretion of H+ as water (H_2O) and carbon dioxide (CO_2).

• *The kidneys*: renal regulation of pH is achieved mostly by retention or excretion of bicarbonate (HCO_3^-).

The lungs and kidneys act in concert such that in the presence of mild renal impairment, increased acid removal is achieved by the lungs and vice versa.

Acidosis/alkalosis

Certain disease states overwhelm these homeostatic mechanisms and result in significant accumulation of acid or base with corresponding deviations from the normal pH. *Acidaemia* occurs when the pH falls below 7.36 and *alkalaemia* when the pH exceeds 7.44. Acidaemia, which signifies an excess of unbuffered hydrogen ions in the blood and body fluids, is the commoner disorder of acid–base balance. The compensatory mechanisms of the body try to normalize the pH in these situations and these are reflected in changes in the blood gas analysis from which the diagnosis of *acidosis* (tendency to low pH) and *alkalosis* (tendency to high pH) is made (Box 6.3).

Blood gas changes

The blood gas analysis also gives the clinician the information as to the metabolic or respiratory origin of the acid–base disturbance in an individual patient. This distinction is based on the relationship between the changes in

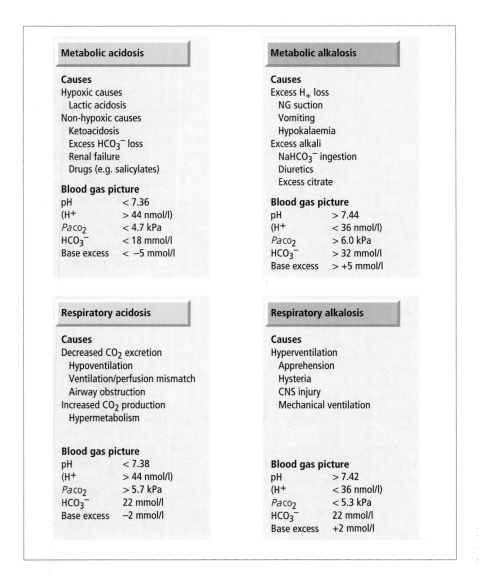

Metabolic acidosis

Causes
Hypoxic causes
  Lactic acidosis
Non-hypoxic causes
  Ketoacidosis
  Excess HCO_3^- loss
  Renal failure
  Drugs (e.g. salicylates)

Blood gas picture
pH	< 7.36
(H+	> 44 nmol/l)
Pa_{CO_2}	< 4.7 kPa
HCO_3^-	< 18 mmol/l
Base excess	< −5 mmol/l

Metabolic alkalosis

Causes
Excess H+ loss
  NG suction
  Vomiting
  Hypokalaemia
Excess alkali
  $NaHCO_3^-$ ingestion
  Diuretics
  Excess citrate

Blood gas picture
pH	> 7.44
(H+	< 36 nmol/l)
Pa_{CO_2}	> 6.0 kPa
HCO_3^-	> 32 mmol/l
Base excess	> +5 mmol/l

Respiratory acidosis

Causes
Decreased CO_2 excretion
  Hypoventilation
  Ventilation/perfusion mismatch
  Airway obstruction
Increased CO_2 production
  Hypermetabolism

Blood gas picture
pH	< 7.38
(H+	> 44 nmol/l)
Pa_{CO_2}	> 5.7 kPa
HCO_3^-	22 mmol/l
Base excess	−2 mmol/l

Respiratory alkalosis

Causes
Hyperventilation
  Apprehension
  Hysteria
  CNS injury
  Mechanical ventilation

Blood gas picture
pH	> 7.42
(H+	< 36 nmol/l)
Pa_{CO_2}	< 5.3 kPa
HCO_3^-	22 mmol/l
Base excess	+2 mmol/l

Box 6.3 The common causes of acidosis and alkalosis and the blood gas findings typical of each abnormality.

the pH and Pa_{CO_2}. When the pH change occurs in the opposite direction to the Pa_{CO_2} (i.e. pH down and Pa_{CO_2} up), the underlying cause is respiratory impairment. By contrast, in metabolic disturbances, the pH change occurs in the same direction as the Pa_{CO_2} (both up — *alkalosis* — or both down — *acidosis*). The *base excess* is derived from the difference between the patient's standard bicarbonate and the normal mean and is a good indicator of metabolic disturbances. A base deficit of −5 to −10 mmol/l is present with metabolic acidosis. (This is sometimes confusingly expressed as base excess of −5 to −10 mmol/l.) With metabolic alkalosis there is a base excess of +5 to +10 mmol/l. Thus from the blood gas analysis it is possible to work out whether the patient is acidotic or alkalotic and whether the abnormality is metabolic or respiratory.

Clinical classification

In practice acid–base disorders are classified as:
- respiratory acidosis (retention of CO_2);
- respiratory alkalosis (excess elimination of CO_2);
- metabolic acidosis (excess production or retention of acid metabolites, and rarely excess ingestion of acids); and
- metabolic alkalosis (abnormal loss of hydrogen ions, excess ingestion of alkali and hypokalaemia).

However, at times the picture is mixed, e.g. mixed metabolic and respiratory acidosis.

Management

The treatment of all acid–base abnormalities entails treatment of the underlying condition, thus allowing the body's buffering and regulatory systems to clear the abnormality and return the pH to the normal range. However, occasionally sodium bicarbonate has to be administered to counter severe metabolic acidosis, e.g. after cardiac arrest. Metabolic alkalosis is treated by intravenous isotonic chloride solutions and correction of hypokalaemia if present. The management of respiratory acidosis and alkalosis entails correction of the underlying ventilatory disturbance.

7 Systemic Inflammatory Response Syndrome

A free radical is a highly active moiety which has been likened to a convention delegate away from his wife — it will combine destructively with anything that is around. (Dr Alex Comfort)

Introduction

Over the last 20 years improvements in early resuscitation following major injury have meant that many very ill patients survive the initial traumatic insult (e.g. ruptured abdominal aortic aneurysm) and are managed thereafter in intensive care units. Many of these patients subsequently develop a hypermetabolic state similar to that seen with septic shock which leads to sequential organ failure involving the following:

- the lungs (adult respiratory distress syndrome; ARDS);
- the kidneys (acute renal failure);
- the gastrointestinal tract (liver failure, stress ulceration);
- the central nervous system (confusion);
- the blood (disseminated intravascular coagulation; DIC);
- the heart (cardiac depression).

The response to injury which occurs in the body and leads to this hypermetabolic state is called the *systemic inflammatory response syndrome* (SIRS) and the sequence of failing end-organs is referred to as *multiple organ dysfunction syndrome* (MODS).

Pathophysiology

The pathophysiology of SIRS/MODS is complex but it appears that one or more of many *initiating factors* (see below) causes a systemic *hyperinflammatory response* and it is the uncontrolled activity of this response that leads to organ failure (Fig. 7.1).

Initiating factors

No single initiating factor for the hyperinflammatory response has been isolated but a few suspects have been identified. It is likely that the clinical syndrome of SIRS results from the interaction of a number of the proposed initiating mechanisms. Infection has long been known to cause a systemic inflammatory response (i.e. septic shock) but the realization that many patients in 'septic shock' had no focus of infection led to the idea that other initiating factors could precipitate a similar syndrome. It appears that the presence of large areas of damaged or necrotic tissue can mimic an infectious focus.

Infection

Uncontrolled infection accounts for 50% of cases of MODS. *Sepsis* has been defined as the presence of micro-organisms or their toxins (e.g. endotoxin) in the bloodstream together with the resultant host response. It has long been recognized that severe infection can lead to septic shock with profound effects on haemodynamics and tissue perfusion. While most forms of circulatory shock induce cellular changes secondary to hypoxia, *Gram-negative septic shock* is associated with primary cellular dysfunction induced by bacterial endotoxins which are composed of lipopolysaccharides (LPS) in the bacterial cell wall. LPS stimulates macrophages and endothelial cells to release cytokines which mediate the inflammatory response (Fig. 7.2). *Gram-positive* organisms (e.g. *Staphylococcus aureus*) release cytokines by adherence to macrophages while their toxins act as superantigens reacting directly with T cells, causing massive cytokine release.

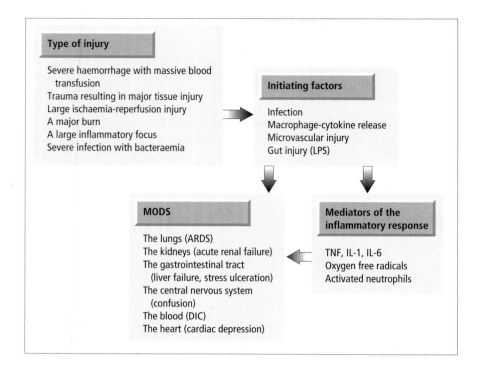

Figure 7.1 Pathophysiology of systemic inflammatory response syndrome (SIRS).

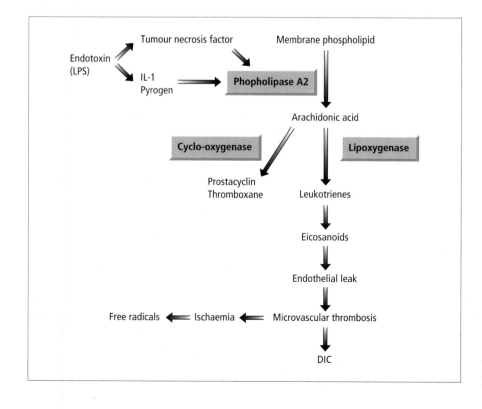

Figure 7.2 The role of endotoxin in promoting an inflammatory response.

Macrophage–cytokine release

Tumour necrosis factor (TNF) is detected in the serum of most patients with SIRS. TNF is a principal mediator of the inflammatory response and it is released with interleukin-1 (IL-1) and interleukin-6 (IL-6) from macrophages. It is thought that persistent stimulation of the release of these cytokines leads to the inflammatory response and tissue injury.

Microcirculatory injury

Ischaemia reperfusion may induce a systemic inflammatory response. Reperfusion of tissues after a period of ischaemia causes the release of toxic oxygen radicals (superoxide, O_2^-, hydrogen peroxide, H_2O_2, and the hydroxyl radical, OH^-) which cause tissue damage by lipid peroxidation. The resulting endothelial damage causes release of cytokines initiating a systemic inflammatory response and end-organ failure.

Gut injury

The normal intestinal mucosa is an effective barrier against microorganisms and endotoxin. A number of adverse changes take place in the septic state which allow bacterial translocation (i.e. the passage of bacteria from the gut to the systemic circulation) to occur.
• The nature of the microflora changes, especially in the presence of antibiotics, to a more pathogenic and more resistant pattern.
• Barrier function is lost through disappearance of tight junctions between epithelial cells, loss of mucus and increase in mucosal permeability.
• The Kupffer cells in the liver, which act as part of the reticuloendothelial system providing the next line of defence, lose their filtering ability and allow bacteria and endotoxin to enter the portal and systemic circulations.
• The hepatocytes in the liver may also be damaged with evidence of jaundice.
• *Candida* normally present in the gastrointestinal tract may migrate to the bloodstream and lungs, particularly when antibiotics are in use.

The gut has been called the 'motor' of SIRS/MODS as it provides a reservoir of bacteria and endotoxin to keep the inflammatory response going. The inflammatory response in turn causes further intestinal injury. The absorptive power of the gut may also be lost because of damage to intestinal villi. Whenever possible, enteral feeding (to avoid further mucosal atrophy) should be the preferred mode of nutritional support in SIRS patients. However, if enteral feeding cannot be sustained, intravenous feeding (total parenteral nutrition; TPN) with its additional hazards is necessary.

Hyperinflammatory response

The interaction between initiating factors (endotoxin, ischaemia/reperfusion, etc.) and the host-mediated response results in changes in cellular metabolism with increased glucose and amino acid utilization. Mediators such as TNF (also called *cachectin*), IL-1 and IL-6 are released, resulting in a cascade of responses including:
• fever from endogenous pyrogen;
• priming of neutrophils to release reactive oxygen intermediates;
• promoting adherence of phagocytes to endothelium;
• activation of complement and release of prostaglandins and thromboxane A_2.

The mechanism by which the systemic inflammatory response causes end-organ failure is slowly being elucidated. The initial events occur at the microvascular endothelium. Thus, oxygen free radicals are released, neutrophil chemotactic factors are produced and surface adhesion molecules are expressed that enhance neutrophil adhesion and migration into the tissues. Further tissue damage is caused by release of destructive molecules from the trapped neutrophils (more oxygen radicals, elastase, collagenase and proteases). As a result, microthrombi are formed, interstitial oedema occurs and organ function deteriorates. Damage to cell membranes allows the free passage of calcium into the cell; this is toxic to mitochondrial function with impairment of oxidative phosphorylation and ultimately cell death.

Clinical features

The patients at risk are those who have sustained a major biological insult, such as:
• severe haemorrhage requiring massive blood transfusion (e.g. liver trauma);
• trauma resulting in major tissue injury (e.g. crush injury);
• large ischaemia reperfusion injury (e.g. reperfusion of a limb following embolectomy);
• a major burn;
• a large inflammatory focus (e.g. peritonitis, pancreatitis); and
• severe infection with bacteraemia (e.g. ascending cholangitis).

Typically the patient seems to do well following resuscitation but after 2 or 3 days develops the characteristic hypermetabolic picture. In the early phase the blood pressure remains normal, peripheral vascular resistance is lowered and there is an increase in the cardiac output. Later on, with the development of shock the blood pressure falls, peripheral resistance decreases further and the cardiac output remains high. There is a metabolic acidosis with a compensatory respiratory alkalosis. Typically there will be a leukocytosis (or leukopenia), thrombocytopenia and hyperglycaemia. Finally, cardiac output decreases with a profound fall in blood pressure and an exacerbation of the metabolic acidosis; oxygen consumption falls, indicating inadequate oxygen perfusion.

The diagnosis of SIRS is made when two or more of the following are present:
- tachycardia;
- tachypnoea or hyperventilation; and
- fever and leukocytosis.

When two or more end-organs fail a diagnosis of MODS is made (Table 7.1).

Table 7.1 Features of end-organ dysfunction.

System	Features
Respiratory (ARDS)	Increasing minute ventilation, Decreased pulmonary compliance Arterial hypoxaemia and hypercapnoea Diffuse fluffy pulmonary infiltrates on chest radiograph
Renal (ARF)	Oliguria Rising urea and creatinine
Liver	Jaundice Decreased protein synthesis (hypoalbuminaemia, prolonged PT)
Gastrointestinal	Gastric stress ulceration Adynamic ileus Acalculous cholecystitis Pancreatitis
Haematology	Leukopenia Disseminated intravascular coagulopathy
Central nervous system	Confusion Decreasing Glasgow coma score

ARDS, Adult respiratory distress syndrome; ARF, acute renal failure; PT, prothrombin time.

Management

The best form of therapy is prevention and every effort should be made during resuscitation to avoid hypotension and gross sepsis (e.g. during bowel surgery) and to ensure adequate oxygenation and urinary output. The general aims of therapy are to:

- treat infection;
- ensure adequate tissue oxygenation;
- maintain nutritional support; and
- minimize systemic inflammation.

Management of the failure of the various end-organs must also be undertaken. This is largely supportive and has been discussed in Chapters 3–5.

Treat infection

Eradication of the source of infection is a priority. Removal of necrotic tissue or drainage of abscesses is essential. Nosocomial (hospital-acquired) infection must be prevented by aggressive physiotherapy, pulmonary toilet and care of central lines. Wounds must be kept clean and debrided, if necessary. Although no localized source of infection may be identifiable in SIRS, blood cultures are positive in one-third of patients. Antibiotic therapy is initiated on the basis of the most likely infecting organisms until the results of blood culture are available, when more specific antibiotic treatment can be initiated.

Adequate tissue oxygenation

Circulatory support with intravenous fluids is important with constant monitoring of urine output and pulmonary artery pressure. Diuretics may be required to maintain urinary output but should only be used when adequate hydration has been achieved. Inotropic support with dopamine and dobutamine is indicated in situations where atrial filling pressure is low because of poor cardiac function. Ventilatory support may be necessary with supplementary oxygen or mechanical ventilation in severe cases. Oxygen delivery must be high as SIRS is associated with increased consumption of oxygen.

Nutrition

Adequate nutrition is essential in the management of patients with SIRS. Nutritional support restores the barrier function of the gut and should thereby reduce bacterial translocation. Whenever possible, enteral feeding is preferred because the enterocyte receives its energy substrates primarily from the gut lumen. However, if enteral feeding cannot be sustained intravenous feeding (TPN) is necessary.

Minimize the systemic inflammatory response

- Corticosteroids have been used in the management of septic shock. However, their role is, at best, uncertain. A reduction in the damaging effects of the inflammatory response can be achieved with corticosteroids but only if given prior to the onset of sepsis so that the practical applications are limited.

• Prevention of free oxygen radical generation by blocking the enzyme xanthine oxidase with allopurinol or scavenging toxic radicals with superoxide dismutase has been shown to be beneficial in a number of experimental models and may be of future value in the clinical situation.

• Anti-TNF and anti-LPS monoclonal antibodies are among the newer approaches which show promise. They function by interrupting the inflammatory mediator cascade which is responsible for the persistent injurious response of the immune system to sepsis.

• Other experimental treatments include the use of the opioid receptor antagonist naloxone which may improve patient haemodynamic response in shock which has been inhibited by the release of β-endorphins in response to stress. Non-steroidal anti-inflammatory agents, by inhibiting the arachidonic acid cascade, should theoretically improve the situation and are currently under investigation.

Prognosis

Overall, the prognosis for patients with SIRS is poor. Factors influencing survival are:

• age — the very young and the very old have a poor outcome;

• severity of the initial insult — the more severe the initial illness, the greater the chance of dying;

• cardiac output — the ability to increase cardiac output during the hypermetabolic state is associated with better survival;

• infection — identification of a septic source carriers a better prognosis;

• end-organ failure — the more end-organs that fail, the worse the outlook.

Patients with three or more end-organ failures almost never survive.

B) Trauma

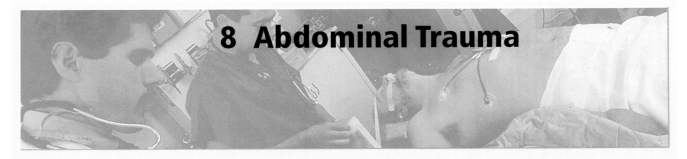

8 Abdominal Trauma

The abdomen is the reason why man does not easily take himself for a god. Friedrich Nietzsche (1844–1900)

Introduction

Injuries to the intra-abdominal organs may result from blunt, penetrating (stab, missile) or blast trauma. *Blast injury* is rare in civilian practice and is usually the result of explosions from gas leakage or faulty household appliances. *Penetrating trauma* is not uncommon and results frequently from knife wounds and more rarely from bullet wounds. *Blunt trauma* remains one of the major public health problems. The vast majority of incidents are caused by road traffic accidents (RTAs). Blood alcohol level exceeding 100 mg/l is found in 25% of drivers involved in automobile accidents. Improved vehicle design, speed restrictions, road testing of old vehicles, breath analyser testing for alcohol and mandatory wearing of seatbelts have reduced the fatal injury rate. However, in the UK, 40 individuals still die every day from accidents, the vast majority being RTAs. In addition to the suffering, disfigurement and disability of the injured individual, trauma incurs a significant financial burden on the state. Not only are valuable health service resources used to treat the patients initially but, as most trauma victims are young active individuals at the height of their earning potential, there is a considerable loss of national revenue in lost years of productivity.

Mechanism of injury in blunt trauma

In blunt trauma, the energy dissipated on impact is distributed over a wide surface area. As the tissues offer different resistance to sudden movement (differential inertia), extreme degrees of *strain* are produced, particularly at points of anatomical fixation. The strain may occur along the *longitudinal axis*, resulting in a stretch or compression injury, or across it (*shear strain*), causing fracture of bones and tearing of soft tissues and organs. The third component of blunt trauma is due to the acute *direct deformity* of tissue at the point of contact. The extent of damage produced by the three components is determined by the kinetic energy (mass × velocity) expended at the time of impact.

Profile of trauma deaths

The profile of trauma deaths plotted against time is given in Fig. 1 on page 37. The first peak, which accounts for half the deaths, is composed of victims who die immediately or very soon after the accident from fatal injuries. The second peak is encountered within hours of the injury and results from haemorrhage and hypoxia. Many of these deaths are preventable if these patients receive adequate on-site resuscitation and are transported rapidly to hospitals which have the necessary expertise and facilities to deal with these injuries — trauma centres. Regrettably, in the UK, unlike other countries, the trauma service lacks this basic organization. The third peak represents deaths occurring as a result of complications of major injuries: uncontrollable sepsis and multiple organ dysfunction syndrome (MODS).

Surgical anatomy of abdominal injuries

In relation to trauma, the abdomen is divided into four components: intrathoracic, true abdominal, pelvic and retroperitoneal (Table 8.1).

Table 8.1 The contents of the 'trauma' compartments of the abdomen.

Intrathoracic	True abdominal	Pelvic	Retroperitoneal
Diaphragm	Small and large intestine	Sigmoid colon	Kidney and ureters
Liver	Pregnant uterus	Rectum	Duodenum
Spleen	Distended urinary bladder	Small-bowel loops	Pancreas
Stomach		Bladder	Aorta
		Urethra	Inferior vena cava
		Ovaries and uterus	

- The intrathoracic abdomen is contained within the lower ribcage and its contents are the diaphragm, liver, spleen and stomach. All may be injured in blunt abdominal trauma but the spleen and the liver are the most frequently affected organs and both present with evidence of internal haemorrhage.
- The true abdomen contains the small and large intestine, the urinary bladder (when distended) and the pregnant uterus. The clinical picture of these injuries is dominated by the development of peritonitis.
- The pelvic abdomen, which is surrounded by the bony pelvis, contains the rectosigmoid, the urinary bladder, urethra, several loops of ileum and the female genital organs. The soft-tissue injuries often arise on a background of severe pelvic fractures when the clinical picture is mixed with evidence of internal bleeding and the development of peritonitis.
- The retroperitoneal abdomen has the kidneys and ureters, pancreas, the second and third parts of the duodenum and the great vessels: aorta and vena cava. Initially, physical findings may be minimal, although there is the ever-present risk of sudden vascular decompensation due to intra-abdominal rupture of a major retroperitoneal haematoma.

Management of trauma

History and examination

The initial management of all trauma patients is to ensure an adequate airway, arrest any bleeding and restore organ circulation. Assessment of injury depends on a detailed history of the trauma from the patient or witnesses and careful physical examination followed by haematological, urinary and radiological investigations. Investigation and management are carried out concurrently and the degree of initial investigation is determined by the stability of the patient.

The type and extent of trauma suffered by the patient determines the type of injuries he or she is likely to have sus-

tained. The height of a fall and the manner of landing, the speed of the car and the use of seatbelt and type of penetrating injury are important facts to determine. The abdomen, pelvis and genitalia must be examined in detail. Generalized abdominal pain or tenderness may indicate a perforated viscus, free intraperitoneal blood or intraperitoneal urine. The presence of peritonism is an indication for peritoneal lavage and subsequent laparotomy if this is positive (see below). Contusions or subcutaneous haematomata may indicate deeper injuries to the pelvis or retroperitoneum. Rib fractures may be associated with splenic, hepatic or renal injuries whilst pelvic fractures may be associated with bladder or urethral injuries. Perineal haematomata may be associated with urethral injuries. Blood at the external urinary meatus indicates a urethral injury unless proven otherwise. Gross or microscopic haematuria in a voided or catheter specimen suggests genitourinary tract injury and requires immediate assessment. The degree of haematuria does not correlate with the severity of the injury.

Resuscitation and urgent surgical intervention

The first priority in all injured patients is *resuscitation* — ensuring that there is an adequate airway, effective breathing and a circulation (Chapters 3 and 4). The circulatory volume must be restored rapidly with crystalloid or colloid solutions while blood is being cross-matched and invasive monitoring should be established (urinary catheter and central venous line). Further management depends on the clinical picture which is assessed as resuscitation proceeds.

The unstable patient

Immediate surgical intervention is essential if the patient is shocked and unstable, and in the presence of positive signs indicative of an acute abdomen. The management flow chart of this clinical situation is outlined in Fig. 8.1.

Patients with massive intra-abdominal haemorrhage often reach the emergency room almost moribund with profound hypotension, a grossly distended tense abdomen

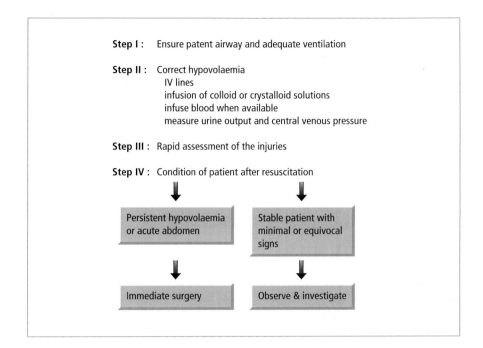

Step I :   Ensure patent airway and adequate ventilation

Step II :   Correct hypovolaemia
            IV lines
            infusion of colloid or crystalloid solutions
            infuse blood when available
            measure urine output and central venous pressure

Step III : Rapid assessment of the injuries

Step IV :   Condition of patient after resuscitation

Persistent hypovolaemia or acute abdomen

Stable patient with minimal or equivocal signs

Immediate surgery

Observe & investigate

Figure 8.1 Management flow chart for unstable patients with abdominal injuries.

and blotchy lower limbs (due to compression of the iliac veins). They remain hypotensive (blood pressure <80 mmHg) despite rapid volume replacement. The cause is either a major vascular (vena cava, aorta, iliac artery) or organ injury (liver, spleen) and, less commonly, fracture of the pelvis. Laparotomy in these patients is usually fatal as the sudden decompression leads to the final fatal exsanguination. Some of these patients can be saved by prompt cross-clamping of the descending thoracic aorta performed through a left anterolateral thoracotomy.

The stable patient

Frequent repeat clinical assessments are required in patients who are stable following resuscitation and in whom the abdominal signs are equivocal. Either peritoneal lavage or laparoscopy is nowadays performed routinely in many centres, particularly when diagnosis is difficult. Computed tomographic (CT) scanning is preferred in the paediatric age group.

Peritoneal lavage

Peritoneal lavage is performed in patients with equivocal physical signs, depressed levels of consciousness from head injury or alcohol, spinal injury and penetrating trauma below the nipple line. It is performed by inserting a dialysis catheter under local anaesthetic into the peritoneal cavity through a small incision made in the midline below the umbilicus. A litre of saline or Ringer's lactate solution is infused over 5–10 min. The perfusate is then siphoned out by placing the empty perfusate bag below the level of the peritoneal cavity. The siphoned perfusate is then examined. The criteria for a positive test are:
- red blood cells >100 000/ml;
- white blood cells >500/ml;
- amylase >110 u/100ml;
- the presence of bile, bacteria or food particles in the peritoneal effluent.

The overall diagnostic accuracy of percutaneous peritoneal lavage in the detection of intra-abdominal trauma is 90%. One disadvantage of this test is the high false-positive rate (15–20%). This is due to minor lesions such as small lacerations which stop bleeding spontaneously by the time laparotomy is performed.

Laparoscopy

A small laparoscope (minilaparoscope) with an external diameter similar to that of the dialysis catheter can easily be inserted into the peritoneal cavity under intravenous sedation and local anaesthesia. Laparoscopy reliably excludes intra-abdominal injury and minor lacerations which do not require laparotomy and which often yield a positive result with abdominal lavage. This technique is used in injured patients with a diminished level of unconsciousness, stab

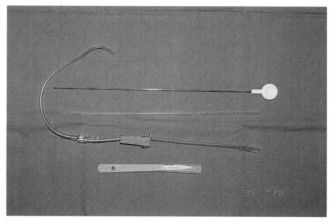

(a)

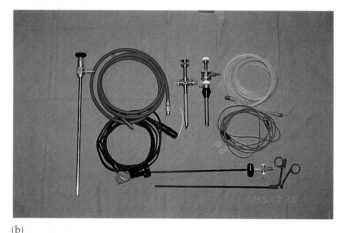

(b)

Figure 8.2 Equipment used for (a) peritoneal lavage and (b) diagnostic laparoscopy.

wounds and in patients with equivocal abdominal signs. The equipment used for peritoneal lavage and diagnostic laparoscopy is shown in Fig. 8.2.

Ultrasound scanning

Because haemoperitoneum and haematomata provide liquid–solid interfaces, high-resolution real–time ultrasonography is an extremely sensitive and accurate method of detecting intra-abdominal injury. Lesions of the liver and spleen give heterogeneous echo patterns. Haematomata appear as sonolucent (transparent) areas while the presence of haemoperitoneum is identified by the crescent-moon sign.

CT scanning

Contrast-enhanced CT scanning of the abdomen is used in the detection of abdominal injuries provided the patient is haemodynamically stable (because the examination takes 45–60 min). It is particularly helpful in children where it is now the diagnostic procedure of choice. In children blunt abdominal injury, even with haemoperitoneum, is frequently treated non-operatively.

Angiography

The use of angiography in the diagnosis of solid organ damage has declined since the introduction of CT scanning, although it is still valuable in confirming significant active bleeding and major disruption of the vascular pedicle of an organ. Isotope scintigraphy was used to detect injury to the solid organs but has been largely superseded by CT and ultrasound scanning of the abdomen.

Antibiotics in abdominal trauma

Systemic antibiotic therapy active against both aerobes and anaerobes is administered to patients with abdominal injuries. The risk factors for the development of infective complications are shock, missile/penetrating aetiology, colon injuries and old age. The most common causative aerobes are *Enterococcus*, *Escherichia coli* and *Klebsiella pneumoniae*, whereas the most commonly cultured anaerobes belong to the *Bacteroides* species. The highest incidence of wound infection, abdominal abscess and mortality is encountered in colon injuries.

Specific intra-abdominal injuries

Hepatic injuries

Injuries to the liver include minor lacerations, which do not require surgical treatment, moderately sized tears which need liver suture and severe injuries which are accompanied by extensive trauma to one or both lobes. The latter are life-threatening because of haemorrhage and other associated injuries. Stable patients with minor injuries are treated conservatively in the first instance. These patients are best followed up by serial CT scanning to monitor resorption of haemoperitoneum and the pattern of healing of intrahepatic lesions. Surgical exploration is necessary if there is evidence of continued blood loss. Simple suture and resectional debridement are the two measures necessary for the control of bleeding due to moderate injuries. In major injuries with bleeding from the vena cava or hepatic veins, the supracolic compartment of the abdomen is packed with gauze rolls. This usually controls the bleeding and allows resuscitation and transfer to a specialized hepatobiliary unit for definitive treatment.

Splenic injuries

Injuries to the spleen are usually sustained by blunt abdominal trauma and the spleen is the most commonly injured organ in RTAs. The injuries may consist of incomplete parenchymal tears, complete lacerations or severe fragmentation with avulsion of the hilar vessels. The clinical features of splenic injury include abdominal tenderness, hypotension and left lower rib fractures. Haematuria may be present. Left shoulder-tip pain, often stressed as a symptom of splenic injury, is in fact rare, being found in only 5% of patients. Associated chest injuries are very common. If in doubt, diagnosis can be confirmed by peritoneal lavage, minilaparoscopy or abdominal ultrasound scanning.

The surgical management of splenic injuries varies. The emphasis in recent years has been on splenic preservation whenever possible because of the risk of overwhelming postsplenectomy infection by encapsulated organisms, particularly *Streptococcus pneumoniae* (see Box 8.1). In this respect, splenic preservation is particularly indicated in children who are more at risk of this complication than adults. Indeed, some of these children are managed conservatively in the first instance, surgery being undertaken only if there is evidence of continued or renewed bleeding. In those patients who require surgery because of active bleeding, splenic preservation (by special suturing and haemostatic techniques) is attempted only if the condition of the patient is stable and there is no contamination of the peritoneal cavity. Otherwise splenectomy is performed; in which case, autotransplantation of splenic slices in omental pouches may be undertaken in an attempt at preserving the splenic immune function. All patients undergoing splenectomy should be vaccinated.

Diaphragmatic injuries

Injuries to the diaphragm are more commonly associated with abdominal than chest injuries. The majority follow RTAs but some are caused by crushing injuries and sharp localized blows such as a kick from a horse. The left diaphragm is more commonly injured than the right. Minor tears are usually unrecognized and may present several years later with incarcerated diaphragmatic hernia. More severe injuries are associated with multiple injuries and ex-

Protection for patients following splenectomy

People who have had a splenectomy are at increased risk of severe post-splenectomy infection. The risk is twelve times that expected in people with a normal spleen and children are the most vulnerable. The greatest period of risk is during the first 2 years after splenectomy but persists throughout life. The common pathogen is *Streptococcus pneumoniae*, but other bacteria with polysaccharide capsules, e.g. *Haemophilus influenza, Neisseria meningitidis* and malaria parasites also pose a significant risk. Patients who become infected may develop septicaemia with frightening speed and die within 24 hours.

Prophylaxis against infection is achieved by vaccination and antibiotics. Three vaccines are now recommended (Pneumococcal vaccine, Haemophilus influenza type b (Hib) vaccine and Meningococcal Groups A and C vaccine) and should be administered prior to or soon after splenectomy. Antibiotic prophylaxis should be given to children until the age of 16 and to everyone for 2 years following splenectomy (e.g. amoxycillin 500 mg daily for adults and 250 mg daily for children, patients allergic to penicillin should be given erythromycin). Some physicians recommend lifelong antibiotic prophylaxis. Asplenic patients travelling to endemic malarial areas should take antimalarial chemoprophylaxis as well as the usual physical anti-mosquito precautions, e.g. insect repellents, screens at night, etc.

Box 8.1

tensive herniation of the abdominal viscera — stomach, colon, omentum, small bowel and spleen on the left side and liver on the right. Massive herniation leads to mediastinal shift, which causes respiratory distress and hypotension from a reduced cardiac output.

Pancreatoduodenal injuries

Injuries to the duodenum and head of the pancreas are more often due to penetrating than blunt abdominal trauma and usually give rise to peritonitis. Diagnosis is usually confirmed by peritoneal lavage, the effluent fluid from which will contain amylase. They are serious injuries and are accompanied by a high mortality and carry a substantial morbidity from the development of intra-abdominal sepsis and duodenal fistula. All these injuries require immediate surgical intervention. The vast majority of pancreatic fistulae which may complicate pancreatic injuries dry up within a short time following treatment with long-acting somatostatin, which has considerably simplified the management of this complication. Blunt injury to the upper abdomen may compress the pancreas against the vertebral column, leading to a traumatic pancreatitis and even transection.

Small intestinal injuries

Intestinal injury following blunt trauma may be due to:
- crushing of the intestinal loops between the vertebrae and anterior abdominal wall;
- a sudden increase in the intra-luminal pressure of the bowel;
- tears at relatively fixed points along the attachment of the intestinal mesentery.

Preoperative diagnosis can be established by peritoneal lavage. The small bowel is more commonly injured than the colon. Associated intra-abdominal injury, most commonly spleen or liver, is present in 40% of patients. Early diagnosis and prompt surgical intervention are the most important determinants of a successful outcome. Surgical treatment consists of resection of devitalized segments of bowel and primary anastomosis. This is followed by thorough saline/antibiotic lavage of the peritoneal cavity before closure of the abdomen. The skin and subcutaneous tissues are left unsutured and packed with acriflavin gauze. Delayed primary suture is undertaken 5–7 days later.

Colonic injuries

Blunt injuries of the colon and rectum are rare and comprise 5% of all blunt injuries to the abdomen. As the force required to produce large-bowel injury needs to be considerable, associated injuries (e.g. liver, spleen, head, chest, pelvis and lower extremity) are common and adversely affect survival. The transverse colon is the most commonly affected segment, followed by the right colon, left colon and rectum. The lesions may consist of incomplete lacerations (seromuscular tears), haematoma or contusion with variable degrees of involvement of the adjacent mesentery or omentum, complete lacerations with faecal spillage and avulsion from the mesentery with full-thickness necrosis.

The operative management depends on the severity of the injury. Minor injuries are closed with primary suture with or without proximal defunctioning colostomy, depending on the extent of faecal contamination and colonic loading (Fig. 8.3a). Severe injuries are excised with exteriorization of the two ends (proximal end-colostomy and distal mucous fistula (Fig. 8.3b). Restoration of continuity is performed a few months later. Following the definitive repair a thorough peritoneal lavage with saline is necessary before closure. As with small-bowel injuries, the skin and subcutaneous tissues are left unsutured and packed; secondary suture is performed 5–7 days later.

Intra-abdominal genitourinary trauma

Approximately 10% of trauma patients seen in the accident and emergency department will have genitourinary trauma to a greater or lesser degree. Prior to catheter insertion the external urinary meatus must be examined for blood, which indicates the presence of urethral injury and the need for retrograde urethrography. When the catheter is passed, or if the patient voids spontaneously, the urine must be tested for blood immediately. Haematuria, gross or microscopic, is present in all patients with bladder or urethral injuries and about 70% of patients with renal or ureteric injuries. In these patients retrograde cystography is performed prior to intravenous urography to rule out a bladder injury. Intravenous urography cannot reliably exclude a bladder injury.

Where a renal injury is suspected intravenous contrast should be injected once the intravenous lines have been erected. A plain abdominal film at the time of injection, 5, 10 and 15 min after injection will establish the presence of two kidneys, their function and any injury present. Urinary extravasation on these films indicates the need for nephrotomograms. It is essential to establish the number of functioning kidneys prior to any surgical exploration. If a CT scan is readily available a contrast study will more thoroughly delineate renal injury than an intravenous urogram. In the case of renal injury with urine extravasation which is being managed conservatively, ultrasonography is a useful means of follow-up.

Renal injuries

Injuries to the kidney are the most common injuries of the urinary system and account for approximately 50% of all genitourinary trauma. More than half these injuries involve patients under the age of 30 years and men are affected four times as frequently as women. Patients with renal abnormalities, such as hydronephrosis, are more prone to renal injury. Children are also at increased risk of renal injury because their kidneys are relatively larger than adults. Blunt trauma from RTAs and sporting mishaps account for 85% of renal injuries. Associated injury to other intra-abdominal organs occurs in approximately 40% of cases. Penetrating injury secondary to gunshot or stabbing occurs less frequently but associated organ injury occurs in approximately 80% of these patients. High-speed vehicle collisions may result in major renal vascular injury due to rapid deceleration.

Classification of renal injuries

Renal injuries are classified as minor, major and vascular:
- *Minor renal injury* (85% of all cases): These injuries consist of renal contusion (bruising), subcapsular

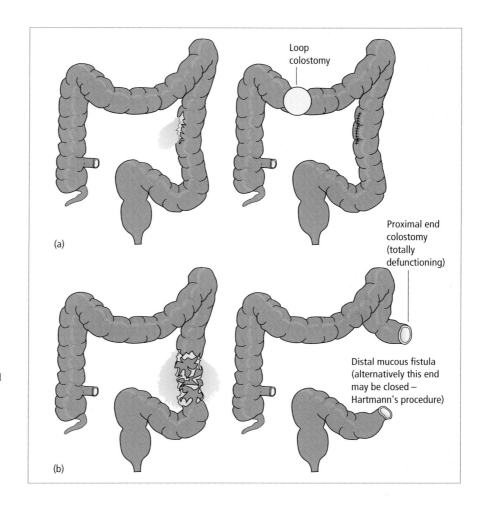

Figure 8.3 (a) Minor colonic injuries are closed with primary suture with or without proximal defunctioning colostomy depending on the extent of faecal soiling and colonic loading. (b) With major colonic injuries the injured colon is excised, the proximal end is exteriorized as an end-colostomy and the distal end exteriorized as a mucous fistula. Alternatively, the distal end may be closed and left intra-abdominally (Hartmann's procedure).

haematoma or superficial lacerations of the cortex not involving the collecting system. Most instances of blunt trauma result in minor renal injuries and approximately 40% of penetrating trauma produces similar injuries.

• *Major renal injury* (14% of all cases): These injuries consist of deep lacerations and are associated with retroperitoneal and perinephric haematomata. If the laceration extends into the collecting system urine extravasation with a perirenal urine collection (urinoma) results. In their severest form deep renal lacerations may cause complete disruption of the kidney.

• *Renal vascular injuries* (1% of all cases): These uncommon but very serious injuries are more frequent with penetrating trauma. They range from intimal tears with subsequent renal artery thrombosis to avulsion of segmental arteries or veins to partial or complete avulsion of the main renal pedicle.

Diagnosis

Any penetrating injury to the flank should be suspected of causing renal injury, whether or not haematuria is present. Blunt injury associated with flank or abdominal tenderness, fractured lower ribs or vertebral transverse bodies or producing haematuria should be suspected of causing renal injury. It is important to remember that haematuria, gross or microscopic, only occurs in 70% of renal injuries and that the degree of haematuria does not correlate with the severity of the injury. A rapid deceleration injury should be suspected as a potential cause of renal vascular injuries. Intravenous urography is the key to diagnosis and staging. If urine extravasation is noted, nephrotomograms are required to delineate further the injury. If the patient is stable a contrast CT scan may be the investigation of choice as it gives a greater degree of detail with respect to the renal injury and may also be used to assess possible associated organ injuries. If there is non-visualization of a kidney renal vascular injury must be suspected and urgent arteriography is indicated.

Treatment

Minor renal injuries are managed conservatively by strict bedrest, antibiotics and monitoring the vital signs, haematocrit and the injured kidney. Patients with major renal injuries pose difficult management questions. Most cases can be managed conservatively as described without significant problems. Indications for surgical intervention are:
- signs of continued blood loss such as falling haematocrit;
- increasing size of retroperitoneal or perinephric haematoma; and
- marked urine extravasation or vascular injury.

The presence of associated organ injury may also call for surgical intervention. Smaller urinomas may be managed conservatively by frequent measurement using ultrasound examination to ensure decreasing size. Larger urinomas should be drained percutaneously and a urinoma that becomes infected (abscess) may require open surgical drainage. Where possible, exploration of renal injury due to blunt trauma should be avoided as the end-result is usually nephrectomy. In contrast, penetrating injuries almost always require surgical exploration.

Complications

- Bleeding at the time of injury and delayed bleeding within the first month of injury are important complications. In most cases bleeding ceases with conservative management but persistent bleeding or later heavy gross haematuria may require exploration.
- Urinomas and haematomas may result in fibrosis leading to obstruction (hydronephrosis) requiring corrective surgery.
- Later complications include hypertension, arteriovenous fistula, hydronephrosis, stone formation, pyelonephritis and decreased function.

For these reasons, careful follow-up of patients following renal trauma is necessary. Thus, patients should have an intravenous urogram 6 months after injury and blood pressure should be monitored regularly for a year after injury.

Ureteric injuries

Ureteric injuries are uncommon but their early recognition is critical as the nephrectomy rate may be as high as 30% when there is a delay in diagnosis. Most ureteric injuries are iatrogenic, with penetrating trauma the second most frequent cause. Blunt trauma to the ureter is rare and usually involves disruption of the ureteropelvic junction after rapid deceleration injuries and most commonly occurs in chil-

dren. The most common cause of iatrogenic injury is pelvic surgery, especially hysterectomy. Surgery for carcinoma of the colon or rectum may be complicated by ureteric injury, especially where the tumour is extensive or ureteric abnormalities exist. Increasingly, endoscopic manipulation of stones with a basket or ureteroscope is being recognized as a potential cause of ureteral perforation or avulsion.

Injury to the ureter may be recognized at the time of surgery or may present in the postoperative period as pyrexia, flank or lower quadrant pain, paralytic ileus or fistula. Haematuria, gross or microscopic, is present in 90% of cases but diagnosis rests on intravenous urography. Delayed excretion with hydronephrosis is the commonest finding but extravasation may also be noted. A retrograde ureterogram will demonstrate the exact site of the obstruction or extravasation.

Early treatment is essential to preserve renal function. Stenting of ureteric repairs is an important determinant of a successful outcome. With prompt surgical intervention a satisfactory outcome can be anticipated in most cases.

Bladder injuries

Bladder injury complicates 10–15% of cases of fractured pelvis. About 90% of bladder injuries are associated with pelvic fractures. Other causes include direct trauma to the lower abdomen in a patient with a full bladder, iatrogenic injuries (endoscopy and pelvic surgery), penetrating injuries and, very rarely, spontaneous rupture of an overdistended bladder. When the pelvis is fractured, fragments may perforate the bladder, resulting in extravasation of urine into the retropubic space (extraperitoneal rupture). If the bladder is full and subjected to trauma the perforation occurs at the weakest point, which is the dome, with extravasation of urine into the peritoneal cavity (intraperitoneal rupture).

Diagnosis

There is a history of blunt abdominal trauma. The patient may be unable to urinate or, if voiding occurs, gross or microscopic haematuria will be apparent. On examination the patient may be shocked due to blood loss from the pelvic fracture or associated organ injury. An acute abdomen, i.e. pain, tenderness and guarding progressing to rigidity, suggests a perforated viscus or free intraperitoneal blood or urine. Urine must be obtained for testing. If haematuria is present a urethral or bladder injury is likely but associated renal injuries may also coexist. For this reason all patients with haematuria after trauma must have an intravenous urogram (Box 8.2). If the patient has not voided spontaneously a catheter is passed after inspecting the external urinary meatus for blood. If blood is present at

Plain abdominal radiography
This will show fractures of the ribs or transverse processes of the vertebra indicating severe trauma and the possibility of associated renal injuries. Loss of the renal outline, loss of the psoas shadow, displacement of bowel gas suggesting a retroperitoneal haematoma or urinoma are other subtle manifestations of urinary tract injury. Pelvic fractures will also be seen and should raise the suspicion of bladder or urethral injuries.

Retrograde urethrogram
Prior to catheterization, the meatus should be inspected for blood. The presence of blood or difficulty in passing a catheter in the absence of blood at the meatus suggests a urethral injury and the need for a retrograde urethrogram. A size 12F Foley catheter is inserted to the fossa navicularis and the balloon inflated with 2–3 ml of water to hold the catheter in place. Twenty ml of water-soluble contrast is gently injected through the catheter to outline the urethra.

Retrograde cystography
This is indicated in all patients with gross or microscopic haematuria on the voided or catheter specimen on urine. Three hundred ml of contrast is infused through the catheter and a film of the distended bladder is taken. The bladder is allowed to drain by gravity and a second film is taken. This second picture is important to show small amounts of extravasation.

Intravenous urography
After setting up the intravenous lines in a patient in whom renal injury is suspected, a bolus injection of contrast (2 ml/kg) is given. Films are taken at the time of injection and at 5 min intervals for 15–20 min. This investigation will establish the presence of two kidneys and their function. If urinary extravasation is present, nephrotomograms are necessary to delineate the degree of injury. If non-function is present then absent perfusion due to a renal vascular injury must be considered and urgent arteriography is necessary.

Computed tomography (CT)
Computed tomography with intravenous contrast gives a better definition of renal injuries than intravenous urography and may also assess the degree of associated intra-abdominal injuries. However, in the emergency situation intravenous urography will suffice.

Ultrasonography
This investigation does not provide significant additional information in the immediate assessment of the trauma patient but it may be used to monitor patients with urinomas who are being managed conservatively.

Box 8.2 Radiological investigations in the management of genitourinary trauma.

the meatus a retrograde urethrogram is necessary to rule out urethral injury before proceeding. If this is normal a cystogram is performed by infusing 300 ml of constrast medium and taking an X-ray. A further exposure is taken after gravity drainage of the contrast through the catheter as small perforations may be missed on the full film. A cystogram may reveal compression of the bladder by pelvic haematoma (teardrop bladder) on the first film with extravasation on the drainage film in extraperitoneal rupture. In intraperitoneal rupture contrast will outline the loops of bowel. In patients with intraperitoneal rupture the serum urea rises with a normal creatinine level due to reabsorption of urea across the peritoneum.

Treatment

Extraperitoneal rupture Very minor ruptures in patients who do not have infected urine may be treated conservatively by catheter drainage alone. However, careful observation is necessary as the pelvic haematoma may become infected, resulting in a pelvic abscess. For the majority of cases, urgent surgical intervention is indicated. The bladder is repaired transvesically by suturing the tear with absorbable sutures, inserting suprapubic and urethral catheters and placing a drain in the retropubic space. A small hole may be made in the peritoneal cavity to inspect the intra-abdominal fluid. If this is blood-stained, full laparotomy is required. Drainage is maintained for 10 days to 2 weeks and a cystogram is performed prior to removal of the suprapubic catheter.

Intraperitoneal rupture Intraperitoneal ruptures are approached transperitoneally. The bladder is drained by urethral and suprapubic catheters and the tear closed in layers with an absorbable suture. The peritoneal cavity is washed out to remove all urine and drained also. Bladder integrity is checked by cystogram prior to removing the suprapubic catheter on the tenth postoperative day.

Recognition of bladder injury is important if mortality and morbidity are to be minimized. A fractured pelvis with haematuria indicates the need for urgent retrograde cystography.

Penetrating abdominal trauma

Stab wounds to the abdomen

The vast majority of stab wounds are inflicted by knives and may be abdominal or thoracoabdominal. A high degree of suspicion of associated diaphragmatic laceration and pleuropulmonary injury is necessary in stab wounds of the upper abdomen as the direction of the knife thrust is often cephalad. Less commonly, stab wounds occur from impale-

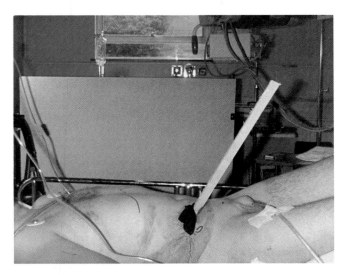

Figure 8.4 Impalement injury to the abdomen. Surprisingly, very little damage was caused by this injury. The caecum was perforated by the stake but the ureter and major vessels escaped injury. A right hemicolectomy was performed and the patient made an uneventful recovery.

ment injuries and these are usually serious and associated with major intra-abdominal trauma (Fig. 8.4).

The management of abdominal stab wounds has changed in recent years to selective surgical intervention depending on the clinical state of the patient, the nature of the wound, and the results of specific investigations, i.e. peritoneal lavage or laparoscopy. The following are the indications for laparotomy following a stab wound:
- hypovolaemia shock;
- peritonitis;
- evisceration of viscera or omentum through the wound;
- gastrointestinal bleeding;
- free air on abdominal films.

Wound exploration is useful in the management of the stable patient. In the absence of fascial penetration, wound toilet and primary suture are performed and the patient can usually be discharged from hospital after a short period of observation. Patients in whom wound exploration shows fascial penetration should have an abdominal lavage or laparoscopic examination followed by immediate laparotomy if indicated by the findings of either test.

Gunshot wounds to the abdomen

Gunshot wounds are considerably more serious than stab wounds and five times as lethal. Gunshot wounds to the abdomen are important because of their rising incidence worldwide and because they are often accompanied by visceral injuries which occur in the majority of cases. Some, especially those inflicted by high-velocity missiles, may not be initially accompanied by physical signs. For this reason all gunshot wounds of the abdomen should be explored as physical examination and peritoneal lavage are unreliable in this situation. The propensity to visceral damage is directly related to the impact velocity and the mass of the projectile. Thus, high-velocity missiles (usually from military weapons) impart a considerable amount of kinetic energy and produce extensive tissue damage, often remote from the site of injury. External contaminants are frequently introduced into the depth of the high-velocity missile wounds. Close-range shotgun injuries (favoured by bank robbers!) result in highly lethal injuries and carry a reported mortality of 90% at less than 3 m.

Emergency laparotomy for abdominal injuries

This must not be delayed unduly, particularly if volume replacement proves difficult, suggesting significant active intra-abdominal bleeding. An adequate reserve of cross-matched blood must be available to cover the procedure. Adequate intravenous lines capable of rapid acceleration of inflow must be in place before the patient is anaesthetized. A further fall in blood pressure is often witnessed with muscle relaxation as the tamponade effect of the abdominal wall is diminished and this is entirely lost as the surgeon opens the abdomen.

The operation is usually performed through a midline incision, as this can be readily extended from xiphoid to symphysis pubis and converted to a thoracoabdominal one when necessary. The first priority is control of haemorrhage. The next step concerns the operative treatment of hollow visceral injuries, especially those involving the colon, in order to minimize contamination. The abdominal exploration must be thorough with a systematic inspection of all the quadrants and retroperitoneum (especially the second part of the duodenum) in order to avoid missed injuries. On completion, the peritoneal cavity is thoroughly lavaged with several litres of warm isotonic saline, especially in the presence of contamination from intestinal damage. Closure of the musculoaponeurotic layer of the abdominal wall is affected by non-absorbable monofilament material. The skin and subcutaneous tissues are left unsutured and the wound packed with acriflavin gauze if the peritoneal cavity had been contaminated by leakage of intestinal contents.

Pelvic genitourinary injuries

Urethral injuries

Urethral injuries are uncommon and usually occur in men in association with straddle injuries or pelvic fractures with disruption of the pelvic ring. Urethral injuries are rare in women.

Injuries to the bulbar urethra

These injuries result from straddle injuries (e.g. falling astride a bicycle crossbar) or a direct kick to the perineum. Self-instrumentation or iatrogenic instrumentation may occasionally be responsible for injury to the bulbar urethra. These injuries vary from a simple contusion or bruise of the urethra to laceration. In addition to the history of direct trauma, bleeding from the urethra and perineal haematoma will be evident. No attempt should be made to pass a urethral catheter under any circumstance. A retrograde urethrogram is indicated to delineate the severity of the injury. If the urethra is intact (no extravasation), a urethral catheter may be passed. If extravasation is present on the retrograde urethrogram a laceration of the bulbar urethra has occurred. A percutaneous suprapubic catheter may be inserted in those patients in whom bladder injury is not suspected. The catheter is left *in situ* for 3 weeks and a micturating cystourethrogram is performed prior to its removal to ensure resolution of the injury. A urethral stricture may develop subsequently at the site of injury.

If there is a possibility of associated bladder injury then formal suprapubic cystostomy with inspection of the bladder and repair of any bladder laceration is necessary. The suprapubic drainage is maintained for 3 weeks and a voiding cystourethrogram performed prior to removal of the suprapubic catheter.

Injuries to the prostatomembranous urethra

Injuries to this portion of the urethra usually result from blunt trauma which causes pelvic fractures with disruption of the pelvic ring. Because of the nature of the trauma, bladder injuries are often present in addition. Patients complain of lower abdominal pain and are unable to void. On examination urethral bleeding with a large, often palpable, pelvic haematoma will be noted. Rectal examination may reveal superior displacement of the prostate (gland impalpable) due to complete disruption of the membranous urethra. A urethral catheter should not be passed under any circumstances. A retrograde ure-throgram is urgently indicated. Free extravasation of contrast into the perivesical space indicates complete disruption of the membranous urethra. Incomplete disruption, which is less common, manifests itself as minor extravasation with some contrast material passing into the bladder. A urinary catheter should not be passed in these cases as it may convert an incomplete disruption into a complete one.

The management of these injuries is somewhat controversial. However, most would agree that primary repair is a poor option because of the increased incidence of complications (stricture, impotence, incontinence) compared with delayed repair. Initial management consists of formal, i.e. operative, suprapubic cystostomy with inspection of the bladder for associated injuries. The suprapubic catheter is left *in situ* for 3 months. At that time a cystogram and urethrogram are performed to determine the extent of the resulting urethral stricture. The stricture is repaired by excision and anastomosis of the bulbar urethra to the apex of the prostate. This may be achieved through a perineal or transpubic approach. The suprapubic catheter is left *in situ* for a further month before repeating the radiological assessment of the urethra.

Complications occur in a small percentage of patients with this management protocol. Stricture at the anastomosis site occurs in approximately 5% of patients and can be dealt with by urethrotomy. Impotence may occur in 10–15% of patients. Incontinence after repair is uncommon and usually resolves slowly. In contrast, primary repair is associated with strictures in about 50% of patients, impotence in 50% of patients and incontinence in 30% of patients.

Penile injuries

Most penile injuries result from accidents during sexual intercourse resulting in a torn frenulum or fracture of the penile shaft. A torn frenulum presents as penile pain and bleeding after intercourse and is best dealt with by elongation of the frenulum (frenuloplasty). Penile fractures occur due to bending during sexual intercourse, resulting in a large and painful haematoma. Surgical correction of the tear in the tunica albuginea will minimize future penile deformity. Penetrating injuries and avulsion injuries occur much less frequently.

Scrotal and testicular injury

Blunt trauma to the scrotum may cause scrotal contusion alone or may also involve the testes. Abnormal testes, such as those with carcinoma, are more prone to trauma and this should be remembered when patients present with testicular injury after minimal trauma. In addition to the history of blunt trauma, examination will reveal a scrotal haematoma. Often the testis is impalpable and all such patients should have an urgent scrotal ultrasound. If ultra- sonography confirms testicular injury, surgical exploration and repair are necessary. It is worthwhile noting that orchidectomy is a distinct possibility in these patients.

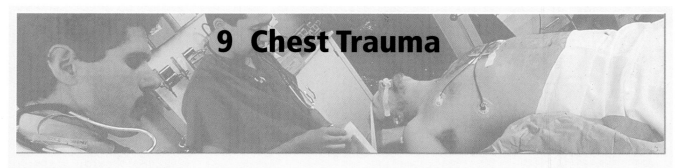

9 Chest Trauma

Fifteen men on a dead man's chest
Yo-ho-ho and a bottle of rum.   (Robert Louis Stevenson 1850–94)

Introduction

Chest injuries are common and in civilian life are sustained by the same mechanisms as abdominal trauma (Chapter 8). Not infrequently the injuries are thoracoabdominal. The majority are caused by blunt trauma from road traffic accidents, although stab and missile injuries are on the increase. Whereas minor injuries involve only the ribcage without significant adverse consequences, major injuries are associated with injury to the vital organs, i.e. lungs, trachea and major bronchi, great vessels and the heart. The full spectrum of thoracic injuries is outlined in Table 9.1.

Air in the pleural cavity is referred to as a *pneumothorax*, while the presence of blood in the pleural cavity is a *haemothorax*. Not uncommonly, both blood and air (*haemopneumothorax*) are found together in the pleural space following severe chest trauma. These conditions are considered fully in Chapter 19.

Specific chest injuries

Fractured ribs

Fractured ribs constitute the commonest chest injury. The lower ribs (fifth to ninth) are usually involved. Fractures of the first four ribs are produced by major external violence; they are always serious and often associated with major intrathoracic injuries to the great vessels, brachial plexus or tracheobronchial tree. Minor fractures are confined to one or two ribs, the exact site depending on the direction and distribution of the force. When three or more ribs are fractured, each in more than one place, a *flail segment* of the chest wall results. This moves paradoxically with respiration (bulges with expiration and becomes depressed with inspiration) and leads to a defective bellows action with diminished lung expansion and impaired gas exchange leading to hypoxia (Fig. 9.1; see also Chapter 3).

Sternal fractures

Sternal fractures are produced by severe trauma (high-speed accidents) and occur most commonly near the manubriosternal junction. They are often associated with flail chest and major intrathoracic (cardiovascular and pulmonary), abdominal and spinal injuries. An electrocardiogram (ECG) and cardiac enzymes should always be obtained in patients with a fractured sternum.

Table 9.1 The spectrum of thoracic injuries.

Chest wall trauma
Fractured ribs
Flail chest
Fractured sternum

Pleuropulmonary injury
Pneumothorax: simple, tension, sucking
Haemopneumothorax: intercostal vessels and lung laceration
Pulmonary contusion
Pulmonary haematoma
Pulmonary laceration
Tracheobronchial disruption

Cardiovascular injury
Cardiac injuries
Aortic rupture and large-vessel injury (innominate, subclavian)

Diaphragmatic injuries

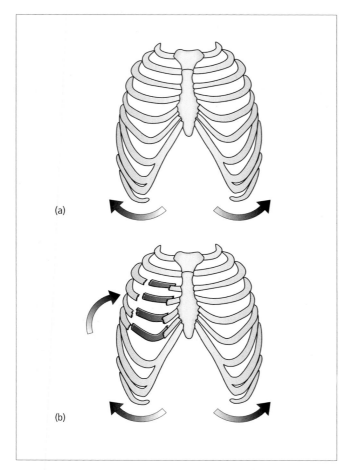

Figure 9.1 (a) Normally, inspiration expands the chest wall by an outward motion of the ribcage. (b) When there is a loose or flail segment (i.e. a loose section of chest wall between anterior and posterior fractures of the same ribs), inspiration causes the flail segment to be sucked inwards while the rest of the chest wall moves outwards. On expiration the flail segment moves outwards while the chest wall chest wall moves inwards. Thus there is paradoxical movement in the flail segment. A row of fractures on either side of the sternum produces the same effect.

Lung injuries

Parenchymal lung lesions include pulmonary contusion, pulmonary haematoma and pulmonary laceration. Contusion consists of an area of traumatic haemorrhagic oedema without laceration (Fig. 9.2). It is often associated with hypoxaemia and haemoptysis and, when severe, may progress to adult respiratory distress syndrome (ARDS). Pulmonary haematoma is rare and follows a localized parenchymal disruption caused by a penetrating chest injury. Pulmonary laceration is caused either by

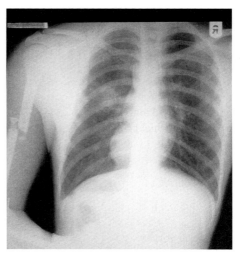

Figure 9.2 Posteroanterior chest film showing pulmonary contusion (localized 'white-out') in left hilar region in a patient following a road traffic accident. Note also the fractures of the left clavicle and mid-shaft of humerus.

fractured ribs or penetrating trauma and results in a pneumothorax.

Diaphragmatic injuries

Injuries to the diaphragm are more common after abdominal trauma and are dealt with in Chapter 8.

Pneumomediastinum

The clinical sign accompanying air in the mediastinum (*pneumomediastinum*) is *surgical emphysema* of the chest wall, head and neck (see Fig. 1.7, page 12). The feel of surgical emphysema has been likened to feeling cracked eggshells under the skin. A systolic crunching sound may be heard over the heart, especially in the left decubitus position (Hamman's sign). Extensive surgical emphysema can give rise to the 'Michelin man' appearance. Pneumomediastinum may be caused by ruptured oesophagus, tracheobronchial disruption or major pulmonary laceration.

Tracheobronchial disruption

Injuries severe enough to cause tracheobronchial disruption carry a high mortality. The majority occur near the carina. Clinically, the manifestations include respiratory distress, large pneumothorax, mediastinal and subcutaneous emphysema.

Management of chest injuries

The initial management follows the principles outlined in Chapter 3, with emphasis on ensuring a patent airway, breathing support and maintenance of an adequate circulation. Following clinical examination and resuscitation, essential investigations include a portable X-ray and blood gas analysis if the patient is cyanosed.

• Correctable lesions such as pneumo- or haemothorax are treated by insertion of underwater seal drainage in the first instance (Chapter 19). Thoracotomy for haemothorax is required if the initial drainage is >1000 ml or there is continued bleeding of > 250 ml/h in the first 4–5 h or >2000 ml in the first 24 h. At thoracotomy, injuries to small arteries are dealt with by suture ligation; lung parenchymal injuries may require local resection but hilar vessel damage often warrants pneumonectomy.

• The immediate management of a flail chest is by compression with the palm of the hand or by placing a sandbag on the flail segment. Most patients with flail chest require endotracheal intubation and positive-pressure ventilation until the chest wall stabilizes. Open surgical fixation of the flail segment is only performed in those patients who require a thoracotomy to deal with major intrathoracic trauma.

• Fractures of the first rib are frequently associated with aortic or oesophageal injury and one should have a high index of suspicion for these injuries when faced with a first rib fracture. The presence of a widened mediastinum or fluid in the chest would mandate further investigation, e.g. contrast-enhanced computed tomographic (CT) scan or arch arteriography.

• The major intrathoracic injuries are referred for specialist treatment in cardiothoracic units once the patient is relatively stable.

• Uncomplicated fractured ribs should not be strapped but are simply treated with injection of the fracture site with long-acting local anaesthetic and administration of adequate amounts of oral analgesics. The local anaesthetic agent should be infiltrated into the angle of the fractured ribs and the normal rib above and below the fracture. A maximum of five to six ribs should be injected. Especially in elderly patients, rib fractures may become complicated by pulmonary collapse and infection due to the shallow breathing involuntarily adopted by these patients, as deep inspiration necessary for alveolar filling is painful.

10 Musculoskeletal Trauma

Sticks and stones may break my bones, but words will never hurt me.   (folk phrase)

Introduction

Fractures are a common medical problem and few people have not broken or do not know someone who has broken a bone. Bones are familiar to us all as inert things which are important for body structure. In reality, however, bones are dynamic living tissues with a very rich blood and nerve supply. The immediate consequences of fracture, therefore, are *severe pain* and *blood loss* and the strategy of the early management is to minimize pain with splints and analgesics and to anticipate the effects of blood loss, i.e. hypovolaemic shock. In the longer term the rich blood supply must be re-established before bone will heal and so from the outset the state of the soft tissues becomes of central importance. Finally, it must be remembered that patients do not die from broken bones but from the results of associated injuries to the chest, head and abdomen and so fractures are not one's first consideration when treating the injured patient.

History-taking after trauma

There are two principal reasons for taking a careful history after trauma:
- clinical; and
- medicolegal.

The clinical history

Bones may be broken in many ways, including simple domestic accidents — which are the most common — high-velocity transport accidents and, more rarely, after battle injuries. The following questions must be asked and answered:

- *What happened?* Once admitted to hospital, most fractures look the same whatever the mechanism of injury. However, there is a world of difference in sustaining a fracture from slipping off a step compared to being hit by a car; the first involves little energy transfer to the affected part of the body while in the second quite a lot of energy is absorbed by the part. The amount of energy transferred to the body in an accident determines not only the bony injury but also the soft-tissue damage and the extent to which the blood supply is disrupted. Therefore, it is important to find out from the victim (*direct history*) and witnesses (*collateral history*) what exactly happened.

- *How did it happen?* How it happened can also help because injuries tend not to occur randomly but in some sort of pattern. For example, a pedestrian hit by a car tends to receive leg injuries from the bumper, pelvic and abdominal injuries from the bonnet and head injuries from the door pillar. Knowing something about these patterns permits the examiner to predict potential injuries and if we think about them we are less likely to miss them.

- *Where and when did it happen?* It is also useful to know how, when and where it happened as a long delay between injury and treatment may limit options in treatment.

- *What was the patient like before it happened?* Once the circumstances of the injury is appreciated then the patient should have a full medical history taken. This is of course secondary to essential treatment required to protect the airway, and control haemorrhage. It is important to establish as much as possible about the patient's previous general medical state. Often medical conditions may be associated with an injury. For example, the patient may have had a fit or collapsed with a hypoglycaemic attack. In the elderly, presentation with a fracture may represent a fall secondary to a myocardial infarction or a cerebrovascular accident. Of course, many patients with fractures will need an anaesthetic and so the state of the cardiovascular and respiratory system must be established. The last time the patient ate or drank should be confirmed so that if possible surgery can be delayed until the stomach is empty, so reducing the risk of aspiration of vomit.

- *Who is the person?* Finally, the social history is extremely important. This may be obtained after the immediate treatment of the fracture has been carried out or may be obtained from a relative. The status of patients before injury must be established. Where do they live and with whom? Do they have stairs to climb into the house or flat or within the home? Can the older patient go to relatives after any hospital stay to rehabilitate (Fig. 10.1)?

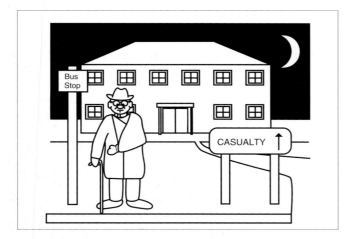

Figure 10.1 It is very important to elicit a social history from the patient. The planning of recovery starts with the admission and not as an afterthought just before discharge. Sending an old person home to a cold top-floor flat with no heating and no relatives on a Friday night with no social provision is of no benefit to the patient, however well the fracture has been treated in hospital.

Medicolegal aspects

Accidents have all sorts of consequences. They affect the patient and the patient's family. They often result in insurance claims and litigation, not infrequently directed at the doctors and nurses who cared for the patient immediately after the accident. It is important therefore to keep meticulous notes and make them at or as soon after events as possible. This is particularly important when it is realized that it is often months or years before one may be called to give an account of an accident. For all concerned, legible and complete notes are essential.

Examination of the traumatized patient

All patients need to have a full physical examination. Priorities should be established in the examination process which may be expressed as listed below.
1 Examine vital areas.
2 Examine injured areas.
3 Examine other areas at risk.
4 Do a general examination.

Vital areas

For patients with multiple injuries, airway protection and cardiorespiratory viability take precedence over everything else. However, for most patients with a single or few injuries, the examination will concentrate on the injured part and the fitness of the patient for anaesthetic.

The injured area

Examination of the fracture site

The suspicion that a patient has sustained a fracture will have been raised from the history. The diagnosis should be confirmed by physical examination of the injured part and only rarely are radiographs needed to make the diagnosis. The signs of fracture are:
- deformity;
- tenderness;
- swelling;
- discoloration or bruising;
- loss of function; and
- crepitus.

Crepitus is perceived as a grating or grinding of the broken bone ends, but this sign should not be purposefully elicited as it will cause intense pain to the patient.

Examination of surrounding tissues

- The *skin* may be partially damaged and present with or subsequently develop *blisters*. Such skin is only partially viable and may not tolerate being incised as part of an operation. If the skin has been breached, the fracture is described as *an open fracture* (see below).
- The *subcutaneous fat* will almost certainly be damaged and later necrosis may cause reddening of the skin with firmness and tenderness; this is easily mistaken for infection.
- The *surrounding muscle* will be damaged to some degree, contributing to limb swelling. If swelling is severe the patient may develop a full-blown compartment syndrome (see below and Chapter 18).
- Damage to *major vessels* is surprisingly rare, except in extensive open injuries where there has been a lot of direct violence. Certain specific fractures (supracondylar elbow fractures and dislocated knee) are often accompanied by arterial damage. Vessels are also at risk from compression (see compartment syndrome) and from damage to the intima. The features of vascular trauma are described in Chapter 18.
- Complete or incomplete division of *nerves* is rare except in penetrating wounds, in association with severe open fractures or with specific trauma (brachial plexus injury). Stretching, or neuropraxia, however, is not uncommon. The nerves are sometimes stretched around deformed fragments and this is sometimes exacerbated by swelling.

Other areas at risk

Certain types of injury are classically associated with other specific injuries and the discovery of one injury should alert the examiner to the possibility of the associated injury. Examples are:

- *Head and spinal injuries.* The possibility that a patient with a head injury also has a spinal injury should constantly be borne in mind. If a blow is sufficient to render a patient unconscious then the same violence could have broken the cervical spine, especially where it joins the head (at the atlas and axis) or where it joins the trunk (at the thoracocervical junction). If a patient is unconscious following a head injury, it is best to assume that he or she has a spinal injury until proven otherwise. Patients should be nursed with a collar and turned correctly (all in one piece and not twisted).
- *Rib fractures and pneumothorax.* The presence of fractured ribs should always raise the possibility of pneumothorax. The possibility of traumatic aortic dissection should be considered in a patient with a fractured left first rib following blunt trauma (see Chapter 18.1).
- *Femoral and pelvic injuries.* Pelvic injuries are sometimes seen in association with major long bone injuries in the lower limb. Dislocation of a hip sometimes accompanies femoral fracture and ligamentous injuries to adjacent joints are always possible in any long bone fracture.
- *Small injuries with big injuries.* It is wise to re-examine the patient on two or three occasions, including the next day, when small injuries are often discovered. It is often small injuries which lead to long-term problems and it is a shame to see, for example, a patient with a well-treated long bone fracture still not at work because of an unrecognized and untreated fracture of some metatarsals.

Investigation of fractures

Plain radiography of the injured area

An X-ray must show the part under investigation and it must be of diagnostic quality. The responsibility of achieving this rests solely with the clinician ordering the film. Dark films are dangerous and vital information may be missed. Equally, it is important to make sure the whole of the site of injury is included in the investigation and so it is safest to include the joint above and the joint below the area in question.

Two films are usually taken at mutual right angles. Conventionally an *anteroposterior* and a *lateral* view are taken. In this way, by always viewing conventional films the examiner recognizes deviations from normal patterns more easily. However, some injuries (e.g. hand injuries) are best seen on *oblique* views (Fig. 10.2).

The radiographic features of a fracture include:
- lucencies at the site of fractures;

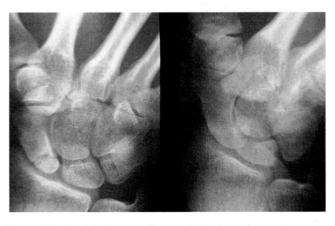

Figure 10.2 Special views are often required when a fracture is suspected. In this case an oblique view clearly shows that the scaphoid is fractured (left picture) but the fracture is not obvious on the conventional anteroposterior view (right picture).

How to describe a fracture

- Which bone is broken and on which side?

- Is the fracture open or closed?

- Where on the bone is it broken?   Intra-articular
                                     Mid-shaft
                                     Proximal or lower third

- What shape is the fracture?   Spiral
                                     Oblique
                                     Transverse

- How many fragments?   Simple
                                     Butterfly
                                     Comminuted

- Position of the distal fragment?
    Displacement: anterior – posterior
                     medial   – lateral
    Angulation: anterior – posterior
                     varus   – valgus
    Rotation: internal – external

Box 10.1

- a discontinuity in the cortex or surface of a bone or joint.

These features may be very obvious or quite subtle. The essence however is an index of suspicion and only rarely should the examiner be surprised by what is revealed by X-ray (Box 10.1).

Radiography of other areas

- Other films may be taken where injury to other areas is contemplated (see above). For example, if the skull is fractured it is wise to X-ray the cervical spine and if the patient is unconscious this is mandatory.
- If the patient is to have an anaesthetic a chest film will help exclude a small pneumothorax which may become lethally significant if the patient is intubated and given positive-pressure ventilation.
- In a case of multiple lower limb injuries it is wise to take a radiograph of the pelvis.
- On occasions it is useful to take radiographs of the opposite normal limb. This is particularly so in children where epiphyseal centres of ossification can produce confusing pictures with many apparently free-floating 'blobs' of bone. A comparison with analogous films of the other side may reveal a displaced fragment, often lying in the joint.
- It is also useful sometimes to X-ray the patient on two separate occasions. For example, scaphoid fractures are frequently invisible on an initial radiograph, only to be re-

vealed on a film taken 2 weeks later. This improvement in a fracture image is almost certainly caused by the hyperaemia in the surrounding bone, which occurs in the acute inflammatory phase following fracture.

Tomography

An alternative to waiting for radiolucency through hyperaemia is to take tomograms. This is a particular radiographic technique whereby the X-ray beam and the film rotate around the limb so that only one point of the limb (the place that is potentially fractured) will be constantly in focus (see Chapter 2). In this way a detailed view of a small area of interest may reveal pathology. A good example is fracture of the odontoid peg, which is often lost amongst confusing shadows at the base of the skull.

Computed tomography (CT)

CT scans are essentially an extension of ordinary tomograms but repeated thousands of times and assembled into a single image by a computer. They represent a section of the body of a few millimetres' thickness and are usually taken in the transverse plane. They are most useful in determining the extent of an injury and are less useful in primary diagnosis. In detail they are of value in planning an operation or determining the stability of a fracture, e.g. the spine.

Magnetic resonance imaging (MRI)

MRI images are produced by aligning the body's hydrogen atoms (protons) in a magnetic field and bombarding them with radiofrequency (RF) waves. The RF waves cause the hydrogen atoms to spin as they acquire energy. Removal of the RF waves causes the protons to release the energy they have acquired. This energy release is picked up by detectors and converted into a grey-scale image. Each tissue produces a characteristic signal; compact bone gives off little or no signal while soft tissue generally gives a good signal. MRI therefore has little place in the management of most fractures but is important for the assessment of spinal cord and spine trauma (see also Chapter 2).

Other investigations

In acute injuries few investigations apart from the plain radiograph are necessary.
- *Ultrasound* of a joint may help in elucidating an effusion.
- When there is doubt, *radioisotope bone scanning* can help in determining whether a bone is fractured or not. This is most useful at about 2 weeks from the injury. It is a highly sensitive test but does not of course tell us anything about the fracture except that it is there. A useful example is the

scaphoid fracture which may be seen on a second X-ray at 2 weeks, but there can still be doubt. A negative scan is a very positive reassurance in such a situation and may help to allay lingering clinical doubt.

Fracture architecture

Why is it important to describe the shape and degree of fragmentation of a fracture? In general, the shape of a fracture tells us about the amount of energy which has caused the damage and so helps us understand it and how we may treat it. In general, *spiral fractures* occur through twisting, which is a common low-energy mode of injury. Such injuries are usually associated with little soft-tissue damage and so the blood supply to the bone is preserved and therefore healing is unlikely to be a problem. In contrast, *oblique* and *transverse fractures* are caused by buckling or direct injury to the bone and involve a lot of energy with soft-tissue stripping and damage to the blood supply. Such injuries will require a lot more consideration when the choice of treatment is being made. The types of fractures are summarized in Fig. 10.3.

How do fractures heal?

Bone has a natural tendency to heal and, unlike any other connective tissue, it has a remarkable repair mechanism which ultimately results in bone regeneration and structural integrity; it is literally 'as good as new'. The pathology of fracture healing is summarized in Fig. 10.4.

This remarkable process and its mechanism remain poorly understood but there are a number of points worth noting.

- First, bones heal in the presence of some movement. This is clear from the example of broken ribs which unite efficiently (albeit painfully!) with prodigious external callus formation. It appears that movement stimulates union but the movement must be small and must not be in certain directions. Essentially, bones are stimulated by micromovement directed along their axis and heal least efficiently if subjected to shearing forces or large movements.
- The converse also holds true, that although bones will heal if there is no movement, then they do so very slowly and by an entirely different process which does not utilize natural external callus formation. This alternative method of fracture healing appears to be similar to the normal remodelling processes of bone, which are slow but sure.

Management of fractures

Immediate management

Pain relief

- *Systemic pain relief* for fractures requires the use of *opiates* given in adequate doses in combination with an antiemetic to offset the side-effects of opiates. In injured patients intravenous rather than intramuscular opiates should

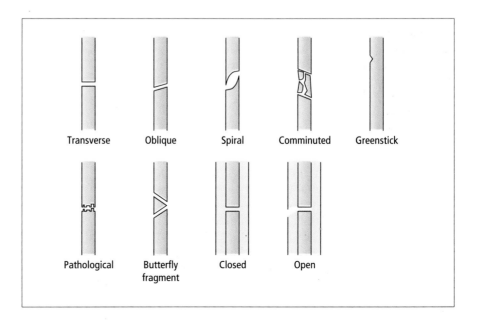

Figure 10.3 Fracture architecture.

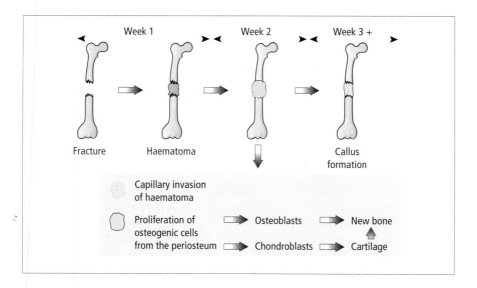

Figure 10.4 The pathology of fracture healing.

be used. Clinicians, particularly when new, are often afraid to give adequate doses of opiates in the fear of affecting consciousness and clinical signs. In general, however, when serious head or visceral injury has been excluded, they may be used generously and early.

• *Local anaesthetic nerve blocks* are frequently effective. A femoral nerve block, for example, can remove the need for systemic drugs following femoral fracture, although the anxiolytic benefits of central nervous system agents should not be underestimated.

• *Splintage* can be applied to most fractures before arriving at hospital. This alone can relieve most intolerable pain. In general, a splint should encompass the joint above and below an injury. Simple expedients such as binding the arm to the chest, with or without a sling, or simply binding the legs together is often sufficient.

• An alternative to splintage is *traction*, which may be used early to relieve muscle spasm, which is a major component of postfracture pain. This is particularly useful for fractures of the femoral neck where splintage is almost impossible to apply.

Blood loss

For most upper limb and peripheral lower limb fractures, blood loss is small and is tolerated even by the elderly. However, blood loss may be significant with major pelvic fractures (6+ units) and long bone fractures, particularly the femur (2–3 units) and the tibia (1 unit). In general, all patients with long bone injuries should be cross-matched for blood and a good-sized venous line established as soon as possible to ensure adequate resuscitation (see Chapter 4). For pelvic fractures two lines may be needed and a central venous line established to ensure transfusion is keeping up with loss.

Open fractures

Open (or, less meaningfully, *compound*) fractures are serious injuries (Fig. 10.5). Considerable violence is re-

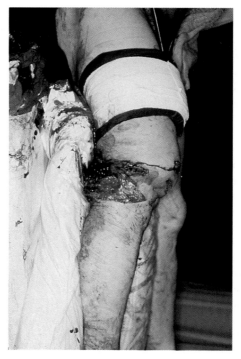

Figure 10.5 An open fracture of the tibia.

quired to cause this type of injury and because there is a break in the skin, bacterial contamination of the bone occurs. The strategy of treatment is to clean the wounds as soon as possible and remove all dead tissue (*debridement*), thus preventing the development of infection. Open fractures are surgical emergencies and, provided that the patient's general condition permits, formal surgical wound debridement should be performed as soon as possible. Wounds are better left open if there is any doubt that closure cannot be achieved without tension on the skin. This means that the vast majority should be left open and closed either as a secondary procedure after a few days or left to heal spontaneously. Such patients all need supplementary broad-spectrum antibiotics and some form of *tetanus prophylaxis*, i.e. tetanus toxoid booster to those with a previous immunization record or human antitetanus globulin for those with no previous active immunity.

Definitive management

The essential strategy of long-term fracture management must be *to return patients to their preinjury level of function by the safest means*. Functional requirements vary from individual to individual depending on many factors, including age, physical health and the patient's occupation. For example, a fractured wrist in a frail elderly patient with poor osteoporotic bone might be managed differently from a young fit, right-handed craftsman. In the former a less than ideal reduction under local anaesthesia might be acceptable, allowing for early discharge and early mobilization of the wrist; the young patient may be prepared to spend many months ensuring a perfect result because that is what is required for his long-term health and employment security. The basic goals of management are: *reduction, immobilization* and *rehabilitation*.

Reduction of fractures

In order to achieve acceptable function a fracture should be reduced and held so that the anatomy of the bone is returned to as near normal as possible.
- If the fracture passes into a joint then the anatomy should be restored accurately if acceptable function is to be achieved.
- If a fracture occurs through the shaft of a long bone, then it is desirable to return the anatomy to normal but the margin for error is much greater and something less than perfect is acceptable.

Closed reduction may be achieved by traction on the distal fragment and then a relocation of that distal part back on to the proximal fragment by manipulation (e.g. Colles fractures are reduced by closed reduction). In order to achieve a reduction, adequate analgesia must be given; this is achieved by general or regional anaesthesia. The manipulative procedure usually involves reversing the direction of the deforming force. If closed reduction is unsuccessful, then *open reduction* may be required, whereby the fracture site is opened surgically and the fragments are relocated directly under vision (e.g. unstable fracture of both forearm bones).

Immobilization of fractures

Once the fracture is adequately realigned, then it must be held in the normal position until the bone has become strong enough to support itself (*united*) and then protected until it is strong enough to bear some load (*consolidated*). Methods of immobilizing fractures are listed below.
- *Casting*: After the fracture has been manipulated, it may be held simply and effectively in a *plaster of Paris* cast until union occurs. The fracture must be held in a position which maintains it in three dimensions (tilt, twist and shift) and it must be the proper length. In order to ensure complete control of all dimensions of the fracture, it is necessary to control the joint above and below the fracture as otherwise joint movement may result in distortion in one or more dimensions. Plaster of Paris is relatively brittle, messy and very difficult to apply well. It is heavy and awkward, particularly in the elderly, and takes up to 3 days to dry fully. For these reasons strong and light *glass fibre* and *polyurethane resin* materials have been developed. These are not as versatile as plaster of Paris and are better for secondary casts which are applied after a week or two when the fracture swelling has settled.
- *Functional bracing*: Casts have a number of disadvantages. They are heavy, immobilize the joints and prevent access to the fracture site. The immobility imposed on a limb by a cast results in muscle wasting and joint stiffness. It is possible to overcome these disadvantages by the technique of functional bracing, i.e. freeing the joints whilst maintaining alignment at the fracture site. In order to maintain three-dimensional control of the fracture it is necessary to support the cast at the joints by a combination of accurate moulding and the provision of hinges, which permit motion in one direction, usually flexion and extension. Functional bracing is highly dependent on a very accurate fit and it is to be used only after a few weeks when pain and swelling have settled. In practice, functional bracing is used in the management of fractures of the tibia and fibula.
- *Internal fixation*: Where accurate reduction and holding of fractures are required, internal fixation is performed. However, internal fixation is technically very demanding, has many complications and, most important of all, it

prevents natural healing. If fixation is to be used it can be achieved in a number of ways.

(a) *Apposition*: Once fractures are realigned they may only need to be held in apposition for healing to proceed satisfactorily. This is particularly true in children. Apposition can be achieved simply by using semiflexible wires known as 'K' (for Kirschner) wires. They hold position without producing immobility and so healing occurs by natural callus formation. They can be left standing proud of the bone and so can easily be pulled out once union is established and before consolidation.

(b) *Interfragmentary compression* (Fig. 10.6) is usually achieved by screws or occasionally by tension band wires. These achieve great accuracy and are particularly valuable in cancellous bone around joints. They are also useful in long bones, particularly in the upper limb, but in these situations extra support is required from an onlay device.

(c) *Onlay devices* consist of metal plates which are used to buttress weak structures around joints and to fix long bones in the upper limb. These very rigid systems inhibit natural bone union and, although they permit early movement, they ultimately delay healing and full load-bearing.

(d) *Intramedullary or inlay devices* are the most satisfactory method of fixation. They achieve alignment without unduly disturbing natural bone healing. They are a relatively inaccurate method of restoring anatomical position and so are not useful around joints. Their great strength makes them ideal devices for treating long bone fractures, particularly in the lower limb.

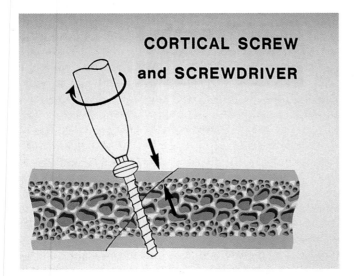

Figure 10.6 Interfragmentary compression is achieved by screwing the two bone fragments together.

• *External fixation*: When fractures are open and associated with extensive soft-tissue damage and contamination, neither plaster casting nor internal fixation is appropriate. Plaster splints are unsuitable because the wounds become inaccessible for inspection and dressings, while internal fixation is hazardous because of the very high risk of wound infection.

A compromise solution is to apply an external fixation device which consists of a strong metal rod (or series of rods) which runs parallel to the fractured bone and is attached to the bone by a series of pins (Fig. 10.7). Such a device stabilizes the fracture and gives access to the soft tissues for dressings and secondary surgery such as skin grafting. A disadvantage of external fixators is the risk of infection at the pin sites.

• *Traction* may be used to hold a fracture in a reduced position. Traction is achieved by the application of a relatively small weight (10–15 lb; 4.50–7 kg) to a limb. The weight exerts a pull along the axis of the broken bone, thus stimulating muscle contraction. The increased muscle tone acts like a splint, holding the broken bone in the position achieved at reduction. In practice, traction is static, dynamic or balanced.

(a) *Static traction* is used for relatively short periods where the pull is applied against another part of the body (e.g. the initial management of a fractured neck of femur uses static traction applied via a Thomas splint).

(b) *Dynamic traction* is used where joints are still permitted to move but by means of pulleys the pull is maintained along the axis of the body. In this case weights provide the traction and the counterforce is achieved by tilting the bed so that friction and the weight of the body prevent the patient being pulled out of bed.

(c) *Balanced traction* is used where fixed traction is in danger of causing damage to a part of the body through pressure. In effect the affected part is isolated by the traction device which is offset by a counterweight to neutralize pressure effects. Traction may be applied either to the skin or via a pin inserted through the bone. The main problem with long-term traction is that the patient is tied to the bed, making hospital stay prolonged and nursing care difficult (Fig. 10.8).

Rehabilitation

Immobilization causes muscle atrophy and joint stiffness which, if not treated aggressively, may lead to contractures and posttraumatic syndromes (e.g. posttraumatic sympathetic dystrophy). Therefore, patients require intensive rehabilitation programmes to help them use their joints as soon as possible after the fracture, to exercise their muscles and begin to use and build up strength in the injured limb.

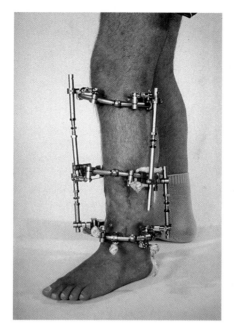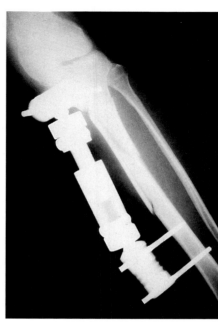

Figure 10.7 (a) An external fixation device has been applied to a fractured tibia. The device in this case consists of two strong metal rods which externally support the tibia. (b) They are attached to the tibia by a series of pins.   (a)   (b)

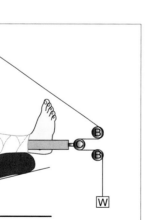

Figure 10.8 A schematic representation of balanced traction.

Most of this work will be done under the supervision of physiotherapists and occupational therapists (see also Chapter 32).

Common fractures and joint injuries

The common fractures encountered in clinical practice are listed in Table 10.1. This list is not exhaustive but these

are the fractures any doctor or student should know about.

Upper limb fractures

Hand injuries are common and cause considerable morbidity if not dealt with correctly. Fractures and dislocations of the fingers are usually caused by direct trauma and are managed by reduction and splinting; the fingers are conveniently splinted to the adjacent fingers while aluminium splints hold hand fractures in place. Displaced fractures can be reduced and held in position with small pins. A *Bennett's fracture* is a fracture of the base of the first metacarpal bone with proximal displacement of the thumb. It is commonly caused by punching and may be treated by closed reduction and POP or by internal fixation. Tendon and nerve injuries are frequently seen following hand trauma and are dealt with in Chapters 11 and 21. The goal in treating any hand injury is early rehabilitation to achieve a good *functional* result.

Falls on the outstretched hand may cause several different types of wrist fracture. A diagnosis of *scaphoid fracture* (Fig. 10.9) is made clinically by eliciting tenderness in the anatomical snuffbox. Oblique views usually demonstrate the fracture on X-ray and treatment is by scaphoid plaster for 6 weeks. Avascular necrosis of the proximal fragment is a well-recognized complication of this fracture and is treated by excising the necrotic bone. A *Colles fracture* is

Table 10.1 Some common fractures and their management.

Site	Mechanism of injury	Management	Specific complications
Upper limb			
Scaphoid	Fall on dorsiflexed hand	POP for 6 weeks	Avascular necrosis
Colles	Fall on dorsiflexed hand	Closed reduction POP 6 weeks	Posttraumatic (reflex) sympathetic dystrophy
Forearm bones	Twisting force or direct blow. Often 'greenstick' in children	Greenstick fracture — above-elbow POP 6 weeks. Others — open reduction and plates	Hand ischaemia
Humerus			
Supracondylar	Fall on hand with the elbow bent, posterior dislocation of distal fragment	Closed reduction with posterior plaster slab with collar and cuff	Brachial artery injury Volkmann's ischaemic contracture
Mid-shaft	Fall on hand or elbow	Collar and cuff (± U-plaster)	Radial nerve injury
Neck	Fall on outstretched hand	Sling for 3 weeks	Stiff shoulder
Clavicle	Fall on outstretched hand	Sling for 3 weeks (rarely, axillary loops)	Malunion
Lower limb			
Calcaneum	Fall from a height	Functional treatment (elevation and early mobilization)	Chronic sickness
Ankle	Abduction, adduction or external rotation	Open or closed but perfect reduction is essential	Ankle stiffness
Tibia and fibula	Direct trauma	Closed fracture — reduction and POP Open fracture — external fixation	Delayed or non-union
Femur			
Supracondylar	Direct violence	Internal fixation	Arterial damage
Mid-shaft	Fall, direct trauma, pathological	Internal or external fixation	Knee stiffness
Neck	Fall in elderly	Internal fixation	Blood loss
Pelvis	Direct trauma, e.g. RTA	Stabilize with external fixation, internal fixation later	Blood loss
Spine	Trauma from fall or RTA	Compression fracture of vertebral body — analgesia/rest Traumatic fracture/dislocation — paraplegia Stabilize and mobilize early	

POP, Plaster of Paris; RTA. road traffic accident.

the commonest of all fractures and produces the classical dinner-fork deformity (Fig. 10.10) with the radial fragment shifted and tilted backwards and radially and impacted (Fig. 10.11). This is usually accompanied by a fracture of the ulnar styloid. Occasionally, forwards displacement of the radial fragment occurs and this is referred to as a *Smith's fracture*. Treatment of both types of fracture is by disimpaction and immobilization in POP for about 6 weeks. Shoulder stiffness (from disuse) is a common complication. Rarely, spontaneous rupture of the extensor pollicis longus tendon may occur and some patients develop posttraumatic (reflex) sympathetic dystrophy (see below).

Fractures of both forearm bones occur as a result of twisting forces or direct trauma. In children the result is a greenstick fracture which simply needs realignment and an above-elbow POP. Adults frequently require internal fixation to achieve good reduction. Fractures of one forearm bone are frequently accompanied by dislocation of the radioulnar joints. A *Monteggia fracture* is a fracture of the ulna with dislocation of the proximal radioulnar joint (Fig. 10.12) while a *Galeazzi fracture* is a fracture of the radius with dislocation of the distal radioulnar joint (Fig. 10.13).

Fractures around the elbow include fractures of the *olecranon* and *head of radius*. However, the most important elbow injury is the *supracondylar fracture* with backward displacement, seen in children (Fig. 10.14). This has to be reduced carefully and it is essential to ensure that there has

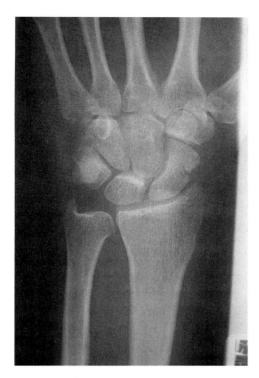

Figure 10.9 Scaphoid fracture.

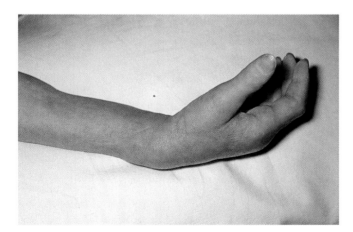

Figure 10.10 Typical 'dinner-fork' deformity seen in a patient with a Colles fracture.

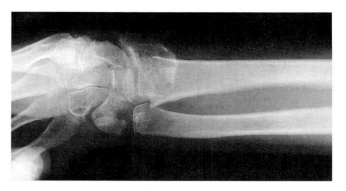

Figure 10.11 In a Colles fracture the radial fragment is shifted and tilted backwards and radially and impacted. There is usually also a fracture of the ulnar styloid.

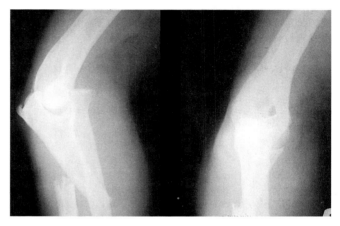

Figure 10.12 A Monteggia fracture is a fracture of the ulna with dislocation of the proximal radioulnar joint.

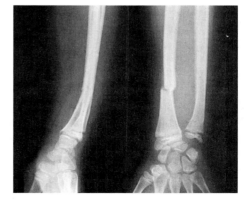

Figure 10.13 A Galeazzi fracture is a fracture of the radius with dislocation of the distal radioulnar joint.

been no injury to the brachial artery, as this may lead to a compartment syndrome and Volkmann's ischaemic contracture (see below). Other fractures of the humerus (*midshaft, neck*) are simply treated with a collar and cuff or sling with early mobilization to avoid shoulder stiffness. *Fractures of the clavicle* are managed similarly.

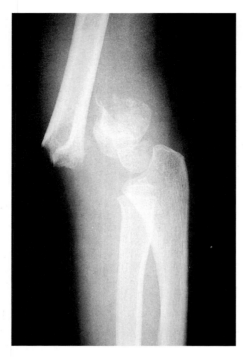

Figure 10.14 A supracondylar fracture of the humerus with backward displacement is a very serious injury, commonly seen in children. There is a very high risk of brachial artery injury with this fracture.

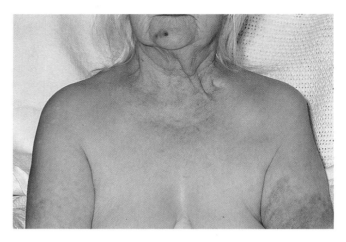

Figure 10.15 This patient has an anterior dislocation of the left shoulder. The arm is held in slight abduction and there is flattening of the deltoid prominence with a depression below the acromium where the head of the humerus should normally be felt. The dislocated humeral head can be seen anteriorly.

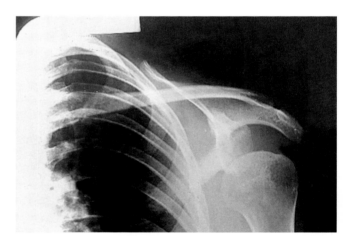

Figure 10.16 A radiograph of a patient with shoulder dislocation reveals the head of the humerus in the subglenoid position.

Upper limb joint injuries

Finger dislocations are common, especially in sport and are easily reduced under digital local anaesthetic block with lignocaine (remember, do *not* use adrenaline!). *Elbow dislocation* may occur following a fall on the hand. The forearm is pushed backwards and the ulna dislocates posteriorly behind the lower end of the humerus. Most elbow dislocations can be reduced by closed techniques under general anaesthesia, after which the patient wears a collar and cuff for 3 weeks.

Anterior dislocation of the shoulder is a very common injury, again caused by a fall on the hand. The humerus is driven forwards tearing the capsule of the shoulder joint. Typically, the patient supports the arm in slight abduction and on examination there is flattening of the deltoid prominence with a depression below the acromium where the head of the humerus should normally be felt (Fig. 10.15). It is possible to feel the humeral head anteriorly but this may be difficult in an obese patient. The patient will not be able to move the arm.

Injury to the circumflex nerve as it passes around the neck of the humerus is a well-recognized complication of anterior shoulder dislocation and this injury should be sought by testing for a patch of anaesthesia over the deltoid muscle prior to reducing the dislocation. The nerve injury, however, is usually a neuropraxia (see Chapter 11) which recovers spontaneously. Radiographs reveal the displaced humeral head in the subcoracoid or subglenoid positions (Fig. 10.16). Reduction under anaesthesia is usually easily achieved but a number of techniques which require only analgesia have evolved for treating this common condition (Box 10.2).

Following reduction the arm is held to the side with the arm flexed across the abdomen and no attempt at abduction

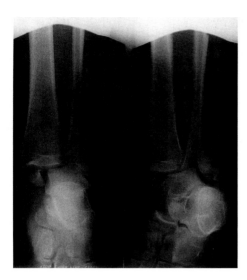

Figure 10.17 A bimalleolar fracture of the ankle with lateral displacement.

Management of anterior dislocation of the shoulder

Hippocratic manoeuvre
The surgeon places his stockinged foot in the patient's axilla while simultaneously pulling on the patient's arm, thus levering the head of the humerus back into position.

Milch manoeuvre
The patient lies prone on a couch with the injured arm hanging vertically. If spontaneous reduction does not occur a bucket is attached to the arm with a bandage and traction increased by filling the bucket with water.

Kocher's manoeuvre
The surgeon pulls on the flexed elbow, rotates the humerus laterally, then adducts it while rotating it medially.

Box 10.2

should be made for a few weeks. In elderly patients, mobilization of the shoulder is begun after 2–3 weeks. In a number of patients recurrent shoulder dislocations occur, often with trivial injury, and these require surgical or arthroscopic treatment.

Lower limb fractures

Fractures and dislocation of the *phalanges* and the *metatarsals* are managed similarly to their equivalent injuries in the hand and early mobilization is encouraged. Fractures of the *talus* and *calcaneum* are usually caused by falls from a height and one should always exclude spinal injury when a patient presents with calcaneal fractures. Dis-

placed talar fractures are managed by open reduction and internal fixation. The talus is, like the scaphoid, also liable to avascular necrosis. Calcaneal fractures are usually treated symptomatically with elevation, analgesia and early physiotherapy and mobilization. Stiffness is a common problem following these fractures.

Ankle fractures are common and are caused by a variety of forces (external rotation, abduction and adduction) applied to the ankle, usually while the foot is fixed. Such trauma results in a number of possible ankle injuries described as malleolar (i.e. fracture of either medial or lateral malleolus), bimalleolar (both medial and lateral malleolus fractured; Fig. 10.17) and trimalleolar (both medial and lateral malleoli and the posterior rim of the tibia, the posterior malleolus). It is important to remember that there may also be ligament injuries associated with a malleolar fracture. Stable ankle fractures may be treated by a cast for 6–8 weeks while unstable fractures require internal fixation.

Tibial fractures are usually caused by direct violence to the bone, e.g. car bumper injury, while twisting forces result in spiral fractures of both tibia and fibula. Because there is so little tissue covering the tibia, these fractures are frequently open and require stabilization with an external fixator (Fig. 10.7). The wound is then debrided and left open. A muscle flap may be required to achieve adequate coverage. Closed undisplaced tibial fractures may be managed with a plaster of Paris cast but instability demands internal fixation with an intramedullary nail or plate and screws. Tibial fractures involving the knee joint (tibial plateau fractures) require careful manipulation and reduction, often by internal fixation.

Supracondylar fractures of the femur are usually caused by direct violence. As with supracondylar humeral fractures, the artery (this time the popliteal artery) is at risk of injury (Fig. 10.18). These fractures are now managed by open reduction and internal fixation. Quadriceps exercises are encouraged from the start. *Fractures of the femoral shaft* may be transverse, spiral or comminuted and are usually associated with considerable blood loss. A transverse fracture following moderate trauma in older patients should raise the suspicion of a pathological fracture. Emergency treatment consists of internal fixation with intramedullary nails, but if the fracture is open an external fixator may be used.

Fractures of hip and proximal femur are common and can conveniently be classified as *intracapsular* and *extracapsular* (Fig. 10.19) depending on the relationship of the fracture to the capsule of the hip joint. Young patients sustain these fractures in road traffic accidents but fractured hips occur more frequently after falls in elderly people with osteoporotic bones. Almost all hip fractures are now

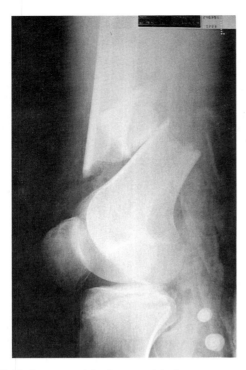

Figure 10.18 A supracondylar fracture of the femur.

managed by internal fixation. Pins and plates are used for extracapsular (trochanteric) fractures while intracapsular

fractures may be plated in the young or treated by total hip replacement or just replacement of the femoral head (Austin-Moore prosthesis) in the elderly. The blood supply to the head of the femur comes from arteries which are reflected from the capsule on to the neck of the femur. These are frequently damaged with intracapsular fractures and therefore it is not surprising that avascular necrosis is a well-recognized complication of these fractures (Fig. 10.20).

Lower limb joint injuries

Ligamentous ankle injuries are extremely common. Usually the lateral collateral ligament is damaged by a sudden inversion force applied to the foot. Clinically there is local tenderness and swelling and, if severe, bruising may develop. Radiographs are indicated to exclude an ankle fracture. Occasionally stress films are required to assess ankle stability. Treatment for most minor ankle sprains is by strapping, elevation and analgesia.

Ligamentous injuries of the knee joint are extremely serious and a considerable cause of morbidity. These are discussed in detail in Chapter 22. Considerable force is required to *dislocate a hip joint* but when it occurs the head of the femur usually dislocates posteriorly (Fig. 10.21). Car accidents which result in the driver's or passenger's knee striking the dashboard are frequently the cause of this injury. Anaesthesia and muscle relaxation are required for

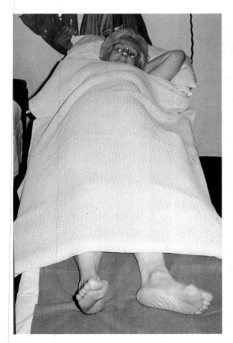

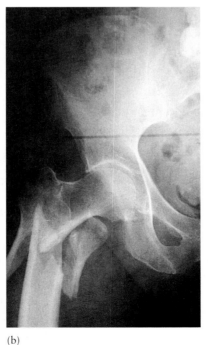

Figure 10.19 The diagnosis of extracapsular fracture of the neck of the femur can be made from the end of the bed. (a) The patient's foot is externally rotated. (b) Radiographs reveal the typical appearances of a transtrochanteric fracture of the neck of the femur.

(a)   (b)

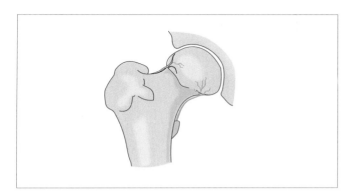

Figure 10.20 Blood supply to the head of the femur.

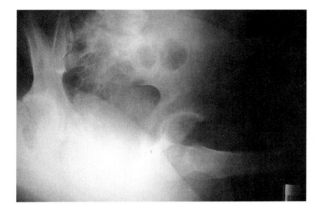

Figure 10.21 Bilateral dislocation of the hip joints and a fractured pelvis in a patient following a road traffic accident.

reduction and the hip needs to be rested for about 3 weeks following the injury. Fractures of the acetabulum often accompany hip dislocation.

Complications of fractures

Early complications may occur either as a direct consequence of the injury or in association with the treatment. Late complications are generally related to the fracture but a few are unfortunately precipitated by treatment (or lack of it). The common complications encountered after a fracture are listed in Table 10.2.

Infection

Bone infection (osteomyelitis) may occur after open fractures or after internal fixation: it is notable that the com-

Table 10.2 Common complications of fractures.

EARLY	
Primary (as a consequence of injury)	*Secondary (as a consequence of treatment)*
Blood loss	Immobility
Infection (open)	Infection
Fat embolism	Plaster disease
Renal failure	Compartment syndrome
Soft-tissue injury	Renal stones
Compartment syndrome	

LATE	
Primary (from the fracture)	*Secondary (from the treatment)*
Non-union	Malunion
Delayed union	Infection
Malunion	
Growth arrest	
Arthritis	

monest cause of bone infection in the western world is surgery! Although infection may delay or prevent union, it is not inevitable that this will be so. Provided a fracture is held stable then it will unite despite infection. If there is movement and infection then non-union is most likely. This phenomenon is poorly understood but if a fracture is infected, provided it is stable, it may be treated by drainage of pus and antibiotics until union has occurred.

Fat embolism

After fracture of a long bone, usually in men under the age of 20, a small number of patients suffer from fat embolism characterized by an increasing degree of respiratory distress, leading to adult respiratory distress syndrome (see Chapter 19). The cause of fat embolism remains unclear. It was originally said to be due to the precipitation of fat from the marrow of the fractured long bone in the lungs. However, an alternative view is that there is a breakdown of tissue fats to free fatty acids which precipitate a pneumonitis. The symptoms (initially *tachypnoea* and *mild confusion*) usually commence within 2–5 days of injury. The patient may have a *petechial rash* on the chest, neck and conjunctiva but this is not a universal finding. Fat globules may be found in the urine and sputum and occasionally are seen in the retinal vessels on fundoscopy. Early diagnosis is dependent on a high index of suspicion and appropriate investigation.

Blood gases will show a hypoxaemia (PaO_2 4.7–6.7 kPa) and respiratory alkalosis (from hyperventilation) and a chest radiograph diffuse opacities which increase to complete 'white-out' over the next few days. In severe cases the respiratory distress increases to the point where positive-pressure ventilation and positive end-expiratory pressure are required (see Chapter 3), but even with this level of support the condition carries a significant mortality. Unfortunately, younger men are more prone to the full-blown syndrome. Early diagnosis and treatment with oxygen and chest physiotherapy are helpful.

Renal failure

Persons with massive soft-tissue injury who are trapped for prolonged periods, particularly where they are shocked or the trapped limbs are relatively ischaemic, are prone to develop acute tubular necrosis. Again the key is to recognize the possibility and be prepared to support such patients with renal dialysis. The cause is purported to be the release of myoglobin and this material is found in abundance in the renal tubules (see Chapter 5).

Compartment syndrome

Compartment syndromes may occur in the upper and lower limbs following a fracture with excessive localized soft-tissue swelling. Classically it occurs in the forearm where it leads to Volkmann's ischaemic contracture, although any muscle compartment lined by a stout fascial sheath may be at risk (e.g. the calf muscles). This condition is discussed more fully in Chapter 18.

Immobility

After injury the injured part needs a short period of rest followed by motion to aid in rehabilitation. The whole person does not need to be immobilized and patients must begin to move and rehabilitate as soon after the injury as possible. Injury results in patients going into negative nitrogen balance and they will lose lean body mass. The effects can be minimized by early mobilization, which will also discourage disuse osteoporosis and the migration of calcium to the blood stream which can precipitate renal stone formation.

Plaster disease

The combination of muscle wasting, stiffness and skin sores is often termed fracture or plaster disease, which is a poor concept. These problems can be minimized or eliminated by early mobilization and it is vital that patients understand that this is their responsibility, only to be aided by therapists and medical staff.

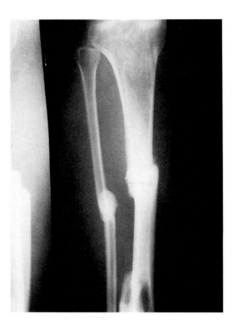

Figure 10.22 Non-union occurs most commonly in the tibia. If a tibial fracture has failed to heal at 20 weeks, a diagnosis of non-union is made. On X-ray, the fracture is still visible and the bone ends are sclerosed.

Delayed and non-union

About 2% of all fractures fail to unite. This is known as non-union (Fig. 10.22). Delayed union is when fractures fail to unite within the expected time. If left to heal naturally, upper limb fractures heal in 6 weeks or so and lower limb fractures in 12 weeks. This rule of thumb is useful but must not be too strictly adhered to and will be modified depending on the degree of violence involved and how the fracture was treated. However, we may say non-union is established at 20 weeks in the lower limb and 10 weeks in the upper. These are arbitrary but practical figures. Delayed union is even less specific and it is really a period between expected union and accepted non-union when the decision to intervene is contemplated. Non-union is commonest in the tibia but may occur at any site. Why fractures go on to non-union is not fully understood but several factors have been implicated:
- excess movement;
- too little movement, e.g. rigid internal fixation;
- soft-tissue interposition;
- poor blood supply;
- infection;
- unstable fracture;
- excessive traction or separation of bone ends; and
- intact fellow bone, e.g. fibula.

Treatment for non-union relies on removing any underlying cause, and then stimulating union. Stabilizing the fracture sufficiently and then adding bone graft seems to stimulate union but how bone graft does this remains an enigma. Bone graft is usually autologous, being taken from the iliac crest and placed next to the fracture. It contains cells and minerals and is probably mediated by humoral factors. It appears to be able to 'switch on' the hitherto deficient mechanism.

Malunion

Malunion implies that the fracture has been allowed to heal in a position that precludes normal function. It usually implies failure of treatment or neglect. Regular review is the mainstay of fracture management and frequent radiological and clinical examination is essential to ensure that all is going well.

Growth arrest

Children have a great capacity to remodel malunited fractures, although they will not remodel rotatory deformities. However, if a fracture breaches the germinal layer of the epiphyseal growth plate, distorted bone growth may occur. These are rare injuries and difficult to manage. All parents of children with epiphyseal injuries must be warned of this possibility if misunderstandings are to be avoided.

Fractures at a glance

DEFINITIONS

- A *fracture* is a break in the continuity of a bone
- Fractures may be *transverse*, *oblique* or *spiral* in shape
- In a *greenstick* fracture only one side of the bone is fractured; the other simply bends
- A *comminuted* fracture is one in which there are more than two fragments of bone
- In a *complicated* fracture some other structure is also damaged (e.g. a nerve or blood vessel)
- In a *compound* fracture there is a break in the overlying skin
- A *pathological* fracture is one through a bone weakened through disease, e.g. a metastasis

CAUSES

Fractures occur when excessive force is applied to a normal bone or moderate force to a diseased bone, e.g. osteoporosis

CLINICAL FEATURES

- Pain
- Loss of function
- Deformity, tenderness and swelling
- Discoloration or bruising
- (Crepitus — should not be elicited!)

INVESTIGATION OF A FRACTURE

- Radiographs in two planes (look for lucencies and discontinuity in the cortex of the bone)
- (Tomography, CT scanning, MR scans — rarely)
- Ultrasonography and radioisotope bone scanning

MANAGEMENT

General
- Look for shock/haemorrhage and check Airway, Breathing and Circulation
- Look for injury in other areas at risk (head and spine, rib fracture and pneumothorax, femoral and pelvic injury)

The fracture

Immediate
- Relieve pain (intravenous opiates, nerve blocks, splints, traction)
- Establish good intravenous access and send blood for group and cross-match
- Open (*compound*) fractures require debridement, antibiotics and tetanus prophylaxis

Definitive
- Reduction (closed or open)
- Immobilization (casting, functional bracing, internal fixation, external fixation, traction)
- Rehabilitation (aim to restore patient to preinjury level of function with physio- and occupational therapy)

COMPLICATIONS

Early	Late
- Blood loss	- Non-union
- Infection	- Delayed union
- Fat embolism	- Malunion
- DVT and PE	- Growth arrest
- Renal failure	- Arthritis
- Compartment syndrome	- Posttraumatic sympathetic (reflex) dystrophy

DVT, deep venous thrombosis; PE, pulmonary embolism.

Posttraumatic (reflex) sympathetic dystrophy

This is a poorly understood syndrome characterized by persistent pain, swelling, hyperaesthesia, stiffness and disuse of a limb following an injury. If it persists, disuse osteoporosis may be seen on X-ray. Treatment consists of physiotherapy with active and passive exercises and pain control. Chronic cases are extremely difficult to treat but pain clinics, vigorous rehabilitation and sympathectomy (in some patients) have been found to be helpful.

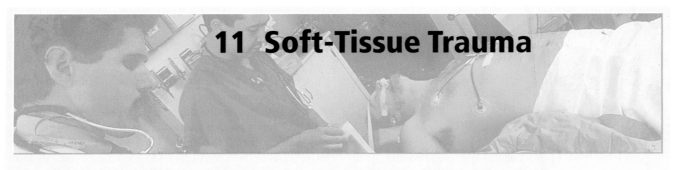

11 Soft-Tissue Trauma

Nobody is on my side, nobody takes part with me: I am cruelly used, nobody feels for my poor nerves.

(Jane Austen, 1775–1817)

Introduction

Although not usually life-threatening, soft-tissue injuries (i.e. injuries to ligaments, tendons, muscles and nerves) are important because they are common and they result in morbidity for the patient and have important economic consequences through loss of work. Whenever the body receives a blow, the energy is transmitted through the soft-tissue layers and the bones to be dissipated as disruption, sound and heat. At low velocity such blows seldom break normal bones but will damage cells and tear soft tissues, causing bleeding followed by an acute inflammatory reaction. Acute inflammation is a physiological response to trauma and is associated with swelling, hyperaemia and pain. First aid consists of actions designed to reduce the effects of acute inflammation and to reduce pain. This may be achieved by applying:

Rest;
Ice;
Compression; and
Elevation.

Ice should be wrapped in a cotton towel before being applied to the injured area as direct contact with the skin may lead to thermal injury. Compression of an injured limb should be supervised and not prolonged or performed without elevation; care should be taken to avoid hindering the circulation (see also compartment syndrome, Chapter 18). Elevation of the affected limb above the heart requires the patient to lie down and have the limb raised or sit with the whole arm elevated (Fig. 11.1). These simple measures can be applied to any injury and

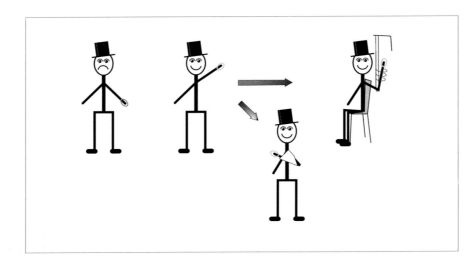

Figure 11.1 Immediate treatment of soft-tissue injury consists of RICE (rest, ice, compression and elevation).

113

can reduce swelling effectively, thus facilitating definitive treatment.

Pain relief

The application of RICE, besides reducing swelling, will also help reduce pain. Simple oral analgesia often provides very effective pain relief and the anti-inflammatory properties of non-steroidal anti-inflammatory drugs (NSAIDs) make them particularly effective in soft-tissue injury. If used early and at relatively higher doses than normal, NSAIDs also help to reduce swelling and inflammation. Occasionally, opiates are required to provide pain relief. However, inordinate pain should alert the clinician to the possibility that some more serious condition such as a fracture or an impending compartment syndrome may have been missed.

Injuries to specific soft tissues

Fat and skin

Most superficial injuries to the fat and skin manifest themselves as bruising (*ecchymosis*) and blisters. The bruising may track along tissue planes but this is natural and simply an effect of gravity. Occasionally, fat necrosis causes an intense red reaction on the skin like an infection or cellulitis. If the patient is well and apyrexial, such reaction should not be treated with antibiotics. Haematomata in these layers may liquefy and cause fluid collections which can be aspirated.

Muscle

Dead muscle cells cannot regenerate. Healing following muscle injury is, therefore, by fibrosis with compensatory hypertrophy of the surrounding muscle cells. However, deposition of fibrous tissue in muscle leads to stiffness. This process cannot be altered but early rehabilitation through movement will minimize stiffness and encourage muscle hypertrophy. Following muscle injury physical therapy within the limits of pain should be instituted as soon as possible. Other techniques such as ultrasound may enhance recovery by dissipating the fibrous tissue.

Ligaments

Incomplete ligament injuries are referred to as *sprains*. Complete injuries are known as *ruptures* or *tears*.
• A sprain is caused by rupture of some, but not all, of the fibres of a ligament. A sprain generally does not cause the associated joint to become unstable but will cause dys-

function through pain. It should also be appreciated that the proprioceptive function of the ligament will be disrupted and this will add to the problems of recovery. Sprains do not require surgical intervention and, following the application of the first-aid measures described above (RICE), recovery is encouraged by exercise — initially non-weight-bearing exercises, rapidly progressing to gradual loading. Most sprains recover in a few weeks depending on the severity of injury and individual requirements, e.g. an athlete may require longer to achieve a high level of performance.
• Ruptures may render a joint unstable and also proprioceptively insensitive in certain planes of movement. Complete ruptures often present with less severe pain than sprains, presumably because of the associated nerve damage. Surprisingly, surgical intervention is seldom required except in specific cases (e.g. cruciate ligament injuries). If joint motion is controlled by splintage early in treatment then most ligaments will heal spontaneously.

Tendons

Tendon injuries generally arise from penetrating trauma, although they may be ruptured by excessive force. They occasionally rupture in middle and old age when subjected to normal forces. In these situations the tendon has undergone degenerative change either due to intrinsic collagen abnormalities or due to abnormal 'wear' against an osteophyte from an adjacent degenerative joint. Tendons usually require surgical repair, which can be technically challenging if function is to be restored. Postrepair physiotherapy to restore movement requires a balance between movement and a reduction in loading so that any repair is not damaged.

Nerves

Nerves may be injured by stretching, crushing or cutting. Stretching or crushing may result in temporary loss of function. Such injuries may be associated with a fracture or a direct injury through pressure. Application of tight bandages or casts around a limb may cause nerve injury through pressure. It is important to document nerve injuries prior to treatment so that the relationship of the injury to the initial trauma is established and the clinician is not exposed to accusations that nerve injury has been caused by treatment.

Types of nerve injury

• *Neurotmesis*: Neurotmesis is complete anatomical division of a nerve with Wallerian degeneration. The nerve tissue distal to the division degenerates and only the support cells survive. New nerve tissue grows back as a series of processes from the damaged cells and so recovery can be prolonged and is usually never completed. Mixed sensory and motor nerves have a particularly poor prognosis and simple sensory nerves such as those found in the fingers are most likely to recover well. *Tinel's sign* is used clinically to mark the level of nerve regeneration. The course of the nerve is percussed with a patella hammer from distally to proximally. A tingling sensation is felt when the level of regeneration is reached.

Complete division of a mixed peripheral nerve results in motor, sensory, vasomotor, sudomotor and trophic symptoms in the anatomical distribution of the nerve. Electromyography is useful in identifying the paralysed muscle groups. Cutaneous sensation is usually lost only over the area of skin *exclusively* supplied by the nerve. For most sensory nerves this area is quite small, as much of the nerve territory is overlapped by supply from adjacent nerves. Destruction of a mixed nerve leads to vasomotor and trophic disturbances, probably related to damage to sympathetic fibres. The anaesthetic skin is dry, does not produce sweat and, when injured, heals slowly. Oedema and cold sensitivity are also recognized. After complete division recovery is enhanced by surgical repair using fine sutures and magnification. However, even with most careful surgery, results are often disappointing.

• *Axonotmesis*: an injury in which the connective tissue survives but most of the axons of the nerve are damaged and Wallerian degeneration occurs. These injuries produce symptoms similar to neurotmesis but their prognosis is better.

• *Neuropraxia*: a minimal lesion producing paralysis without peripheral nerve degeneration. The commonest cause is pressure. As the nerve remains in continuity and tissue damage is incomplete, recovery occurs fairly rapidly. It is important that the muscles and joints in the distribution of the nerve distal to injury are kept mobile so that rehabilitation, once recovery is established, is feasible.

The factors which influence recovery following nerve injury are summarized in Table 11.1.

Specific nerve injuries

Examination of all peripheral nerves can be considered under three headings: sensory loss, motor loss and trophic changes. An understanding of the anatomy of nerve supply is essential to understanding the lesions produced. The common upper limb nerve injuries are summarized in Table 11.2.

Table 11.1 Factors which adversely affect nerve recovery following injury.

Older patients
More proximal levels of nerve injury
Injury caused by excessive trauma
Injuries to mixed nerves
Increasing distance between the nerve ends at the time of repair
Need to use nerve graft in repair

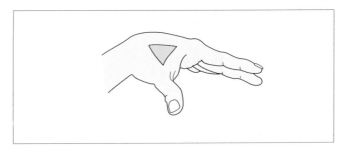

Figure 11.2 In radial nerve injury there is a characteristic wristdrop due to paralysis of the extensors of the wrist. There is only a very small area of anaesthesia at the base of the thumb and index finger as there is considerable sensory overlap from the median and ulnar nerves.

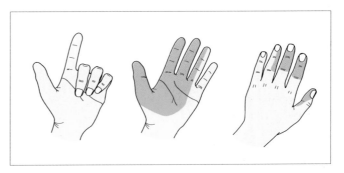

Figure 11.3 In high median nerve lesions the flexors of the wrist and fingers will be paralysed, except those supplied by the ulnar nerve, i.e. flexor carpi ulnaris and the medial half of flexor digitorum profundus. Thus, when the patient attempts to flex the fingers, the index finger remains extended (the pointing sign). With high and low lesions there will be failure to abduct and oppose the thumb, resulting in a simian or ape-like hand. Wasting of the muscles of the thenar eminence will be pronounced in all median nerve lesions. There will be sensory loss to the palmar surface of the lateral $3\frac{1}{2}$ fingers and from the proximal interphalangeal joint distally on the dorsal surface of the same fingers.

Table 11.2 The clinical features of some common upper limb peripheral nerve injuries.

	Cause	Motor	Sensory	Trophic
Brachial plexus injury				
Complete	Motor cycle accidents	Complete arm paralysis	Complete arm anaesthesia	Muscle wasting
Upper (C4–6; Erb/Duchenne)	Motor cycle accident/ obstetric injury	Limb assumes 'waiter's tip' position	Decreased sensation over outer upper arm	Muscle wasting
Lower (C7, 8, T1; (Klumpke)	Cervical rib/shoulder dislocation	Paralysis of the small muscles of the hand (may be a Horner's syndrome)	Sensory loss of inner side forearm and medial $3\frac{1}{2}$ fingers	Wasting of muscles in hand
Radial nerve injury (see Fig. 11.2)				
	Mid-shaft fracture of humerus 'Saturday night' palsy (falling asleep with arm draped over the back of a chair!)	Wristdrop	Anaesthesia of a small area at the base of the thumb and index finger	Minimal wasting of long wrist extensors
Median nerve injury (see Fig. 11.3)				
At the elbow	Fracture of lower end of humerus Elbow dislocation	'Pointing' index finger and 'simian hand' (loss of abduction and opposition of the thumb)	Sensory loss over all palmar aspect and distal dorsal aspect of radial $3\frac{1}{2}$ fingers	Thenar eminence wasting
At the wrist	Lacerations	Simian hand		Thenar eminence wasting
Ulnar nerve injury (see Fig. 11.4)				
At the elbow	Fracture of medial epicondyle of the humerus	Claw hand (*main en griffe*)	Palmar and dorsal medial $1\frac{1}{2}$ fingers	Wasting of all
At the wrist	Lacerations	Marked claw hand	Palmar and dorsal medial $1\frac{1}{2}$ fingers	small muscles of the hand apart from the thenar eminence

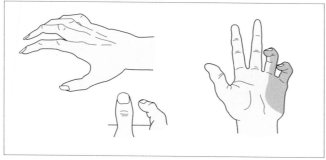

(a)

Figure 11.4 (a) Injury to the ulnar nerve produces a classical deformity known as claw hand or *main en griffe*. This occurs with both high and low lesions but the deformity is much more pronounced with *low* lesions. The clawed appearance results from the unopposed actions of the long extensors and flexors of the fingers. Wasting of all of the small muscles of the hand (except the muscles of the thenar eminence) occurs and is seen most easily on the dorsum of the hand. (Weakness of the adductor pollicis accounts for *Froment's sign*: if the patient holds a piece of paper between the thumb and fingers, the terminal phalanx of the thumb of the affected hand flexes due to the unopposed action of flexor pollicis longus.) Sensory loss is to the medial $1\frac{1}{2}$ fingers and affects both the dorsal and palmar surfaces.

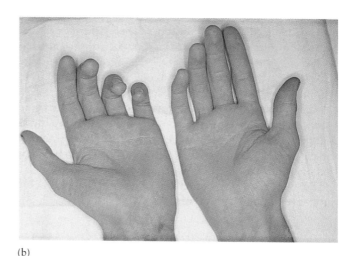

(b)

Figure 11.4 (b) A typical low ulnar nerve lesion. Note the scar at the wrist.

Sciatic nerve injuries

The sciatic nerve may be injured by penetrating trauma (e.g. an 'intramuscular' injection) or a posterior dislocation of the hip. There is paralysis of the hamstring muscles and all of the muscle groups below the knee. Only the muscles of the anterior compartment of the thigh are unaffected (as they are supplied by the femoral nerve). Sensory loss is also extensive, with complete anaesthesia below the knee except for a narrow strip along the medial side supplied by the long saphenous branch of the femoral nerve.

The common peroneal branch of the sciatic nerve is at risk of injury as it winds around the neck of the fibula. Unfortunately, this nerve often suffers iatrogenic injury either from too tight a plaster cast or from inadequate protection from pressure while the patient is under anaesthesia. Clinically, the patient has footdrop and anaesthesia on the dorsum of the foot. Most pressure-induced injuries are neuropraxias and as long as the paralysed part is managed carefully (by skin care, massage, passive joint movement and the use of spring-loaded 'lively' splints), a good outcome can be expected.

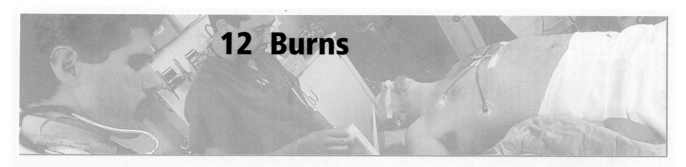

12 Burns

The Lord himself is thy keeper: the Lord is thy defence upon thy right hand;
So that the sun shall not burn thee by day: neither the moon by night.   (The Book of Common Prayer, Psalms cxxxi.5)

Introduction

Burns and scalds are commonly seen in Accident and Emergency departments throughout the UK. The actual incidence can only be estimated from data published by the Department of Health. However, in 1981 over 10 000 people required hospital admission for burns in England and Wales, of whom approximately half were children. More recently, a national burns database has been commenced which should give a more accurate picture.

In casualty departments and in burns centres it is now possible to treat all burned patients aggressively, so that they survive the shock period. However, where there is a significant risk of an individual (of any age) succumbing from the burn injury (see Prognosis, below), an overall assessment should be made to determine whether treatment should be aggressive or symptomatic. Important factors to be taken into account include:
- age and sex of the patient;
- life expectancy of the patient;
- the distribution of the burn;
- the likely outcome in terms of quality of life; and
- family and social circumstances.

In some instances it may be more humane to treat the patient symptomatically and allow him or her to die with dignity rather than attempting a futile, aggressive approach. However, such a decision should be made by senior, experienced personnel, and only after wide consultation.

Causes of burns

Thermal injury

Burns may be caused in a variety of ways. The most commonly encountered aetiology is by thermal energy, which is of two types:
- *Dry heat*: Direct contact with a hot object, e.g. the glowing element of an electric fire, or from a flame (Fig. 12.1).

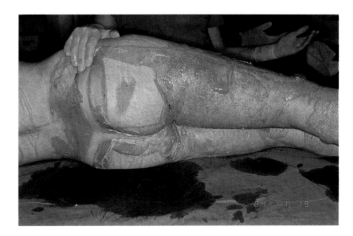

Figure 12.1 Superficial burns of buttocks and legs sustained when the patient's clothing caught fire.

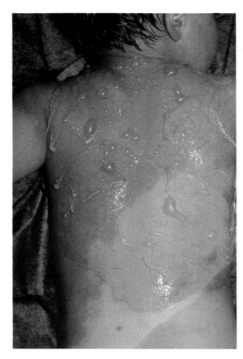

Figure 12.2 An extensive scald from hot water on the back of a child.

• *Moist heat*: Hot liquids (or vapours such as steam) give rise to scalds (Fig. 12.2).

Electrical burns

The majority of electrical burns are caused by accidents in the home involving the domestic electricity supply at

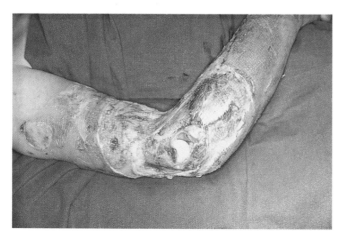

Figure 12.3 An electrical burn through the elbow joint. Note the extensive tissue destruction.

220–250 V. High-voltage injuries are less common, but in all cases several factors have to be considered (Fig. 12.3).

• Flash burns can occur when there is no actual contact with the electricity supply, and are usually superficial.

• When there has been contact, the damage caused is from passage of the current through the body. The severity of the injury depends on the *strength of the current*, the *duration of contact* and the *electrical resistance* of the body. Thus, the injury will be greater when there is a strong current, with prolonged contact and decreased electrical resistance (e.g. if the body is wet).

• The current passes through the body via an entry and exit point. Sometimes only one of these points is obvious, and so the entire body surface should be examined if both points are not immediately apparent, to avoid missing a significant burn in an area hidden by clothing or on the undersurface of a limb.

• As the current passes from the skin surface into the deeper tissues, progressively less damage is inflicted, although structures such as vessels, and especially nerves, can conduct the current more effectively, with potentially serious sequelae.

• The conducting system of the heart may be affected, and in all cases an electrocardiogram should be taken. In some cases cardiac monitoring will be required.

• Unlike thermal burns, electrical burns do not have a clear zone of demarcation. Surrounding the area of visible damage there is a zone of less obvious damage, which may not be necrotic, but the healing ability of this tissue is impaired. Surgical excision of the electrical burn will frequently involve debridement of deeper tissues along the track of the burn, and excision of a rim of tissue around the edges to incorporate the zone of partial damage.

• Appropriate flap cover or reconstruction is generally required for all but the smallest burns.

Chemical burns

Industrial accidents are the usual cause of chemical burns. Rarer causes are domestic accidents (e.g. spilling of caustic cleaners) and chemical warfare. When dealing with chemical burns, it is essential that the substance involved be quickly removed from the affected area, and then the area washed thoroughly under running water. Once this has been done, enquiries can be made regarding a suitable antidote. Some substances, especially alkalis, can penetrate into the skin and deeper tissues and cause continuing injury. These burns are best treated by early surgical excision.

Radiation burns

Radiation burns may be seen after accidental overdosage of radiotherapy or after accidents involving nuclear power.

Unlike thermal burns, there may be a delay before radiation burns become apparent.

- In the acute stage (during the first few days) there may be erythema and blistering of the skin similar to a partial-thickness thermal burn. These burns usually heal, albeit slowly, over a period of several weeks or months.
- With more severe radiation exposure, a chronic injury develops after months or years; the tissues become pale, hard and atrophic, and multiple telangiectases develop in the affected skin. Ulceration, which may become chronic and indolent (with potential for malignant change), may occur. Treatment involves excision of the damaged tissues and cover with a vascularized flap.

Evaluation of burns

History

An accurate history is important when assessing a burn. The history may be available from the patient, from relatives or friends, or from the emergency services. Points to note in the history are:

- the precise time of burning;
- the temperature of the burning agent;
- the length of contact with the burning agent; and
- the possibility of smoke inhalation, or respiratory burns from hot gases.

With scalds it is useful to ask whether the water was freshly boiled or not; if the scald was from tea or coffee, was it black or had it been cooled by the addition of milk?

Physical examination

There should always be a quick initial assessment of severity of the burn, taking in depth, size and distribution (see below). At this time, it should be noted whether there is evidence of burning in areas requiring special consideration:

- soot in the nose, singed nostril hairs: smoke inhalation/respiratory burn;
- carbonaceous sputum: smoke inhalation/respiratory burn;
- burns inside the mouth, hoarse voice: need for intubation/tracheostomy;
- burns to the eyes or eyelids: ophthalmological opinion/early surgery;
- circumferential burns or eschar: need for escharotomy.

Burn depth

Burns in the past have been described in various ways. First-, second- and third-degree burns was one popular categorization, but unfortunately there are now several classifications

with a varying number of degrees, ranging from two to six. To overcome this confusion a simple descriptive terminology has evolved:

- a *partial-thickness* burn indicates a superficial burn that will heal with conservative measures;
- a *full-thickness burn* indicates a burn that will require new skin cover by surgical intervention.

However, life is never that simple! Partial-thickness burns can be subdivided into *superficial* and *deep dermal* burns and a mixed picture of full- and partial-thickness burns (*mixed-thickness burns*) can also be seen.

Partial-thickness burns

Superficial burns Simple erythema (e.g. sunburn) always indicates a superficial burn, and will settle spontaneously without scarring. Slightly more thermal damage produces blistering with loss of the superficial layers of the skin. However, the skin remains pink and moist and sensation will be intact. The pinprick test is used to determine whether the nerve endings in the skin have (full-thickness burn) or have not (partial-thickness burn) been damaged. Unfortunately, this test is not absolutely reliable; a positive test shows that living cells must be present but a negative test is not always indicative of a full-thickness burn. A completely dependable method of assessing burn depth is still not available and even in the most experienced hands the depth of a burn can be misjudged.

Superficial burns heal by re-epithelialization of the area from surviving germinal layer cells or from epithelial structures such as hair follicles and sweat glands. An excellent cosmetic result can usually be expected with minimal or no scarring.

Deep dermal burns A deep dermal burn is a partial-thickness burn that extends into the dermis, but is not actually a full-thickness burn; only deeper hair follicles or sweat glands remain. The burn usually has a whitish appearance initially (Fig. 12.4). The diagnosis becomes clearer at 10–14 days when the slough begins to separate. At this stage mottling and 'fat-domes' (i.e. areas where the subcutaneous tissue protrudes through holes in the dermis) become visible. Deep dermal burns will eventually heal on their own, but with a scar that may become hypertrophied. They often do better with tangential excision and skin grafting.

Mixed-thickness burns The majority of burns consist of areas of partial- and full-thickness injury, reflecting gradations in the intensity and distribution of the thermal injury. Classically, these burns were treated by dressings for 2–3 weeks to allow superficial areas to heal and deeper areas to

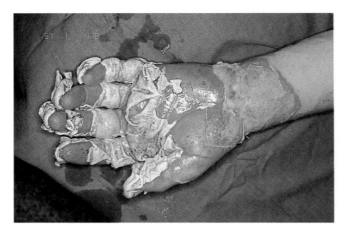

Figure 12.4 Deep dermal burn of the left hand. As the white slough separates, healthy but delicate new skin is exposed underneath.

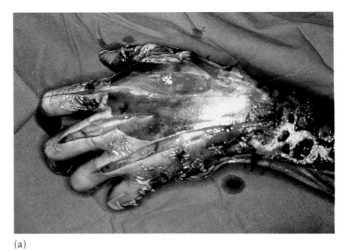

(a)

(b)

Figure 12.5 (a) Full-thickness burn of the left hand with escharotomies. (b) A charred leg following burning in a house fire.

demarcate. This approach ensured that excision of potentially viable tissue was kept to a minimum. However, some surgeons advocate early tangential excision and skin grafting, pointing to the advantages of reduced time to healing, reduced hospital stay and a superior final result. Early tangential excision and grafting are currently used in special areas such as hands, although with improvements in surgical techniques, skin culture and use of homo- and xenografts, this treatment may become more widespread in the future.

Full-thickness burns

By definition the whole thickness of the skin is destroyed in a full-thickness burn, but deeper structures such as fat, muscle and even bone can be involved if the causal agent or circumstances are of sufficient severity. On examination, there is characteristically a numb, hard, leathery, yellow-brown eschar with thrombosed veins (Fig. 12.5). Granulation tissue forms under the slough, and epithelialization can only occur by ingrowth from the wound edges. In time, scar tissue is laid down, and wound contracture takes place, resulting in deformity that can be severely disabling, in both appearance and function.

Unless the area involved is small, surgical excision and skin grafting are essential (Fig. 12.6).

Burn area

Assessment of the burn size is important; patients with a burn of 15% of the total body surface area (10% in the case of children) require resuscitation and intravenous fluids. An approximate estimate of burn size can be rapidly made using the rule of nines devised by Wallace in 1951 Fig. 12.7).

Simple erythema should not be included in the calculation, and it is useful to remember that the palm and closed fingers of the patient's hand represent approximately 1% of total surface area. Lund and Browder charts are widely available, and these allow an accurate estimation of burn size, taking into account varying percentages for the head and lower limb in children, and incorporating recording of the proportion of partial- to full-thickness burn.

Investigations

In general, no special investigations need to be performed on burned patients unless an inhalational injury is suspected. A full blood count and urea and electrolytes (U & E)

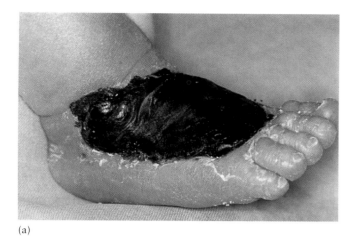

(a)

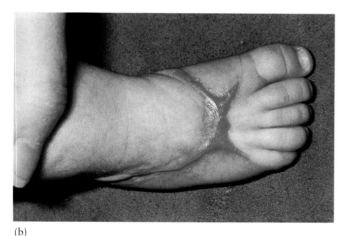

(b)

Figure 12.6 (a) Full-thickness burn on the dorsum of a child's foot. (b) The burn eschar was removed and the wound allowed to heal, leaving hypertrophic scars and scar contracture on the dorsum of the foot.

will probably indicate dehydration with a high haemoglobin, haematocrit and urea. Serum should be sent for grouping and cross-matching as blood may be required later. A chest X-ray, blood gases and carbon monoxide estimation should be obtained for suspected inhalational injury and bronchoscopy may also be indicated in these patients. Patients who have sustained electrical burns require an electrocardiogram and cardiac enzyme estimation.

Management of burns

The criteria for admission of a patient with burns to hospital or a burns unit are given in Box 12.1.

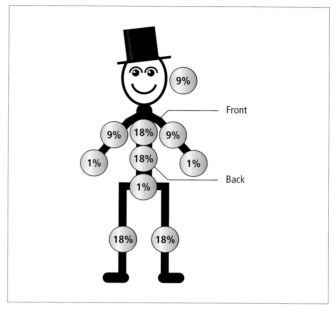

Figure 12.7 Rule of nines.

Admission criteria for a patient with burns

Major burn injury
- Should be treated in a burns unit
- Partial-thickness burns > 25% of body surface area in adults
  > 20% of body surface area in children
- Full-thickness burns > 10% of body surface area
- Burns involving sensitive areas: hands, feet, face, eyes, perineum
- Burns with significant inhalational injury
- Electrical burns

Moderate burn injury
- Should be admitted to hospital but not necessarily a burns unit
- Partial-thickness burns 15–25% of body surface area in adults
  10–20% of body surface area in children
- Full-thickness burns 2–10% of body surface area

Minor burn injury
- Can be treated as an outpatient
- Partial-thickness burns < 15% of body surface area in adults
  < 10% of body surface area in children
- Full-thickness burns < 2% of body surface area

Box 12.1 Criteria for admission of a patient with burns to hospital or a burns unit.

Minor burns

A minor burn is one that does not require intravenous resuscitation or emergency measures. However, a patient with a minor burn may still require hospitalization, e.g. if the dressings cannot be managed at home, or the burn is in an awkward area requiring specialist assistance or monitoring. There are broadly two methods of treating burns: by exposure and with dressings.

Exposure

After local cleaning and removal of loose skin, the area of the burn is left exposed to the air and allowed to dry. For this type of therapy it is essential that the treatment environment should be clean, and often this means admitting the patient to a special burns unit bed. Most departments treat burns of the face in this way, and sometimes awkward areas such as the perineum are treated similarly.

Dressings

Dressings are applied to burns for a number of reasons:
- absorption of burn wound exudate;
- application of antibiotic/antiseptic to the wound surface; and
- to act as a mechanical barrier to infection.

Two dressings commonly used for the management of burns are:
- *Tulle gras impregnated with chlorhexidine* which is placed against the burn surface and surrounded by an absorptive bandage incorporating gauze and wool. The outer layer can be changed as necessary when the exudate soaks through.
- *Silver sulphadiazine* cream applied directly to the burn surface surrounded by an absorptive layer of gauze. This preparation has good antibacterial activity against Gram-negative organisms, particularly *Pseudomonas aeruginosa*, and has the added advantage of providing topical analgesia to the burned area. Disadvantages include the fact that the skin can become macerated and discoloured with deposition of silver, giving rise to difficulty in burn depth assessment, and that fairly frequent dressing changes are required. Burns of the hands (and often feet) are now invariably treated by placing the hand in a polythene bag after local application of silver sulphadiazine cream. This retains the cream in contact with the burn while simultaneously allowing optimal mobilization of the digits.

Surgery

Areas of full-thickness or deep partial-thickness burns are debrided using a skin-graft knife or dermatome and split-skin grafts are then applied. Skin grafts are normally inspected for 'take' and stability at 5 days, unless there is sufficient cause for concern (e.g. from infection) to prompt inspection earlier. The skin grafts are usually perforated using a mesher before application. This improves contouring of the graft to the bed, allows blood and exudate to escape between the interstices of the mesh, and if necessary allows the graft to be expanded by opening up the interstices and allowing a larger area of the wound to be covered than would otherwise have been possible.

Major burns

Burns can be considered to be major when they require urgent intravenous resuscitation, or emergency procedures to be carried out, or both. In adults, a 15% surface area burn and in children a 10% surface area burn require intravenous resuscitation.

Burn shock

After sustaining a major burn, a patient can arrive at the hospital in a relatively good condition. This can be deceptive and resuscitative measures should be instituted without delay to prevent 'burn shock' from developing.

The surface of the skin may be destroyed to a varying extent from the thermal injury, but beneath this there will be a zone of injury where cells have not been completely devitalized. This results in inflammation, oedema, increased capillary permeability and fluid loss in the form of exudate. This fluid is similar in composition to plasma, but with less protein. Rapid fluid shifts and fluid losses can occur, resulting in *hypovolaemic shock* (see Chapter 4). The main clinical features to look for are:
- complaints of feeling cold;
- intense thirst;
- pallor and sweating;
- hypotension with a weak, thready, rapid pulse; and
- 'air hunger'.

Initial resuscitation

Patients with a major burn require a number of procedures and investigations upon arrival at the hospital, and these should be performed without delay:
- The airway should be checked and intubation (rarely, tracheostomy) performed if necessary.
- Reliable intravenous access should be obtained and an infusion commenced (see below). Occasionally a central venous line is necessary, particularly in cases with suspected renal damage. However, central lines are not utilized routinely because of the risk of introducing infection.
- A urinary catheter should be passed to monitor hourly urinary output. Urine concentration measurements (osmo-

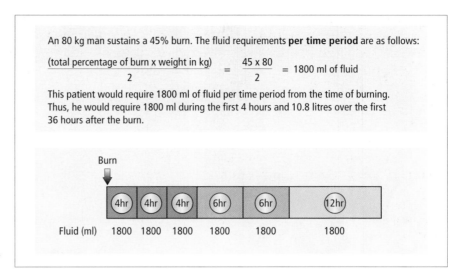

An 80 kg man sustains a 45% burn. The fluid requirements **per time period** are as follows:

$$\frac{(\text{total percentage of burn x weight in kg})}{2} = \frac{45 \times 80}{2} = 1800 \text{ ml of fluid}$$

This patient would require 1800 ml of fluid per time period from the time of burning. Thus, he would require 1800 ml during the first 4 hours and 10.8 litres over the first 36 hours after the burn.

Burn

4hr	4hr	4hr	6hr	6hr	12hr

Fluid (ml)   1800   1800   1800   1800   1800   1800

Figure 12.8 Muir and Barclay formula for fluid requirements of a burned patient.

lality) can be useful. The presence of haemoglobinuria is indicative of deep burns, and/or renal damage.

• The burn wound should be quickly assessed, and then as soon as possible, covered with a sterile dressing to minimize contamination and to prevent further damage. Saline or povidone-iodine (Betadine)-soaked gauze is satisfactory, and also helps to relieve pain.

• The temperature, pulse rate and blood pressure should be ascertained and recorded. The investigations listed above should be performed.

• Intravenous analgesia should be given, especially if the patient is restless.

• The use of antibiotic prophylaxis is disputed, but there is a mortality associated with staphylococcal toxic shock syndrome, particularly in children, and this has led to a wider acceptance of the early use of antibiotics, even in smaller burns.

• If the patient has nausea and vomiting, a nasogastric tube should be passed, and subsequent hourly aspirates recorded.

Fluid therapy

The time at which the burn occurred should be ascertained, and all calculations are derived from this, not from the time of arrival at the hospital. Various formulae have been developed in order to aid assessment of fluid losses and the requirement for fluids during the resuscitation period. All these formulae are guides only, and the clinician should frequently reassess the condition of the patient. The prime objective of resuscitation in all forms of shock is to restore and maintain tissue perfusion. The fluid that is being lost in the burn exudate is similar to plasma, and there is controversy as to whether the replacement fluid should be colloid, crystalloid, or a mixture of the two.

One commonly used formula is the Muir and Barclay formula (Fig. 12.8), in which the immediate postburn period is divided into six intervals or rations, during which equal volumes of fluid, usually colloid, are given.

The patient described in the example in Fig. 12.8 would require 1800 ml of fluid over the first 4 h after injury, at an hourly rate of 450 ml/h. However, it is important to remember that the fluid requirement has to be estimated *from the time of the burn*. Thus, if the patient was admitted to hospital 2 h after the burn, there would be a $(450 \times 2) = 900$ ml deficit to be made up. Hence the calculated rate of infusion for the first hour after *admission* would be:

900 ml deficit + 450 ml for the third hour itself = 1350 ml/h

The rate of infusion for the second hour after admission (fourth hour from injury) will be 450 ml/h. From this simple example it is obvious that substantial volumes of fluid need to be given to patients after major burns, and while the formula provides a rule-of-thumb guide to the fluid requirements, it is no substitute for close haemodynamic monitoring and frequent assessment.

Composition of the resuscitation fluid

There is some controversy as to what fluid should be used when resuscitating a burned patient. The exudate from the burn resembles plasma but has a slightly lower protein content. Therefore, one would assume that the ideal resuscitation fluid would be plasma. However, plasma is not always easily obtained and it is expensive. Thus, several regimes consisting of varying proportions of crystalloid

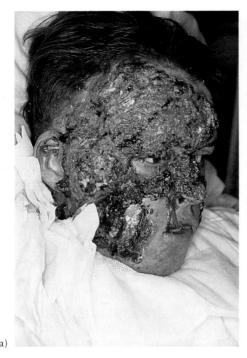
(a)

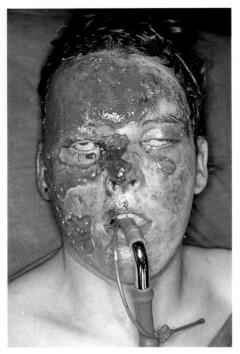
(b)

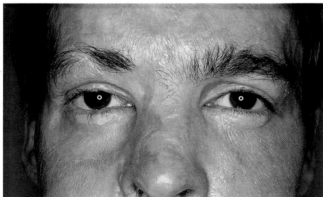
(c)

Figure 12.9 (a) Infected eschar following burns to the face; (b) the eschar has now been excised completely and the wound is ready to be grafted; (c) final result 2 years later.

(Ringer lactate) and colloid (plasma or 4.5% human albumin solution) have been proposed. Many burns in North America are managed with a mixture of crystalloid and colloid; the crystalloid is given over the first 24 h and the colloid (often plasma) after that. Most burns units in the UK utilize the Muir and Barclay formula as a guide to resuscitation and use more colloid than crystalloid. Human albumin solution (HAS) is the most commonly used colloid.

• The daily (metabolic) water requirement of the patient should not be forgotten and other fluid losses, such as from nasogastric aspiration, should be replaced, in addition to the burn fluid requirements calculated via the formula.

• Inevitably, red cells are lost from a burn and need to be replaced. Unfortunately, there is no easy guide to replacement but a general rule-of-thumb is to give 1 unit of blood for every 10% of deep burn area.

• Burned patients become hypermetabolic and require supplemental feeding, usually administered as enteral feeding.

Management of the burn wound

As with all potentially shocked patients, analgesia should be administered *intravenously*. Burned patients are usually in a lot of pain and opiates will often be required to achieve adequate pain relief. After resuscitation the burn wound should be washed with water and loose tissue and blisters debrided. A topical antimicrobial agent should be applied and the wounds treated in a suitable environment. As soon as possible (i.e. when the patient is stable at about 48 h postburn), full-thickness burns should be excised and grafted (Fig. 12.9). However, with very large burns the extent of excision may be limited by the availability of autologous donor skin for grafting. In this situation the skin graft mesher is particularly useful (Fig. 12.10). Physiotherapy should be commenced early in the management of the burned patient so that function is maintained and contractures are avoided.

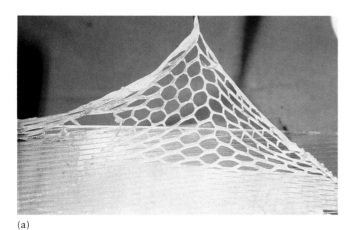

(a)

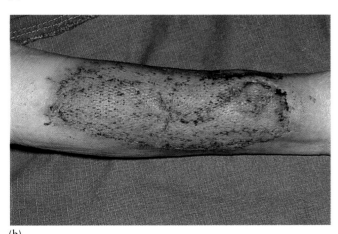

(b)

Figure 12.10 (a) Meshed split-skin graft. Following harvesting of split-skin graft, the graft is passed through a skin graft mesher. The graft mesh can easily be expanded to cover large areas of skin loss. (b) Recently applied meshed skin graft.

Complications of burns

Infection in burns

Infection is a major hazard in burned patients. As a result, superficial burns can be converted into full-thickness burns, split-skin grafts can be destroyed (especially by Streptococci) and systemic infection can be life-threatening. In most burns units regular inspection and swabbing of wounds are now undertaken and invasive infection is diagnosed when 10^6 or more microorganisms are present in the wound. Some units give systemic antibiotics (e.g. penicillin) routinely to burned patients, while others rely on topical antimicrobial agents (e.g. silver sulphadiazine cream) and only give systemic antibiotics if an invasive infection is diagnosed. Early excision and grafting of the burn would minimize the risk of wound infection.

In the past, tetanus was sometimes seen following burns and it should be remembered that all burned patients should receive appropriate tetanus prophylaxis (see Chapter 30).

Limb ischaemia

Circumferential full-thickness burns act like a tourniquet on a limb and can compromise the circulation to the limb distal to the burn. If there is any doubt about the perfusion of the limb, the circumferential burn should be divided by making an incision through the full thickness of the wound on the medial and lateral aspects of the extremity. This is known as *escharotomy* (Fig. 12.5a).

Curling's ulcer

In the past gastric and duodenal ulcers and erosive gastritis were common in patients with burns. The association between these ulcers and burns was first made by Curling in 1842. The incidence of this problem is very low today because of better resuscitation of the burned patient, avoidance of sepsis and appropriate prophylaxis (i.e. administration of antacids or H_2 blockers; see also Chapter 28).

Burns contractures

Contractures are common after serious burn injury and, if not managed aggressively, may lead to serious loss of joint function, e.g. burns of the hand (Fig. 12.11) or around the axilla frequently cause contractures such that abduction of the arm and movement of the shoulder are seriously impeded. The best way to prevent contractures is by a programme of physiotherapy instituted almost immediately

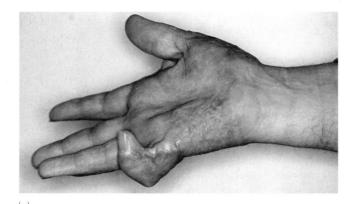

(a)

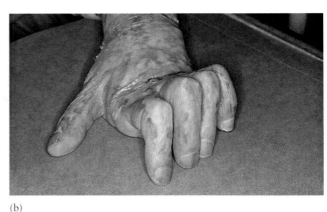

(b)

Figure 12.11 (a) Severe contracture following a burn to the dorsum of the hand; (b) very bad scar contracture of the little finger following a full-thickness burn.

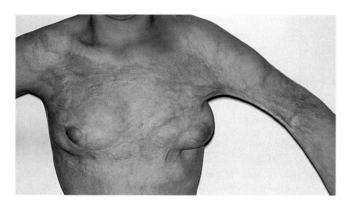

Figure 12.12 Scar contractures of the axilla frequently impede shoulder movement. Vigorous physiotherapy started almost immediately after the burn may help to modify the extent of contracture.

after the burn (Fig. 12.12). Hypertrophic scars may also develop following burns (Fig. 12.13). These may be prevented by the application of compression garments during the recovery period.

Prognosis

The prognosis following a burn depends on:
- the depth and extent of the burn;
- the age of the patient; and
- the development of complications.

Thus, the very old and the very young do badly. Patients over 65 years with a 25% burn have a very poor prognosis.

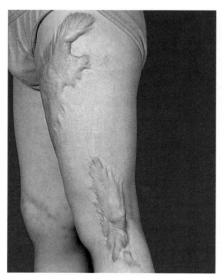

(a)

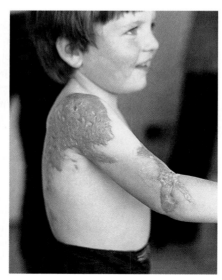

(b)

Figure 12.13 Hypertrophic scars on (a) a leg and (b) around the axilla following burns.

Some young patients have survived a greater than 70% burn but this is the exception rather than the rule. An approximate rule-of-thumb is to *sum the percentage of the burn* and the *age of the patient in years* to give the probability of death. For example, the probable mortality from a 25% burn in a 35-year-old patient would be approximately 25 + 35 = 60% or 0.6. From this, it can be seen that in the elderly, even quite trivial burns can be fatal, although

death may not be immediate, as the probability figures indicate the likelihood of eventual demise of the burned patient.

For those who do survive a major burn, life is not easy. Most are disfigured and have problems with contractures. However, with multidisciplinary rehabilitation programmes 90% of patients have been able to return to gainful employment and achieve a good quality of life.

Burns at a glance

DEFINITION

A *burn* is the response of the skin and subcutaneous tissues to thermal injury. A *partial-thickness* burn is a superficial burn which usually heals with conservative management. A *full-thickness* burn requires excision and skin grafting

CAUSES

- Thermal injury from dry (flame, hot metal) or moist (hot liquids or gases) heat sources
- Electricity (deep burns at entry and exit sites, may cause cardiac arrest)
- Chemicals (usually industrial accidents with acid or alkali)
- Radiation (partial-thickness initially but may progress to chronic deeper injury)

CLINICAL FEATURES

General
- Pain
- Swelling and blistering

Specific
- Evidence of smoke inhalation (soot in nose or sputum, burns in the mouth, hoarseness)
- Eye or eyelid burns (early ophthalmological opinion)
- Circumferential burns (will need escharotomy)

INVESTIGATIONS

- FBC, U&E
- If inhalation suspected:
  (a) Chest X-ray
  (b) Arterial blood gases
  (c) Carbon monoxide

- Group and cross-match
- ECG/cardiac enzymes with electrical burns

MANAGEMENT

General
- Start resuscitation (**ABC**, set up good IV lines, give oxygen)
- Assess size of burn (Wallace rule-of-nines)
  (a) Major > 15% burn in adult, > 10% in child
  (b) Minor < 15% burn in adult, < 10% in child

Major burns
- Monitor pulse, BP, temperature, urinary output, give adequate analgesia IV, pass nasogastric tube, tetanus prophylaxis
- Give IV fluids according to Muir/Barclay formula:
  $$\frac{\% \text{ burn} \times \text{weight in kg}}{2} = \text{one aliquot of fluid.}$$
  Give six aliquots of fluid over first 36 h in 4–4–4–6–6–12 h sequence from time of burn. Crystalloid and colloid solutions are used
- The burn wound is treated as for minor burns (see text)

Minor burns
- Rx by exposure–debride wound and leave exposed in special clean environment
- Rx by dressings–cover with tulle gras impregnated with chlorhexidine or silver sulphadiazine under absorptive gauze dressings
- Debridement of eschar and split-skin grafting

COMPLICATIONS

- Infection (beware the streptococcus). Treat established infection (10^6 organisms present in wound biopsy) with systemic antibiotics
- Limb ischaemia from circumferential burn (prevent by escharotomy)
- Stress ulceration (Curling's ulcer; prevent with antacid or H_2-blocker prophylaxis)
- Contractures—avoid by early physiotherapy

PART 3 General and Specialist Surgery

13 Digestive Tract Disorders

To eat is human, to digest divine. (Charles T. Copeland, 1860–1952)

Introduction

Diseases of the gastrointestinal tract are very common and almost everyone will have symptoms of gastrointestinal upset at some time during life. It has been estimated that digestive diseases account for more hospital admissions than any other disease category. Gastrointestinal symptoms may indicate relatively benign disease (e.g. rectal bleeding with haemorrhoids) or may be the herald of serious pathology (e.g. rectal bleeding with rectal carcinoma). The surgeon must therefore obtain a thorough history from the patient, perform a detailed physical examination and form a differential diagnosis. A logical plan of investigation should then be initiated to reveal the underlying pathology. Management strategy will depend on what is revealed.

Evaluation of the patient with gastrointestinal disease

Evaluation of the patient

Clinical assessment

When dealing with a patient with a suspected gastrointestinal disorder it is best to let the patient give the story of the problem before asking about specific symptoms. General points to be considered in the history are:
- past and family history;
- smoking and alcohol history;
- foreign travel;
- urinary symptoms (Chapter 20); and
- menstrual and gynaecological history.

Symptoms

The main symptoms of gastrointestinal disease are given in Table 13.1.
- *Dysphagia*: This term is used to signify difficulty in swallowing. The patient usually indicates that food sticks somewhere retrosternally and often will volunteer a history of specific foods (usually solids) causing dysphagia. The common causes of dysphagia are given in Table 13.2.
- *Heartburn and regurgitation*: Heartburn is usually described as a substernal burning sensation, often occurring after meals and often associated with an acidic or bitter

Table 13.1 Symptoms of gastrointestinal disease.

Dysphagia
Heartburn and regurgitation
Retrosternal pain
Abdominal pain
Weight loss and anorexia
Nausea and vomiting
Altered bowel habit
Rectal bleeding and perianal symptoms
Jaundice

Table 13.2 Common causes of dysphagia.

Tumours of the oesophagus or cardia
Peptic oesophagitis with stricture
Corrosive stricture
Primary motility disorders of the oesophagus
Scleroderma
Extrinsic compression from bronchial tumours
Pharyngeal pouch

taste in the mouth (regurgitation). Lying or stooping tends to exacerbate the symptoms. Heartburn is a manifestation of gastro-oesophageal reflux or peptic ulcer disease.
- *Retrosternal pain*: This symptom is classically associated with cardiac disease but patients with oesophageal disease (primary motility disorders and gastro-oesophageal reflux) may also present with severe retrosternal pain.
- *Abdominal pain*: This is a common symptom of gastrointestinal pathology and most diseases of the abdominal organs are associated with abdominal pain. Abdominal pain may be acute or chronic and three types of pain are recognized: visceral, somatic and referred pain. *Visceral pain* is caused by stretching or contracting hollow organs and is usually colicky in nature. *Somatic pain* is produced by irritation of the parietal peritoneum and is usually continuous. *Referred pain* is the perception of pain in an area of the body distant to the site of origin of the pain, e.g. lower abdominal pain with testicular torsion.

A number of specific pieces of information need to be obtained when taking a history from a patient with abdominal pain:

(a) *Type of pain* Colicky pain usually indicates hyperperistalsis which may be caused by an obstructive process (e.g. intestinal obstruction, biliary colic, ureteric colic) or an infective process (e.g. gastroenteritis). Typically, colicky pain comes in waves, mounts to a crescendo and then passes off for a period (usually minutes) before the cycle starts again. Colicky pain is often associated with nausea, vomiting or diarrhoea and is not relieved by altering position. It makes the patient restless.

Continuous pain usually indicates parietal peritoneal irritation (e.g. peritonitis) and may be described as 'burning', 'boring', 'sharp' or 'stabbing' by the patient. Nausea and vomiting may occur and the pain is usually made worse by shifting positions. Thus, the patient tends to lie still.

(b) *Onset of pain* The onset of pain may give important clues as to its origin. A perforated viscus will produce sudden intense continuous pain; an episode of pancreatitis will induce continuous pain of gradual onset while ureter colic will produce sudden severe colicky pain. Intestinal obstruction usually induces gradual-onset colicky abdominal pain.

(c) *Site of pain* The site of onset of the pain often gives a clue as to the anatomical structure most likely to be involved (Fig. 13.1).

In general, foregut structures cause upper abdominal pain, midgut structures produce central abdominal pain, while hindgut structures give rise to lower abdominal pain. Often visceral-type pain precedes somatic pain so that the site of pain may change with the progress of the disease, e.g. diverticulitis may initially present with lower abdominal pain which later becomes localized to the left iliac fossa.

Diffuse abdominal pain is not uncommon and in this situation the patient is unable to localize the pain to any one area. There are several causes for diffuse abdominal pain,

e.g. peritonitis (see below), non-specific abdominal pain, mesenteric adenitis, mesenteric ischaemia, sickle-cell crisis, leukaemia, porphyria and diabetes mellitus.

(d) *Radiation of pain* Radiation of pain from its site of onset to other areas often gives important clues as to the cause. Biliary pain radiates from the right upper quadrant around the back on the right side. Pain extending into the back indicates retroperitoneal pathology, e.g. pancreatitis, a penetrating posterior duodenal ulcer, leaking abdominal aortic aneurysm. Renal or ureteric pain radiates from the loin into the groin and genitalia while testicular pain may radiate to the iliac fossa and be confused with appendicitis.

(e) *Duration and periodicity* Acute abdominal pain is defined as pain for less than 6 h. Such pain is usually severe and usually has a fairly obvious cause. The elucidation of the cause of chronic abdominal pain is much more difficult and often requires great clinical skill. Periodicity refers to the time pattern of the pain — monthly, twice-yearly with no pain in between, etc. Peptic ulcer pain classically exhibits periodicity. The patient complains of pain for days or weeks with long painfree spells, usually lasting months.

(f) *Relieving and exacerbating factors* Position, food and drugs are the three factors usually involved. *Position* has no effect on colicky pain and in fact patients with colicky pain keep altering their position in an attempt to relieve the pain. Patients with somatic pain tend to find the most

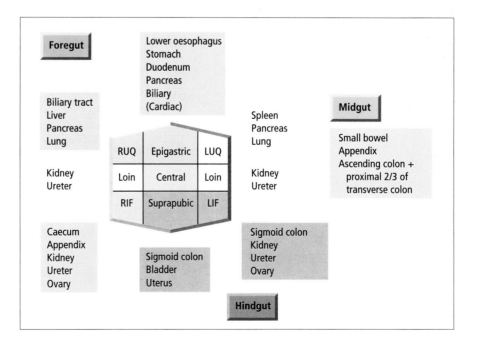

Figure 13.1 Clinical regions of the abdomen.

comfortable position and remain in that position; classically patients with pancreatitis find that sitting forward gives the most comfort. *Food* may exacerbate (e.g. gastric ulcer) or relieve (e.g. duodenal ulcer) pain and certain foods may provoke an episode of pain (e.g. fatty foods may induce biliary colic). Pain lasting for a number of hours after eating any meal may indicate mesenteric ischaemia (mesenteric angina). *Drugs* may affect pain. Anti-inflammatory drugs will exacerbate peptic pain but dull the pain of malignancy, while antacids and H_2-receptor antagonists usually relieve peptic ulcer pain.

(g) *Associated symptoms* Associated symptoms such as nausea, vomiting, change in bowel habit, weight loss, anorexia and symptoms of chronic anaemia should be sought.

• *Weight loss and anorexia*: Involuntary weight loss of more than 5% is usually serious and requires investigation. There are several causes of weight loss which must be considered (Table 13.3). However, in spite of extensive investigation no cause can be found for weight loss in a percentage of patients. *Anorexia* is the term used for loss of appetite and is usually found in association with weight loss.

• *Nausea and vomiting*: Nausea is defined as a feeling of an impending desire to vomit while vomiting is the forceful ejection of gastrointestinal content through the mouth. There are numerous causes for nausea and vomiting, some

Table 13.3 Common causes of weight loss.

Gastrointestinal
Malignancies, e.g. carcinoma of the stomach or pancreas
Inflammatory bowel disease, e.g. Crohn's disease
Malabsorption syndromes, e.g. pancreatic disease

Endocrine
Thyrotoxicosis
Diabetes mellitus
Addison's disease

Chronic infection
Hepatitis
Tuberculosis
Fungal and helminthic infections

Immunological
Lymphoma
AIDS

Psychiatric
Depression
Eating disorders, e.g. anorexia nervosa

AIDS, Acquired immunedeficiency syndrome.

Table 13.4 Some common causes of nausea and vomiting.

Any obstruction to the alimentary tract
Visceral pain
Poor gastric emptying, e.g. after surgery
Gastroenteritis
Viral hepatitis
Metabolic disorders, e.g. uraemia
Drugs, e.g. morphine
Vestibular disturbances
Pregnancy
Psychogenic

of which are listed in Table 13.4. Often there are associated symptoms which give a clue as to the cause.

• *Altered bowel habit*: 'Normal' bowel habit varies widely from individual to individual but alterations in bowel habit (i.e. constipation or diarrhoea) are two of the most frequent manifestations of digestive disease.

Constipation is difficult to define but a person who passes easily a formed stool one to three times per day is not constipated. The important fact to note in the history is a *change in pattern* for a given individual. The causes of constipation are myriad but there are a number of common causes:

(a) Acute constipation is usually caused by intestinal obstruction (e.g. due to a bowel carcinoma), which when complete causes absolute constipation (i.e. neither bowel motion nor flatus is passed) and is associated with abdominal distension and vomiting.

(b) Patients with acute anal disease, such as anal fissure (which was probably the result of constipation), will avoid defecation because of pain and thereby set up a vicious cycle.

(c) Chronic constipation may be due to colonic dysmotility (e.g. Hirschsprung's disease, laxative abuse), abnormal defecation (e.g. rectal intussusception) or drugs such as iron or codeine.

Diarrhoea is defined as an increase in the volume, frequency or fluidity of stool. Most people have experienced diarrhoea which lasts for hours or days but diarrhoea lasting for more about 2 weeks is significant. Causes of diarrhoea include:

(a) inflammatory bowel disease (ulcerative colitis and Crohn's disease);

(b) diverticular disease and colon cancer;

(c) infections: bacteria (*Shigella*, *Salmonella*, *Vibrio cholerae*, *Escherichia coli*); parasitic (amoebiasis, giardiasis);

(d) peptides from tumours (vasoactive intestinal polypeptide, serotonin, substance P, calcitonin);

(e) bile acid irritation of the colon after ileal resection;

(f) blind-loop syndrome;

(g) laxative abuse and drugs.

Spurious diarrhoea is diarrhoea in the presence of obstruction. It is commonly seen in patients with faecal impaction. Liquefied stool passes around the obstruction and the patient paradoxically presents with diarrhoea and not constipation.

Steatorrhoea is the passage of stools which contain large amounts of fat. Typically the stool is loose, bulky and offensive. It tends to float and is difficult to flush away. Various malabsorption syndromes are associated with steatorrhoea.

• *Rectal bleeding*: The passage of blood from the back passage is a significant symptom and should be investigated. The commonest cause of rectal bleeding is *haemorrhoids* and typically the blood will be bright red and seen on the toilet tissue or on the toilet bowl. Small amounts of bright red blood associated with excruciating pain while defecating are classical of a *fissure-in-ano*. The most sinister cause of rectal bleeding is a *carcinoma* in the terminal bowel (anus, rectum, sigmoid colon). It may be associated with passage of mucus or pus and often the patient has a sense of incomplete evacuation of the bowel. Inflammatory bowel disease, particularly ulcerative colitis, is often associated with rectal bleeding and tumours sited more proximally in the bowel may also give rise to bleeding (caecal carcinoma frequently presents with an iron-deficiency anaemia secondary to occult chronic blood loss). The passage of fluid, black, offensive stool is *melaena* and indicates rapid blood loss from the proximal gastrointestinal tract (e.g. bleeding peptic ulcer).

• *Perianal symptoms*: Anal or *perianal pain* is caused by perianal abscess, anal fissure, thrombosed external piles or true haemorrhoids if they become strangulated. *Perianal discharge* may be caused by a *fistula-in-ano* or *pilonidal* sinus while rectal pathology may cause *anal discharge*. Prolapsing haemorrhoids or rarely a prolapsing pedunculated polyp may give a sensation of *something coming down* from the rectum during defecation. Rectal prolapse gives a sensation of something hanging down from the anus continuously. *Pruritus ani* or *perianal itching* is a common symptom resulting from local skin irritation exacerbated by scratching. There are numerous causes for the initial irritation ranging from poor hygiene, sensitivities to foodstuffs, drugs and soaps, and anal or perianal pathology. In children, threadworms are a common cause of perianal itching, which is worse at night time. *Tenesmus* is a painful desire to defecate. The patient feels that the rectum is full; but when attempting to defecate nothing happens. The sensation of fullness is caused by a space-occupying lesion (usually a carcinoma) in the rectum.

Table 13.5 Classification of jaundice.

Prehepatic	Surgical implications
Haemolytic anaemias	Pigment gallstones
Transfusion reactions	
Absorption of haematoma	e.g. after repair of ruptured abdominal aortic aneurysm
Hepatic	
Congenital syndromes	
Gilbert's disease	
Crigler–Najjar	
Dubin–Johnson	
Hepatitis	
Viral	Surgeons at high risk for hepatitis B
Alcoholic	
Drug-related	
Cirrhosis	Gastrointestinal haemorrhage from varices
	Liver transplantation
Tumours	Resection of primary and secondary liver tumours
Sepsis	Cholestatic jaundice is commonly seen as part of multiple organ dysfunction syndrome (MODS)
TPN	Frequently used in surgical patients
Posthepatic	
Extrahepatic biliary obstruction	All these problems are treated by surgeons
Gallstone obstructing the CBD	
Pancreatitis	
Tumours	
Secondaries at porta hepatitis	
Bile duct tumours	
Carcinoma of head of pancreas	
Tumours of ampulla of Vater	
Duodenal tumours	
Benign stricture of the CBD	Incidence has increased with laparoscopic cholecystectomy

TPN, Total parenteral nutrition; CBD, common bile duct.

• *Jaundice*: Jaundice is a yellow discoloration of the skin, mucous membranes and sclera due to the presence of excess bile pigments in the tissues. The itching that often accompanies jaundice is due to deposition of bile salts in the tissues. There are numerous causes of jaundice which can be broadly classified as prehepatic, hepatic and posthepatic (Table 13.5). Patients with posthepatic (obstructive) jaundice are the group most often seen by surgeons. Failure of absorption of the fat-soluble vitamin K in this group can result in prolongation of the prothrombin time and haemorrhagic complications, especially during surgery.

Table 13.6 Examination of a patient with a suspected gastrointestinal disorder.

Inspection	Palpation	Percussion	Auscultation
Hands			
Palmar crease (anaemia)	Palmar fascia (Dupuytren's contracture)		
Finger ulcers (Raynaud's with scleroderma)			
Koilonychia (anaemia)			
Palmar erythema (liver disease)			
Face and neck			
Conjunctiva (anaemia)	Supraclavicular fossa (nodes)		
Sclera (jaundice)			
oral mucosa (anaemia, jaundice, aphthous ulcer)			
Spider naevi (liver disease)			
Abdomen			
Movement/contour	*Acute*: guarding/rigidity/tenderness	Tenderness	Bowel sounds
Surface markings/abnormalities	*Non-acute*: tenderness/enlarged organs	Size of organs Distinguish liquid from gas distension	Bruits Succussion splash
Hernial orifices	Intra-abdominal masses		
Genitalia			
Penis (phimosis/ penile tumours)	Scrotum/two testes Tenderness/scrotal mass/can you get above it?/transillumination	–	–
Rectum and anus			
Sentinal pile (fissure)	Rectal examination tenderness/impaction/ empty rectum/rectal wall (tumour), prostate (size consistency)	–	–
Sinus (Crohn's disease/fistula-*in-ano*)			
Pilonidal sinus	Haemoccult test for occult blood		
Perianal inflammation	gastrointestinal bleeding		

Physical examination

A detailed description of examination of the abdomen has already been given in Chapter 1. However, the main features of physical examination for a patient with suspected gastrointestinal disease are summarized in Table 13.6.

Investigations

Numerous investigations are now available to the surgeon for assessment of patients with suspected gastrointestinal disease. These include laboratory investigations, several imaging techniques and endoscopy. Often biopsies are required to make a definite diagnosis of gastrointestinal disease.

Laboratory investigations

The laboratory investigations commonly used are given in Table 13.7.

Imaging the gastrointestinal tract

Plain films

A *chest radiograph* may give a lot of information about the gastrointestinal tract:
- pulmonary shadowing due to aspiration;
- air/fluid level behind the heart shadow due to a hiatus hernia;
- air under the right hemidiaphragm from a perforated viscus;

Table 13.7 Laboratory investigations available for assessment of patients with gastrointestinal disease.

Investigation	Abnormality	Pathology	Example
Haematology			
Full blood count	Anaemia		
	Iron deficiency	GI blood loss	Oesophagitis/cancer of the caecum
	Megaloblastic	B_{12}/folate deficiency	Gastrectomy/ileal disease
	Polycythaemia	Dehydration	Vomiting/diarrhoea
	Leukocytosis	Bacterial infection	Acute appendicitis
	Thrombocytosis	Postsplenectomy	Trauma
	Thrombocytopenia	Hypersplenism	Portal hypertension, DIC
Prothrombin time	Prolonged	Obstructive jaundice	Impacted CBD stone
Biochemistry			
Urea	Elevated	Dehydration	Vomiting
Sodium	Elevated	Water deprivation	Total dysphagia
	Decreased	Sodium loss	Vomiting, diarrhoea, sweating
Potassium	Decreased	Potassium loss	Diarrhoea, vomiting, diuresis
Calcium	Elevated	Malignancy	Primary liver cancer
	Decreased	Ca^{2+} precipitation	Acute pancreatitis
	Decreased	Osteomalacia	Vitamin D deficiency
Proteins	Hypoalbuminaemia	Failure of albumin production in liver	Lack of amino acid intake in diet, malabsorption
	C-reactive protein	Non-specific increase with inflammation	Crohn's disease
Arterial blood gases	Metabolic alkalosis	Loss of gastric HCL	Pyloric stenosis
	Metabolic acidosis	Lactic acidosis	Mesenteric ischaemia
Bilirubin	Elevated	Liver and biliary disease	Obstructive jaundice
Liver enzymes	Alkaline phosphatase transaminases	Bile duct and liver disease	Obstructive jaundice and hepatitis
Microbiology			
Stool examination	Helminth/protozoa	Gut infestation	Amoebic colitis from *Entamoeba histolytica*
	Bacteria	*Salmonella, Shigella, Escherichia coli*	All cause diarrhoea
	Bacterial toxin	*Clostridium difficile*	Causes antibiotic-induced enterocolitis
	Viruses	Rotavirus	Diarrhoea

GI, Gastrointestinal; DIC, disseminated intravascular coagulation; CBD, common bile duct; HCL, hydrochloric acid.

- air/fluid under the diaphragm with a subphrenic abscess.

A *plain abdominal radiograph* is a very useful examination when assessing the acute abdomen:
- Dilated loops and air fluid levels are seen with intestinal obstruction.
- Air-filled loop occupying most of the abdomen indicates a sigmoid volvulus.
- A distended featureless air-filled colon is seen in a patient with toxic megacolon from ulcerative colitis.
- 10% of gallstones may be seen on a plain abdominal X-ray.

Ultrasonography

Ultrasonography is very simple to use, relatively cheap and safe. It has a role in the diagnosis of gallbladder, liver and pancreatic disease and is used to guide needles precisely to obtain biopsies or aspirate intra-abdominal collections.

- It is very sensitive at demonstrating gallstones within the gallbladder but not good at detecting common bile duct stones.
- It is the investigation of choice to distinguish between extrahepatic biliary obstruction and hepatocellular causes of jaundice. Ultrasound is also used to confirm hepatomegaly, to assess further the cause of an abnormal isotope scan and to detect the presence of hepatic metastases.
- It is useful to diagnose and monitor the size of cysts and pseudocysts in the pancreas and can also detect, but not as reliably, solid lesions in the pancreas.

Bowel contrast studies

Barium sulphate is a radiodense substance which is used to outline the gastrointestinal tract. It is insoluble in water and is not absorbed. X-rays taken as it passes along the alimentary tract provide information on the anatomy and pathology of the various sections of the bowel. Barium swallow, meal and follow-through are used to assess the oesophagus, stomach, duodenum and small intestine, while a barium enema outlines the large bowel.

A *barium swallow* is useful in demonstrating a hiatus hernia with reflux, but the patient has to be tilted head-down to demonstrate reflux. Cineradiology is also used occasionally to demonstrate motility disorders of the oesophagus.

A *barium meal* is used to outline the stomach and the best results are obtained if a double-contrast technique is used, i.e. barium and gas (the gas is usually generated by effervescent tablets or carbonated drinks). Peptic ulceration and gastric neoplasms are detected by barium meal.

Barium follow-through studies attempt to outline the small bowel but this can be a difficult examination because of the length of the small bowel and the fact that the loops are overlying one another. Occasionally a *small-bowel enema* is performed to demonstrate the small bowel. This is done by placing a tube into the duodenum and infusing large amounts of barium. These techniques can be valuable in detecting Crohn's disease in the small bowel.

A *barium enema* is performed by placing a catheter into the patient's rectum and infusing barium to outline the colon. Patients need bowel preparation (i.e. purgation) prior to barium enema and the double-contrast technique where air as well as barium is insufflated into the bowel gives the best results. Polyps, carcinoma of the bowel and diverticulitis are all detected by barium enema.

A *defecating proctogram* is performed by imaging the rectum and anal canal while the patient evacuates barium which has been instilled into the rectum. This investigation is very useful in the investigation of patients with anal incontinence.

Biliary contrast studies

An *oral cholecystogram* is obtained by taking X-rays of the gallbladder which has been outlined by an iodine-containing contrast material. The patient swallows iodine-containing tablets the day before the examination. The contrast is absorbed from the gut, excreted in the bile and concentrated in the gallbladder. Images are taken before and after a fatty meal so that gallbladder emptying can be assessed. Failure to see an image could be due to failure of absorption of the contrast rather than gallbladder disease and occasionally a double-dose study is attempted. The study is contraindicated in jaundice as no excretion of contrast occurs. A study is abnormal when the gallbladder fails to opacify or when gallstones, which are seen as mobile filling defects, are detected. Ultrasound examination (see above) has displaced oral cholecystography as the first line of investigation of the gallbladder.

Intravenous cholangiography has had somewhat of a revival with the advent of laparoscopic cholecystectomy. An iodine-containing substance which is injected intravenously is concentrated in the bile. X-rays including tomograms, demonstrate the gallbladder and the common bile duct. Intravenous cholangiography is also contraindicated in patients with jaundice and occasionally anaphylactic reactions occur.

Endoscopic retrograde cholangiopancreatography (ERCP) is a technique where a catheter is passed into the bile and pancreatic ducts via a side-viewing endoscope. The papilla of Vater is cannulated and contrast is injected into the two ducts. ERCP is indicated in patients suspected of having biliary tract disease (e.g. stones in the common bile duct, cholangiocarcinoma) or pancreatic disease (e.g. chronic pancreatitis, pancreatic cancer) and has the advantage that further diagnostic (e.g. biopsy, manometry) and therapeutic procedures (papillotomy, placement of stents) may be performed simultaneously. Sepsis and pancreatitis are the two major complications of ERCP.

Percutaneous transhepatic cholangiography (PTC) is another technique for direct opacification of the biliary tree in the jaundiced patient. In this study the liver is punctured percutaneously with a small (Chiba) needle and under fluoroscopic control an intrahepatic bile duct is penetrated and contrast injected. PTC is particularly useful for proximal bile duct obstruction (e.g. hilar cholangiocarcinoma) and diagnostic and therapeutic procedures can also be performed.

Operative cholangiograms are obtained during cholecystectomy to assess whether or not stones are present in the common bile duct. If stones are detected they are removed by opening the common bile duct and the duct is closed over a T-tube. Prior to removing the T-tube 7 days later a *T-tube cholangiogram* is performed to ensure that no stones have been left behind.

Radionuclide imaging

Technetium 99m (^{99m}Tc) is an isotope used to label colloid preparations, e.g. sulphur colloid. ^{99m}Tc colloid is injected intravenously and a γ-camera is placed over the patient to detect the radioactivity emitted by the isotope. This investigation is indicated in patients with occult gastrointestinal bleeding where the extravasated blood gives an area of high radioactivity. Focal disease in the liver (e.g. neoplasm, pyogenic abscess) is indicated by discrete areas of low radioactivity against a background of high activity, while diffuse decrease in density is indicative of generalized parenchymal disease. Occasionally ^{99m}Tc is given to patients in a burger and its passage from the stomach is monitored to measure gastric emptying.

Technetium-labelled imido-diacetic acid (^{99m}Tc HIDA) scanning is used to demonstrate the biliary tree. In a normal scan the liver, bile ducts, gallbladder and upper small bowel are seen in rapid succession as the isotope is excreted into the bowel. Non-opacification of the gallbladder is strong evidence of gallbladder disease.

^{99m}Tc pertechnetate is concentrated in gastric mucosa and this scan is useful in the diagnosis of haemorrhage from a Meckel's diverticulum.

^{67}Ga (gallium) is an isotope which is concentrated in areas of acute inflammation and this scan is sometimes used to detect abscesses such as liver abscess or subphrenic abscess.

Other imaging techniques

Computed tomography (CT) is a technique whereby a cross-section of the body is irradiated by an external X-ray source which rotates around the body to produce an image which represents a transverse cut through the body. In this way anatomy and pathological anatomy can be studied in great detail. In the gastrointestinal tract CT scans are used:
• to 'look at' areas difficult to detect in other ways, e.g. mediastinal lymphadenopathy, retroperitoneal tumours, pelvic lesions;
• to demonstrate liver tumours and biliary disease in those in whom ultrasound proves unsatisfactory;
• to assess organ damage in abdominal trauma; and
• to guide needles for biopsy or aspiration.

In *magnetic resonance imaging* (MRI) an externally applied magnetic field causes protons in tissues to align in the direction of the magnetic field. By applying a radiofrequency pulse perpendicular to the magnetic field, the alignment of the protons is disrupted and the changing magnetization induces a voltage in a receiver coil which can be magnified and detected to produce an image. MR scans are used as an adjunct to CT scans.

Endoscopy

Upper gastrointestinal endoscopy

Oesophagogastroduodenoscopy The upper gastrointestinal tract, from the upper oesophagus to the second part of the duodenum, is easily examined using a forward-viewing fibreoptic gastroscope. Direct inspection of the mucosa, photography and biopsy are all facilitated by this technique. Landmarks to be noted when performing endoscopy are the squamocolumnar (i.e. oesophagogastric, pale pink/orange red) junction, the angulari incisura, the pylorus

and the first (and sometimes) second part of the duodenum. On withdrawing the scope the cardia is viewed by the J-manoeuvre.

A number of therapies are also possible via the gastroscope:
• dilatation of oesophageal stricture;
• placement of tubes for palliation of oesophageal neoplasia;
• injection of varices;
• removal of foreign bodies from oesophagus and stomach;
• placement of percutaneous endoscopic gastrostomy (PEG);
• polypectomy; and
• control of upper gastrointestinal bleeding by injection, bipolar cautery, heater probe or Nd-YAG laser (photocoagulation).

ERCP (see above).

Lower gastrointestinal endoscopy

Proctoscopy This is used to examine the anal canal and the lower rectum. A proctoscope is a short metal tube to which a light is attached (Fig. 2.12). It is inserted into the rectum with an obturator which is removed once the scope is in place. The patient lies in the left lateral position for this investigation. Proctoscopy is used to examine the anus for fissure and haemorrhoids, which may be injected or banded. Inflammatory bowel disease involving the rectum (e.g. ulcerative colitis) is easily seen on proctoscopy and biopsies can be obtained.

Sigmoidoscopy Rigid sigmoidoscopy allows direct inspection of the rectum and sigmoid colon to 25 cm from the anal margin while flexible sigmoidoscopy permits examination to 60 cm. Most (but not all) colonic neoplasms will be found in this area. Sigmoidoscopy is performed in the left lateral or the knee–elbow position and the patient requires some bowel preparation (e.g. phosphate enema) prior to the study. Sigmoidoscopy is indicated in patients with rectal bleeding to detect the cause, e.g. carcinoma, inflammatory bowel disease. If a polyp is discovered it may be removed for histological examination.

Colonoscopy Fibreoptic colonoscopy permits direct inspection of the entire colon and occasionally the terminal ileum. Good bowel preparation is essential for a satisfactory study and the procedure is performed under sedation in the left lateral position. As well as polyps and neoplasms, angiodysplasia and diverticular disease are readily diagnosed on colonoscopy.

Laparoscopy

Laparoscopy permits views of the liver, gallbladder, peritoneum and pelvic organs. This technique is useful for detecting liver and peritoneal secondaries when other less invasive diagnostic modalities have failed. It also provides a more accurate diagnosis of lower abdominal pain, especially in young women and recently a number of surgical operations have been performed laparoscopically (cholecystectomy, hiatus hernia repair, bowel resection).

Specialized investigations

- *Oesophageal manometry* is performed by passing fine perfused tubes connected to pressure transducers into the stomach and withdrawing them into the oesophagus. Pressure recordings are taken in the stomach, gastro-oesophageal junction and oesophagus during and between swallowing. Oesophageal manometry is very helpful in the diagnosis of achalasia and other motility disorders of the oesophagus.
- *pH Studies* Continuous pH monitoring can be performed by placing an electrode 4–5 cm above the oesophagogastric junction. The patient keeps a diary of symptoms which can be correlated with changes in pH in the oesophagus. Whether the symptoms are due to reflux oesophagitis or not can be assessed in this way.
- *Pentagastrin test* This is the standard investigation in a patient in whom hypergastrinaemia is suspected. A nasogastric tube is passed and gastric secretions are collected for an hour — basal acid secretion. A synthetic gastrin analogue (pentagastrin) is then administered and the acid secretions are collected again for another hour. Pentagastrin should stimulate maximum acid secretion and the second collection is the maximal acid secretion. In patients with hypergastrinaemia basal and maximal acid secretions will be identical.
- *Electromyography (EMG)* and *anorectal manometry* are physiological tests used to assess patients with anal incontinence. EMG is performed by inserting a fine-needle electrode into the puborectalis muscle and the external sphincter. Maximum contraction of the sphincter should produce action potentials in the muscles. Pelvic floor muscle function is often deranged in patients with anal incontinence. Anorectal manometry is performed by placing an open or balloon-tipped catheter in the anal canal. Resting anal pressure and pressure during maximum external sphincter contraction are measured. By inflating a second balloon catheter in the rectum, the rectosphincteric reflex and the internal sphincter relaxation response can be assessed.

The oesophagus, stomach and small intestine

Thought depends absolutely on the stomach; but, in spite of that, those who have the best stomachs are not the best thinkers. (Voltaire, in a letter to d'Alembert)

The oesophagus

Anatomy

The oesophagus extends from the pharynx to the gastric cardia and measures 25–30 cm in length. It has an upper sphincter, the cricopharyngeus, and a lower sphincter derived from its circular muscle fibres. The cricopharyngeal sphincter lies opposite the sixth cervical vertebra about 15 cm from the upper incisor teeth. The arch of the aorta crosses and indents the oesophagus on its left side at 22 cm from the incisor teeth and the left main bronchus crosses it at 27 cm. The oesophagus is a midline structure which deviates to the left in its cervical portion, to the right in its thoracic course and inclines anteriorly and to the left as it passes through the diaphragmatic hiatus.

The outer muscular layer is longitudinal and the inner layer circular. The mucosal lining is squamous epithelium. The oesophageal nerve supply is composed of sympathetic preganglionic fibres from the spinal cord segments T5 and T6 and postganglionic fibres from the cervical, paravertebral and coeliac ganglia. The parasympathetic nerve supply is from the glossopharyngeal, recurrent laryngeal and vagus nerves. A myenteric plexus of ganglia and nerve fibres lies between the muscle layers.

The arterial blood supply is from the inferior thyroid artery, bronchial arteries and direct small branches from the aorta. Branches from the left gastric artery and inferior phrenic artery supply the lower end. Venous drainage is to the inferior thyroid vein, the azygos and hemiazygos system in the chest and to the left gastric or coronary vein in the lower third. Lymphatic drainage is to regional lymph nodes and thence to the supraclavicular deep cervical and coeliac lymph nodes.

Physiology

Swallowing is initiated by tongue movements which force a bolus into the oropharynx. Simultaneously the soft palate is elevated to close the nasopharynx and the epiglottis assumes a horizontal position to protect the larynx. When the bolus enters the oropharynx the pharyngeal constrictor muscles undergo involuntary contraction. This is accompanied by relaxation of the cricopharyngeus which allows the bolus to enter the oesophagus. The upper sphincter (cricopharyngeus) resumes the contracted state and a peristaltic wave is initiated in the oesophagus which propels the bolus down the oesophagus until it reaches the lower sphincter. When the peristaltic wave reaches the lower sphincter the latter relaxes and enables the bolus to enter the stomach.

Gastro-oesophageal reflux

Gastro-oesophageal reflux is now the commonest cause of dyspepsia in western countries. Prevention of reflux is a complex mechanism involving a number of physiological and anatomical factors at the gastro-oesophageal junction. The most important of these are:
• the lower oesophageal sphincter pressure;
• the length of the intra-abdominal segment of the lower oesophageal sphincter;
• the angle of His;
• the sling fibres around the cardia;
• the crural fibres; and
• the mucosal rosette.
  Failure of this mechanism, which is often, but need not be, accompanied by a sliding hiatus hernia (Fig. 13.2), brings about pathological reflux of gastric contents into the oesophagus.

Clinical features

Clinical features cannot be relied upon for diagnosis as symptoms may be simulated by peptic ulcer or gallbladder disease. However, the common symptoms are:
• heartburn;
• retrosternal pain radiating to epigastrium, angle of jaw

and down either arm;
• regurgitation of sour (acid) gastric contents into the mouth and pharynx;
• boring pain in the back which may arise from a penetrating ulcer in a Barrett's oesophagus; and
• dysphagia which may develop due to benign oesophageal stricture.

Investigations

Barium studies (swallow and meal) may reveal:
• a sliding hernia;
• an ulcer in the oesophagus;
• a benign structure.
  Endoscopy allows visualization of the degree of oesophagitis present, although this may correlate poorly with the symptoms. Endoscopy also facilitates biopsy.

pH Monitoring

Twenty-four-hour pH monitoring provides a computerized assessment of the degree of reflux, from which a reflux score can be calculated.

Treatment

General measures include weight loss, avoidance of coffee, alcohol, smoking, chocolate and fatty foods. Tight abdominal garments and positions that exacerbate symptoms (e.g. lying flat) should be avoided.

Medical treatment

Control of acid secretion by H_2-receptor antagonists and the use of alginate to minimize the effects of reflux will help reduce symptoms. Prokinetic drugs, by improving the

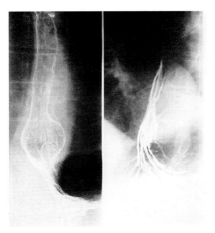
(a)

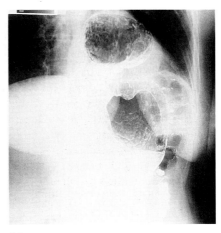
(b)

Figure 13.2 Radiographs of (a) sliding hiatus hernia; (b) rolling hiatus hernia.

clearance of acid from the lower oesophagus, reduce the amount of damage done by reflux. Cisapride and metoclopramide are the drugs most frequently used. Omeprazole, a proton pump inhibitor, is extremely effective in treating gastro-oesophageal reflux because of its powerful suppression of gastric acid secretion.

Surgical treatment

Antireflux surgery is the most effective long-term method of reflux prevention. Side-effects, which are usually temporary, are gas bloat (i.e. an inability to belch) and dysphagia. The most frequently used antireflux procedures are the Nissen fundoplication (Fig. 13.3; which may also be performed laparoscopically; Fig. 13.3c), Hill's posterior gastropexy and Belsey's mark IV procedure (a partial fundoplication).

Benign strictures are probably best treated by a combination of antireflux surgery and dilatation. The safest dilators are those passed over a guidewire such as the Eder-Puestow system or the Celestin or Savary systems (Fig. 13.4). If control of reflux is adequate most strictures will remain patent after a few dilatations. Intractable strictures which are clearly fibrotic may need resection with interposition of a segment of colon or jejunum pedicled on its own vasculature.

Barrett's oesophagus

Barrett's oesophagus (Fig. 13.5) is a metaplastic change in which sheets of columnar epithelium replace the squamous epithelium of the lower oesophagus for a variable distance. It occurs in response to epithelial damage by reflux of acid and probably bile and duodenal secretions also. Its import-

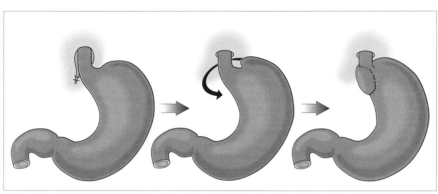

(a)

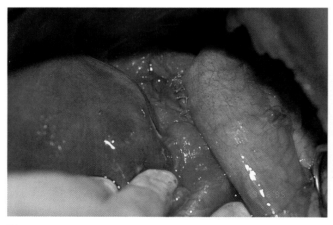

(b)

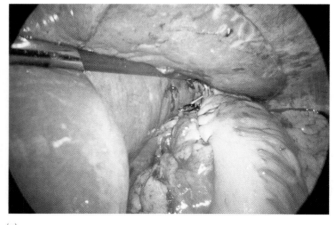

(c)

Figure 13.3 (a) Diagram illustrating the steps in a Nissen fundoplication. The hiatus in the diaphragm is narrowed and the fundus of the stomach is mobilized and wrapped around the lesser curve. The wrap is held in position by a number of sutures.

(b) Operative photograph of a Nissen fundoplication. The fundus of the stomach has been wrapped around but the sutures have not yet been placed. (c) Laparoscopic fundoplication.

ance lies in its malignant potential (40 times greater than normal) and its susceptibility to the complications of stricture and penetrating ulcer (Barrett's ulcer).

Antireflux surgery may promote regression of Barrett's epithelium and may lessen the risk of malignant change.

Barrett's ulcer should be resected if it does not heal promptly with medical treatment or antireflux surgery. Persistent ulcers may bleed or perforate into the mediastinum, with disastrous consequences. Barrett's epithelium may sometimes regress following successful antireflux surgery and this may lessen the risk of malignant change.

Primary motility disorders

The three most important motility disorders of the oesophagus are:
• achalasia;
• diffuse oesophageal spasm; and
• nutcracker oesophagus (symptomatic peristalsis).

The principal symptoms of motility disorders are dysphagia and retrosternal pain. They require full oesophageal investigation but the most significant investigation is manometry, which can discriminate between the three above-mentioned disorders. Scintigraphy is useful as a screening test to identify abnormal oesophageal transit but cannot discriminate between the different dysmotilities.

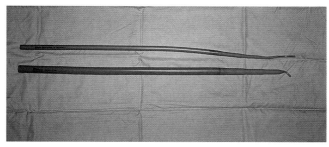

(a)

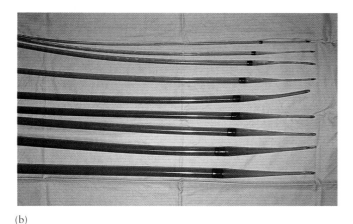

(b)

Figure 13.4 (a) Celestin dilators; (b) Savary dilators.

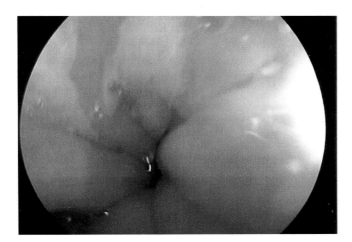

Figure 13.5 Endoscopic view of Barrett's oesophagus.

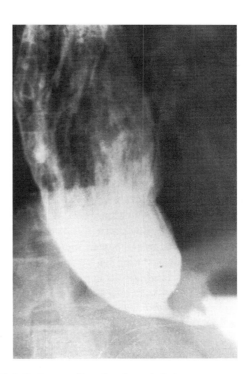

Figure 13.6 Barium swallow showing achalasia.

Gastro-oesophageal reflux at a glance

DEFINITIONS

Gastro-oesophageal reflux is a condition caused by the retrograde passage of gastric contents into the oesophagus resulting in inflammation (*oesophagitis*) which manifests as dyspepsia. A *hiatus hernia* is an abnormal protrusion of the proximal stomach through the oesophageal opening in the diaphragm, resulting in a more proximal positioning of the oesophagogastric junction and predisposition to gastro-oesophageal reflux. *Sliding* (common) and *rolling* or *paraoesophageal* (rare) hiatus herniae are recognized

CAUSES

- Failure of normal mechanisms of gastro-oesophageal continence (lower oesophageal sphincter (LOS) pressure, length of intra-abdominal LOS, angle of His, sling fibres around the cardia, the crural fibres of the diaphragm, the mucosal rosette)
- LOS pressure reduced by smoking, alcohol and coffee

CLINICAL FEATURES

- Retrosternal burning pain, radiating to epigastrium, jaw and arms. (Oesophageal pain is often confused with cardiac pain)
- Regurgitation of acid contents into the mouth (waterbrash)
- Back pain (a penetrating ulcer in Barrett's oesophagus)
- Dysphagia from a benign stricture

INVESTIGATIONS

- Barium swallow and meal — Sliding hiatus hernia / Oesophageal ulcer / Stricture
- Oesophagoscopy — Assess oesophagitis / Biopsy for histology / Dilate stricture if present
- 24-h pH monitoring — Assess the degree of reflux

MANAGEMENT

General
- Lose weight; avoid smoking, coffee, alcohol and chocolate
- Avoid tight garments and stooping

Medical
- Control acid secretion (H_2-receptor antagonists, e.g. ranitidine, or proton pump inhibitors, e.g. omeprazole)
- Minimize effects of reflux (give alginates to protect oesophagus)
- Prokinetic agents (e.g. metoclopramide, cisapride) improve LOS tone and promote gastric emptying

Surgical
- Antireflux surgery (e.g. Nissen fundoplication) which may be performed by laparotomy or laparoscopy

COMPLICATIONS

- Benign stricture of the oesophagus
- Barrett's oesophagus (a premalignant metaplasia of the lower oesophagus in which columnar epithelium replaces the normal squamous epithelium)

Achalasia

Achalasia is a condition in which peristalsis is absent from the lower two-thirds of the oesophagus and the lower sphincter fails to relax. It is associated with degeneration of the myenteric nerve plexus. The dorsal motor nucleus of the vagus may also show abnormalities. In time, the oesophagus becomes grossly dilated (Fig. 13.6). Aspiration of retained contents may occur due to regurgitation. Weight loss is common and retrosternal pain may sometimes occur. Medical treatment is ineffective, although long-acting nitrites may be of symptomatic help. Specific treatment is by forceful dilatation of the cardia with pneumatic dilators (Fig. 13.7) or Heller's myotomy, which involves dividing the lower oesophageal sphincter down to the mucosa (Fig. 13.8). Both are low-risk procedures which give good results. The outcome of Heller's myotomy is more effective and longer-lasting than pneumatic dilatation.

Diffuse spasm

This is a rare condition characterized by dysphagia and retrosternal pain. The symptoms are intermittent and are associated with repetitive simultaneous contractions of the oesophageal body of variable amplitude which are present at least 30% of the time. The appearance on barium swallow is characteristic, showing a 'corkscrew oesophagus' (Fig. 13.9). Long myotomy may provide relief but medical treatment with calcium channel blockers sometimes helps.

Nutcracker oesophagus

Nutcracker oesophagus (symptomatic peristalsis) is the commonest abnormality of oesophageal motility. Also known as symptomatic peristalsis, manometry shows normal peristalsis but with wave amplitudes in excess of 150 mmHg. It is probably the commonest cause of ret-

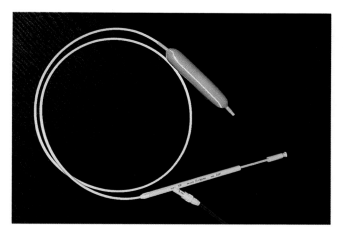

Figure 13.7 Oldbert oesophageal balloon for dilatation of achalasia.

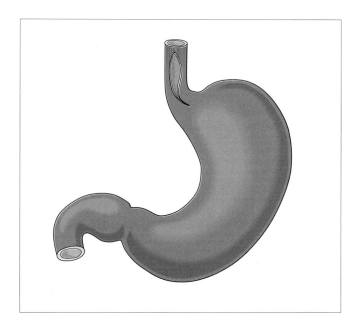

Figure 13.8 Diagram of Heller's myotomy.

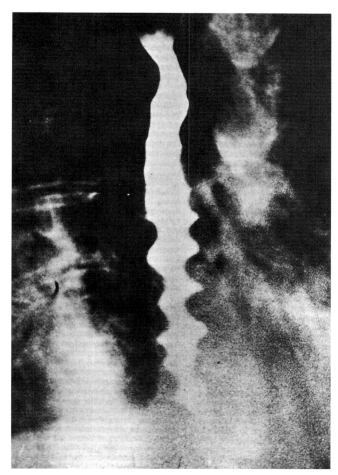

Figure 13.9 Radiograph demonstrating a corkscrew oesophagus.

rosternal angina-like pain and the patient frequently undergoes full cardiac evaluation before being sent for investigation of the oesophagus. Long-acting nitrates and calcium channel blockers have been of some help. Surgical intervention is not usually indicated.

Tumours of the oesophagus

Benign tumours

Benign tumours of the oesophagus are rare. The commonest is the leiomyoma which may cause dysphagia and require surgery. It can be shelled out of the oesophageal wall with good results.

Malignant tumours

Malignant tumours of the oesophagus are mostly squamous in type (Fig. 13.10a). Adenocarcinomas arise in the lower oesophagus and are mainly associated with Barrett's oesophagus (Fig. 13.10b). The incidence of adenocarcinoma is increasing rapidly. In western countries the most significant factors associated with development of

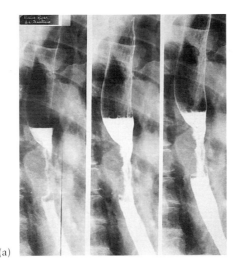

(a)

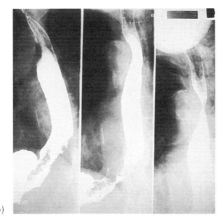

(b)

Figure 13.10 (a) Squamous carcinoma of the middle third of the oesophagus. Note the 'shouldering' at the upper end. (b) Adenocarcinoma of the lower third of the oesophagus.

oesophageal cancer are the abuse of alcohol and tobacco. In high-incidence areas like South Africa and northern China, other factors like mineral deficiencies and nitrosamines may be important.

Symptoms

Progressive dysphagia occurs from the narrowing of the oesophageal lumen by the tumour. Weight loss occurs due to the patient's inability to eat a normal diet. Local spread to perioesophageal tissues and local lymph nodes is common at the time of presentation, although overt metastases to distant organs are not usually seen at that time.

Diagnosis

Barium studies show characteristic narrowing of the oesophageal lumen with shouldering (Fig. 13.10a). Endoscopy reveals a malignant stricture with an ulcerated surface. Biopsy confirms the diagnosis. If an upper-third lesion is present, bronchoscopy is important to exclude invasion of a bronchus.

Treatment

If the prognosis is limited and palliation is the sole aim of treatment, intubation with an Atkinson, Wilson Cooke or Celestine tube (Fig. 13.11) will enable the patient to swallow semisolids. An alternative is laser treatment or the use of iridium wires for intraluminal irradiation. Photo-

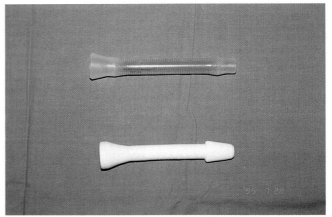

(a)

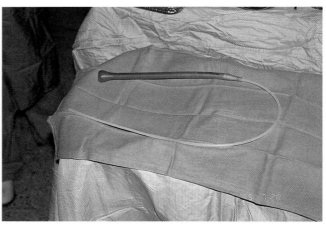

(b)

Figure 13.11 (a) Atkinson (bottom) and Wilson Cooke (top) tubes; (b) Celestine tube.

dynamic therapy may also be employed using a laser and a sensitizer such as haematoporphyrin.

Resection of the lesion with 10 cm clear margins on either side of the tumour will give excellent palliation with some prospect of cure if lymph nodes are not involved. Reconstruc- tion of the oesophagus is either by gastric 'pull-up' or colon transposition (Fig. 13.12). Combination therapy using exter- nal-beam irradiation and chemotherapy prior to surgery is under trial and may improve survival although, perhaps, at the expense of increased morbidity and mortality.

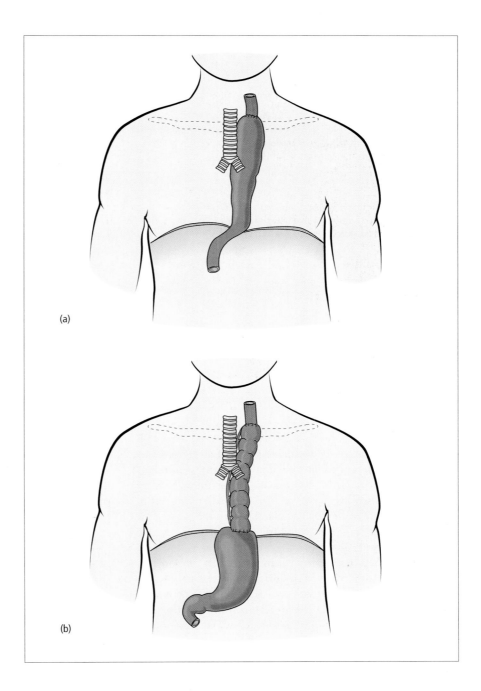

(a)

(b)

Figure 13.12 Reconstruction of oesophagus after oesophagectomy with (a) gastric 'pull-up' or (b) colon transposition.

Carcinoma of the oesophagus at a glance

DEFINITION

Malignant lesion of the oesophagus

EPIDEMIOLOGY

M : F=3 : 1. Age 50–70 years. High incidence in areas of China, Russia, and among the Bantu in South Africa

AETIOLOGY

Predisposing factors
- Alcohol consumption and cigarette smoking
- Chronic oesophagitis and Barrett's oesophagus
- Stricture from corrosive (lye) oesophagitis
- Achalasia
- Plummer–Vinson syndrome (oesophageal web, mucosal lesions of mouth and pharynx and iron-deficiency anaemia)
- Nitrosamines

PATHOLOGY

- Histological type: 60% *squamous carcinoma* (upper two-thirds of oesophagus), 40% *adenocarcinoma* (lower third of oesophagus)
- Spread: lymphatics, direct extension, vascular invasion

CLINICAL FEATURES

- Dysphagia progressing from solids to liquids
- Weight loss and weakness
- Aspiration pneumonia

INVESTIGATIONS

• Barium swallow	Narrowed lumen with 'shouldering'
• Oesophagoscopy	Malignant stricture
• Bronchoscopy	Assess bronchial invasion with upper-third lesions
• CT scanning	Assess degree of spread if surgery is being contemplated

MANAGEMENT

Palliation
- Intubation with Atkinson or Celestin tube
- Intraluminal irradiation with iridium wires
- Laser resection of the tumour
- Surgical excision of the tumour

Curative Rx
- Rarely, surgical resection is curative if lymph nodes are not involved. Reconstruction is by gastric 'pull-up' or colon interposition

Other Rx
- Combination therapy with external-beam radiation, chemotherapy and surgery is under trial

PROGNOSIS

- Following resection, 5-year survival rates are about 15% but overall 5-year survival (palliation and resection) is only about 4%

The stomach

Introduction

The prime function of the stomach is that of a reservoir for ingested food. Its upper part is capable of adaptive relaxation, that is, the musculature relaxes during filling, thereby preventing a significant rise in the intragastric pressure during eating and drinking. The distal part of the stomach is often referred to as the antropyloric pump or mill because its contractions are responsible for churning the food into liquid chyme before delivering it in graduated amounts to the small intestine via the pyloric sphincter. A certain amount of digestion of food occurs in the stomach as a result of the action of hydrochloric acid and pepsin. The other important function of the stomach is the secretion of intrinsic factor which is necessary for the absorption of dietary vitamin B_{12} by the terminal ileum. The important

investigations used in the management of patients with suspected gastric disorders are barium contrast studies and endoscopy with biopsy of any lesions found.

Peptic ulceration (Fig. 13.13)

There are three conditions which fall in this category: chronic duodenal ulcer disease, chronic gastric ulceration and erosive gastritis.

Chronic duodenal ulcer

Pathology

The incidence of chronic duodenal ulcer (Fig. 13.13a) has declined somewhat during the last two decades. The ulceration most commonly involves the duodenal bulb (first part) and is characterized by alternating cycles of healing and relapse, indicating that affected individuals have an innate

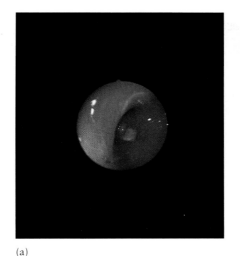

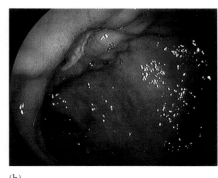

(b)

Figure 13.13 Endoscopic view of peptic ulcers: (a) duodenal ulcer; (b) gastric ulcer on lesser curvature of the stomach.

(a)

diathesis (susceptibility) to recurrent ulceration of the duodenal mucosa. The disease is more common in males, in smokers, alcohol abusers and in individuals who are subject to chronic stress. Duodenal ulceration is associated with hypersecretion of acid by the stomach. There is increasing evidence that infection by the organism *Helicobacter pylori* (Fig. 13.14) is involved in the aetiology of chronic duodenal ulcer. The peak incidence of the disease occurs during the third to fifth decades.

Clinical features

The dominant symptom of active duodenal ulceration is epigastric pain during fasting. This hunger pain, which may wake the patient at night, is relieved by food and antacids only to return several hours later. There is often associated heartburn in many patients. Classically the pain exhibits periodicity. When a chronic posterior wall ulcer penetrates the pancreas, the pain may become persistent without relief by antacids and may radiate to the back. Vomiting may occur. This usually indicates pyloric hold-up due to oedema of the duodenal bulb (reversible) or to fibrotic narrowing, pyloric stenosis, when it is persistent and progressive. The symptom of pyloric stenosis is vomiting of food recognizable by the patient as having been eaten several hours beforehand. The other complications of duodenal ulcer disease are haemorrhage and perforation. The former presents with haematemesis and melaena, the latter with peritonitis. The only finding in a patient with uncomplicated duodenal ulceration is epigastric tenderness. In patients with pyloric stenosis, there is epigastric fullness and the presence of a succussion splash. This must be elicited when the patient has been fasting for several hours. A splash is

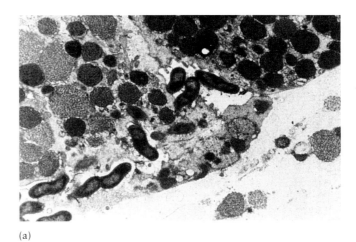

(a)

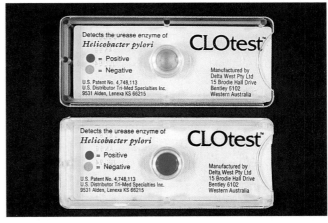

(b)

Figure 13.14 (a) *Helicobacter pylori* in duodenal mucosa (scanning electron micrograph); (b) *Campylobacter*-like organism (CLO) test.

heard as the patient is shaken from side to side by the lower ribcage.

Treatment

The treatment of duodenal ulcer disease is medical in the first instance. The current standard regimen entails the ad-

ministration of *H₂-blocker drugs*. These agents (cimetidine, ranitidine, famotidine, etc.) block the H_2 histamine receptors and result in healing rates approaching 90%. However, indefinite maintenance treatment after the full therapeutic course is essential to prevent relapse. *Colloidal bismuth* (De-Nol), which is bactericidal to *H. pylori*, is followed by similar healing rates and relapse following cessa-

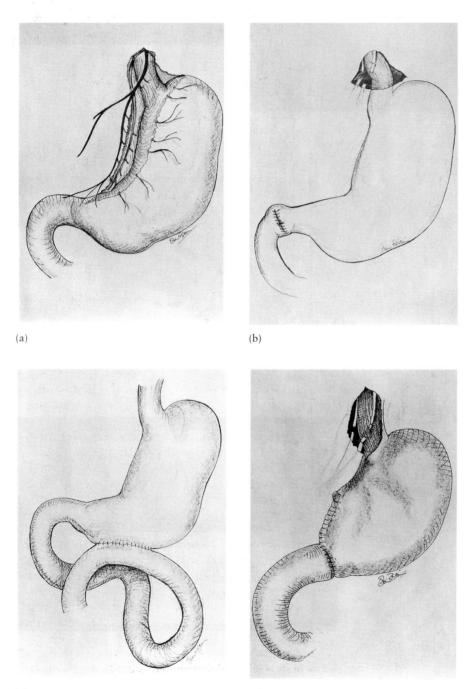

(a)

(b)

(c)

(d)

Figure 13.15 Surgery for peptic ulcer disease: (a) highly selective vagotomy; (b) truncal vagotomy and pyloroplasty (widening of the pylorus); (c) truncal vagotomy and gastrojejunostomy; (d) truncal vagotomy and antrectomy.

tion of therapy is less frequent than that which is experienced after treatment with H_2-blockers. The efficacy of antibiotics such as clarithromycin alone or with proton pump inhibitors (e.g. omeprazole) in healing duodenal ulcers is now established.

Surgical treatment is reserved for failures of medical therapy, for non-compliance with medication and for those patients who develop complications.

• Nowadays the preferred operation for elective surgical treatment of uncomplicated duodenal ulcer disease is highly selective vagotomy (Fig. 13.15a). This procedure denervates only the parietal cells, thereby reducing gastric acid secretion without altering the contractile activity and emptying of the stomach. In this respect, it is superior to the alternative operation of truncal vagotomy which requires gastric drainage (pyloroplasty (Fig. 13.15b) or gastrojejunostomy (Fig. 13.15c)) as, by impairing gastric contractions, it delays emptying. Truncal vagotomy and drainage also impart a significant risk of undesirable postprandial symptoms which may cause long-term disability in some patients (see below). The most effective operation in terms of permanent ulcer healing is truncal vagotomy and antrectomy (Fig. 13.15d), but this procedure carries an even greater risk than vagotomy and drainage of unpleasant long-term side-effects — early vasomotor dumping (fainting after meals), reactive postprandial hypoglycaemia (late dumping), bile vomiting and gastritis and explosive diarrhoea. The varied nature of postgastric surgery complications is outlined in Table 13.8.

• Perforated duodenal ulcer presents with peritonitis and is treated by emergency suture closure of the perforation with

Table 13.8 Postgastric surgery complications.

Nutritional consequences
  Weight loss
  Anaemia
  Milk intolerance
  Bone disease
Vasomotor dumping
Reactive hypoglycaemia
Bile reflux and vomiting
Explosive diarrhoea
Small-stomach syndrome
Mechanical complications
  Obstructions
  Jejunogastric intussusception
  Bezoar
Others
  Cholelithiasis
  Gastric cancer
  Pulmonary tuberculosis

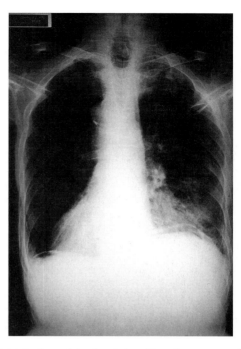

Figure 13.16 Perforated duodenal ulcer. Note the presence of air under the right hemidiaphragm on the chest X-ray.

toilet of the peritoneal cavity. This is followed by full medical treatment (Fig. 13.16).

• The management of upper gastrointestinal haemorrhage is discussed below, but the operation for a bleeding duodenal ulcer is underrunning of the bleeding vessel with a non-absorbable suture. Previously a truncal vagotomy was added for bleeding duodenal ulcers but this is nowadays often omitted in view of the efficacy of antibiotic therapy and omeprazole.

• The treatment of benign pyloric stenosis consists of truncal vagotomy and gastroenterostomy.

Chronic gastric ulcer

Pathology

There are two types of gastric ulcer: type I and type II. Type I gastric ulcers occur in the body of the stomach in patients over 50 years and are associated with atrophic gastritis and hypoactivity (Fig. 13.13b). Type II gastric ulcers develop in the antrum or pyloric canal (prepyloric or pyloric channel ulcers) and have the same clinical and pathological features as duodenal ulcers.

The exact pathogenesis of type I gastric ulcer remains unknown. It is variously attributed to diminished mucosal resistance, delayed gastric emptying, bile reflux and infec-

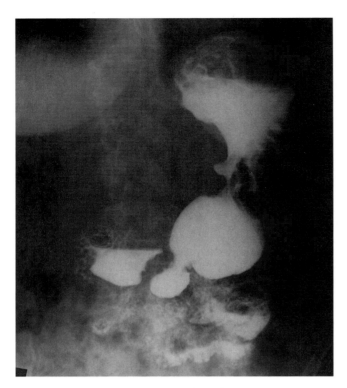

Figure 13.17 Barium meal showing an hourglass contracture due to an ulcer in the middle third of the stomach.

tion with *H. pylori*. It is liable to the same complications as duodenal ulcers: penetration, perforation, bleeding and cicatricial stenosis. Cicatricial stenosis may cause a teapot deformity when the ulcer is situated high up in the lesser curve or an hourglass contracture when located in the middle of the stomach (Fig. 13.17). A posterior chronic gastric ulcer may penetrate the body of the pancreas and erode the splenic artery, causing torrential haemorrhage. A lesser curve ulcer may also penetrate the liver substance.

Clinical features

In addition to occurring in an older age group, the clinical features of a chronic gastric ulcer differ from those of a duodenal ulcer. Epigastric pain is induced by eating and for this reason the patient is afraid to eat and thus exhibits weight loss at presentation. Nausea and vomiting are more common and occur in the absence of stenotic complications of the disease. Although periodicity of symptoms is encountered, this is not as obvious as in patients with duodenal ulcer. Chronic blood loss causing an iron-deficiency anaemia is a very common clinical presentation of patients with type I gastric ulcer.

Treatment

The most commonly used medical treatment for gastric ulcer is H_2-blockers or a proton pump inhibitor. This has replaced other regimens such as the use of Biogastrone. The important practical aspect of management is that the patient should undergo a repeat endoscopic examination after 6–8 weeks of therapy. If the ulcer has not healed, it should be regarded as malignant. Further biopsies are taken and the patient is referred for surgical treatment. Surgical treatment is indicated even if the repeat biopsies are benign.

Elective treatment for chronic gastric ulcer which has failed to heal on medical therapy consists of partial gastrectomy, including the ulcer, with restoration of gastroduodenal continuity (Billroth I gastrectomy; Fig. 13.18a). The stenotic complications are also treated by gastric resection. The emergency treatment of perforated gastric ulcer entails biopsy of the perforation to exclude malignancy followed by suture closure and toilet of the peritoneal cavity.

Erosive gastritis

This is one of the commonest acute gastric disorders encountered in surgical practice. It is a syndrome of varied aetiology (Table 13.9) which results in diffuse oedema and erythema of the gastric mucosa with focal mucosal haemorrhages, erosions (small shallow ulcers) and ulcerations.

The most frequent cause is damage induced by the chronic ingestion of non-steroidal anti-inflammatory drugs (NSAIDs). The condition most commonly presents with severe haematemesis and can progress to perforation. In patients with NSAID-induced disease, coexistent lesions in the upper jejunum are frequently present and may be the cause of bleeding. Perforation of ulcers seems to be more common with steroid-induced disease. The cause of stress-induced erosive gastritis in critically ill patients, e.g. severe head injuries, severe sepsis from any cause, extensive burns, etc., remains unknown.

Upper gastrointestinal haemorrhage

This is a common gastroenterological emergency. The presentation is with haematemesis, which can consist of altered (coffee-ground vomit) or fresh blood, or with melaena or both. If the blood loss is substantial, hypovolaemic shock (Chapter 4) develops and immediate attention is required. The causes of acute upper gastrointestinal haemorrhage are shown in Table 13.10. The commonest cause is erosive gastritis induced by NSAIDs followed by chronic peptic ulceration. Between them, these account for 90% of cases.

The management of patients with upper gastrointestinal bleeding requires a joint medicosurgical team approach.

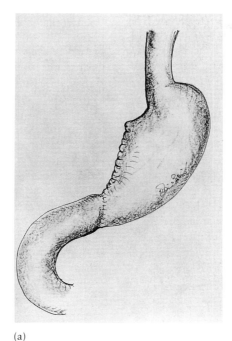 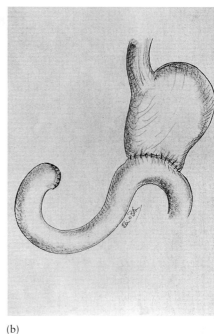

(a)   (b)

Figure 13.18 (a) Billroth I gastrectomy; (b) Polya gastrectomy.

Table 13.9 Causes of erosive gastritis.

Non-steroidal anti-inflammatory drugs
Alcohol abuse
Steroids
Critical illness (stress-induced)
Reflux bile gastritis (after gastric surgery)

Table 13.10 Causes of upper gastrointestinal bleeding (in order of incidence).

Erosive gastritis
Chronic peptic ulceration
Varices (portal hypertension)
Mallory–Weiss mucosal tears at the gastro-oesophageal junction
Others: tumours, vascular malformations, etc.

The initial treatment consists of resuscitation with setting up of an intravenous line for infusion of crystalloids/plasma expander until cross-matched blood is available, insertion of a nasogastric tube with intermittent or continuous drainage, catheterization of the bladder to assess urine output and monitoring of pulse rate and blood pressure. In unstable patients, a central venous line is also inserted for repeat measurements of the central venous pressure.

An upper gastrointestinal endoscopy is performed once the patient is stable. This usually determines the cause. Endoscopic treatment by sclerotherapy is used for both variceal bleeding and chronic ulcer disease. Other forms of endoscopic treatment include coagulation of the bleeding vessel with bipolar cautery, heater probe or Nd–YAG laser (photocoagulation). These endoscopic measures often reduce the need for surgical intervention and the amount of blood transfused. In patients with erosive gastritis, treatment with long-acting somatostatin can be effective in stopping the bleeding. On the other hand, there is no evidence that H_2-blockers are effective in this setting, although they are frequently used.

Surgical treatment is reserved for patients who continue to bleed or in whom bleeding recurs. There are endoscopic features which indicate a high risk of recurrent or continued bleeding. The important ones are active spurters and large visible vessels. In some centres, these patients are treated surgically in the first instance. The nature of the surgical treatment depends on the cause. Bleeding erosive gastritis unresponsive to conservative measures requires a total gastrectomy, bleeding gastric ulcer a partial gastrectomy and bleeding duodenal ulcer underrunning of the bleeding vessel with a non-absorbable suture. Previously a truncal vagotomy was added for bleeding duodenal ulcers but this is now often omitted in view of the efficacy of antibiotic and omeprazole therapy. The emergency treatment of bleeding oesophageal varices includes oesophageal transection using the end to end anastomosis (EEA) stapler if sclerotherapy is unsuccessful.

Zollinger–Ellison syndrome

This syndrome is characterized by severe intractable gastroduodenal ulceration due to gastrin-secreting amine precursor uptake and decarboxylation (APUD) tumour most commonly situated in the pancreas. The tumour is often malignant and may metastasize to the regional lymph nodes and the liver. Even when malignant, the tumour is slow-growing, so that long-term survival is possible despite the presence of metastatic disease if the condition is recognized and treated. The ulcers may be multiple and atypical in position and have a propensity to bleed and perforate. As the disease is due to persistent acid stimulation by a raised plasma gastrin (usually above 400 pg/ml), the basal acid secretion relative to the maximal acid secretion after pentagastrin injection is grossly elevated. Indeed, the disease should be suspected whenever the basal secretion exceeds 60% of the response to pentagastrin. Serum gastrin levels can also be measured by a radioimmunoassay.

A similar condition of intractable ulceration may be caused by two rare conditions: antral G-cell hyperplasia and retained gastric antrum. The latter results after partial Polya gastrectomy when a portion of the antrum is inadvertently retained with the duodenal stump (Fig. 13.18b). The retained antral tissue is now left in a permanent alkaline environment which leads to persistent unchecked secretion of gastrin. There are special provocation tests (calcium infusion, protein meal and secretion challenge) which, by altering the plasma gastrin level, are used to distinguish between

---

Peptic ulcer at a glance

DEFINITION

A peptic ulcer is a break in the epithelial surface of the oesophagus, stomach or duodenum (rarely Meckel's diverticulum), caused by the action of gastric secretions (acid and pepsin) and, in the case of duodenal ulceration, infection with *Helicobacter pylori*. Remember the aphorism, 'no acid, no ulcer'

CAUSES

- Imbalance between acid/pepsin secretion and mucosal defence
- Acid hypersecretion occurs because of increased numbers of parietal cells (or rarely in response to gastrin hypersecretion in the Zollinger–Ellison syndrome)
- Defects in mucosal defence (e.g. mucus secretion)
- NSAIDs and the usual suspects (!): alcohol, cigarettes and 'stress'

CLINICAL FEATURES

Duodenal ulcer (DU) and type II gastric ulcer (i.e. prepyloric and antral)
- M/F=4 : 1, 25–50 years
- Epigastric pain during fasting (hunger pain), relieved by food/antacids, typically exhibits periodicity
- Boring back pain if ulcer is penetrating posteriorly
- Haematemesis from ulcer penetrating gastroduodenal artery posteriorly
- Peritonitis if perforation occurs with anterior duodenal ulcer
- Vomiting if gastric outlet obstruction (pyloric stenosis) occurs (note succussion splash and watch for hypokalaemic hypochloraemic alkalosis)

Type I gastric ulcer (i.e. body of stomach)
- M/F=3 : 1, 50+ years
- Epigastric pain induced by eating

- Weight loss
- Nausea and vomiting
- Anaemia from chronic blood loss

INVESTIGATIONS

- FBC, U&E
- Faecal occult blood
- Oesophagogastroduodenoscopy
- Barium meal

MANAGEMENT

Medical
- Avoid smoking and foods which cause pain
- Antacids for symptomatic relief
- H$_2$-blockers (ranitidine, cimetidine)
- Proton pump inhibitors (omeprazole)
- Colloidal bismuth ⎱ These are effective
- Clarithromycin and omeprazole ⎰ against *H. pylori*
- Re-endoscope patients with gastric ulcer after 6 weeks because of risk of malignancy

Surgical
- Only indicated for failure of medical Rx and complications
- Elective for DU   Highly selective vagotomy
- Elective for GU   Billroth I gastrectomy
- Perforated DU/GU   Simple closure of perforation and biopsy
- Haemorrhage   Endoscopic control by sclerotherapy, undersewing bleeding vessel ± vagotomy
- Pyloric stenosis   Gastroenterostomy ± truncal vagotomy

FBC, full blood count; U&E, urea and electrolytes; DU, duodenal ulcer; GU, gastric ulcer.

the Zollinger–Ellison syndrome and both retained antrum and G-cell hyperplasia.

The treatment of Zollinger–Ellison syndrome varies with the exact details of the tumour in the individual patient. The most effective medical therapy is omeprazole. This proton pump inhibitor which switches off gastric secretion completely must be maintained indefinitely. Patients with a localized operable tumour benefit from surgical excision of the lesion. Since the advent of omeprazole, the need for total gastrectomy has been greatly reduced.

Chronic atrophic gastritis

Two types of chronic atrophic gastritis are recognized.

Type A chronic atrophic gastritis

Type A is associated with achlorhydria, impaired absorption of vitamin B_{12}, the presence of parietal cell antibodies in the serum and the development of pernicious anaemia. The atrophic process involves the body of the stomach with relative sparing of the antrum. Gastrin level is raised and may cause hypertrophy of the enterochromaffin cells within the gastric mucosa with the development of endocrine tumours.

Type B chronic atrophic gastritis

Type B gastritis, though often accompanied by reduced gastric acid secretion, rarely results in achlorhydria and does not usually cause pernicious anaemia. The pathological process develops in the antrum and gradually spreads to involve the rest of the stomach. Type B atrophic gastritis is caused by chronic mucosal damage: dietary salts, viral infections, bile reflux and especially infection with *H. pylori*. The gastritis may undergo metaplasia to intestinal-type epithelium and a change in the nature of the mucin from neutral to the acid sulphated variety. The metaplasia may progress to dysplasia and eventually to carcinoma. Chronic type B atrophic gastritis is often asymptomatic but it may be associated with iron-deficiency anaemia, low vitamin C levels and hypoproteinaemia.

Both type A and type B atrophic gastritis predispose to the development of invasive gastric cancer.

Gastric tumours

Gastric tumours may be benign and malignant. Gastric cancer is much more common than either gastric lymphoma or smooth-muscle tumours.

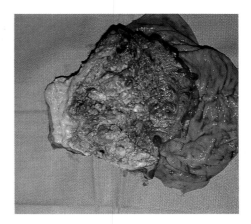

Figure 13.19 Resection specimen showing the presence of a large carcinoma in the antrum of the stomach.

Benign tumours

These include gastric adenomas and various non-neoplastic gastric polyps. The most common type is the regenerative hyperplastic variety which develops in relation to gastritis and peptic ulceration. The hamartomatous polyps of the Peutz–Jeghers syndrome may also occur in the stomach. Gastric adenoma may undergo malignant transformation and for this reason is best removed. This is usually performed endoscopically.

Gastric carcinoma (Fig. 13.19)

Introduction

Gastric carcinoma carries a poor prognosis in western countries largely due to late diagnosis. Although there has been a declining incidence of the disease during the past 30 years, it remains the third commonest gastrointestinal tumour in the UK. It is more commonly encountered in males and the peak age incidence is at 70–80 years. Nutritional factors (spiced salty foods, polycyclic hydrocarbons, high dietary salt, excess nitrates and protein malnutrition), smoking, alcohol abuse and *H. pylori* infection have been implicated on epidemiological grounds. The recognized risk factors for the development of gastric carcinoma are:
- atrophic gastritis with metaplasia and dysplasia;
- pernicious anaemia;
- previous partial gastrectomy;
- familial hypogammaglobulinaemia;
- adenomatous polyps; and
- blood group A.

Pathology

The disease starts in the mucosa as a nodule or depressed ulcer and when confined to the mucosa and submucosa is referred to as early gastric cancer. By the time of diagnosis, the majority of gastric cancers in western countries have invaded the muscularis propria of the stomach wall and have usually metastasized to the regional lymph nodes — advanced gastric cancer. Spread also occurs to the peritoneal cavity, liver omentum, ovaries and to the lungs. Histologically there are various classifications but the important one is the Lauren (DIO) system. According to this, tumours are either of the intestinal (I) or diffuse (D) types. Tumours which do not fit into these two categories are labelled as other (O). Intestinal cancer arises on a background of atrophic gastritis and is a well-circumscribed adenocarcinoma. Diffuse cancer arises from a 'normal' mucosa and is a poorly localized lesion which infiltrates rapidly the walls of the stomach and when extreme leads to a thickened shrunken stomach — leather-bottle stomach (*linitis plastica*). The intestinal cancer is more commonly encountered in the elderly and carries a better prognosis than the diffuse variety.

Clinical features

Early gastric cancer of the intestinal type is asymptomatic but early diffuse cancer may present with dyspepsia simulating peptic ulceration. Irrespective of stage, the most common presentation is that of *recent dyspepsia* in a patient above the age of 50 years. Indigestion is vague and consists of epigastric discomfort, postprandial fullness and loss of appetite. The symptoms may respond to antacid therapy. Therefore it is important that an endoscopy is performed in all these patients before any treatment is prescribed. *Anaemia* is often present at diagnosis. This is usually of the iron-deficiency type from chronic blood loss. An obstructing carcinoma at the cardia will cause *dysphagia*, whereas an antral neoplasm leads to symptoms of pyloric stenosis with *vomiting* after meals.

Curable gastric cancer is associated with a negative physical examination. Physical findings such as enlarged lymph nodes in the left supraclavicular region, epigastric mass, enlarged liver, ascites and jaundice signify advanced incurable disease.

Treatment of gastric cancer

The mainstay of treatment is surgical excision with adequate margins on either side of the neoplasm and the removal of the locoregional lymph nodes. Some of these curative excisions are quite extensive and may involve removal of the spleen and the distal pancreas. Resections may be palliative. These are more limited and provide the best palliation even in the presence of incurable disease. At least one-third of cases are inoperable. Obstructive symptoms in these patients are treated by intubation (for tumours of the cardia) and by anterior gastroenterostomy for antral tumours. Gastric carcinoma does not respond to radiotherapy but worthwhile regression may be achieved with combination chemotherapy using etoposide, epirubicin and cisplatin.

Gastric lymphoma

The stomach is the most common site of primary extranodal lymphomas. Despite this, primary gastric lymphoma is much less common than secondary involvement of the stomach by primary nodal lymphomas and gastric carcinoma. Histologically, primary gastric lymphoma originates from the *mucosa-associated lymphoid tissue (MALT)* and is therefore an example of MALT lymphoma. *H. pylori* infection has also been implicated in the aetiology of gastric lymphoma. The symptoms are similar to those of gastric cancer and include dyspepsia, anorexia, weight loss, nausea and vomiting, and diarrhoea. Some may present acutely with gastrointestinal haemorrhage or perforation. Treatment is surgical resection followed by radiotherapy. The results are generally much better than those for gastric carcinoma. Non-resectable lesions are treated with radiotherapy and combination chemotherapy such as the CHOP regimen.

Smooth-muscle tumours

These may be benign (leiomyoma) or malignant (leiomyosarcoma), although differentiation between the two can be difficult, even on histological grounds. They form solid well-circumscribed masses which can be submucosal or intramural and are commonly situated in the upper two-thirds of the stomach. When large, central necrosis may occur and lead to acute haemorrhage. Small tumours are treated by wedge resection and large ones by partial gastrectomy.

The small intestine

Introduction

The main function of the small intestine is the digestion and absorption of foodstuffs — fats, carbohydrates and proteins. The enzymic digestion to monosaccharides, fatty acids, monoglycerides and amino acids involves the action

Gastric carcinoma at a glance

DEFINITION

Malignant lesion of the stomach

EPIDEMIOLOGY

M/F=2 : 1. Age 50+ years. Incidence has decreased in western world over last 50 years. Still common in Japan, Chile and Scandinavia

AETIOLOGY

Predisposing factors
- Diet (smoked fish, pickled vegetables, benzopyrene, nitrosamines)
- Atrophic gastritis
- Pernicious anaemia
- Previous partial gastrectomy
- Familial hypogamma globulinaemia
- Gastric adenomatous polyps
- Blood group A
- Helicobacter pylori infection

PATHOLOGY

- Histology: adenocarcinoma
- Advanced gastric cancer (penetrated muscularis propria) may be polypoid, ulcerating or infiltrating (i.e. linitus plastica)
- Early gastric cancer (confined to mucosa or submucosa)
- Spread: lymphatic (e.g. Virchow's node); haematogenous to liver, lung, brain; transcoelomic to ovary (Krukenberg tumour)

CLINICAL FEATURES

- History of recent dyspepsia (epigastric discomfort, postprandial fullness, loss of appetite)

- Anaemia
- Dysphagia
- Vomiting
- Weight loss
- The presence of physical signs usually indicates advanced (incurable) disease

INVESTIGATIONS

- FBC, U&E, faecal occult blood
- OGD (see the lesion and obtain biopsy to distinguish from benign gastric ulcer)
- Barium meal (space-occupying lesion/ulcer with rolled edge)

MANAGEMENT

Palliation
- Gastrectomy, gastroenterostomy for malignant pyloric obstruction, intubation for obstructing lesions at the cardia

Curative Rx
- Surgical excision with clear margins and locoregional lymph node clearance

Other Rx
- Combination chemotherapy with etoposide, epirubicin and cisplatin may induce regression

PROGNOSIS

- Following 'curative' resection 5-year survival rates are approximately 20% but overall 5-year survival (palliation and resection) is only about 5%

OGD, oesophagogastroduodenoscopy

---

of activated pancreatic enzymes, those of the succus entericus and brush-border enzymes (in the apical microvilli of the intestinal cells). Bile salts are essential for the absorption of fats. Normally, the absorption of foodstuffs is completed in the jejunum and upper ileum but absorption of the bile salts and vitamin B_{12} occurs in the terminal ileum which has localized transport sites for these substances. Thus, disease or excision of the terminal ileum leads to malabsorption of both vitamin B_{12} and bile salts. The reabsorption of bile salts by the terminal ileum is essential for the maintenance of an adequate bile salt pool which circulates between the liver and the gut (the enterohepatic circulation). Malabsorption of bile salts leads to depletion of the bile salt pool and consequently malabsorption of fat. In addition, the bile salts reach the colon where they are deconjugated and dehydroxylated to form toxic derivatives which irritate the colonic mucosa and cause diarrhoea.

Crohn's disease

Also known as regional enteritis, this is a chronic transmural inflammatory disorder of the alimentary tract. Although it may affect any part of the gastrointestinal tract, the most common site is the terminal ileum and caecum, followed by the colorectal region. The aetiology of Crohn's disease remains unknown. The disease is segmental, with skip lesions interspersed between areas of normal bowel. Macroscopically the bowel becomes oedematous and thickened with a tendency to deep fissure ulcers and fistula formation (Fig. 13.20). There is also marked thickening of the mesentery with the fat of the mesentery riding up on to the bowel wall. Microscopically there is transmural inflammation (involving all coats) which may include non-caseating epithelioid-cell granulomas containing Langhans giants cells. These granulomas, which resemble those found in sarcoidosis, are found in 50% of resected

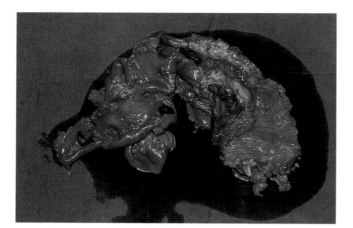

Figure 13.20 Operative specimen showing the presence of a small-bowel stricture in a patient with Crohn's disease of the small bowel.

specimens. The regional lymph nodes are usually enlarged and may contain granulomas.

The complications of Crohn's disease account for the serious nature of this disorder. They include abscess, sinus and fistula formation, intestinal obstruction, prolonged ill health and malnutrition, with growth retardation in children. The peak incidence of the disease is in the third decade. The most common symptom of small-bowel Crohn's disease is abdominal pain. Some present acutely with a picture closely simulating acute appendicitis, or acute obstruction or diffuse peritonitis. Perianal lesions (abscess and sinuses) are often present even in patients without rectal involvement.

The general radiological appearance in Crohn's disease shows fluid levels due to obstruction or internal fistulae. The important investigation is a small-bowel enema which is used to document the presence and location of the small-bowel disease (Fig. 13.21). The specific signs include narrowing of the terminal ileum (string sign of Kantor), stricture formation or perpendicular ulcers. Indium-labelled white blood cell scanning with a γ-camera is useful in assessing the extent of disease and may indicate which parts of the bowel are involved.

The treatment of Crohn's disease is medical in the first instance. This consists of dietary manipulation, use of anti-inflammatory drugs (steroids and salazopyrine), antibiotics and in some patients immunosuppressive agents. Acutely ill patients and those with the short-gut syndrome require parenteral nutrition. The indications for surgical treatment are shown in Table 13.11. Surgical treatment consists of localized resections for florid disease and stricturoplasty for burnt-out stenotic lesions. Unfortunately, recurrence is very common after resection.

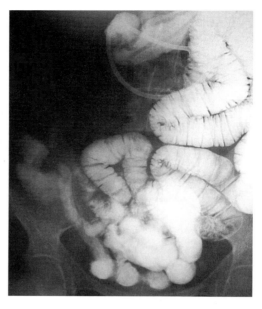

Figure 13.21 Small-bowel enema showing multiple areas of Crohn's disease with intervening normal intestine (slip lesions).

Table 13.11 Indications for surgical treatment in small-bowel Crohn's disease.

Onset of complications
Peritonitis
Obstruction
Abscess
Fistula
Growth retardation

Failure of medical treatment
Severe symptoms
Chronic invalidism

Complications of medical treatment
Steroid side-effects

Short-gut syndrome

Short-gut syndrome follows massive resection (>50%) of the small intestine (Table 13.12). Patients with a residual bowel length of 2 m have a diminished capacity for work and those with less than 1 m have permanent intestinal failure so that nutrition can only be maintained by home parenteral nutrition. To some extent the critical length of residual bowel necessary to prevent failure depends on the site of resection and the presence or absence of the ileocaecal valve. Thus, ileal resections are less well-tolerated than jejunal resections, mainly due to loss of localized transport sites for the absorption of bile salts and vitamin B_{12}.

Crohn's disease at a glance

DEFINITION

Crohn's disease is a chronic transmural inflammatory disorder of the alimentary tract

EPIDEMIOLOGY

M/F=1 : 1.6. Age: young adults. High incidence among Europeans and Jews

AETIOLOGY

- Unknown
- Impaired cell-mediated immunity

PATHOLOGY

Macroscopic
- May affect any part of the alimentary tract
- Skip lesions in bowel (affected bowel wall and mesentery are thickened and oedematous; frequent fistulae)
- Perianal disease characterized by perianal induration and sepsis with fissure, sinus and fistula formation

Histology
- Transmural inflammation
- Non-caseating epithelioid cell granulomas with Langhans giant cells. Regional nodes may also be involved

CLINICAL FEATURES

- Abdominal pain; some present with appendicitis picture; some with intestinal obstruction, fistulae or abscesses

- General ill health, malnutrition, anaemia
- Extra intestinal features:
  - (a) Eye   Episcleritis, uveitis
  - (b) Joints   Arthritis
  - (c) Skin   Erythema nodosum
- Perianal disease, *fissure-in-ano, fistula-in-ano*, perianal sepsis

INVESTIGATIONS

- FBC (macrocytic anaemia)
- Small-bowel enema (narrowed terminal ileum, string sign of Kantor, stricture formation fistulae)
- Abdominal ultrasound (abscess formation)
- Indium-labelled white cell scan

MANAGEMENT

Medical
- Nutritional support (enteral and parenteral feeding)
- Anti-inflammatory drugs (salazopyrine, steroids)
- Antibiotics (only for specific complicating bacterial infections)
- Immunosuppressive agents (azathioprine)

Surgery
- For complications (peritonitis, obstruction, abscess, fistula)
- Failure of medical treatment

PROGNOSIS

Crohn's disease is a chronic problem and recurrent episodes of active disease are common

---

Table 13.12 Lesions which may necessitate extensive resections of the small intestine.

Crohn's disease
Mesenteric infarction
Radiation enteritis
Mid-gut volvulus
Multiple fistulae
Small-bowel tumours

The most common cause nowadays is repeated resections of the small bowel for recurrences of Crohn's disease. Immediately following the resection, there is complete intestinal decompensation so that survival depends on total parenteral nutrition. Subsequently, intestinal adaptation, which consists of dilatation of the residual small intestine and villous enlargement, results in improved absorption and, provided the patient has more than the critical length of 1.0 m, oral nutrition with sup-

plements and intestinal sedative drugs can be resumed in time. These patients are, however, subject to certain complications (Table 13.13).

Blind-loop syndrome

This is also known as the stagnant-loop syndrome and results from bacterial overgrowth in the small intestine as a result of stasis due to stricture, enterocolic fistula, jejunal

Table 13.13 Extraintestinal complications of massive small-bowel resections.

Gastric hypersecretion — peptic ulceration
Cholesterol gallstone formation — reduced bile salt pool
Hepatic disease
Impaired renal function
Urinary stone formation
Metabolic bone disease

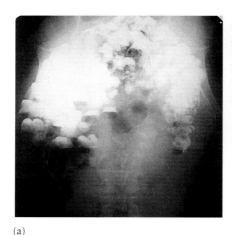

(a)

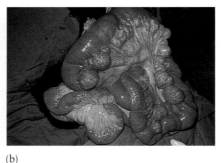

(b)

Figure 13.22 (a) Radiograph and (b) operative specimen showing jejunal diverticulosis which may lead to bacterial overgrowth and the blind-loop syndrome.

diverticulosis (Fig. 13.22) or kinking caused by adhesions of the small-bowel loops. The bacterial overgrowth causes patchy mucosal inflammation and leads to the deconjugation and dehydroxylation of the intraluminal bile salts. As these tertiary derivatives are ineffective in emulsifying dietary fat, absorption of fat and fat-soluble vitamins is impaired. The absorption of carbohydrates and proteins is also impaired, though to a lesser extent. In addition, the bacteria bind vitamin B_{12} and convert it to inactive derivatives which block the ileal receptors for the vitamin as well as intrinsic factor.

The symptoms and signs of bacterial overgrowth include asthenia, nausea and vomiting, excessive bowel sounds and weight loss. Diarrhoea is frequent and is usually watery. Other clinical features include glossitis and stomatitis, anaemia which may be megaloblastic, hypoproteinaemia, hypocalcaemia and peripheral oedema. The treatment of bacterial overgrowth includes surgical correction of the underlying abnormality whenever possible. Otherwise, improvement in both symptoms and nutritional state can be achieved by intermittent courses of oral antibiotics such as tetracycline.

Radiation enteropathy

Both the small and the large intestine may sustain damage from radiotherapy, especially when the dose administered exceeds 40 Gy (4000 rad). Some groups are more susceptible. These include patients who have had previous surgery, those with a history of pelvic sepsis, the elderly and patients with diabetes, hypertension and cardiovascular disease. Radiation enteropathy is characterized by transmural fibrosis and ischaemia due to a proliferative endarteritis and vasculitis. In addition there is obliteration of the intestinal lymphatics. Aside from chronic symptoms such as abdominal pain, diarrhoea and rectal bleeding, intestinal perforation,

acute haemorrhage and infarction may occur. Apart from intestinal sedative drugs to alleviate the diarrhoea, there is no effective medical therapy and, if limited, the condition is treated by resection.

Specific intestinal infections

Many gastroenterological infections are viral but both acute and chronic bacterial infections do occur. The two chronic bacterial infections of surgical importance are intestinal tuberculosis and actinomycosis.

Intestinal tuberculosis

Intestinal tuberculosis is often accompanied by tuberculous peritonitis and may be primary or secondary. Primary intestinal tuberculosis is due to infection by *Mycobacterium bovis* acquired by drinking infected (and unpasteurized) milk. The secondary type is caused by infection by *M. tuberculosis* and is secondary to pulmonary disease. Intestinal tuberculosis usually affects the distal ileum of children and young adults and can be hypertrophic, ulcerative or fibrotic. Chronic systemic symptoms include ill health, anorexia, fever, night sweats, dyspepsia and weight loss. In addition, abdominal pain is often present and, on examination, a tender inflammatory mass is present in the right iliac fossa. The patient may present acutely with intestinal obstruction, perforation or bleeding. The treatment of the uncomplicated disease is medical with antituberculous chemotherapy. Patients with complicated disease require emergency resection of the diseased area together with antituberculous chemotherapy.

Tuberculous peritonitis usually presents with ascites and abdominal distension. It may be secondary to tuberculous mesenteric lymph nodes or intestinal tuberculosis and rarely tuberculous pyosalpinx. *M. tuberculosis* can be cultured from the straw-coloured ascitic fluid and at laparotomy or laparoscopy the peritoneum and omentum are characteristically studded with tubercles which are small white nodules. Treatment is by antituberculous chemotherapy (Chapter 19).

Abdominal actinomycosis

Ileocaecal actinomycosis is rare. The infection is caused by *Actinomycosis israelii* and usually develops several weeks after a perforated appendicitis. It forms an indurated mass in the right iliac fossa with suppuration and sinus formation. The treatment is conservative with penicillin and lincomycin.

Tumours of the small intestine

Tumours of the small intestine are rare and account for less than 10% of all gastrointestinal neoplasms. Benign tumours include adenomas and neurogenic tumours. The adenomas may occur in association with any of the various types of familial polyposis: polyposis coli, Gardner's syndrome (familial polyposis and epidermoid cysts) and Turcot's syndrome (familial polyposis and brain tumours). The commonest presentation of benign small-bowel tumour is intussusception and some may bleed but the majority are asymptomatic. The malignant neoplasms include adenocarcinoma, carcinoid tumours, lymphomas and smooth-muscle tumours. Malignant small-bowel tumours tend to present late, usually with intestinal obstruction and for this reason carry a poor prognosis. Like gastric lymphoma, intestinal lymphoma is derived from the MALT lymphoid tissue.

Carcinoid tumours

These are neuroendocrine APUD tumours which arise from the Kulchitsky cells of the crypts of Lieberkühn (enterochromaffin cells) and are subdivided into foregut, midgut and hindgut tumours. There are staining and secretory differences between these three categories. The fore and midgut carcinoids secrete a variety of hormones in addition to serotonin (5-hydroxytryptamine), whereas the hindgut tumours do not secrete active peptides. The clinical manifestation of jejunoileal carcinoids include diarrhoea, intestinal obstruction, palpable mass, gastrointestinal haemorrhage and, rarely, infarction. The development of the carcinoid syndrome is associated with advanced disease and extensive hepatic involvement. The clinical features of this syndrome include attacks of cutaneous flushing, intestinal colic, diarrhoea, bronchospasm, cardiac lesions (tricuspid insufficiency and pulmonary stenosis) and skin rashes. The diagnosis is confirmed by urinary estimation of 5-hydroxyindoleacetic acid, which is a derivative of serotonin.

Treatment of small-bowel tumours

The treatment of malignant small-bowel tumours is by resection. Lymphomas are also treated by radiotherapy or chemotherapy, usually following resection of the disease, but also as the primary treatment in patients with inoperable tumours. The best agent for the control of carcinoid symptoms is long-acting somatostatin.

Meckel's diverticulum

Meckel's diverticulum is the persistent remains of the vitellointestinal tract and occurs on the antimesenteric border of the terminal ileum in approximately 2.0% of individuals, usually within 60 cm of the ileocaecal valve. It is a true diverticulum and is therefore composed of all the intestinal coats. It may contain heterotopic tissue: gastric, pancreatic, duodenal and colonic. In infants under the age of 2 years, ulcerated ectopic mucosa in a Meckel's diverticulum is the commonest cause of copious rectal bleeding. The other complications include obstructive inflammation, which is clinically indistinguishable from acute appendicitis, perforation and volvulus. All these complications require emergency surgical treatment, which consists of excision of the diverticulum. Usually the appendix is removed at the same time (Fig. 13.23).

The vermiform appendix

Acute appendicitis

This is the commonest surgical emergency in western countries. It is rarely encountered before the age of 2 years, reaches its peak incidence in the second and third decades but may occur at any age. Perforation of the acutely

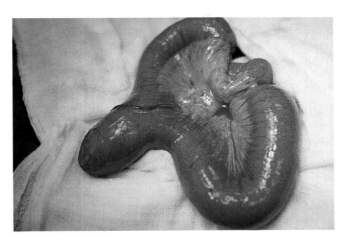

Figure 13.23 Meckel's diverticulum.

inflamed appendix is encountered most commonly in children and the elderly.

Pathology

Acute appendicitis is generally thought to arise from infection superimposed on luminal obstruction from any cause. However, luminal obstruction is not invariably present and mucosal ulceration is frequent. In some patients at least, the disease may be secondary to viral infection which causes lymphoid hyperplasia and ulceration of the mucosa leading to bacterial invasion. Irrespective of exact origin, the infection is a mixed one with both Gram-negative aerobes (*Escherichia coli, Streptococcus faecalis*) and anaerobes (*Bacteroides, Clostridium*).

Clinical features

The clinical features of acute appendicitis are usually characteristic.

History The history consists of the sequential development of periumbilical colicky abdominal pain which is followed by nausea and vomiting. Vomiting is often excessive in children, when the condition may simulate gastroenteritis. Within a few hours, the pain becomes localized to the right iliac fossa. The patient usually has a mild pyrexia on admission to hospital.

Examination On examination the patient is flushed and has a tachycardia, furred tongue and halitosis. Tenderness on mild palpation is maximal over the right iliac fossa over McBurney's point (junction of the upper two-thirds with lower one-third of the line between the anterior superior iliac spine and the umbilicus). This is the most important sign of acute appendicitis. The patient usually experiences pain in the same region when asked to cough. This is equivalent to eliciting rebound tenderness in this region — a physical sign which must be sought with extreme gentleness. If the appendix has perforated, the abdominal signs are those of peritonitis. A rectal examination is important and right-sided pelvic tenderness is elicited in 30% of patients, especially those with a pelvic appendix. Other physical signs (Rovsing, psoas, etc.) are most unreliable and are of historical interest only. A leukocytosis is invariably present.

Appendix mass Some patients may present late and on examination have an inflammatory mass in the right iliac fossa. This is indurated, fixed and tender. The mass consists of the inflamed appendix surrounded by adjacent bowel loops and greater omentum. This inflammatory phlegmon may proceed to the formation of a true abscess or resolve. In

any event, the situation may give rise to diagnostic difficulties. The differential diagnosis then includes Crohn's disease, carcinoma of the caecum with associated appendicitis, ileocaecal tuberculosis and actinomycosis.

Differential diagnosis In the more usual early acute appendicitis, the important differential diagnosis includes mesenteric lymphadenitis in children and pelvic disease in females in whom the diagnosis is often incorrect. The clinical picture of mesenteric lymphadenitis is similar to that of acute appendicitis but the signs are less pronounced and the abdominal tenderness changes with different positions of the patient — shifting tenderness. The important common disorders which may masquerade as acute appendicitis in the child-bearing female are acute salpingo-oophoritis, ectopic pregnancy and ruptured corpus luteum cysts.

Treatment

The treatment of acute appendicitis is appendicectomy carried out as soon as the diagnosis is made (Fig. 13.24). The management of patients with appendix mass is conservative in the first place. These patients are put on antibiotics, intravenous fluids and hourly observations of temperature and pulse rate with repeat abdominal examination. If the condition resolves, an interval appendicectomy is performed a few months later. If the condition deteriorates, surgical treatment is undertaken as a matter of urgency.

Complications

The complications of acute appendicitis include wound infection, intra-abdominal abscess formation, adhesion formation, portal pyaemia (pylephlebitis) and abdominal

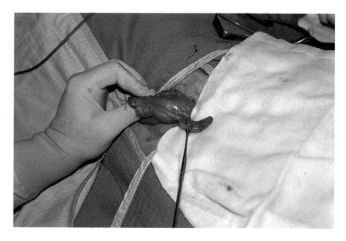

Figure 13.24 Operative photograph of acute appendicitis.

Acute appendicitis at a glance

DEFINITION

Acute appendicitis is an inflammation of the vermiform appendix

EPIDEMIOLOGY

Commonest surgical emergency in the western world. Rare under 2 years, common in second and third decades but can occur at any age

PATHOLOGY

- Infection superimposed on luminal obstruction from any cause
- Viral infection, lymphoid hyperplasia, ulceration, bacterial invasion, appendicitis

CLINICAL FEATURES

- Periumbilical abdominal pain, nausea, vomiting
- Localization of pain to right iliac fossa
- Mild pyrexia
- Patient is flushed, tachycardia, furred tongue, halitosis
- Tender (usually with rebound) over McBurney's point
- Right-sided pelvic tenderness on PR examination
- Peritonitis if appendix is perforated
- Appendix mass if patient presents late

INVESTIGATIONS

- Diagnosis is a clinical diagnosis but WCC (almost always leukocytosis) and CRP (usually raised) are helpful
- Ultrasound for appendix mass and, if in doubt, to rule out other pelvic pathology (e.g. ovarian cyst)

DIFFERENTIAL DIAGNOSIS

- Mesenteric lymphadenitis in children
- Pelvic disease in women (e.g. pelvic inflammatory disease, urinary tract infections, ectopic pregnancy, rupured corpus luteum cyst)
- (More rarely: Crohn's disease, cholecystitis, perforated duodenal ulcer, right basal pneumonia, torsion of the right testis, diabetes mellitus)
- Acute non-specific abdominal pain

MANAGEMENT

- Acute appendicitis – appendicectomy
- Appendix mass – IV fluids, antibiotics, close observation
  (a) If symptoms resolve – interval appendicectomy after a few months
  (b) If symptoms progress – urgent appendicectomy ± drainage

COMPLICATIONS

- Wound infection
- Adhesions
- Abdominal actinomycosis (rare!)
- Intra-abdominal abscess
- Portal pyaemia

PR, Per rectum; WCC, white cell count; CRP, C-reactive protein.

---

actinomycosis. These complications usually occur in patients with perforated disease. Intra-abdominal abscess may occur anywhere in the peritoneal cavity but the commonest is pelvic abscess. The manifestations of this complication include intermittent pyrexia and diarrhoea with the passage of mucus. On rectal examination, a tender boggy mass is palpable. The abscess usually discharges spontaneously into the rectum with healing. Adhesion formation may give rise to recurrent small-bowel obstruction and may cause sterility in the female.

Appendiceal carcinoid tumours

The appendix is the most common site of carcinoid tumours and carcinoid tumour of the appendix is the most common appendiceal tumour. The others include adenocarcinoma, mucinous neoplasms and lymphoma. The vast majority of appendiceal carcinoids are found incidentally at the time of appendicectomy and usually arise from the tip of the organ. Less commonly, they originate from the base of the appendix when they may invade the lumen and cause appendicitis. They rarely metastasize and the prognosis is good.

The colon and rectum

Cancer's a funny thing
I wish I had the voice of Homer
To sing of rectal carcinoma
Which kills a lot more chaps in fact
Than were bumped off when Troy was sacked.
JBS Haldane   (1892–1964)

Diverticular disease

Congenital diverticula

Congenital diverticula may be found in the caecum and may bleed, giving rise to anaemia and melaena. Inflammation of a solitary caecal diverticulum will present like acute appendicitis or as an inflammatory mass resembling an appendix phlegmon or an appendicular abscess. It may also present in a less acute fashion, giving rise to a suspicion of caecal carcinoma.

Acquired diverticulosis

Aetiology

In most western countries the diet is deficient in fibre, thus altering the bulk and consistency of colonic residue. As a result the normal segmental contractions of the colon are more vigorous and prolonged, raising the intraluminal pressure. This eventually leads to herniation of the mucosa through the circular muscle of the colonic wall where the anterior and posterior branches of the marginal artery enter. This gives rise to two rows of diverticula adjacent to the appendices epiploicae. The disease is slightly more common in females and there is an increasing incidence from the fourth or fifth decade onwards.

Pathology

Diverticula are mainly found in the sigmoid colon, although they may also be seen more proximally. They emerge between the taenia coli and may contain faecoliths. The circular muscle of the colon is thickened and the taenia are thickened also, causing shortening of the colon.

Clinical presentation

In the majority of patients diverticular disease is *asymptomatic*. However a number of patients present with one or more of the following complications:
- painful diverticulosis;
- acute diverticulitis;
- perforation of a diverticulum;
- obstruction;
- fistula; and
- haemorrhage.

Painful diverticulosis

A number of patients present with intermittent attacks of pain, principally located in the left iliac fossa and accompanied by either constipation or alternating constipation and diarrhoea with mucus. The pain may be transient or persist for some days and is relieved temporarily by passing flatus. An increase in dietary fibre, although it may initially cause exacerbation of the symptoms, will usually produce relief in a week or so.

Acute diverticulitis

This complication of colonic diverticulosis produces a more generalized picture of malaise, anorexia and fever with local signs of tenderness, rigidity and a palpable mass in the left iliac fossa. Abdominal distension may occur and a sentinel loop of small bowel may sometimes be seen in plain films of the abdomen. Frequency and haematuria are the result of adherence of the inflamed loop of colon to the bladder. Treatment includes bed rest, intravenous fluids, analgesia and antibiotics. In almost all patients the acute attack will subside with this regimen.

Perforation

In some patients acute inflammation may progress to perforation. Such a perforation may become walled-off as a pericolic abscess or may perforate freely into the peritoneal cavity, causing generalized faecal peritonitis. If signs of generalized peritonitis are absent the patient may be treated conservatively but any exacerbation of symptoms is an indication for laparotomy.

Formerly, drainage of local collections of pus, repair of the perforation with an omental patch and a proximal defunctioning colostomy was the recommended treatment. Such treatment was associated with a high postoperative mortality. Nowadays resection of the inflamed and perforated segment is recommended with proximal colostomy and closure of the distal colon. This is known eponymously as Hartmann's procedure. Restoration of colonic continuity is undertaken 6 months later.

Obstruction

An episode of acute inflammation may be complicated by acute large-bowel obstruction due to occlusion of the bowel lumen, but this is likely to subside with resolution of the inflammation. Repeated attacks of inflammation with thickening of the bowel wall and fibrous stricture formation may precipitate recurring attacks of subacute obstruction. Small-bowel obstruction due to adherence of a loop of small intestine to a sigmoid inflammatory mass may also occur (see below). Distinction from colonic cancer may be difficult and the two may co-exist.

Fistula

Adherence of the inflamed colon to adjacent organs may cause fistula into the small bowel, vagina or bladder. A fistula involving the small intestine may cause diarrhoea or subacute obstruction. Communication with the vagina or uterus will be evident from discharge of faecal material through the vagina. Colovesical fistula presents as intractable cystitis and, if the fistula is large enough, with pneumaturia. Resection of the inflamed loop of colon and repair of the fistula is the appropriate treatment.

Haemorrhage

Severe acute haemorrhage may occur in elderly patients with diverticular disease due to erosion of the vessels adjacent to the diverticulum. The haemorrhage usually occurs without warning and is not usually associated with complications of the diverticulosis such as inflammation. The acute bleed is treated conservatively in most cases but resection of the affected sigmoid loop may be necessary to avoid repeated attacks. The bleeding must be distinguished from that caused by angiodysplasia. The location of the bleeding can sometimes be identified at sigmoidoscopy. Angiography is required to demonstrate angiodysplasia.

Diverticular disease at a glance

DEFINITION

Diverticular disease (or *diverticulosis*) is a condition in which many sac-like mucosal projections (diverticula) develop in the large bowel, especially the sigmoid colon. Acute inflammation of a diverticulum causes *diverticulitis*

EPIDEMIOLOGY

M/F = 1 : 1.5 Age 40s and 50s onwards. High incidence in the western world, where it is found in 50% of people over 60 years

AETIOLOGY

- Low fibre in the diet causes an increase in intraluminal colonic pressure causing herniation of mucosa through the coats of the wall of the colon
- Weak areas in wall of colon where nutrient arteries penetrate to submucosa and mucosa

PATHOLOGY

Macroscopic
- Diverticula mostly found in (thickened) sigmoid colon
- Emerge between the taenia coli and may contain faecoliths

Histology
- Projections are *pseudodiverticula* as they contain only submucosa and mucosa and not all layers of intestinal wall

CLINICAL FEATURES

- Mostly asymptomatic
- Painful diverticulosis — LIF pain, constipation, diarrhoea
- Acute diverticulitis — Malaise, fever, LIF pain and tenderness ± palpable mass and abdominal distension
- Perforation — Peritonitis + features of diverticulitis

- Large-bowel obstruction — Absolute constipation, distension, colicky abdominal pain and vomiting
- Fistula — To bladder (cystitis/pneumaturia) To vagina (faecal discharge PV) To small intestine (diarrhoea)
- Lower GI bleed — Distinguish from angiodysplasia

INVESTIGATIONS

- Diverticulosis — Barium enema/colonoscopy
- Diverticulitis ⎱ FBC, WCC, U&E, CXR
- Perforation ⎰ Plain film of abdomen
- Obstruction — Gastrografin or dilute barium enema
- Fistula — MSU, cystoscopy, colposcopy
- Haemorrhage — Colonoscopy, selective angiography

MANAGEMENT

Medical
- High-fibre diet (fruit, vegetables, wholemeal breads, bran)

Surgical
- Usually for complications or, rarely, failed medical treatment
- Elective left colon surgery without peritonitis: resect diseased colon and rejoin the ends (primary anastomosis)
- Emergency left colon surgery with peritonitis: resect diseased segment, oversew distal bowel (i.e. upper rectum) and bring out proximal bowel as end-colostomy (Hartmann's procedure)
- Complicated left colon surgery (e.g. colovesical fistula): resection, primary anastomosis, defunctioning proximal colostomy

PROGNOSIS

- Diverticular disease is a 'benign' condition but there is significant mortality and morbidity from the complications

LIF, Left iliac fossa; PV, per vaginam; MSU, midstream urine

Vascular lesions of the colon

Angiodysplasia

Angiodysplastic lesions of the colon occur in the elderly and give rise to recurrent episodes of severe bleeding or chronic anaemia due to persistent slow blood loss. These anomalous vessels are mostly confined to the caecum and right side of the colon and can only be identified at angiography. Intra-arterial infusion of vasopressin or embolization with injection of Gelfoam into the appropriate vessels may be employed to stop bleeding. Right hemicolectomy may be a more certain means of providing a cure.

Ischaemic colitis

Ischaemic colitis occurs in elderly patients who have arteriosclerosis, blood disorders with increased viscosity, or who have had surgical interference with the colonic blood supply as in resection of an aortic aneurysm. If sufficiently acute and severe, the interference with the blood supply may cause gangrene. If less severe or more chronic, the condition may be transient or the end-result may be stricture.

The patient presents with severe crampy left-sided abdominal pain followed by bloody diarrhoea. The degree of pain and tenderness reflects the severity of the condition. If severe symptoms persist, gangrene should be suspected and laparotomy and resection undertaken. Conservative measures with intravenous fluids and antibiotics are appropriate for less severe forms of ischaemia. When the acute symptoms have subsided, barium studies may show lateral indentations in the column of barium (thumb-printing), indicating mucosal oedema. If later stricture formation occurs, the lesion may resemble a stenosing colonic carcinoma on barium studies. Resection may be required for subacute obstruction.

Volvulus of the colon

Caecal volvulus

Poor fixation of the caecum in the right iliac fossa may result in volvulus. The torsion is clockwise and may cause acute closed-loop obstruction with rapidly supervening gangrene and generalized peritonitis. The condition may resolve spontaneously but more frequently requires surgical intervention with resection of a gangrenous caecum of fixation of the latter to the right iliac fossa if intervention has been early enough.

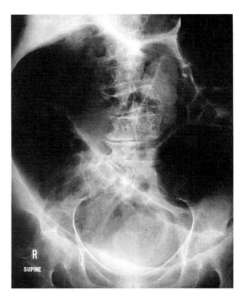

Figure 13.25 Plain abdominal X-ray showing a sigmoid volvulus.

Sigmoid volvulus

Volvulus of the sigmoid colon tends to occur in elderly, constipated institutionalized patients who are mentally defective. In addition to the above interrelated factors there is a redundant sigmoid loop on a narrow mesentery. Torsion occurs around the mesenteric axis. A varying degree of obstruction occurs from chronic to subacute to acute obstruction and strangulation. The patient presents with abdominal distension and tenderness and plain X-rays of the abdomen demonstrate a grossly dilated loop of large bowel (Fig. 13.25). Decompression of the loop with a flatus tube or sigmoidoscope may be possible in subacute obstruction. More often, laparotomy is required. Fixation of the untwisted loop to the left iliac fossa may be sufficient if the bowel is viable. If not, resection should be carried out. It is probably wisest to defer reconstruction of the colon to a later date and limit the emergency operation to a Hartmann's procedure. Resection of the sigmoid loop and end-to-end anastomosis are indicated for recurrent obstruction.

Chronic inflammatory bowel disease

By convention, the term inflammatory bowel disease is confined to two conditions, *ulcerative colitis* and *Crohn's disease* of the colon. Although easily distinguished from one another in their classical presentations, in some patients there is sufficient overlap in symptomatology, radiological findings and histological features to make either diagnosis a possibility — indeterminate colitis. An accurate diagnosis is important, however, as the correct diagnosis has implications for prognosis and treatment.

Ulcerative colitis

In ulcerative colitis the proximal extent of the inflammation is variable but the rectum is almost always involved. The small intestine is not affected except for the backwash ileitis which may occur in patients with proximal colonic disease and an incompetent ileocaecal valve.

Extracolonic manifestations of ulcerative colitis include:
- eye disorders (iritis, interstitial keratitis, retrobulbar neuritis);
- arthritis (sacroiliitis, ankylosing spondylitis);
- skin disorders (pyoderma gangrenosum, erythema nodosum);
- renal calculi and pyelonephritis;
- blood disorders (hypochromic anaemia, deep vein thrombosis and haemolytic anaemia); and
- hepatic disease and cholangitis.

Aetiology

A genetic orgin for the disease is suggested by its ethnic and familial associations and its association with human leukocyte antigen (HLA)-B27 phenotypes. Ulcerative colitis may also have an autoimmune basis. It is no longer seriously regarded as a psychosomatic illness, although psychological stresses may be involved in its onset.

Clinical features

Ulcerative colitis presents in the third and fourth decades and is more common in females. Colonic symptoms are diarrhoea with passage of mucus and pus and rectal bleeding. Abdominal pain is often present. Systematic symptoms include anorexia and weight loss. A low-grade pyrexia usually accompanies the symptoms. The disease may pursue a mild and chronic course and the disease in these patients is usually confined to the distal colon and rectum.

A more severe and progressive form of the disease may run a rapid course and develop complications such as toxic megacolon, perforation and severe bleeding. Fulminant ulcerative colitis may develop *de novo* or occur as an exacerbation of chronic disease. The patient develops profuse diarrhoea and bleeding and rapidly becomes hypovolaemic and shocked and the abdomen becomes distended and painful. Toxic megacolon and perforation may ensue. These patients are desperately ill and in this situation require rapid resuscitation and urgent colectomy.

Investigations

- Plain films of the abdomen are useful in the severely ill patient (Fig. 13.26a). They can demonstrate air under the diaphragm if a perforation has occurred and will show the progressive colonic dilatation in patients with toxic megacolon.
- In chronic ulcerative colitis a *barium enema* will demonstrate loss of haustrations and the rigidity and shortening aptly described as 'lead-pipe' appearance (Fig. 13.26b). Diffuse narrowing can also be noted, as well as a fuzzy appearance at the margins of the barium outline due to mucosal ulceration.
- *Sigmoidoscopy* will demonstrate an inflamed friable mucosa which bleeds easily on contact. Mucosal ulceration is unusual but may be present in severe cases.

Pseudopolyps may also be seen (Fig. 13.26c). Biopsy confirms the diagnosis with an inflammatory infiltrate of lymphocytes, plasma cells, eosinophils and mast cells in the mucosa and submucosa. The crypts of Lieberkühn are inflamed and crypt abscesses develop which coalesce and cause ulceration.

Treatment

Medical treatment

- *Sulphasalazine* (Salazopyrin), which is a combination of a sulphonamide and aminosalicylic acid, may induce remission in acute attacks and is effective in the prevention of relapse. It is less effective than steroids and is used only in mild cases or as maintenance therapy. Side-effects which may inhibit its use are nausea, vomiting and headache, skin rashes and blood dyscrasias.
- Occasionally *azathioprine* is used in combination with sulphasalazine to reduce relapse frequency in resistant cases.
- *Steroids* used topically as Predsol enemas or orally (30–40 mg prednisolone) are probably the treatment of choice in mild ulcerative colitis. For moderately severe cases a higher oral dose is appropriate but with severe acute disease intravenous hydrocortisone is required with transfer to high oral dosage of prednisolone when improvement takes places.
- *High-fibre diet* and bulk-forming agents such as *methylcellulose* may be useful and occasionally antidiarrhoeal drugs such as *codeine phosphate* are required.

Surgical treatment

Indications Surgery is indicated if *medical treatment fails* to control an acute episode or if *relapses are too frequent*. Surgery may also be necessary because of complications

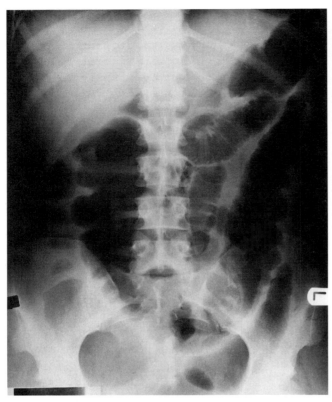

(a)

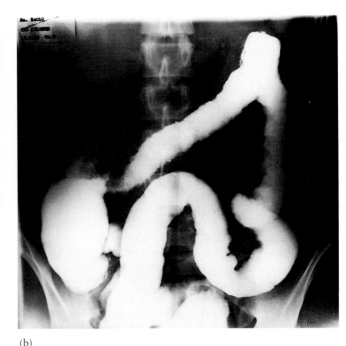

(b)

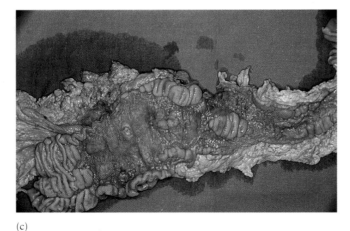

(c)

Figure 13.26 (a) Plain abdominal film of a patient with acute ulcerative colitis. Note the dilated colon, mucosa oedema, 'thumb-printing', thickened haustra, absence of faeces, small-bowel dilatation. (b) Barium enema showing ulcerative colitis. Note the shortened narrow colon, loss of haustrations and the 'lead-pipe' colon. (c) Pathology specimen of ulcerative colitis. Note the presence of superficial ulceration and pseudopolyposis (regenerative tissue from surviving islands of mucosa).

such as *perforation* or *toxic megacolon* and because of the *risk of cancer* in ulcerative colitis of more than 10 years' duration (see below).

Surgery Classically surgery for ulcerative colitis consists of removing the colon, rectum and anus (panprocto-colectomy) and creating a permanent ileostomy. As ulcerative colitis is confined to the large bowel, this procedure is curative but leaves the patient with one of the following ileostomies.

• A well-functioning spout ileostomy (*Brooke ileostomy*; Fig. 13.27) gives very satisfactory results with abolition of all intestinal symptoms and greatly improved general health. Problems may occur with the ileostomy such as re-traction, prolapse or obstruction, and refashioning of the ileostomy may be necessary.

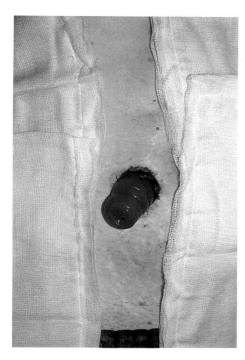

Figure 13.27 Brooke ileostomy. Unlike a colostomy, an ileostomy has a long spout.

• The *Koch ileostomy* provides a continent stoma; this involves the construction of a reservoir and a continent valve with the stoma in the right iliac fossa. Evacuation is carried out by catheter. Disruption of the valve mechanism with incontinence and occasional fistula formation are complications. This procedure is rarely done now.

More recently, surgeons have attempted to preserve the anal sphincters by performing a colectomy but retaining a short rectal stump which is then stripped of its mucosa. To maintain continence a reservoir (ileal pouch) is created from the distal ileum and anastomosed to the anus. The construction of an ileal pouch (usually J-shaped) and pouch–anal anastomosis enables the removal of all diseased mucosa with preservation of sphincter function and anal continence. Stool frequency is high (6–8 motions per day) and continence of flatus not assured. There may also be some soiling at night time.

Complications of ulcerative colitis

• *Perforation.* Perforation may occur during an acute attack or in association with toxic megacolon. The patient develops generalized peritonitis and septic shock but the clinical features may be masked if the patient is on steroid therapy. The mortality is around 30%.

• *Toxic megacolon.* In toxic megacolon the inflammatory process involves the full thickness of the bowel wall with coalescence of crypt abscesses, destruction of the muscle layer and the myenteric plexus and severe dilation of a very friable colon. Signs and symptoms include pyrexia, tachycardia, anaemia, hypovolaemia and electrolyte disturbance. The abdomen is distended, bowel sounds are absent and blood pressure is low. Perforation is imminent and if intense medical treatment does not elicit an immediate response, emergency colectomy is needed. The mortality is 20–30%.

• *Carcinoma.* Patients with extensive ulcerative colitis involving the entire colon in whom the disease has been present for more than 10 years have a significantly higher risk of developing cancer than the general population. Because of the confusion between symptoms of ulcerative colitis itself and symptoms of a tumour, diagnosis is often late and the prognosis is poor. Hence, the need for surveillance in patients at risk.

Crohn's disease

Although originally called regional ileitis because of its classical presentation, Crohn's disease can occur anywhere in the gastrointestinal tract (see above), including the colon and frequently perianally. Its symptomatology is very varied, ranging from chronic diarrhoea, abdominal pain and weight loss to the clinical features of acute appendicitis, pyrexia, vomiting and right iliac fossa pain. It may also present as an abdominal mass, as acute intestinal obstruction and with multiple perianal fissures and abscesses. The extra-alimentary tract manifestations of Crohn's disease are arthritis and skin conditions such as erythema nodosum and pyoderma gangrenosum. Crohn's disease gives rise to chronic ill health and children fail to thrive, have retarded growth and are generally malnourished. The aetiology of Crohn's disease is unknown but heredity and autoimmune reactions may play a part.

Pathology

In contrast to ulcerative colitis, the inflammation of Crohn's disease involves the full thickness of the bowel wall. Crypt abscesses are rare but non-caseating granulomas are present (Fig. 13.28). The bowel serosa is involved, as are the mesentery and regional lymph nodes. Macroscopically the bowel wall is reddened and thickened. The mucosa has a cobblestone appearance with deep fissured ulcers surrounded by oedematous mucosa. The mesentery is shortened and thickened and lymph nodes are enlarged and show a hyperplastic reaction. Fistulae may occur to the skin, to adjacent loops of bowel or to the bladder or vagina.

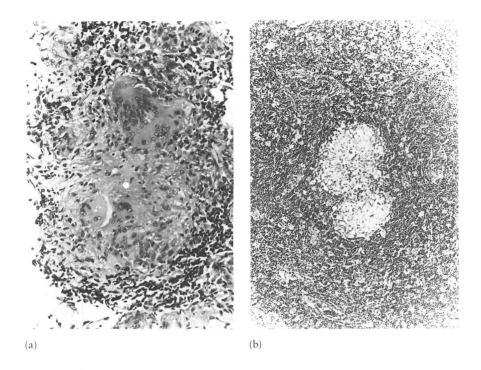

(a)

(b)

Figure 13.28 Non-caseating granuloma. Note the presence of giant cells with multiple nuclei.

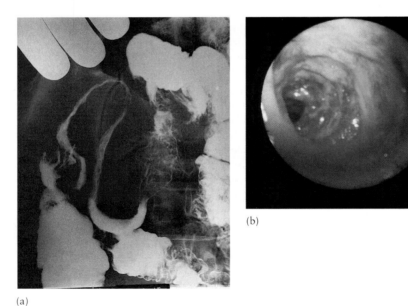

(a)

(b)

Figure 13.29 (a) Barium enema showing Crohn's colitis; (b) endoscopic view of Crohn's colitis.

Investigations

Barium enema may show the extent of the lesions (Fig. 13.29a). Simoidoscopy and colonoscopy allow visualization of Crohn's lesions located in the colon or rectum (Fig. 13.29b). The disease is patchy in distribution and the rectum is often uninvolved. The histological features ob-

tained on biopsy are chronic inflammatory infiltrate with lymphocytes and non-caseating granulomas. The fissured ulcers are narrow and deep.

Treatment of Crohn's disease

Differentiation between ulcerative colitis and Crohn's disease is important as treatment strategies are different in

Table 13.14 Comparison of the features of ulcerative colitis and Crohn's disease.

	Ulcerative colitis	Crohn's disease
Aetiology	HLA-B27 phenotype	Unknown
Pathology		
Macroscopic	Rectum (always), colon, terminal ileum (backwash ileitis)	Any part of GI tract, skip lesions
	Mucosa only, superficial ulceration, pseudopolyps	Full-thickness (hosepipe), fissures, mesentery involved
Microscopic	Crypt abscesses	Non-caseating granulomas
Clinical		
Bowel features	Rectal bleeding, diarrhoea	Abdominal pain and mass, malaise, diarrhoea, perianal disease
Non-GI features	Iritis, arthritis, blood, skin and renal disorders (see text)	Erythema nodosum
		Pyoderma gangrenosum
Complications	Haemorrhage, perforation, toxic megacolon, carcinoma	Stricture, fistulae
Radiology	*Barium enema*	*Barium meal and follow-through, barium enema*
	Shortened narrowed colon, loss of haustrations, 'lead-pipe' colon	Altered mucosal pattern, 'string sign', deep penetrating ulcers
Management		
Medical	Sulphasalazine	Dietary manipulation
	Steroid enema	Sulphasalazine, metronidazole
	Systemic steroids	Systemic steroids, azathioprine
	Azathioprine	
Surgery	Panproctocolectomy and ileostomy	Only for complications and limited to localized resections and
	Ileal pouch	stricturoplasties.

HLA, Human leukocyte antigen; GI, gastrointestinal.

the two conditions, with surgery playing a minor role in the management of Crohn's disease (Table 13.14).

Supplementary diet to correct malnutrition is important in the management of Crohn's disease. Elemental diets may help and supplements of oral iron are needed. In severe malnourished states total parenteral nutrition is required. This may also be useful in accelerating remission of an acute exacerbation. Salazopyrin may be used for acute episodes and maintenance therapy. Metronidazole may benefit patients with perianal disease. Prednisolone may be necessary to induce remission in severe acute attacks of inflammation. Azathioprine may sometimes be of benefit.

The surgical treatment of Crohn's disease is largely the treatment of its complications. Strictures may need to be dilated, adhesions may need to be divided in obstruction and localized segments of small bowel may require resection. Acute regional ileitis should be treated conservatively as it is often due to *Yersinia* infection and will resolve completely. Crohn's disease involving the colon may need resection with ileorectal anastomosis or, if the rectum is involved, may require panproctocolectomy with ileostomy. Sphincter-saving operations or reservoirs are not suitable in Crohn's disease. The treatment of Crohn's perianal disease is essentially the treatment of

abscess by drainage and the laying open of fissures and fistulae. Metronidazole may be beneficial.

Colonic polyps

Polyps may occur anywhere in the gastrointestinal tract. Polyps occurring in the colon or rectum are the hamartomatous lesions of juvenile polyposis, or adenomas and villous papillomas.

Juvenile polyps

Juvenile polyps occur in infants and young children. They may be single or multiple, are pedunculated and found mainly in the rectum and distal colon. There is a familial tendency and they are more common in male children. The polyps are vascular and secrete mucus. They have little malignant potential. When identified they should be removed endoscopically.

Adenomatous polyps

Adenomatous polyps are pedunculated, vary in size from a few millimetres to several centimetres and occur mainly in

Ulcerative colitis at a glance

DEFINITION

Ulcerative colitis is a chronic inflammatory disorder of the colon, beginning in the rectum and extending proximally for a variable extent

EPIDEMIOLOGY

M/F = 1 : 16 Age 30–50. High incidence among relatives of patients (up to 40%) and among Europeans and Jews

AETIOLOGY

- Genetic origin: increased prevalence (10%) in relatives, associated with HLA- B27 phenotype
- May have autoimmune basis

PATHOLOGY

Macroscopic
- Disease confined to colon; rectum always involved; may be 'backwash' ileitis
- Only the mucosa is involved, with superficial ulceration, exudation and pseudopolyposis

Histology
- Crypt abscess, inflammatory polyps and highly vascular granulation tissue. Epithelial dysplasia with long-standing disease

CLINICAL FEATURES

- Diarrhoea, passage of mucus, pus and blood per rectum

Mild or moderate disease
- Abdominal pain, anorexia, weight loss and anaemia
- Extraintestinal features

		% Involved
Joints	Arthritis	25%
Eye	Uveitis	10%
Skin	Erythema nodosum Pyoderma gangrenosum	10%
Liver	Pericholangitis, fatty liver	3%
Blood	Thromboembolic disease	

Severe/fulminant disease
- 6–20 bloody bowel motions per day
- Fever, anaemia, dehydration, electrolyte imbalance
- Colonic dilatation/rupture—*toxic megacolon*

INVESTIGATIONS

- FBC (iron-deficiency anaemia)
- Barium enema — loss of haustrations, shortened lead-pipe colon
- Sigmoidoscopy — inflamed friable mucosa, bleeds to touch
- Biopsy — typical histological features
- Plain abdominal radiograph — colonic dilation or air under diaphragm indicating perforation in toxic megacolon

MANAGEMENT

Medical
- High-fibre diet, antidiarrhoeal agents (codeine phosphate)
- Anti-inflammatory drugs (salazopyrine, steroids)
- Steroid enemas if disease confined to rectum
- Immunosuppressive agents (azathioprine) occasionally

Surgery
Indications
- Failure of medical treatment
- Complications: profuse haemorrhage, perforation/toxic megacolon, risk of cancer (greater with longer disease, more aggressive onset and more extensive disease)
Operations
- Panproctocolectomy with ileostomy (Brooke, Koch)
- Colectomy with preservation of anal sphincter and creation of ileal pouch (e.g. J-shaped pouch)

PROGNOSIS

Ulcerative colitis is a chronic problem that requires constant surveillance unless surgery, which is drastic but curative, is performed

---

the rectum and sigmoid colon (Fig. 13.30). They are often asymptomatic but may produce anaemia from chronic occult bleeding. Rarely they may initiate an intussusception. They may also give rise to crampy abdominal pain. If a lot of mucus is secreted, spurious diarrhoea may occur, but this is more common with villous papillomas. Adenomatous polyps have malignant potential and should be removed when diagnosed.

Villous papilloma

Villous papillomas are sessile lesions which spread around the circumference of the bowel and secrete copious amounts of mucus. The mucus discharge produces spurious diarrhoea. Significant losses of potassium may occur, giving rise to a metabolic acidosis with lethargy, muscle weakness and mental confusion. There is a significant risk of malignant change. Some are small enough to be amenable to endoscopic removal with a snare or diathermy coagulation, but larger masses may need wide excision after infiltration of the submucosa which dilutes adrenaline solution. The cut edges of normal mucosa are then approximated. Where malignant change has occurred in a polypoid lesion, a formal resection of colon or rectum should be carried out.

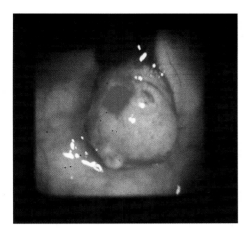

Figure 13.30 Endoscopic view of a colonic polyp of rectum.

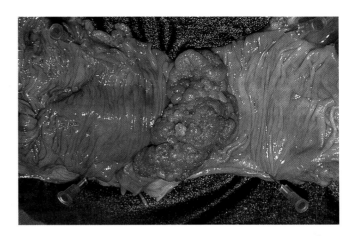

Figure 13.31 Pathology specimen showing circumferential colon cancer.

Familial polyposis

Familial polyposis coli is an inherited autosomal dominant condition in which hundreds of adenomas develop throughout the colon and rectum early in the second decade. The patient may be relatively asymptomatic but bleeding, abdominal pain and diarrhoea are all likely symptoms. The risk of developing carcinoma is virtually 100% within 15 years. The most appropriate treatment is panproctocolectomy with ileal-pouch anal anastomosis.

Gardner's syndrome

In this condition the patient develops multiple colorectal adenomas in association with sebaceous and dermoid cysts, osteomas and desmoid tumours of the abdominal wall. The extracolonic manifestations of the syndrome may predate the colonic adenomas by some years. The risk of cancer is similar to that in familial polyposis. Radical resection is indicated.

Carcinoma of the colon and rectum

Adenocarcinoma of the colon and rectum is one of the most common cancers occurring in the western world (Fig. 13.31). It occurs in both sexes but is somewhat more common in men. Almost half of these tumours occur in the rectum and almost three-quarters are within reach of the flexible sigmoidoscope (60 cm from the anal margin). Hereditary factors, such as familial polyposis coli, are responsible for its development in some cases. Other aetiological factors include ulcerative colitis, colonic polyps and excess bile salts. The high incidence in western countries is attributed to the low-fibre, high-fat diet common in industrialized societies.

Pathology

Carcinoma of the colon or rectum is an adenocarcinoma with a fibrous stroma which may progress in different ways:

- as an exophytic cauliflower-type of growth;
- as an ulcerating lesion penetrating through the bowel wall;
- as an annular constricting growth;
- as a diffuse infiltrating tumour; or
- as the rare colloidal mucus-secreting tumour.

Colorectal carcinoma metastasizes to regional lymph nodes and via the blood stream to the liver. Figure 13.32 shows a skin deposit from a primary bowel cancer.

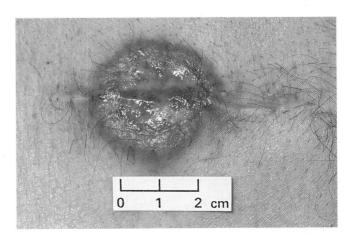

Figure 13.32 Skin deposit from a primary colon cancer.

Clinical features

The clinical presentation reflects the location of the tumour.
• A carcinoma in the caecum progresses silently, the only manifestation being occult blood in the stools and persistent anaemia due to chronic blood loss. This is sometimes mistaken for an appendix mass but its persistence despite treatment invites further investigation, and identification at barium enema or colonoscopy follows.
• A tumour in the ascending colon is likely to behave similarly to caecal carcinoma but may give rise to dyspeptic symptoms or colicky abdominal pain.
• The latter is a constant feature of carcinoma in the transverse or descending colon due to the partial obstruction of an annular constricting lesion. Alteration in bowel habit is also a consequence of a constricting lesion with periods of constipation followed by episodes of diarrhoea. Blood and mucus can be identified in the stool.
• Tumours in the rectum secrete mucus and bleed from the ulcerated surface and the accumulated blood and mucus are passed accompanied by tenesmus as an early-morning bloody diarrhoea.
• A significant percentage present as large bowel obstruction.

Investigation

Digital rectal examination is essential and many rectal tumours can be identified as a craggy ulcerated mass at this examination. More proximal tumours are identified at *sigmoidoscopy* or *colonoscopy*. The rigid sigmoidoscope affords only a limited examination to 30 cm but the flexible sigmoidoscope enables the distal 60 cm of bowel to be examined, which should identify 70% of tumours. Access to the remainder requires full colonoscopy or double-contrast barium enema. *Biopsy* of any lesion visualized is essential. Even if a tumour is seen and confirmed at biopsy, a full colonic examination should always be carried out as 3% of tumours are synchronous. Metachronous tumours occur in 3% of cases also, so follow-up of previously treated tumours should include full investigation.

The appearance of a tumour on *barium enema* is of a constricting filling defect — characteristically an 'apple-core' deformity (Fig. 13.33a). Double-contrast enema will identify smaller tumours and suspicious polyps (Fig. 13.33b).

Treatment

Resection of the tumour with adequate margins and including the regional glands is indicated when the diagnosis has been confirmed. It is advisable to arrange an intravenous urogram prior to operation to exclude involvement of the ureters and bladder. Bowel preparation is undertaken prior

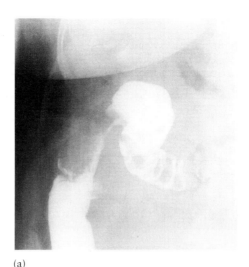

(a)

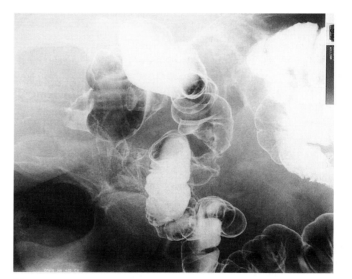

(b)

Figure 13.33 Barium enema showing 'apple-core lesion' at (a) the splenic flexure and (b) the sigmoid colon.

to resecting lesions on the left side of the colon. No preparation is required for right-sided lesions. Appropriate antibiotics to cover Gram-positive (e.g. *Streptococcus faecalis*) and -negative (e.g. *Escherichia coli*, *Klebsiella*, *Proteus*) aerobes and Gram-negative (e.g. *Bacteroides*) anaerobes should be given perioperatively.

Surgical procedures

General principles include early ligation of the vascular pedicle, no-touch technique and avoidance of contamination by bowel content. The procedure varies with the site

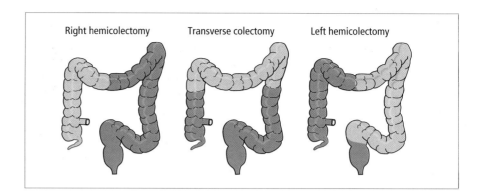

Right hemicolectomy   Transverse colectomy   Left hemicolectomy

Figure 13.34 Surgery for colonic tumours. The area of resection for right hemicolectomy (purple), left hemicolectomy (orange) and transverse colectomy (green) is shown.

of the lesion. Right hemicolectomy with end-to-end ileo-colic anastomosis is indicated for carcinoma of the caecum or ascending colon. Wide resection including hepatic and splenic flexure is indicated in tumours of the transverse colon. In tumours of the descending or sigmoid colon the splenic flexure should be included in the resection (Fig. 13.34).

Low anterior resection is now the standard operation for most rectal tumours. Formerly, the belief that 5 cm distal clearance was necessary and that 5 cm of distal rectum had to be preserved to ensure normal sphincter function meant that if the tumour was within 10 cm of the anal margin, an abdominoperineal resection was mandatory. The subsequent realization that rectal tumours drained proximally and that 2 cm distal clearance was adequate, plus the realization that sphincter control could be maintained with less than 5 cm of rectum, enabled very low anterior resections to be carried out. The advent of circular stapling instruments was of enormous benefit in overcoming the technical difficulties of very low anastomoses. However, abdominoperineal resection with an end-colostomy in the left iliac fossa is still necessary occasionally.

When a patient presents with colonic obstruction or perforation secondary to a carcinoma, a laparotomy is performed and the carcinoma-bearing segment of bowel excised. However, primary anastomosis is inadvisable in this situation. Preliminary defunctioning colostomy may be carried out for obstruction and Hartmann's procedure is appropriate in the presence of perforation with excision of the perforated segment, proximal colostomy and closure of the rectal stump.

Prognosis

The outcome of resection for carcinoma of the colon and rectum depends on the stage of the tumour. Dukes classification, although originally described for carcinoma

Table 13.15 Modified Dukes classification for staging colorectal cancers.

Dukes stage	Extent of pathology	5-year survival (%)
A	Tumour is confined to bowel mucosa	90
B1	Tumour involves the muscle wall but not completely	70
B2	Involves the serosa	60
C1	Tumour involves the muscle wall but not completely Local lymph nodes involved	30
C2	Involves the serosa Local lymph nodes involved	

of the rectum, can be applied to the colon also. A modified Dukes classification is in wide usage (Table 13.15).

Radiotherapy and chemotherapy have a limited role in the management of patients with colorectal cancer, although most patients with Dukes C disease now receive adjunct chemotherapy. Studies have shown that fluorouracil and levamisole given 3–5 weeks after surgery reduce the recurrence rate by about 40% and mortality by 30% in patients followed for a median of 5 years. Liver metastases can be resected with a good prospect of survival if there are fewer than five metastases or the metastases are confined to a lobe of the liver. About 25% of such patients survive for 5 years.

Carcinoma of the anus

Anal carcinoma is uncommon. It is a squamous carcinoma which arises from the squamous epithelium of the lower half of the anal canal. It is a disease of the elderly which presents with rectal bleeding, anal pain, discharge and ulceration. The diagnosis is confirmed by biopsy and metastases are to the inguinal nodes. Treatment now is by combined local radiotherapy and chemotherapy which has displaced abdominoperineal resection. Rarely, malignant melanoma presents as an anal lesion. Early metastases are frequent and this lesion has a well-deserved bad reputation (see Chapter 17).

Benign anal and perianal disorders

Haemorrhoids

Haemorrhoids are also referred to as piles, which comes from the Latin word *pilae*, meaning 'balls'. A haemorrhoid consists of a venous plexus draining into the superior haemorrhoidal vein and a small branch of the superior rectal artery surrounded by areolar tissue. They are classically found at the 3, 7 and 11 o'clock positions when looking at the anus in the lithotomy position (Fig. 13.35a). The venous congestion which produces the haemorrhoid is due to an increase in venous (portal) pressure brought about by straining at stool or to the alteration in haemodynamics during pregnancy, including the obstruction to venous return caused by the fetus. Haemorrhoids are common in western countries because of the lack of dietary fibre which predisposes to constipation and straining. Men are affected more frequently than women. Haemorrhoids are described as *internal* when covered by mucosa only and *external* when

Colorectal carcinoma at a glance

DEFINITION

Malignant lesions occurring in the rectum and colon

EPIDEMIOLOGY

M/F=1.3 : 1 Age 50+ years. Incidence has increased in western world over last 50 years

AETIOLOGY

Predisposing factors
- Diet (low in indigestible fibre, high in animal fat)
- A prior colorectal cancer
- Ulcerative colitis
- Increased faecal bile salts
- Selenium deficiency
- Adenomatous polyps
- Hereditary polyposis coli
- High anaerobic bacterial count in faeces

PATHOLOGY

Macroscopic
- Polypoid, ulcerating, annular, infiltrative
- 75% of lesions are within 60 cm of the anal margin
- 3% are synchronous (i.e. a second lesion will be found at the same time) and 3% are metachronous (i.e. a second lesion will be found later)

Histology
- Adenocarcinoma (10–15% are mucinous adenocarcinoma)
- Staging by Dukes classification:

A	confined to mucosa	B_1	muscle wall but not serosa
B_2	involves serosa	C_1	muscle wall + lymph nodes
C_2	serosa + lymph nodes	D	distant metastases

- Spread: lymphatic, haematogenous (via veins to liver), peritoneal

5FU, 5-fluorouracile.

CLINICAL FEATURES

- Anaemia — caecal cancers often present with anaemia
- Colicky abdominal pain — tumours which are causing partial obstruction, e.g. transverse or decending colonic lesions
- Alteration in bowel habit — either constipation or diarrhoea
- Bleeding or passage of mucus per rectum
- Tenesmus (frequent or continuous painful desire to defecate) — rectal lesions

INVESTIGATIONS

- Digital rectal examination
- FBC, U&E, faecal occult blood
- Sigmoidoscopy (rigid to 30 cm/flexible to 60 cm) and colonoscopy (whole colon; see the lesion, obtain biopsy)
- Double-contrast barium enema ('apple-core lesion', polyp)
- Carcinoembryonic antigen is usually raised in advanced disease

MANAGEMENT

Surgery
- Resection of the tumour with adequate margins and regional lymph nodes
- Procedures: right hemicolectomy (no bowel prep.) for lesions from caecum to splenic flexure; left hemicolectomy (bowel prep.) for lesions of decending and sigmoid colon; low anterior resection for rectal tumours; abdominoperineal resection and colostomy for very low rectal lesions Hartmann's procedure for emergency surgery to left colon

Other Rx
- Adjunct chemotherapy for patient with Dukes C (5FU and levamisole)
- Resection for liver metastases if < 5 are present

Prognosis
- 5-year survival depends on staging: A (80%), B (60%), C (35%), following resection of liver metastases (25%)

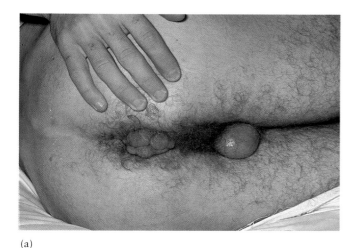

(a)

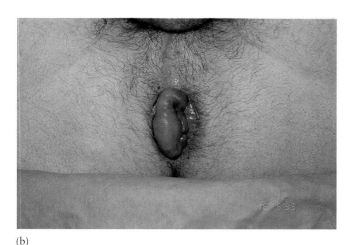

(b)

Figure 13.35 (a) Third-degree haemorrhoids; (b) prolapsed thrombosed piles are extremely painful and usually require surgical treatment.

covered by squamous epithelium of the anal canal because of some degree of prolapse. *First-degree* haemorrhoids are small and do not prolapse; *second-degree* haemorrhoids are small and prolapse during defecation but retract spontaneously. *Third-degree* haemorrhoids remain prolapsed.

Clinical features

Symptoms are intermittent and are precipitated by straining during periods of constipation.

• *Itching* and *perianal irritation* are due to the venous congestion and perianal leakage of mucus.

• *Bleeding* is due to trauma from scybalous stools during defecation. The latter also accounts for the severe pain often experienced during defecation.

• *Prolapse* gives rise to a sensation of pressure and 'something coming down' with increased irritation due to congestion and mucus discharge.

Treatment

• First-degree haemorrhoids may respond satisfactorily to bulk laxatives and an increase in dietary fibre.

• If these simple methods are unsuccessful, most patients with first-degree and second-degree haemorrhoids will benefit from *injections of phenol in almond oil* to the base of the piles. The injection is carried out with a special syringe and shouldered needle so that it can be delivered submucosally into the neck or base of the pile above the dentate line via a proctoscope. One injection into each haemorrhoid base should be sufficient but the procedure may be repeated after a few weeks if necessary.

• *Ligation with rubber bands (Barron's bands)* is also effective with second-degree haemorrhoids. The mucosa at the base is picked up in a special instrument and the pedicle constricted with a rubber band, with subsequent sloughing of the haemorrhoids over a period of 10 days or so. The procedure is painful and requires regular analgesia for the first few days.

• *Freezing of the haemorrhoids* with a cryoprobe has also been used successfully. The probe is applied to the overlying mucosa. Sloughing of the haemorrhoid with mucosal ulceration duly occurs with mucus discharge. Healing takes several weeks and there is considerable pain in the initial postoperative period.

• Stretching of the anal sphincter (*Lord's procedure*) under general anaesthetic may improve venous drainage by breaking down fibrous bands which inhibit normal dilation. The procedure also decreases sphincter tone, thus improving drainage and decreasing the need for straining. However, overstretching may lead to anal incontinence.

• *Haemorrhoidectomy* is necessary for third-degree haemorrhoids either in the uncomplicated state or in the prolapsed thrombosed (Fig. 13.35b) and ulcerated state. The three primary haemorrhoids are excised. The conventional procedure (Milligan–Morgan haemorrhoidectomy) leaves raw surfaces with intervening mucocutaneous bridges so that stenosis is avoided during the healing process. Suture of the mucosa is recommended by many nowadays to accelerate healing.

Complications of haemorrhoidectomy are relatively rare. Haemorrhage may require reoperation to ligate the bleeding vessel. Anal stenosis is a late complication if excess mucosa and skin have been excised.

Rectal prolapse

Incomplete or mucosal prolapse is common in children and rarely requires treatment other than prevention of straining at stool and avoidance of constipation. In adults, prolapse is more likely to be complete, involving the full thickness of the bowel wall.

Aetiology

Rectal intussusception and poor sphincter tone are regarded as precipitating factors as is trauma during child birth.

Clinical features

Mucus discharge and bleeding accompany the prolapse which may occur during defecation or may appear on standing erect. If the sphincter is lax, incontinence may also be a problem.

Treatment

Surgery offers the only prospect of cure and in the most successful operations the rectum is approached from above, mobilized, drawn upwards and held in position by fixing it to the sacrum. These procedures used to require a laparotomy but can now be performed laparoscopically. The operation of choice in the UK is the rectopexy using prolene mesh to keep the mobilized rectum in place. In the USA preference is given to the Ripstein operation in which the mobilized rectum is supported in the hollow of the sacrum with a Teflon sling. The Thiersch operation, in which the anal canal is surrounded by a wire ring or nylon or Teflon tape, is not very satisfactory, being usually too loose or too tight. It is tried in patients who are unfit for anything more extensive. In frail patients the prolapsed rectum may be excised perineally — De Loirme's operation. Patients with severe constipation and rectal prolapse are best treated by anterior resection.

Perianal haematoma

This is a very painful condition which occurs when a small blood vessel ruptures underneath the perianal skin, causing a painful tender blue swelling. The condition resolves spontaneously in 4 or 5 days but if the pain is severe, incision and evacuation of the clot under local anaesthesia will provide instant relief.

Anal fissure

A fissure is a longitudinal tear in the mucosa of the anal canal due to local trauma sustained while evacuating a

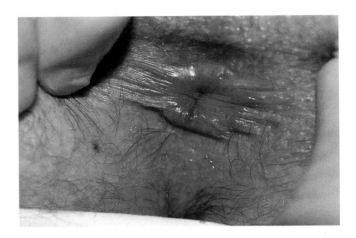

Figure 13.36 Fissure-*in-ano* in the classical position — midline posteriorly.

constipated stool. Almost all fissures occur in the midline posteriorly (Fig. 13.36). At the distal end of a fissure a skin tag, referred to as a *sentinel pile*, can be seen. Fissures are extremely painful due to severe sphincter spasm. The pain is initiated at defecation but persists afterwards. Healing of a fissure is inhibited by sphincter spasm which prevents adequate drainage. While relief can be obtained by local application of anaesthetic cream, definitive treatment requires either sphincter dilatation or lateral sphincterotomy. Either procedure promotes rapid healing of the fissure.

Perianal infections

Perianal infection is extremely common and often presents as an abscess requiring urgent surgical attention. A focus of infection starts in the anal glands which lie between the internal and external sphincters. These glands normally drain into the anal canal at the level of the anal valves. Infection spreads inferiorly and laterally to give rise to ischiorectal and perianal abscesses respectively (Fig. 13.37).
• The commonest problem encountered is a *perianal abscess* which presents as a painful inflamed lump adjacent to the anal margin (Fig. 13.38). Treatment is by urgent incision and drainage, usually using a cruciate incision and excising some of the skin edges to deroof the abscess. Healing is rapid and is encouraged by daily saline baths. If the abscess cavity communicates with the anal canal internally and the perianal skin surface externally, a fistula-*in-ano* may become established (see below).
• An *ischiorectal abscess* is more extensive and more serious and is usually accompanied by constitutional symptoms. It presents as a brawny indurated swelling over the ischiorectal fossa and, as the two ischiorectal fossae

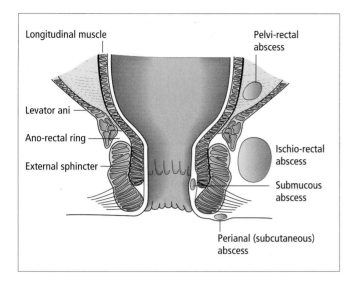

Figure 13.37 The anatomy of perianal infection. From Ellis H. and Calne R. *Lecture Notes on General Surgery*, 8th edn. Oxford: Blackwell Scientific Publicatons, 1993.

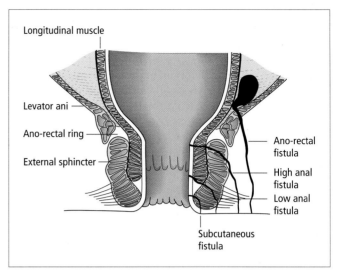

Figure 13.39 Low and high fistula-*in-ano*. From Ellis H. and Calne R. *Lecture Notes on General Surgery*, 8th edn. Oxford: Blackwell Scientific Publications, 1993.

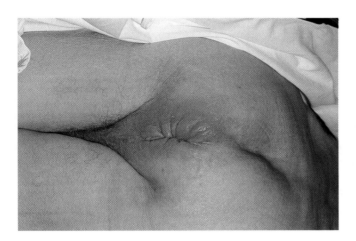

Figure 13.38 Perianal abscess.

communicate via the postsphincteric space, bilateral involvement may occur. Treatment is also by adequate incision and drainage.

- A *pararectal abscess* occurs if there is extension of the infection above the levator ani. This is essentially a pelvic abscess and requires urgent drainage (often performed radiologically now).
- A *pilonidal abscess* occurs in the skin of the natal cleft and represents an infection of an associated pilonidal sinus. Incision and drainage deal with the abscess but the sinus may require further therapy (see below).
- *Perianal warts* are caused by viruses and, as with genital warts (see Chapter 20), are transmitted by sexual activity.

Other sexually transmitted diseases should be considered and treatment consists of topical podophyllin and excision or cauterization of warts in extreme cases.

Fistula-*in-ano*

Perianal abscesses which discharge spontaneously into the anal canal or are inadequately drained are likely to persist as perianal fistulae (fistula-*in-ano*) with persistent discharge of pus both on to the skin and into the bowel (Fig. 13.39). The external orifice (there may be multiple external orifices) is located a few centimetres from the anal margin, the edges are lined with granulation tissue and commonly there is a discharge.

Aetiology

Most infections giving rise to fistulae are non-specific but an association with ulcerative colitis or more particularly with Crohn's disease is well recognized. The latter is prone to develop multiple fistulous openings in the perineum ('watering can' perineum). Tuberculosis may be an occasional cause.

Treatment

Low fistulae are treated by passing a probe through the fistulous track, identifying the internal opening and then laying the entire track open by cutting down on the probe. Continence is not a problem after surgery for low fistulae, although complete control of flatus may be deficient. With high fistulae there is a serious problem with faecal incontinence if the internal sphincter is divided. Defunctioning colostomy as a preliminary procedure may help clear up infection. Division of the deep external sphincter or the puborectalic ring will cause faecal incontinence. Use of a seton, by which an unabsorbable suture is tied tightly around these muscles so that it causes sufficient fibrosis to anchor the muscles as it cuts through them, reduces considerably the risk of incontinence.

Pilonidal sinus

Pilonidal (nest of hairs) sinuses are commonly found in the upper end of the natal cleft, usually in hirsute young men (Fig. 13.40). Congenital and acquired theories of aetiology have been advanced but clinically patients present with a sinus in the natal cleft, from which hairs protrude. The condition is common in truck-drivers and it is thought that the movement of the buttocks while driving encourages the migration of hair into the natal cleft and possibly into a congenital sinus. Pilonidal sinuses are also found in the web spaces between the fingers of hairdressers, caused by implanted hairs from their customers.

A pilonidal abscess occurs when the sinus becomes infected and requires urgent incision and drainage. The sinus is more difficult to treat. Daily baths and regular shaving of the natal cleft area may help some patients but others require surgical ablation of the sinus network. This may be done by excision of the sinus-bearing area, which may be quite extensive. Methylene blue is injected into the mouth of the sinus to outline the network and the entire sinus system is excised. The defect is allowed to granulate, with healing taking several weeks. Alterna-

tively, the sinuses may be deroofed and curetted and phenol applied.

The acute abdomen and intestinal obstruction

The sunken cheeks, the dark rings around the eyes
The beads of sweat which on the forehead rise
The haunted look, all tell at any age
Peritonitis in the latest stage.
Zachary Cope (1949)

The collective term *acute abdomen* is used to describe a group of acute life-threatening intra-abdominal conditions which often lead to peritonitis and require emergency surgical intervention.

Aetiology

The causes of an acute abdomen fall into four main categories: inflammatory, traumatic, obstructive and vascular (Table 13.16).

Inflammatory

The inflammatory intraperitoneal conditions originate either as acute inflammations of specific regions of the

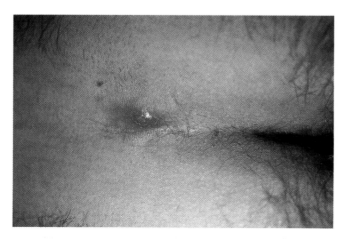

Figure 13.40 Pilonidal sinus and abscess.

Table 13.16 Acute abdomen – disease processes.

Inflammatory
Secondary bacterial peritonitis
Primary bacterial peritonitis

Traumatic
Injury to solid organs — acute intra-abdominal bleeding
Peritonitis secondary to intestinal injury

Obstructive
Acute intestinal obstruction (small bowel)
Chronic intestinal obstruction (colonic)

Vascular
Mesenteric infarction
Strangulated external /internal herniae
Volvulus (small or large intestine)

Benign anal and perianal disorders at a glance

HAEMORRHOIDS

Definition
- A haemorrhoid (pile) is a submucosal swelling in the anal canal that consists of a venous plexus, a small artery and areolar tissue

Aetiology
- They are caused by increased venous pressure from straining (low-fibre diets) or altered haemodynamics (e.g. during pregnancy)
- They are found at the 3, 7 and 11 o'clock positions in the anal canal

Clinical features
- First-degree (1°; bleeding/itching only), second-degree (2°; prolapse during defecation), third-degree (3°; constantly prolapsed)

Treatment
- 1°: Bulk laxatives and high-fibre diet, injection sclerotherapy
  2°: Injection sclerotherapy, Barron's bands, cryosurgery
  3°: Haemorrhoidectomy (complications: bleeding, anal stenosis)

RECTAL PROLAPSE

Definition
- Condition characterized by protrusion to a variable degree of the rectal mucous membrane from the anus

Aetiology
- Precipitating factors: rectal intussusception and poor sphincter tone

Clinical features
- Mucus discharge, bleeding, obvious prolapse

Treatment
- Rectopexy (rectum is 'hitched' up on to sacrum and held in place with a prolene mesh)

PERIANAL HAEMATOMA

Definition
- Very painful subcutaneous haematoma caused by rupture of small blood vessel in the perianal area. Evacuation of the clot provides instant relief

ANAL FISSURE

Definition
- Longitudinal tear in the mucosa of the anal canal, in the midline posteriorly (90%) or anteriorly (10%)

Aetiology
- Caused by local trauma during passage of constipated stool

Clinical features
- Exquisitely painful on passing bowel motion. Small amount of bright red blood on toilet tissue. Severe sphincter spasm. Skin tag at distal end of tear (sentinel pile)

GA, General anaesthesia; TB, tuberculosis.

Treatment
- Lateral sphincterotomy, anal dilatation (Lord's procedure) under GA

PERIANAL INFECTIONS

Definition
- Bacterial infections presenting as abscesses in the perianal region

Aetiology
- Focus of infection starts in anal glands and spreads to cause:
  (a) Perianal abscess: adjacent to anal margin
  (b) Ischiorectal abscess: in ischiorectal fossa
  (c) Pararectal abscess: above levator ani

Clinical features
- Painful, red, tender, swollen mass ± constitutional symptoms

Treatment
- Incision and drainage, antibiotics

FISTULA-*IN-ANO*

Definition
- Abnormal communication between the skin in the perianal region and the anal canal

Aetiology
- Track connecting skin and anal canal becomes established and persists following drainage of a perianal abscess. May be associated with Crohn's disease (multiple fistulae), ulcerative colitis and TB

Clinical features
- Chronic perianal discharge. External orifice of track with granulation tissue is easily seen perianally

Treatment
- Probing and laying open the track. Complex high fistulae may need colostomy and a seton.

PILONIDAL SINUS

Definition
- A blind-ending track containing hairs in the skin of the natal cleft

Aetiology
- Movement of buttocks promotes hair migration into a (?congenital) sinus

Clinical features
- Usually present as abscess (Rx incision and drainage). Sinus is in midline posterior to anal margin with hair protruding from orifice

Treatment
- Good personal hygiene. Excision of sinus network may be required

gastrointestinal tract, e.g. acute appendicitis, acute diverticulitis or as primary perforations of the gastro-intestinal tract either as a consequence of benign disease (e.g. perforated duodenal ulcer) or malignant tumours (per-forated gastric lymphoma, caecal carcinoma, etc.). All the conditions in this category invariably lead to a localized or generalized peritonitis.

Traumatic

Intra-abdominal injuries may be due to blunt or penetrating abdominal trauma (Chapter 8). When solid organs such as the liver and spleen are involved, the clinical picture is dominated by acute hypovolaemia due to massive internal haemorrhage. By contrast, when the pancreas or gastro-intestinal tract is traumatized, the symptoms and signs are those of peritonitis.

Obstructive

Obstructions of the gastrointestinal tract may involve the small intestine (acute) or the large bowel (chronic). The clinical picture of acute intestinal obstruction is dominated by vomiting, colicky abdominal pain and dehydration due to fluid and electrolyte losses, whereas chronic obstructions present with absolute constipation and marked abdominal distension. Unless the integrity of the wall of the obstructed bowel is compromised (as may happen in patients in whom the diagnosis is delayed), there is no peritoneal contamination and therefore signs of peritonitis are absent.

Vascular

Acute intestinal ischaemia leading to infarction of segments of the gastrointestinal tract may be due to thrombotic or embolic occlusion of the mesenteric vessels, to volvulus (twisting) of loops of small or large intestine, and external compression of the blood supply by bands or adhesions or the neck of external/internal herniae. Intestinal infarction is a serious condition which carries a high mortality. The clinical picture is dominated by severe pain, peritonitis, shock and, in some patients, rectal bleeding.

Peritonitis

Peritonitis is inflammation of the peritoneum and may be divided into three types.

1 *Secondary peritonitis*: The majority of the morbid processes outlined above lead to a breach of the integrity of the wall of the gastrointestinal tract with transmigration of intestinal bacteria to the peritoneal cavity or actual escape of intestinal contents with substantial contamination of the peritoneal space. The consequence is an acute secondary bacterial peritonitis.

2 *Primary peritonitis*: Primary bacterial peritonitis is a much rarer condition which is the result of primary infection of the peritoneal lining by streptococcal organ-isms, usually in females. Another type of primary bacterial peritonitis occurs in cirrhotic patients with ascites, where the infection may be caused by a variety of bacteria, including Gram-negative aerobic organisms.

3 *Chemical peritonitis*: In some situations, the peritoneal inflammation is initially chemical in nature, e.g. early stages of perforated duodenal ulcer, extravasation of uninfected urine (bladder injuries) or bile (after biliary operations). This is sometimes referred to as chemical peritonitis but un-treated it invariably merges into acute secondary bacterial peritonitis.

Clinical manifestations

Irrespective of the exact aetiology, established peritonitis is usually accompanied by well-recognizable systemic and local symptoms and signs.

• The *systemic manifestations* emanate from the presence of a serious infection: the patient looks ill, is toxic with a high metabolic rate, pyrexia, tachycardia and leukocytosis. If the bacteria have invaded the blood stream (bacteraemia, septicaemia), attacks of rigors (shivering) are encountered; the patient feels cold although his or her temperature is elevated above 38°C. The combination of fluid and electrolyte losses (vomit, fluid inside the oedematous intestinal loops and peritoneal exudate which is sequestrated) and the enhanced insensible loss caused by the pyrexia, lead to dehydration with dry mouth, loss of skin turgor and collapse of the peripheral veins.

• *Local symptoms*: The pain of acute peritonitis is due to irritation of the somatic nerves supplying the parietal peritoneum. Its extent and exact location depend on whether the peritonitis is generalized or localized to a particular quadrant of the intra-abdominal cavity. It is always severe, constant and aggravated by movement (passive or active) and thus the patient lies still in the supine position and may at times draw up the knees to relax the abdominal musculature.

• *Local signs*: The local or abdominal signs are elicited by a methodical sequence of inspection, palpation, percussion and auscultation of the abdomen and a digital rectal examination.

(a) *Inspection*: On inspection of the normal abdomen, the abdominal wall is seen to move with respiration; it bulges with inspiration as the diaphragm descends. This normal excursion is often absent in patients with peritonitis as the abdominal muscles over the area of peritoneal inflammation undergo reflex spasm.

(b) *Palpation*: The same phenomenon accounts for the tight feel of the abdominal musculature noted during light palpation and often referred to as *guarding*. When marked, the abdominal muscles actually feel rigid (*rigidity*), although descriptions of board-like rigidity are exaggerated and have conveyed the wrong impression that deep palpation is necessary to elicit this sign. In fact, deep palpation is absolutely contraindicated in all patients with acute abdomen as it serves no purpose other than to inflict severe pain on the patient and thereby lose his or her confidence. Tenderness on light palpation elicited over the affected region is a most useful and reliable sign. *Rebound tenderness* is experienced by the patient when pressure of the palpating hand is released. Considerable store has been laid on this physical sign in the past. More recent studies have cast some doubt on its value in clinical practice. Certainly, it must be elicited with great gentleness.

(c) *Percussion*: A more humane way to evoke rebound tenderness is to tap gently the affected area, or better still, ask the patient to cough, which, by moving the inflamed viscera against the inflamed parietal peritoneum, reproduces the localized pain.

(d) *Auscultation* of the abdomen in patients with peritonitis reveals a silent abdomen (no identifiable borborygmi) due to absence of the normal peristaltic activity. At times tinkling bowel sounds may be heard. These are due to passive movement of fluid within dilated loops of inflamed gut and signify the presence of a paralytic ileus.

(e) *Digital rectal examination*: No examination of a patient with an acute abdomen is complete without a rectal examination. Although this is best carried out in the left lateral position, if the patient is in severe pain it may be conducted in the supine posture with flexion and abduction of the hip joints. The specific findings on digital rectal examination may include pelvic tenderness, boggy swelling in the rectovesical pouch and tenderness caused by movement of the cervix in the female.

Haemoperitoneum

Haemoperitoneum means free blood in the peritoneal cavity. It may arise:
- from intra-abdominal injuries;
- as a complication of intra-abdominal operations;
- from gynaecological disorders:
  (a) ruptured ectopic pregnancy;
  (b) ruptured corpus luteum cyst;
- from severe acute necrotizing pancreatitis;
- from advanced peritoneal carcinomatosis; or
- from spontaneous rupture of primary liver tumours (rare).

Clinical types

In the clinical context haemoperitoneum is best considered in two categories: progressive and stable.

- *Progressive haemoperitoneum* implies active continued intra-abdominal bleeding and is most commonly encountered with injuries to the solid organs (liver and spleen) or as an early complication after abdominal surgery. In addition to obvious signs of hypovolaemic shock, there is progressive distension of the abdomen which in severe injuries involving major vessels (e.g. hepatic veins) may become so tense as to obstruct the lower limb vessels in the groin. Postoperative bleeding is due either to slipping of a ligature on a blood vessel or to reactionary bleeding. The latter occurs from cut small blood vessels which were missed at operation because the operative field was dry but which bleed subsequently as the blood pressure rises after recovery from surgery and anaesthesia.

The signs and symptoms of progressive haemoperitoneum are dominated by the rapid loss of circulating blood volume with the development of hypovolaemic shock. In this respect, the local abdominal signs, apart from the increasing abdominal distension, are of minor importance. The patients will only survive with prompt resuscitation and immediate surgical intervention.

- A *stable haemoperitoneum* implies that the lesion which caused the haemoperitoneum in the first instance is no longer actively bleeding. Given time, the blood may track along tissue planes to appear in the flank (Grey Turner sign found in patients with necrotizing pancreatitis; Fig. 13.41) or in the periumbilical region (Cullen's sign, also found associated with necrotizing pancreatitis and rarely with missed ruptured ectopic pregnancy).

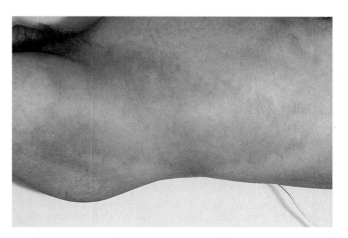

Figure 13.41 Grey Turner sign in a patient with pancreatitis.

The manifestations of patients with stable peritoneum are not always clearcut. The patient may appear clinically anaemic but this is best confirmed by haemoglobin estimation. Although free peritoneal blood acts as an irritant, the pain is not marked and tenderness is mild or absent. At times the patient complains of shoulder-tip pain when lying supine. This is the result of diaphragmatic irritation. In equivocal cases raising the foot of the bed, thereby encouraging any free blood present to flow into the subdiaphragmatic spaces, enhances shoulder tip-pain. The abdomen may be distended and may have a doughy feel. Shifting dullness can sometimes be elicited.

Initial management of a patient with acute abdomen

The key considerations which influence both the nature of the immediate resuscitation and the definitive surgical treatment of a patient with an acute abdomen are:
- a history of trauma;
- the presence of cardiovascular instability; and
- clinical evidence of sepsis.

The examination of these patients must be quick but thorough and include an assessment of the vital signs.

Hypovolaemic shock

If there is evidence of shock from internal haemorrhage, immediate volume replacement via an adequate intravenous line and infusion of colloid solutions or isotonic saline is given priority. Blood samples are taken for blood grouping and rapid cross-matching. Cross-matched blood should be available within 30 min in most hospitals nowadays. The urinary bladder is catheterized in these patients to enable hourly measurement of the urine output (see Chapter 4).

Sepsis

If the patient is stable but toxic, dehydrated and in pain, an intravenous line is set up for fluid and electrolyte replacement and opioid analgesia administered intravenously or intramuscularly without delay. The view that analgesia should be withheld initially in these patients because it may mask physical signs is incorrect. Aside from being unkind, it reduces patient cooperation and confidence. A nasogastric tube is inserted in patients with peritonitis and intestinal obstruction. The nasogastric tube is left draining continuously into a bag and the patency of the tube checked by syringing and aspirating every hour by the nursing staff.

Antibiotics are administered in all patients with evidence of intra-abdominal sepsis. If the infection is thought to be arising from the upper gastrointestinal or hepatobiliary tract, a cephalosporin (active against Gram-negative aerobes) is sufficient, but if the peritonitis is generalized or the disease is thought to be originating from the colon, additional cover for Gram-negative anaerobes must be provided. This usually entails the administration of metronidazole in addition to the cephalosporin or aminoglycoside. The exact antibiotic regimen may be changed in the individual patient subsequent to clinical progress, bacterial culture and sensitivity tests.

If immediate surgery is not undertaken in any of these patients after they have been assessed by the more senior surgical staff, careful monitoring of their progress with pulse, temperature, blood pressure, urine output charting and repeated physical examination of the abdomen is carried out. Provided the patient is improving, conservative management is continued, but if deterioration is observed or the condition remains static, then further special tests or exploratory laparotomy is carried out.

Investigations

The basic investigations which are necessary in all patients with an acute abdomen are listed in Table 13.17. The essential blood investigations will give information on the degree of hydration (haemoglobin (Hb), packed cell volume (PCV), white blood cells (WBCs)), electrolyte imbalances (urea and electrolytes), the presence of hyperamylasaemia (pancreatitis, perforated peptic ulcer, intestinal strangulation and infarction) and the presence of sepsis (WBC, blood cultures). The chest X-ray is important, especially in the detection of free air under the diaphragm, which is always indicative of intestinal perforation or laceration (see Fig. 13.16). The abdominal films will detect the presence and indicate the site of intestinal obstruction.

Table 13.17 Investigations in patients with acute abdomen.

Essential
Haemoglobin, white blood cells, packed cell volume
Urea, electrolytes and amylase
Chest X-ray and abdominal scout films (erect/supine)
Blood cultures for high fever and pyrexia

Special
Ultrasound and computed tomography examination
Peritoneal lavage
Minilaparoscopy

There are a number of special investigations which may be carried out in patients admitted with blunt abdominal trauma or acute undiagnosed abdominal pain. These include ultrasound examination, abdominal CT scan, peritoneal lavage and minilaparoscopy. These tests are only performed in trauma patients if the cardiovascular system is stable, i.e. the patient is not shocked.

- *Ultrasound examination and abdominal CT scanning* are both very useful in the detection of intraparenchymal haematomas, free fluid in the peritoneal cavity and localized inflammation and oedema.
- *Peritoneal lavage* is carried out after the insertion of a peritoneal dialysis catheter in the immediate subumbilical region. If blood or blood-stained fluid emerges immediately through the catheter, the test is positive. Otherwise, a litre of Hartmann's solution is infused and then aspirated for examination. The test is considered positive if:
  (a) the fluid returns heavily blood-stained;
  (b) the red blood cells (RBCs) >100 000/ml;
  (c) the WBC >500/ml;
  (d) the amylase >110 u/100 ml; or
  (e) bile, bacteria or food particles are present.

Peritoneal lavage is most commonly used in the diagnosis of suspected blunt intra-abdominal trauma. Its one disadvantage is a 15–20% false-positive rate due to minor lesions which stop bleeding and do not require laparotomy.

- *Minilaparoscopy* More recently, patients with suspected intra-abdominal injuries or patients with undiagnosed acute abdominal pain are being subjected to minilaparoscopy under local anaesthesia and intravenous sedation with midazolam. This procedure allows the inspection of the peritoneal cavity and its contents after insufflation with nitrous oxide. Both traumatic and inflammatory lesions can be diagnosed in this fashion and decisions as to the need or otherwise for emergency surgical intervention determined.

Complications of acute abdomen

The complications which may arise in these patients are outlined in Table 13.18.

The acute complications develop early, usually during the same hospital admisson. The most common is wound infection which may be minor or major, i.e. requiring opening of the skin and subcutaneous tissue to drain the collection which is necessary for healing by granulation (secondary intention). A more serious but less common early wound complication is total wound dehiscence, i.e. complete disruption of the abdominal wall. Often the skin edges remain approximated by the skin sutures, but an

Table 13.18 Complications of acute abdomen.

Acute (early)
Wound infection
Wound dehiscence
Abscess formation
Fistula formation
   External
   Internal

Chronic (late)
Incisional hernia
Wound sinus
Adhesions
   Recurrent small-bowel obstruction
   Bacterial overgrowth (blind loop)

obvious bulge is present in the subcutaneous layer with exudation of copious serosanguineous discharge. The treatment of wound dehiscence is immediate surgical intervention. The extravasated loops are washed and replaced in the peritoneal cavity and the abdominal wall closed in a single layer with large bites of non-absorbable sutures.

Intra-abdominal abscesses may be located in the various compartments of the subphrenic region (on the right or left side), in the pelvis or between loops of the small intestine. The systemic manifestations of intraperitoneal abscesses include malaise, weight loss, intermittent pyrexia (Fig. 13.42) and persistent leukocytosis. There may or may not be any localizing signs. A subphrenic abscess may cause shoulder tip pain. Intraloop abscesses (often multiple) induce a prolonged ileus and a pelvic abscess (most commonly encountered after a perforated appendicitis) causes rectal tenderness and diarrhoea. These abscesses are easily located by either ultrasound or CT examination and many are drained percutaneously avoiding the need for surgical intervention.

Intestinal fistulae may be external (enterocutaneous) or internal (between adjacent hollow viscera). Fistulae arise either from breakdown of an intestinal closure or anastomosis or because of delayed recognition or treatment of an intra-abdominal abscess which then bursts either between bowel and abdominal wall or between adjacent hollow viscera (e.g. colovesical fistula). An external high small-bowel fistula is a serious complication because most of the gastrointestinal secretions are lost through the fistulous opening (high-output fistula). As well as significant daily fluid and electrolyte losses, these fistulae lead to profound excoriation of the abdominal wall as this is digested by the activated pancreatic enzymes. These patients are managed by total parenteral nutrition and careful isolation of the

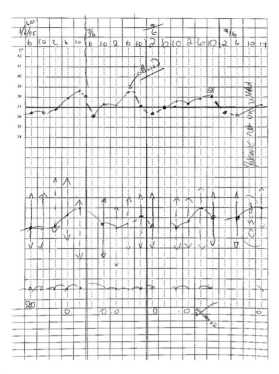

Figure 13.42 Pulse and temperature chart in a patient with intra-abdominal abscess.

fistulous discharge with the use of skin barriers and efficient sump suction drainage. Provided there is no distal obstruction or residual intra-abdominal abscess, the fistula usually heals with this conservative management. Colonic fistulae are much less serious and generally have a lower output. The same principles of management are adopted, except that nutrition is maintained enterally with low-residue or elemental diets.

The chronic complications include incisional herniae, usually in patients who developed a postoperative wound infection and the formation of intraperitoneal adhesions. When significant, the latter cause considerable chronic disability from recurrent attacks of small-bowel obstruction and the development of bacterial overgrowth (blind-loop syndrome) in the kinked small-bowel loops. The bacterial overgrowth results in malabsorption, anaemia and diarrhoea. A common chronic wound complication is the development of a persistent wound sinus. This is related to infection around a non-absorbable suture used in wound closure. Unless this is removed surgically, the sinus and the discharge persist, although one sinus may heal temporarily and then recur.

Intestinal obstruction

Definitions and types

Intestinal obstruction may be complete (total blockage of the lumen) or incomplete (partial blockage). It may present acutely (acute intestinal obstruction) with dramatic symptoms when the obstruction is situated at any point between the second part of the duodenum and the caecum. Alternatively, the presentation may be more insidious — over several weeks, when the obstruction is located in the colon and is referred to as chronic intestinal obstruction. If the blood supply to the obstructed segment is not jeopardized, the obstruction is referred to as simple or mechanical, to distinguish it from those obstructions in which the blood supply is compromised at an early stage — strangulating intestinal obstructions.

Aetiology and pathophysiology

The various causes of mechanical intestinal obstructions can be grouped as extramural, intramural and intraluminal (Table 13.19).

Extramural obstructions are due to extrinsic compression of the walls of the gut by bands, adhesions or tumours (particularly secondary deposits in lymph nodes). Adhesive small-bowel obstruction secondary to previous peritonitis or surgical intervention is nowadays the commonest cause of intestinal obstruction.

Intramural obstructions are caused by lesions (neoplastic or inflammatory or cicatricial) arising from the wall of the intestine. The most common cause of this type of obstruction is carcinoma, usually of the colon.

Table 13.19 Causes of mechanical intestinal obstruction.

Extramural
Adhesions, bands
Herniae: external and internal
Compression by tumours (nodal tumour deposits)

Intramural
Inflammatory disease: Crohn's disease
Tumours: carcinomas, lymphomas, etc.
Strictures

Intraluminal
Faecal impaction
Swallowed foreign bodies
Bezoars
Gallstone

Although intraluminal small-bowel obstructions are rare, chronic colonic intraluminal obstruction by impacted faeces in constipated elderly patients is quite common. The small-bowel lumen may be blocked by a swallowed object (children, mentally subnormal individuals) or a bolus made up of indigestible material (orange pith or hair bezoar, particularly in gastrectomized patients) or a gallstone. The latter arises when a large gallstone in a chronically inflamed gallbladder which has become adherent to the duodenum erodes through the two organs by a process of pressure necrosis, thus entering the duodenum and becoming impacted lower down in the small intestine, usually the terminal ileum. The condition is known as gallstone ileus. By virtue of its origin it is always accompanied by a cholecystoduodenal fistula, which allows reflux of enteric contents and air into the biliary tract.

Specific types of intestinal obstruction

Mechanical obstruction

Following the onset of the obstruction, the distal bowel empties to a collapsed state, whereas the proximal bowel becomes hyperactive with vigorous peristaltic contractions in an effort to overcome the obstruction. These cluster contractions are the cause of the severe colicky abdominal pain experienced by these patients. Additionally, the bowel proximal to the obstruction dilates. The dilatation is due to the accumulation of swallowed air and increased intestinal secretions. The interface between the air and fluid in the dilated loops accounts for the fluid levels seen in the erect abdominal film of these patients. The wall of the obstructed gut becomes oedematous. This is the result of increased transudation across the capillary membrane as the venous drainage of the affected segments is impaired by the distension. The fluid and electrolytes which accumulate in the lumen of the obstructed bowel and within its wall are effectively lost (sequestrated third-space losses) and contribute (together with vomiting) to the fluid and electrolyte deficit of these patients. Bacterial overgrowth occurs within the obstructed loops of intestine. Unless the distension is relieved, there is progressive occlusion, by stretching, of the intestinal intramural vessels such that, untreated, a mechanical intestinal obstruction leads to ischaemia and eventually necrosis with perforation of the bowel.

Strangulating obstruction

Here, in addition to the luminal obstruction, the viability of the gut is compromised because of impairment of its blood supply at an early stage. Common examples include strangulation caused by bands, adhesions and tight hernial sacs (strangulated herniae). There are special forms which merit separate attention: these include intussusception, volvulus, closed-loop obstruction and mesenteric infarction.

Intussusception This consists of telescoping of a loop of bowel inside itself (ileoileal = ileum inside ileum; ileocolic = ileum inside caecum or ascending colon; Fig. 13.43a). It may or may not originate from a lead point, which is usually a swelling of the mucosa or submucosa (e.g. inflamed Peyer's patch, mucosal adenoma, submucosal lipoma, etc). Intussusception occurs most commonly in infants and children usually between 3 and 18 months of age, but may be encountered in adults. The blood supply of the involved bowel is compromised at an early stage and unless the intussusception is reduced early (e.g. by barium enema or surgery), infarction and peritonitis supervene (Fig. 13.43b).

Volvulus Volvulus is a 360° twist of a loop or loops of intestine. The rotation causes early obstruction of the vascular pedicle supplying the affected portion. Risk factors for small-bowel volvulus (which may affect the whole of the midgut) include adhesions or bands between the antimesenteric aspect of the bowel and the anterior abdominal wall and congenital malrotation of the gut. Volvulus of the sigmoid colon is encountered in the elderly, in patients with chronic constipation and those with a redundant pelvic mesocolon (Fig. 13.25). Unless recognized early, volvulus leads to intestinal infarction which often involves large segments of the gut.

Closed-loop obstruction Although volvulus is an example of this type of obstruction, i.e. segment of the affected bowel closed at proximal and distal ends, the term closed-loop obstruction is usually reserved for a complete obstruction of the left colon (usually by an annular carcinoma of the descending or sigmoid colon) in the presence of a competent ileocaecal valve. This prevents the proximal distended colon from decompressing into the small intestine. Meanwhile, small-bowel contents may continue to pass into the caecum through the one-way ileocaecal valve. The result is a rapid build-up of pressure in the colon with the brunt being taken by the caecum which becomes markedly distended to the point of ischaemia when it perforates, usually through a clearcut hole — pistol-shot perforation.

Mesenteric infarction In this serious condition, there is primary occlusion of the blood supply to the intestine from thrombotic or embolic disease of the mesenteric vessels. Most commonly, the superior mesenteric vessels are occluded with infarction of the entire midgut from the level of the mid-duodenum to the junction of the proximal with the

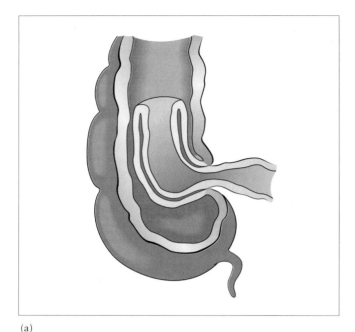

(a)

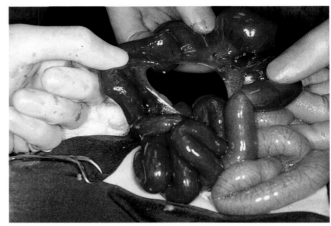

Figure 13.44 Infarcted midgut.

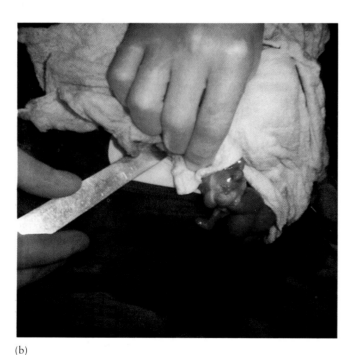

(b)

Figure 13.43 (a) Diagram of ileocolic intussusception; (b) operative photograph of reduction of an ileocolic intussusception. The ileum, which is a slightly dusky colour, is being milked back out of the caecum.

distal two-thirds of the transverse colon (long-loop infarction; Fig. 13.44). The condition, which affects patients who are elderly and suffer from cardiac and atheromatous vascular disease, is usually fatal. At times the extent of the infarction is less extensive, when resection may be followed by survival but the patient has insufficient small bowel for digestion and absorption and develops the short-gut syndrome. There is another type of small-bowel infarction which is encountered in patients with chronic hypoxia (chronic pulmonary disease, heart failure, etc.) and is due to hypoperfusion. The ischaemia is patchy and the mesenteric vessels appear patent, the block occurring in the small intramural vessels of the intestine (microcirculation). This variant is known as non-occlusive mesenteric infarction.

The same occlusive process may involve the vessels supplying the colon and lead to ischaemic colitis. This tends to affect predominantly the left colon and presents with a picture of acute inflammation not dissimilar from acute colonic diverticulitis. Fortunately the affected colon, although oedematous and inflamed, does not usually infarct and the process subsides with conservative management. However, a stricture of the left colon commonly situated just distal to the splenic flexure develops some weeks to months later.

Paralytic ileus

This term is used to describe a syndrome in which intestinal obstruction is due to absence of the normal peristaltic contractions. Although often abbreviated to ileus, this is incorrect as this word, which is of Greek derivation, means to 'roll'. Adynamic ileus is most commonly encountered after intra-abdominal surgery, when it is short-lived (few days) and often referred to as physiological ileus. The temporary cessation of intestinal motor activity is due to handling and exposure of the intestinal loops. On occasions, it is pathologically prolonged, when it is associated with postoperative intra-abdominal sepsis and fibrinous adhesion formation — postoperative ileus. In this setting the differentiation between mechanical and paralytic obstruction is difficult and often the clinical picture is mixed.

Paralytic ileus may also be caused by spinal injuries and by the accumulation of retroperitoneal blood or irritant exudates which disturb the functional activity of the coeliac plexus and splanchnic nerves — retroperitoneal haematoma from renal injuries, ruptured abdominal aneurysms, acute pancreatitis, etc. Haemoperitoneum may also be accompanied by some loss of intestinal peristaltic activity. Infective paralytic ileus is the most serious and is secondary to peritonitis from any cause.

Clinical features of intestinal obstruction

Symptoms

The cardinal symptoms of mechanical bowel obstruction are:
- vomiting;
- colicky abdominal pain;
- abdominal distension;
- absolute constipation.

Notwithstanding, the symptomatology may be varied and the clinical picture of acute small-bowel obstruction is quite different from that of chronic (colonic) obstruction.

Vomiting is a marked feature of high small-bowel obstruction but is rarely encountered in colonic obstruction. Initially, the vomit consists of food followed by bile-stained fluid which later on becomes faeculent. This is caused by the bacterial overgrowth in the obstructed small intestine. Vomiting, together with the sequestration of fluid in the dilated loops, rapidly leads to dehydration with significant water and electrolyte deficits, particularly Na+ and Cl-. The dehydration leads to raised packed cell volume and prerenal azotaemia with elevation of the blood urea and reduced urine output.

The *pain* in mechanical small-bowel obstruction is colicky in nature, situated in the centre of the abdomen around the umbilicus and accompanied by hyperperistaltic rushes which can easily be heard by the stethoscope. In colonic obstruction the pain is more of a discomfort and is situated in the suprapubic region. However, in the presence of closed-loop obstruction with marked caecal dilatation and impending perforation, localized pain is present in the right iliac fossa. Constant severe pain is ominous and indicates either infarction of the bowel or the onset of peritonitis. Paralytic ileus in itself is painless, except when secondary to peritonitis, when the pain is generalized and constant.

Abdominal distension becomes progressively more marked the lower the obstruction is situated and may reach extreme degrees in low colonic obstruction and paralytic ileus. It is caused by accumulation of gas and fluid within the obstructed bowel.

Following the onset of mechanical obstruction, the patient may have a bowel motion as the distal segment empties. Thereafter, there is *absolute constipation* (no passage of either flatus or faeces).

Physical signs

The physical signs of intestinal obstruction are usually clearcut. Dehydration is accompanied by loss of skin turgor. Pyrexia is mild unless there is infarction and peritonitis. Fluid and electrolyte losses cause a reduction of circulating blood volume with some hypotension and persistent tachycardia. The distended abdomen is resonant to percussion on the anterior aspect but is dull towards the flanks. Auscultation confirms the presence of excessive peristaltic activity (borborygmi) which coincide with attacks of colic. In paralytic ileus bowel sounds are not heard; instead these are replaced by tinkling high-pitched sounds due to passive movement of fluid within the dilated loops.

Tenderness and rebound tenderness are indicative of ischaemic bowel or developing peritonitis (due to imminent or established perforation). It is usually accompanied by a deterioration in the general condition of the patient and change in the character of the pain, which becomes severe and constant.

Rectal examination in small-bowel obstruction usually confirms an empty rectum. In colonic obstruction the findings are available: empty rectum, gross faecal loading (in obstruction due to faecal impaction) or a low neoplasm can be palpated by the examining finger.

Investigations in intestinal obstruction

The essential investigations in patients with intestinal obstruction are Hb, PCV, WBCs, urea and electrolytes, chest X-ray, plain erect and supine abdominal films.

Both the Hb and the PCV are elevated because of the haemoconcentration. The raised blood urea is the result of an element of prerenal failure due to the hypovolaemia. The WBC count is usually normal or slightly elevated unless there is bowel infarction and/or peritonitis. The serum Na+ and Cl- are low. Hyperkalaemia may be observed in patients with infarcted intestine.

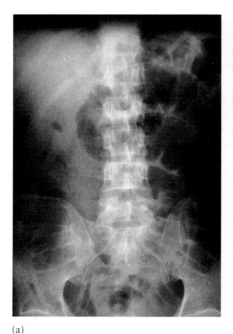

(a)

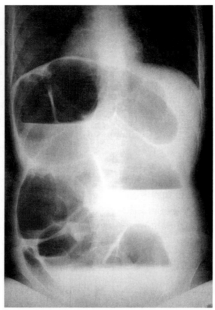

(b)

Figure 13.45 (a) Valvulae conniventes. Supine film showed a dilated jejunum in mechanical small-bowel obstruction. The soft-tissue markings extend the whole length of the dilated segment. The obstructed ileum is relatively featureless. (b) Haustral soft-tissue markings in colonic obstruction. They do not extend across the whole width of the affected segment. Note the presence of air–fluid levels.

The chest X-ray shows an elevated diaphragm which is secondary to the abdominal distension. In addition there may be free air underneath the right diaphragm in patients with infective paralytic ileus (secondary to intestinal perforation). The erect abdominal film is taken to outline air–fluid levels. These are multiple and centrally placed in a ladder fashion in small-bowel obstructions. In large-bowel obstruction they are less numerous and located in the flanks and suprapubic regions (Fig. 13.45b). The supine film is used to assess the distension of the intestine and helps to differentiate small from large intestine. Dilated jejunum often exhibits parallel soft-tissue shadows which extend the whole width of the involved segment (due to the folds of the small-bowel mucosa — valvulae conniventes; Fig. 13.45a), whereas in the obstructed colon the haustra cause crescentic soft-tissue shadows which do not traverse the entire width of the bowel (Fig. 13.45b). Also, the obstructed colon has a sacculated outline. The obstructed ileum is relatively featureless.

Other investigations which may be necessary are contrast examinations (Gastrografin swallow and meal, gentle barium enema) and sigmoidoscopy.

Management of intestinal obstruction

The management of intestinal obstruction is based on four principles:
• decompression of the obstructed gut;

• replacement of the fluid and electrolyte losses;
• special conservative measures in certain situations;
• surgical intervention.

Decompression

Although various long tubes were used in the past, decompression is nowadays achieved by the insertion of a nasogastric Ryle's tube. This is aspirated at least every hour and left draining into a bag in the intervening periods. The daily aspirate is measured and the amount used in calculating the daily fluid and electrolyte requirements (see Chapter 6). If the intestinal obstruction responds to conservative management, the daily amount of aspirate gradually reduces and its nature changes to clear, often bile-stained fluid.

Fluid and electrolyte therapy

Fluids and electrolytes are given through a peripheral venous line. As the major losses are water, sodium and chloride, the usual crystalloid solution consists of isotonic saline and 5% dextrose solution. Initially, large amounts are administered (1.0 l every 3–4 h) to replace the losses. Thereafter, maintenance intravenous fluid therapy is continued until return of normal bowel function. The usual daily requirements of K+ (40–120 mmol) are met by infusing 60–80 mmol of potassium chloride in divided doses over 24 h. If hypokalaemia is severe, up to 40 mmol may be infused over 1 h in 500 ml of fluid. It is important to remember that potassium must always be administered slowly and never given as a bolus injection because of the risks of cardiac arrhythmias and arrest.

Special conservative measures

For certain types of intestinal obstruction, additional specific measures may result in rapid relief of the obstruction, thereby avoiding surgical intervention. Examples include the passage of a rectal tube or flexible sigmoidoscope to deflate a sigmoid volvulus, barium contrast enema to reduce an early intussusception in an infant and manual removal of faeces and/or oil retention enema to deal with obstruction caused by faecal impaction.

Assessment of progress

It is important that the patient is assessed at frequent intervals to establish progress on conservative management. This is confirmed by relief of symptoms (vomiting

and pain), improvement of the general condition and vital signs (pulse rate, temperature and blood pressure) and certain observations: reduction in the amount of aspirate and abdominal girth, and return of normal bowel sounds.

Surgical intervention is undertaken if:
- the underlying disease needs surgical treatment — obstructed hernia, obstructing carcinoma, etc. In this respect, intestinal obstruction due to adhesions often settles with conservative management and therefore is not initially treated surgically unless there is clinical evidence of strangulation;
- if the patient does not improve with conservative treatment;
- if there are signs of strangulation or peritonitis.

Intestinal pseudo-obstruction

This is sometimes referred to as Ogilvie's syndrome as he first described the condition in two patients with advanced

Intestinal obstruction at a glance

DEFINITIONS

Complete intestinal obstruction indicates total blockage of the intestinal lumen, whereas *incomplete* denotes only a partial blockage. Obstruction may be *acute* (hours) or *chronic* (weeks), *simple* (mechanical), i.e. blood supply not compromised, or *strangulated*, i.e. blood supply is compromised. A *closed-loop obstruction* is an obstruction of the colon in the presence of a competent ileocaecal valve

CAUSES

- *Extramural:* Adhesions, bands, volvulus, herniae (internal and external), compression by tumour (e.g. frozen pelvis)
- *Intramural:* Inflammatory bowel disease (Crohn's disease), tumours: carcinomas, lymphomas, strictures, paralytic (adynamic) ileus, intussusception
- *Intraluminal:* Faecal impaction, foreign bodies, bezoars, gallstone ileus

PATHOPHYSIOLOGY

- Bowel distal to obstruction collapses
- Bowel proximal to obstruction distends and becomes hyperactive. Distension is due to swallowed air and accumulating intestinal secretions
- The bowel wall becomes oedematous. Fluid and electrolytes accumulate in the wall and lumen (third-space loss)
- Bacteria proliferate in the obstructed bowel
- As the bowel distends, the intramural vessels become stretched and the blood supply is compromised leading to ischaemia and necrosis

CLINICAL FEATURES

- Vomiting, colicky abdominal pain, abdominal distension, absolute constipation (i.e. neither faeces nor flatus)

- Dehydration and loss of skin turgor
- Hypotension, tachycardia
- Abdominal distension and increased bowel sounds
- Empty rectum on digital examination
- Tenderness or rebound indicates peritonitis

INVESTIGATIONS

- Hb, PCV: elevated due to dehydration
- WCC: normal or slightly elevated
- U&E: urea elevated, Na+ and Cl- low
- CXR: elevated diaphragm due to abdominal distension
- Abdominal X-rays: erect film demonstrates air–fluid levels; supine film gives a clue as to whether obstruction is in small (central distension/valvulae conniventes shadows cross entire width of lumen) or large (peripheral distension/haustral shadows do not cross entire width of bowel) bowel
- Contrast studies, sigmoidoscopy to show site of obstruction

MANAGEMENT

- Decompress the obstructed gut — pass nasogastric tube
- Replace fluid and electrolyte losses — give Ringer's lactate or NaCl with K+ supplementation
- Relieve the obstruction surgically if:
  (a) underlying cause needs surgical treatment (e.g. hernia, colonic carcinoma)
  (b) patient does not improve with conservative treatment (e.g. adhesion obstruction)
  (c) there are signs of strangulation or peritonitis

cancer and involvement of the subdiaphragmatic auto-nomic plexus and postulated an imbalance between sym-pathetic and parasympathetic activity as the underlying cause. It is now thought to result from impairment of the reflex circuits within the enteric nervous system which ensure normal peristaltic progression. The syndrome is characterized by massive dilatation of the colon, suggesting distal organic colonic obstruction. This rare functional obstruction is usually encountered in elderly patients with severe extra-abdominal illness or injury (heart failure, sepsis, trauma, etc.). Other documented associations include chronic administration of hypnotics and sedatives, lead toxicity, hypothyroidism and various neurological dis-orders. The diagnosis is made by exclusion of organic disease. Air–fluid levels are often absent in this condition. Untreated the dilatation is progressive and when this exceeds 10 cm in the caecum, rupture with peritonitis may ensue. Treatment involves correction of the underlying cause, supportive management and decompression of the colon by passage of a rectal tube, sigmoidoscope or colonoscope.

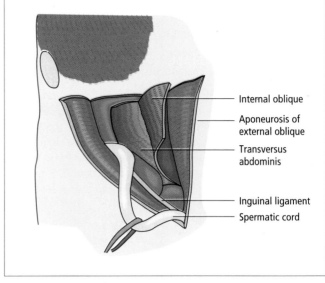

(a)

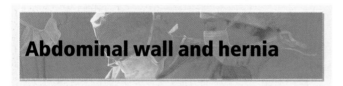

Abdominal wall and hernia

Anatomy

The inguinal canal

The anterior wall of the inguinal canal is formed by the aponeurosis of the external oblique and in its lateral half by the internal oblique and transversus abdominis muscles. The floor of the canal is formed by the inguinal ligament and the roof of the canal by the conjoint tendon, which con-sists of the fused inferior borders of internal oblique and transversalis abdominis. The posterior wall of the canal consists of the transversalis fascia with a portion of the medial end formed by the insertion of the conjoint tendon (Fig. 13.46a).

At its lateral end the transversalis fascia is penetrated at the deep inguinal ring by the spermatic cord with the inferior epigastric artery passing upwards and medial to it. Thus an indirect inguinal hernia as it emerges through the deep ring within the spermatic cord has the conjoint tendon laterally and above it, the inferior epigastric artery medially and the inguinal ligament inferiorly.

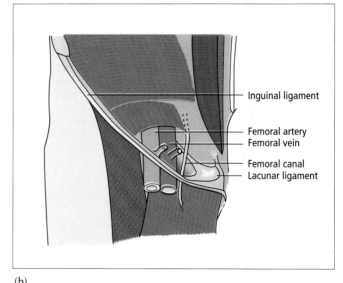

(b)

Figure 13.46 Anatomy of (a) the inguinal and (b) the femoral canal.

The femoral canal

The femoral canal is bounded anteriorly by the inguinal ligament, posteriorly by the fascia over the pectineus muscle, medially by the lacunar ligament and laterally by the femoral vein. The canal often contains a named lymph gland (of Cloquet; Fig. 13.46b).

Table 13.20 Common abdominal herniae and their management.

Name	Site of defect	Treatment
Umbilical	Umbilicus	Observe
Paraumbilical	Just above umbilicus	Surgical repair (Mayo)
Epigastric	Midline between umbilicus and xiphisternum	Surgical repair
Inguinal		
Indirect	Deep inguinal ring	Infant: herniotomy only
		Adult: herniotomy/herniorrhaphy (Sholdice, Darn; occasionally truss)
Direct	Posterior wall	Herniorrhaphy
Femoral	Femoral canal	Surgical repair (femoral, Lotheissen, McEvedy)
Incisional	Previous abdominal wound	Surgical repair (occasionally Marlex mesh)

Disorders of the abdominal wall

Haematoma of rectus sheath

A haematoma of the rectus sheath presents as a swelling in the anterior abdominal wall, usually below the umbilicus, and associated with sudden abdominal wall strain such as sneezing or coughing. This causes a tear in a branch of the inferior epigastric artery and the rapid formation of a haematoma. Clinically the patient experiences severe abdominal pain with nausea and vomiting accompanied by pyrexia and leukocytosis. The abdominal wall swelling is tender and takes several weeks to resolve. No intervention is needed if the diagnosis is certain. If not, the haematoma should be evacuated and the artery ligated.

Desmoid tumour

These slow-growing non-metastasizing tumours arise from the rectus abdominis muscles and may attain a very large size. The histology of the tumour is variable and it may resemble a low-grade fibrosarcoma. It is easily palpated and is rendered more prominent by contraction of the abdominal muscles. It may be associated with Gardner's syndrome and may be related to childbirth injuries.

Common abdominal herniae

A hernia is defined as the protrusion of a viscus or part of a viscus through an abnormal opening. Herniae may occur in the brain (e.g. after head injury), in muscle through its fascial covering, internally in the abdomen (internal hernia) or externally through a weak normal opening (inguinal and femoral hernia) or an abnormal opening (e.g. incisional hernia) in the abdominal wall. The common external abdominal herniae are presented here (Table 13.20; Figs 13.47 and 13.48).

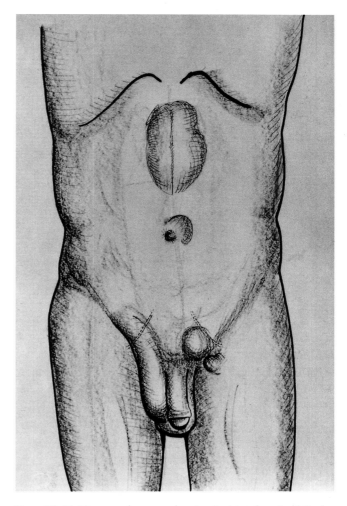

Figure 13.47 Diagram of common herniae. Incisional, periumbilical, indirect inguinoscrotal (right), direct inguinal and femoral (left) herniae are shown.

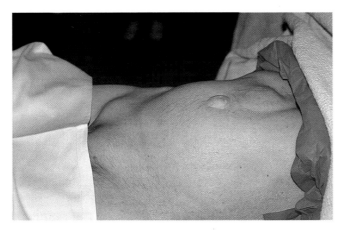

Figure 13.48 Femoral (right), inguinal (left), paraumbilical and incisional herniae all in the one patient. Courtesy of Mr K. Mealy.

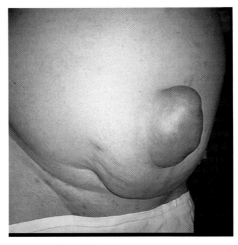

Figure 13.50 Paraumbilical hernia

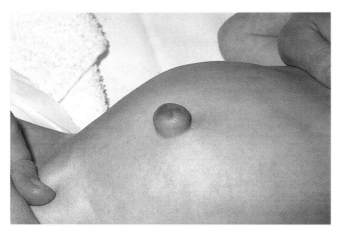

Figure 13.49 Congenital umbilical hernia.

Umbilical hernia

True umbilical hernia is common in infants (especially in Africans) and is due to a persistent defect in the abdominal wall at the umbilicus. The majority close spontaneously and surgical closure is rarely necessary. Intervention is necessary in the unlikely event of strangulation or incarceration (Fig. 13.49).

Paraumbilical hernia

These herniae occur in obese adult women and are prone to strangulate. The defect occurs through the midline just above the umbilicus (Fig. 13.50). The sac may contain omentum or small intestine or both, and because of the narrow neck, strangulation is relatively common. With long-standing herniae, adhesions occur between the con-

tents and the wall of the sac so that the hernia becomes irreducible.

Strangulated herniae are repaired as an emergency. Long-standing herniae should be repaired electively. The Mayo repair is commonly used. With this technique the contents of the sac are freed from its walls and reduced. The sac is excised. The fascial defect is repaired transversely with the upper flap overlapping the lower, thereby doubling the strength of the repair.

Epigastric hernia

These usually small but often quite painful swellings occur in the midline between xiphisternum and umbilicus. The swelling most frequently consists of herniation of extra-peritoneal fat through a small defect in the linea alba. Sometimes it carries a peritoneal sac with it which may contain omentum but this is rare. Pain is localized to the site with tenderness on pressure but it may also simulate peptic ulcer symptoms. Clinical examination reveals a tender swelling in the midline. Sometimes incarcerated fat becomes devascularized and necrotic.

Treatment is surgical and may be carried out under local anaesthesia, enlarging the defect, excising the fat and suturing the defect with unabsorbable sutures.

Inguinal hernia

Inguinal hernia is a common complaint, occurring mostly in men. It is twice as frequent as femoral hernia and in males more than 90% of herniae are inguinal.

Inguinal hernia may occur at any age. In children they are generally associated with developmental disorders such as

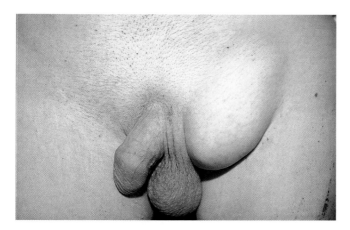

Figure 13.51 Inguinal hernia

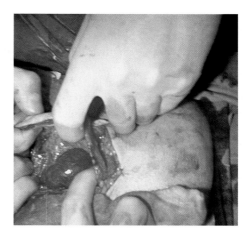

Figure 13.52 Strangulated inguinal hernia (operative photograph).

persistent processus vaginalis or testicular maldescent. Inguinal hernia is also common in young adult males and this is also related to a congenital defect such as a persistent processus, which may be precipitated from potential to actual existence by physical effort (Fig. 13.51).

An *indirect inguinal hernia* occurs when a sac develops by emerging through the deep inguinal ring and passing through the inguinal canal in the spermatic cord adjacent to the vas deferens and surrounded by the coverings of the cord. The sac, if sufficiently large, may emerge through the external inguinal ring or descend into the scrotum. It may contain omentum or small bowel and has the potential to become irreducible and strangulate. On examination an indirect inguinal hernia is detectable above and medial to the pubic tubercle. The latter may be detected by palpating laterally along the pubic ramus or by invaginating the scrotum in the male, when it can be felt underneath and just lateral to the spermatic cord. Unless incarcerated, an inguinal hernia has an impulse on coughing and if reducible can be controlled by pressure over the internal inguinal ring, which is situated at the mid inguinal point 1 cm above the pulsation of the femoral artery.

A *direct inguinal hernia* occurs as a result of a weakness in the transversalis fascia and is common in the elderly. Aetiological factors such as chronic cough, chronic strain during micturition because of prostatic hypertrophy, or chronic constipation make it more common in the elderly. A direct hernia usually appears as a diffuse bulge which cannot be controlled by pressure over the internal ring. It is above and lateral to the pubic tubercle and does not enter the scrotum. A direct inguinal hernia has a wide neck, in contrast to the narrow neck of the indirect hernia. In consequence, a direct hernia is much less likely to strangulate.

Strangulation

Strangulation of an inguinal hernia develops when constriction occurs at the neck of the sac cutting off the blood supply of the contents. Initially the venous blood supply is obstructed. This causes swelling of the contents (omentum or bowel) and eventually a combination of oedema and constriction cuts off the arterial blood supply and gangrene supervenes in the strangulated loop (Fig. 13.52).

These changes are accompanied by severe local pain with irreducibility of the hernia and tenderness. The symptoms of small-bowel obstruction are also evident, with colicky abdominal pain, nausea and vomiting.

When the hernia first becomes obstructed it is possible to reduce it by manipulation. It is important, however, to ensure that the hernia is not reduced *en masse* into the abdominal cavity with the contents still strangulated by the constricting neck of the sac. An irreducible hernia *per se* does not indicate strangulation and may be *incarcerated* with an adequate blood supply but completely irreducible.

Management of inguinal hernia

Ideally all inguinal herniae should be repaired by elective surgical operation. Surgery is usually performed under general anaesthesia but local or regional anaesthesia is also used. Surgical repair classically consists of two elements: excision of the hernial sac (*herniotomy*) and repair or buttressing of the weakness in the posterior inguinal canal (*herniorrhaphy*). In infants (always indirect herniae) the internal and external rings are superimposed and only a herniotomy is required for effective treatment. Laparoscopic repair of adult inguinal hernia is also performed by some surgeons.

Complications of hernia repair include:
- haematoma, which may be in the wound or scrotum;
- acute urinary retention; this frequently follows bilateral repair;
- wound infection — this should be rare as hernia repair is a *clean* operation, but in practice an infection occurs in 5–8%;
- chronic pain — trapping of the ilioinguinal nerve;
- testicular pain and swelling followed by atrophy usually means that the repair is too tight and the testicular artery is compromised. Testicular atrophy will occur when the swelling subsides;
- recurrence of hernia occurs in about 5% of patients but the rate is higher when surgical technique is poor.

Occasionally a *truss* may be used to control an inguinal hernia if the patient is unfit for or refuses surgery. However, trusses are unsatisfactory, do not treat the hernia and the patient is still at risk of incarceration and strangulation.

Femoral hernia

A femoral hernia emerges through the femoral canal and may be felt as a soft swelling below and lateral to the pubic tubercle (Fig. 13.53). It is a protrusion of peritoneum through the femoral canal, below which it emerges subcutaneously. It is usually a small sac and may contain omentum or small bowel. Because of its position below the inguinal ligament it must be distinguished from a saphena varix, which disappears on pressure or on lying down and has a cough impulse. It must also be recognized instead of femoral artery aneurysm, enlarged lymph nodes or, on very rare occasions, a psoas abscess.

Strangulation

Femoral herniae often strangulate. Because of their small size, femoral herniae do not provide local signs and symptoms comparable to inguinal hernia and the swelling of a strangulated femoral hernia may be impalpable. However, there is evidence of small-bowel obstruction and this should stimulate a careful search for a hernia.

Management of femoral hernia

Femoral herniae are more likely to lead to strangulation than inguinal herniae and therefore should always be repaired without delay. A truss should not be used. Surgically the hernia may be approached from below (femoral approach) or above (via the inguinal canal — *Lotheissen approach* — or via the rectus abdominus muscle — *McEvedy approach*). The contents of the sac are emptied, the sac is excised and the femoral canal is obliterated with three interrupted non-absorbable sutures.

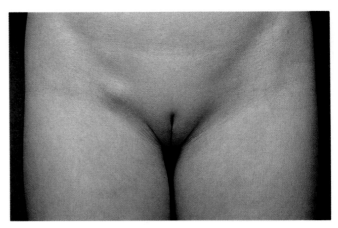

(a)

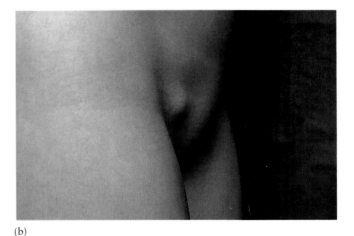

(b)

Figure 13.53 Femoral hernia: (a) anterior and (b) lateral views.

Incisional hernia

This is a hernia which occurs through a defect in an old abdominal wound. Wound infection predisposes to incisional hernia. The margins of the defect in the abdominal wall under the old incision can often be felt and the hernia is easily demonstrated by asking the supine patient to raise his or her head off the pillow (thus tensing the abdominal muscles; Fig. 13.54). An incisional hernia often contains bowel which is adherent to the peritoneal sac. Surgical repair requires excision of the sac, identification and apposition of the margins of the hernia. Occasionally, with a very large incisional hernia, it is not possible to bring the muscle edges together and sometimes a polypropylene mesh (Marlex) has to be inserted to close the abdominal wall defect.

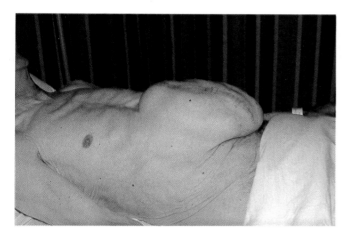

Figure 13.54 Large incisional hernia.

Unusual herniae

Inguinal variations

• *Sliding hernia (hernia en glissade)*: Some inguinal hernias are sliding hernias, which means that retroperitoneal structures, e.g. large bowel, herniate into the inguinal canal and scrotum, dragging their overlying peritoneum with them. Thus the peritoneal sac itself is empty and the contents of the hernia lie behind the sac. These can often be quite difficult to repair.

• *Littre's hernia*: This is an unusual hernia in which the sac of an inguinal hernia contains a Meckel's diverticulum.

• *Maydl's hernia (hernia-en-W)*: In this rare form of inguinal hernia, two loops of intestine are incarcerated in the sac. The intervening loop of small intestine which remains in the abdominal cavity becomes strangulated by compression of its mesenteric vessels at the neck of the sac.

Richter's hernia

A Richter's hernia is a variant of strangulated hernia. When a Richter's hernia is present, only part of the circumference of the small bowel is strangulated. As a consequence, while the patient is still able to pass flatus, he or she experiences colicky abdominal pain and vomiting and radiological evidence of small-bowel obstruction is present.

Spigelian hernia

This is an interstitial hernia of the abdominal wall. The defect occurs at the lateral border of the rectus abdominis, emerging through a defect in the transversus and internal oblique fascia halfway between the umbilicus and the pubic

symphysis. The swelling is diffuse and difficult to palpate as it is covered by the external oblique. It may be identified by its position above and medial to the location of an inguinal hernia.

Obturator, gluteal and lumbar hernia

These are excessively rare herniae which occur with herniation through the obturator foramen, the gluteal and lumbar regions. It is likely that most doctors will never see any of these herniae.

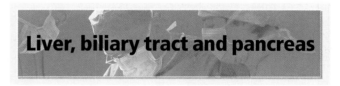

Liver, biliary tract and pancreas

The liver

Overview of hepatic disease

The liver is the largest organ of the body and consists of two lobes which are made up of eight segments. The liver has important metabolic, synthetic, detoxification and defence functions. Acute hepatic disease can be due to infections, usually by viral agents (hepatitis A, B and C, etc.) or may be induced by drugs (Table 13.21), alcohol and other poisons or toxic metabolites of certain anaesthetic agents such as halothane.

Acute hepatitis may be a mild to moderate disease or severe with massive liver cell necrosis leading to fulminant hepatic failure. Both can progress to chronic liver disease (chronic hepatitis) which, when aggressive, is characterized by ongoing piecemeal necrosis and fibrosis. Alcohol-related liver disease is a serious and common problem in many western countries. It can lead to an acute disorder (acute alcoholic hepatitis) or to chronic liver disease, which often

Table 13.21 Drug-induced liver disease.

Type of injury	Drug causing injury
Fatty infiltration	Tetracycline
Hepatitis	Halothane, monoamine oxidase inhibitors
Cholestasis	Carbamazepine, chlorpropramide
Necrosis	Paracetamol, isoniazid
Tumours	Oestrogens and androgens

Abdominal herniae at a glance

DEFINITION

- A hernia is the protrusion of a viscus or part of a viscus through an abnormal opening

TYPES

- Umbilical
- Paraumbilical
- Epigastric
- Inguinal (direct and indirect)
- Femoral
- Incisional

PATHOPHYSIOLOGY

- The defect in the abdominal wall may be congenital (e.g. femoral canal) or acquired (e.g. an incision) and is lined with peritoneum (the sac)
- Raised intra-abdominal pressure further weakens the defect, allowing some of the intra-abdominal contents (e.g. omentum, small-bowel loop) to migrate through the opening
- Entrapment of the contents in the sac leads to incarceration (unable to reduce contents) and strangulation (blood supply to incarcerated contents is compromised)

CLINICAL FEATURES

- Patient presents with a lump over the site of the hernia
  - (a) femoral herniae are below and lateral to the pubic tubercle
  - (b) inguinal herniae are above and medial to the pubic tubercle
  - (c) indirect inguinal herniae can be controlled by digital pressure over the internal inguinal ring
  - (d) direct inguinal herniae protrude through Hasselbach's triangle (inguinal ligament, lateral border of rectus, inferior epigastric artery)
  - (e) incisional herniae bulge on tensing the recti
- Patient may present with a complication (incarceration, intestinal obstruction, strangulation)

MANAGEMENT

- Surgical repair should be undertaken unless patient is very unfit
- Herniotomy = excision of the hernial sac (children)
- Herniorrhaphy = repairing the defect (adults)

COMPLICATIONS OF SURGERY

- Haematoma (wound or scrotal)
- Acute urinary retention
- Wound infection
- Chronic pain
- Testicular pain and swelling leading to testicular atrophy
- Hernia recurrence (about 5%)

progresses to cirrhosis. The specific histological hallmarks of both acute and chronic alcoholic liver disease are fatty change and hyaline deposits (Mallory's hyaline).

Cirrhosis of the liver may develop on a background of known liver disease but often the primary agent or disease remains undetermined, when the condition is referred to as cryptogenic cirrhosis. In some patients, the cirrhosis is the result of chronic biliary tract obstruction and this may be a primary condition (primary biliary cirrhosis) or secondary to long-standing extrahepatic obstruction by strictures (secondary biliary cirrhosis). Other less common non-malignant disorders of the liver include haemochromatosis due to iron overload and sclerosing cholangitis, which is a condition of unknown aetiology characterized by fibrous obliteration of the intra- and extrahepatic biliary tract.

In western countries, the commonest liver tumours are secondary deposits; primary liver neoplasms are relatively rare.

Assessment of liver disease

The assessment of liver disease is based on history, physical examination and specialized tests. In the physical examina-

tion, the stigmata of chronic liver disease are important (Table 13.22).

Severe acute or end-stage chronic liver disease is always associated with varying degrees of diminished level of consciousness and specific changes are observed on the electroencephalogram (EEG). Advanced disease is also accompanied by muscle wasting, ascites and portal hypertension with splenomegaly.

Table 13.22 Stigmata of chronic liver disease.

Important	Less important
Jaundice	Parotid enlargement
Spider naevi	Palmar erythema
Hepatomegaly	Dupuytren's contracture
Splenomegaly	Breast enlargement
Bleeding tendency	Testicular atrophy
Muscle wasting	Flapping tremor
Ascites and oedema	Foetor hepaticus
Neuropsychiatric manifestations	
Portal hypertension	

Table 13.23 Laboratory tests performed in patients with liver disease.

Haematological	Haemoglobin and platelet count
Biochemical tests	Bilirubin, transaminases and bile ductular enzymes (alkaline phosphatase or gammaglutamyl transpeptidase)
Clotting studies	Prothrombin and kaolin cephalin times
Viral studies	Detection of viral antigens and antibodies

Table 13.24 Causes of portal hypertension.

Prehepatic inflow obstruction
Portal vein thrombosis
Occlusion by extrinsic compression

Intrahepatic obstruction
Presinusoidal
    Periportal fibrosis
    Schistosomiasis
Postsinusoidal
    Cirrhosis

Extrahepatic outflow obstruction
Veno-occlusive disease
Budd–Chiari syndrome

Increased arterial blood flow to portal venous system
Arteriovenous fistula

The laboratory tests performed routinely in a patient with suspected liver disease are shown in Table 13.23.

Imaging of the liver parenchyma is carried out by ultrasound and CT scanning. Specialized angiographic studies of the hepatic arterial and portal venous system are needed in patients with portal hypertension and in patients with liver tumours. A liver biopsy may be required to elucidate the nature of chronic liver disease.

Cirrhosis of the liver

Cirrhosis is defined as disordered fibrosis with regenerative nodules. Two broad categories are described depending on the size of the nodular change: micronodular and macronodular. Cirrhosis is an irreversible state and is clinically accompanied by jaundice and the other stigmata of chronic liver disease. When due to alcohol, the course is variable, with progression of the disease being halted if the patient breaks the alcohol habit. Primary biliary cirrhosis is an autoimmune process which results in progressive destruction of the intrahepatic bile ducts and parenchyma. It usually affects middle-aged women and is accompanied by elevation of serum immunoglobulin M and the presence of circulating antimitochondrial antibodies. Another feature of the disease is the fatty deposits around the eyes (xanthelasma) and over the extensor surface of the large joints.

The important surgical complications of cirrhosis are the development of portal hypertension and hepatoma. The only effective definitive treatment of cirrhosis is liver transplantation.

Portal hypertension

Portal hypertension signifies an elevated portal pressure (>15 mmHg). It results either from inflow or outflow obstruction to the portal blood flow (Table 13.24). Rarely, portal hypertension is caused by increased blood flow into the portal venous system due to an arteriovenous fistula between the portal vein and the hepatic artery.

Irrespective of aetiology, obstruction to portal venous flow leads to congestion, opening up of collateral venous pathways and splenomegaly. The enlarged spleen traps the circulating platelets, leading to thrombocytopenia of increasing severity. Collateral veins form around the falciform and round ligaments, leading to an enlarged periumbilical leash of veins (*caput medusae*). However, the most important collateral pathway is the communication between the tributaries of the left gastric vein and the azygos vein in the lower oesophagus. These enlarge to form dilated veins (varices) in the submucosal plane and around the oesophagus. These oesophageal varices (Fig. 13.55) may burst at any time, leading to severe life-threatening variceal haemorrhage. The situation is further aggravated by three factors:

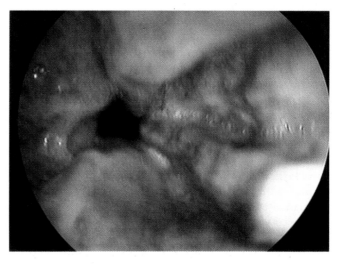

Figure 13.55 Oesophageal varices (endoscopic view).

1 Impaired clotting and thrombocytopenia often associated with chronic liver disease.

2 Defective hepatocyte function which deteriorates further because of hypovolaemia secondary to haemorrhage.

3 The blood in the gastrointestinal tract is broken down by bacteria with the formation of large amounts of ammonia which is absorbed and contributes to the development of encephalopathy, an almost invariable finding in these patients.

Management of bleeding varices

The management of patients with bleeding varices includes:
- immediate resuscitative measures to restore the blood volume;
- assessment of the liver and clotting function;
- methods to arrest the bleeding; and
- measures to prevent the development of encephalopathy.

Some agents, such as terlipressin (Glypressin) and somatostatin, administered by intravenous infusion, can arrest the bleeding by lowering the portal venous pressure. More usually, however, severe variceal bleeding requires more active intervention by sclerotherapy and balloon tamponade. Sclerotherapy is performed during flexible endoscopy and is very effective in controlling variceal bleeding. If not, or should the haemorrhage recur, balloon tamponade using a trilumen tube (Fig. 13.56) is used. This invariably stops the bleeding but the tamponade cannot be continued much beyond 12 h because of the risk of pressure necrosis and oesophageal perforation. If bleeding recurs on deflation of the tamponade, emergency surgical intervention is needed. This consists of oesophageal transection using the EEA stapler gun (Fig. 13.57).

Nowadays, portosystemic shunts are only performed electively and in patients with good liver function. Shunting effectively reduces portal hypertension by allowing the portal blood to drain directly into the systemic circulation but, because the detoxification process of the liver is bypassed, encephalopathy often occurs. Usually a selective shunt is carried out. In contrast to total shunts such as portocaval anastomosis, selective shunts do not take away all the portal blood flow from the liver and, for this reason, are followed by a reduced incidence of chronic encephalopathy. More recently, a radiological technique of intrahepatic shunting has been developed. This is achieved by passing a metallic stent via the internal jugular vein through the vena cava into a hepatic vein and, having developed a track through the substance of the liver between a hepatic vein branch and a portal vein branch, the stent is deployed to keep the track open, thus creating an intrahepatic shunt. This technique is called transjugu-

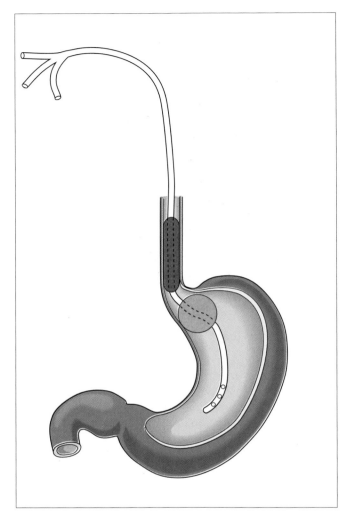

Figure 13.56 Balloon tamponade of the oesophagus by a trilumen tube (Sengstaken or Blakemore or Minnesota). From Ellis H. and Calne R. *Lecture Notes on General Surgery*, 8th edn Oxford: Blackwell Scientific Publications, 1993.

lar intrahepatic portosystemic shunt, or TIPS for short (Fig. 13.58).

The measures used to minimize or prevent the development of hepatic encephalopathy in patients with bleeding varices are the administration of oral lactulose or neomycin (not both) to reduce ammonia formation and absorption, and daily magnesium sulphate enemas to empty the colon of blood.

Hepatic tumours

- *Benign hepatic tumours* are rare and include *adenomas* and *focal nodular hyperplasia*, which may be induced by oestrogen therapy, including the contraceptive pill. With-

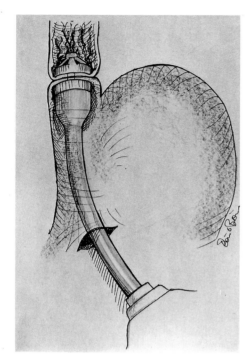

Figure 13.57 Diagrammatic representation of oesophageal transection for oesophageal varices using the EEA stapling gun.

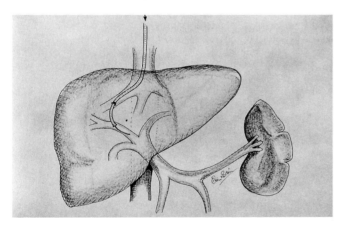

Figure 13.58 Trans jugular intrahepatic portosystemic shunt (TIPS). A metallic stent is placed percutaneously via the internal jugular vein to establish a communication between a portal vein and a hepatic vein tributary in the substance of the liver.

drawal of oestrogen may be followed by regression. *Haemangiomas* can also occur in the liver and usually do not require any active treatment. Benign tumours are commonly discovered accidentally during the course of investigation for some other complaint but they may give rise to pain and hepatic adenomas may rupture spontaneously,

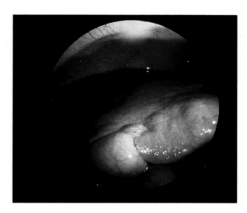

Figure 13.59 Laparoscopic view of secondary deposits in the liver.

especially during pregnancy, and present with massive intraperitoneal bleeding.

• *Secondary tumours*: The most common tumours encountered in the liver are secondary deposits from primary tumours of the breast, lung, stomach, colon, pancreas and prostate (Fig. 13.59). Virtually any tumour can metastasize to the liver. Hepatic deposits when extensive lead to progressive jaundice and are invariably fatal, although the survival varies considerably from a few weeks to several months. Most are untreatable but when involvement is minimal, treatment with local excision, chemotherapy (systemic or regional through the hepatic artery) or embolization may result in worthwhile palliation and increased survival.

• *Primary liver cell carcinoma (hepatoma)* (Fig. 13.60) may arise from normal liver or on a background of cirrhosis (cirrhomimetic). The most important aetiological factor is hepatitis B virus infection which results in integration of the viral genome into the host DNA. The clinical features include dragging pain, usually in the right hypochondrium or lower chest, anorexia and vomiting, fever and a palpable liver. The α-fetoprotein is usually elevated and the liver function tests are abnormal. Primary hepatomas may rupture, causing massive haemoperitoneum. Unless diagnosed early and treated by the appropriate hepatic resection, the prognosis is poor. One particular type of well-differentiated primary hepatoma arising in a normal liver (fibrolamellar carcinoma) occurs in young adults of both sexes and carries a better prognosis. This type is nowadays treated by hepatic transplantation.

Subphrenic and hepatic abscesses

In western countries hepatic intraparenchymal abscesses are rare, whereas perihepatic subdiaphragmatic abscesses

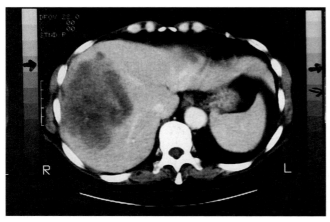

(a)

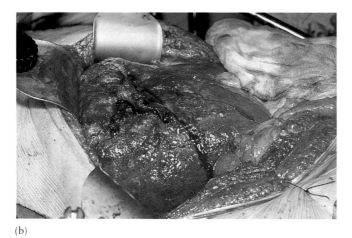

(b)

Figure 13.60 (a) Computed tomographic and (b) operative views of a primary liver cell carcinoma.

are relatively common. There are two main types of hepatic abscess: pyogenic and amoebic.

• The *pyogenic* type is most commonly the result of septic cholangitis and is often multiple, the infection being caused by a mixture of Gram-negative aerobic and anaerobic bacteria.

• *Amoebic* abscess is secondary to intestinal amoebiasis caused by *Entamoeba histolytica*. It may form a huge cavity with liquefaction necrosis of the liver parenchyma. The fluid content is described as resembling chocolate-coloured anchovy sauce. Both types of abscess are more frequent in the right lobe.

The clinical features of hepatic abscess include toxicity with high intermittent fever, sweating, anorexia, nausea and vomiting, jaundice and pain. The pain is aggravated by movement and coughing. On examination, a tender hepatomegaly is found. In addition, there is an associated leukocytosis and an anaemia. An amoebic liver abscess may rupture through the diaphragm into the bronchial tree with expectoration of large amounts of 'anchovy-sauce' pus.

Perihepatic subdiaphragmatic abscesses may occur in any of the six recognized subdiaphragmatic spaces. They are secondary to peritonitis (residual infection) from any cause or abdominal operations on the gastrointestinal and biliary tract (contamination or leakage of gut biliary contents) and may also follow splenectomy (infected haematoma). Clinically, they may manifest soon after surgery or treatment of peritonitis during the same hospital admission or present subsequent to discharge from hospital. The clinical features include toxicity with intermittent fever, failure of progress, asthenia, lethargy and, at times, episodes of rigors due to bacteraemia. Breathlessness may be present and is due to splinting of the diaphragm on the affected side and to the frequent presence of a sympathetic ipsilateral pleural effusion. The diagnosis is established by screening for diaphragmatic movement by fluoroscopy or ultrasound, and documentation of the fluid collection by ultrasound or CT scan of the upper abdomen. Many of these abscesses can now be treated by percutaneous drainage or aspiration under CT or ultrasound control together with systemic antibiotics. Open surgical drainage is reserved for multiloculated abscesses with large amounts of thick pus containing slough.

Hepatic cysts

Hepatic cysts are of various types. The commonest is the *simple solitary cyst* which forms a well-encapsulated surface lesion containing serous fluid without any communication with the biliary tract. These lesions are usually asymptomatic and generally discovered accidentally during investigation by ultrasound. Unless large or secondarily infected, they require no treatment. Gross cystic replacement of the hepatic parenchyma with similar cysts occurs in patients with *polycystic disease* of the liver and kidneys. Multiple intrahepatic bile duct cysts are a feature of a congenital disease of the biliary tract, which is accompanied by hepatic fibrosis (*Caroli's disease*). The clinical picture of this rare condition is dominated by recurrent attacks of cholangitis. Finally, *hydatid cysts* due to infestation by *Echinococcus granulosus* or *E. multilocularis* are common worldwide. Humans are the secondary host for these parasites and acquire the condition from dogs which carry the adult worm. The pathogenic potential of hydatid cyst is high. They may become secondarily infected or rupture into the biliary tract or intraperitoneally. Treatment of hydatid cysts of the liver includes specific medical therapy with mebendazole or albendazole together with surgical excision.

Hepatic failure

The liver is the largest organ in the body. In addition to its key role in carbohydrate, steroid and fat metabolism, it is essential for synthesis of various proteins, including blood-clotting factors and for the detoxification of both endogenous metabolites and ingested or parenterally administered substances and drugs. The Kupffer cells form an integral part of the reticuloendothelial system which mops up any particulate matter and bacteria, thereby providing an important defence mechanism against infection. Failure of this organ is therefore accompanied by profound changes: synthetic failure (proteins), gross metabolic derangement, severe bleeding tendency, accumulation of toxic metabolites and false neurotransmitters which impair the level of consciousness, diminished resistance to bacterial invasion and water and salt retention.

Hepatic failure and hepatic encephalopathy are often used synonymously. Strictly speaking, encephalopathy refers to the neuropsychiatric syndrome characterized by mental impairment, neurological signs (apraxia, hyperactive stretch reflexes) and diminished level of consciousness from mild confusion to stupor and deep coma. The encephalopathy is more severe and less frequently recoverable in acute fulminant liver failure than in chronic liver disease.

Acute liver failure

Acute fulminant liver failure is defined as severe encephalopathy occurring within 6–8 weeks of the onset of the illness. Essentially, this consists of acute massive hepatocellular damage in a previously normal liver caused by poisoning such as paracetamol, viral infections (A, B, C), halothane anaesthesia and mushroom poisoning (*Amanita phalloides*). The disease carries a high mortality. Biochemical evidence of massive liver cell necrosis in these patients includes marked elevations of the transaminases and deepening jaundice. The coma is accompanied by gross cerebral oedema with raised intracranial pressure. There is multisystem involvement with clotting failure, renal impairment, fall in the peripheral resistance, pulmonary insufficiency and an increased susceptibility to serious infections.

Treatment

The treatment of fulminant liver failure is supportive and carried out within the setting of an intensive care unit. The useful therapeutic measures include ventilatory support, haemofiltration, extraction of poisons, reduction of cerebral oedema by 20% mannitol infused intravenously, antibiotics for established infections, etc. Increasingly, liver transplantation is being used to treat these patients.

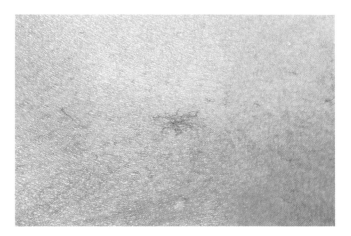

Figure 13.61 Spider naevi in a patient with alcoholic cirrhosis.

Chronic liver failure

This arises on a background of chronic liver disease (cirrhosis) which may be caused by alcohol or other hepatic disorders such as biliary atresia or hypoplasia (children), chronic hepatitis, primary biliary cirrhosis, sclerosing cholangitis, etc. The patient therefore exhibits the stigmata of chronic liver disease (Table 13.22). The important ones are jaundice, spider naevi, hepatosplenomegaly, ascites and oedema, muscle wasting, bruising, neuropsychiatric manifestations and portal hypertension.

Spider naevi are subcutaneous endarterioles (Fig. 13.61) and therefore, when emptied by compression, fill from the centre outwards (centripetally). They appear in the distribution of the superior vena cava. *Splenomegaly* is accompanied by a thrombocytopenia and the extent of the impairment of the clotting function reflects the severity of the hepatic decompensation. In addition to *reduced clotting factors*, abnormal anticoagulant substances are present and these compound the bleeding tendency. *Water and salt retention* results in ascites (Fig. 13.62) and peripheral oedema. It is in part due to the renin–aldosterone response but other factors are involved: reduced effective extracellular fluid volume because of the sequestrated ascitic fluid (third-space losses), diminished glomerular filtration rate and reduced sensitivity to the atrial natriuretic peptide. Water and salt retention is often accompanied by *hypokalaemia* and *alkalosis*. *Muscle wasting* is an important feature of chronic liver disease and is often overlooked by clinicians. The serum *albumin*, is *reduced* and the level reflects the severity of the disease. Unless there is ongoing piecemeal necrosis, the transaminases are not grossly elevated. In alcoholic patients the gammaglutamyl transpeptidase is elevated.

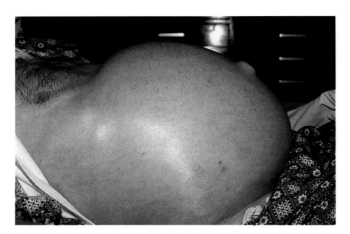

Figure 13.62 Gross ascites and muscle wasting in chronic liver disease.

In addition to these changes, encephalopathy may develop with progression of the disease: behavioural changes, mental impairment, inability to concentrate and sleepiness are particularly common. Coma may occur spontaneously or be induced by drugs. It may complicate an episode of gastrointestinal variceal bleeding or portosystemic shunting. The encephalopathy of chronic liver disease is often recoverable with treatment. Progression to terminal liver failure is evidenced by renal decompensation (hepatorenal syndrome), foetor hepaticus, coma and flapping tremor of the hands when these are dorsiflexed.

Treatment

Chronic liver disease is managed medically in the first instance and this is aimed at halting the progress of the disease. Abstinence from alcohol is essential in patients with alcoholic cirrhosis. Dietary measures include salt restriction, control of dietary protein intake and the administration of fat-soluble vitamin supplements. The protein intake is adjusted to the level which the patient can tolerate without causing encephalopathy. Itching when present is controlled by oral cholestyramine. The ascites and oedema are treated with salt restriction, antialdosterone drugs (spironolactone) and loop diuretics. Tapping and drainage of ascites (paracentesis), although practised are inadvisable as this may precipitate encephalopathy and introduce infection into the peritoneal cavity. If ascites becomes unresponsive to medical measures, surgical treatment with peritoneovenous shunting often provides symptomatic relief. The management of encephalopathy associated with bleeding varices has been outlined. En-

cephalopathy itself is treated by the correction of hypokalaemic alkalosis, magnesium sulphate enemas to empty the colon of blood and nitrogenous residues and oral lactulose or neomycin.

The only definitive treatment in patients with chronic hepatic failure is liver transplantation. Nowadays this is performed before the patient has reached the end-stage of the disease, provided the criteria for acceptance to a transplant programme are present in the individual patient.

The biliary tract

The intrahepatic biliary tree drains through the right and left hepatic duct which join just outside the liver in the porta hepatis to form the common hepatic duct. This receives the cystic duct draining the gallbladder and, as the common bile duct, runs down the hepatoduodenal ligament before traversing the head of the pancreas to terminate in the duodenal papilla situated on the medial wall of the second part of the duodenum. The important common disorders of the biliary tract are gallstone disease and tumours (cholangiocarcinoma). Other conditions such as parasitic infestations are rare in western countries.

Jaundice

One of the most common presentations of hepatic and biliary disease is jaundice. The term is derived from the French word *jeune*, meaning yellow. This pigmentation is due to accumulation of bilirubin in the blood and tissues. Thus, jaundice signifies hyperbilirubinaemia. The elevated bilirubin has to exceed 35–40 µmol/l before the yellowish pigmentation (icterus) can be recognized clinically. Thus overt clinical jaundice detected in the sclera, conjunctivae, skin, etc. is always significant. The causes of jaundice are outlined in Table 13.25.

Table 13.25 Clinical classification of jaundice.

Type	Mechanism
Haemolytic/congenital hyperbilirubinaemias	Excess production of bilirubin
	Defective bilirubin uptake or secretion by hepatocyte
Hepatocellular	Defective secretion of conjugated bilirubin into the bile canaliculi
Cholestatic/obstructive (intra- or extrahepatic)	Impairment of bile flow subsequent to secretion of conjugated bilirubin by hepatocyte

Bilirubin metabolism

This classification is based on the normal metabolism of bilirubin and an awareness of this process is essential to the proper understanding of the pathophysiology and management of jaundiced patients. Bilirubin is produced in the reticuloendothelial system from the enzymic breakdown of haem, which is derived from the effete red blood corpuscles. This unconjugated bilirubin is water-insoluble and is therefore carried in the plasma attached to albumin. On reaching the liver, the bilirubin moiety is taken up by the hepatocytes where it is conjugated by a specific enzyme (glucuronyl transferase) to the water-soluble bilirubin glucuronide (conjugated bilirubin) and then excreted into the bile canaliculi and thence to the biliary tract and duodenum. In the intestine, the conjugated bilirubin is degraded by bacteria to derivatives collectively known as urobilinogen. Some urobilinogen is reabsorbed into the portal circulation and re-excreted in the bile. A small amount of the reabsorbed urobilinogen escapes into the systemic circulation and is excreted in the urine. Most urobilinogen is excreted in the faeces as stercobilin, which is the pigment that stains the faeces the normal brownish colour (Fig. 13.63).

Bilirubin abnormalities in jaundice (Table 13.26)

Haemolytic jaundice

In haemolytic jaundice excess production of unconjugated bilirubin is such as to exhaust the ability of the liver to conjugate this extra load; the faeces are normal in colour and the urine does not contain bilirubin as the unconjugated bilirubin–albumin complex is not filtered through the glomeruli. However, excess urobilinogen is formed by the intestinal bacteria and this appears as excess urobilinogen in the urine.

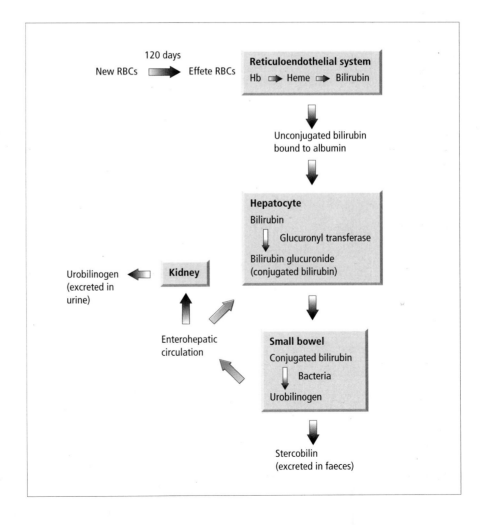

Figure 13.63 Bilirubin metabolism.

Hepatocellular jaundice

In hepatocellular jaundice the hepatocyte is injured and the picture changes as the disease progresses. Initially the reabsorbed urobilinogen cannot be re-excreted by the damaged hepatocytes and is therefore excreted in the urine. So in the initial stages urobilinogen levels rise in the urine. As the disease progresses swelling and oedema cause intrahepatic cholestasis and the serum conjugated bilirubin levels rise and bilirubin appears in the urine. As little bile is now getting into the intestine the production of urobilinogen falls and urobilinogen disappears from the urine.

Obstructive jaundice

Any lesion, disease process or drug which blocks the release of conjugated bilirubin from the hepatocyte or stops its delivery into the duodenum results in cholestatic (obstructive jaundice) with the accumulation of excess conjugated bilirubin and an elevation of the alkaline phosphatase activity. This type of jaundice is therefore accompanied by pale stools and the presence of dark frothy urine containing bilirubin as the conjugated bilirubin which accumulates in excess is water-soluble. Because no bile is reaching the intestine, bile salts are not available for the emulsification and absorption of fat. The important consequence of this is malabsorption of vitamin K which occurs in all patients with cholestatic jaundice and leads to defective synthesis of all the vitamin K-dependent clotting factors by the liver with prolongation of the prothrombin time. The absence of bilirubin in the intestine results in the lack of production of stercobilin by the colonic bacteria and, therefore, the stools are pale and frothy (unpigmented and high in fat).

Investigation of the jaundiced patient

The investigation of a patient with jaundice follows a set pattern which is outlined in Table 13.27. If this is fol-

Table 13.26 The changes in bilirubin metabolism in different types of jaundice.

| Type of jaundice | Serum bilirubin | | Urinary | |
	Unconjugated	Conjugated	Bilirubin	Urobilinogen
Haemolytic	Elevated	Normal	Absent	Elevated
Hepatocellular				
Early	Normal	Normal	Absent	Elevated
Late	Normal or elevated	Elevated	Present	Absent
Obstructive	Normal	Elevated	Present	Absent

Table 13.27 Investigations of jaundiced patients.

History and physical examination
Contacts, drugs, transfusion, alcohol, travel
Pale stools, dark urine (cholestasis)
Bilirubin present in urine (cholestasis)
Stigma of liver disease (hepatocellular)
Palpable gallbladder (cancer of the head of pancreas)

Screening for viral infections
Hepatitis A, B, C

Biochemical studies
Bilirubin, alkaline phosphatase or gammaglutamyl transpeptidase, transaminases and albumin

Haematological
Evidence of haemolysis (haemolytic jaundice)
Prothrombin time (elevated in cholestatic and hepatocellular jaundice)

Ultrasound (US) examination of the liver
Dilatation of the biliary tree (cholestasis):
    Endoscopic retrograde cholangiopancreatography
    Percutaneous transhepatic cholangiography
Details of hepatic parenchyma
Gallstones (gallbladder and bile ducts)
Pancreatic lesions

Contrast visualization of the biliary tract (indicated in patients with dilatation on US)
Endoscopic retrograde cholangiopancreatography
Percutaneous transhepatic cholangiography

Liver biopsy (indicated in patients without dilatation on US)

lowed, the exact cause is elucidated in every case. Visualization of the biliary tract by special contrast studies is essential in all patients with dilatation of the biliary tract demonstrated by ultrasound (US) examination. Endoscopic retrograde cholangiopancreatography (ERCP) (Fig. 13.64a) is generally preferred to percutaneous transhepatic cholangiography (PTC) (Fig. 13.64b) as it is accompanied by a lower incidence of complications such as bleeding and bile leakage into the peritoneal cavity.

Perioperative management of jaundiced patients undergoing surgery

Patients with obstructive jaundice who require surgery are prone to the development of certain specific complications. The important ones are:
• bleeding due to diminished synthesis of clotting factors;
• infections because of reduced resistance to bacterial invasion;

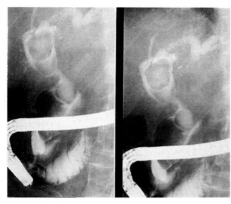

(a)

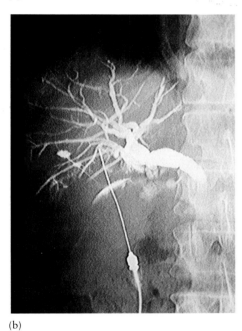

(b)

Figure 13.64 (a) Endoscopic retrograde cholangiopancreatography showing ductal calculi; (b) percutaneous retrograde cholangiography demonstrating a bile duct stricture.

• renal failure which is associated with the presence of endotoxinaemia following absorption of endotoxin from the gut (hepatorenal syndrome).

Thus, specific prophylactic measures are needed when considering surgery in a jaundiced patient. Parenteral vitamin K analogue is administered to correct the elevated prothrombin time before surgery and systemic antibiotic therapy active against Gram-negative aerobic bacteria given with induction. Prophylaxis against renal failure includes adequate hydration with intravenous fluids and the administration of an osmotic or loop diuretic with induc-

tion of anaesthesia. All these patients must have a catheter inserted into the urinary bladder to monitor hourly urine output.

Gallstone disease

Gallstone disease is common worldwide except in Africa. Prevalence rates in western countries vary considerably, from 5 to 38%. Females are twice as commonly affected as males. Gallstones are classified in accordance with their chemical composition:
• predominantly cholesterol;
• predominantly bilirubinate (pigment); or
• predominantly calcium compounds.

In most western countries cholesterol stones form the majority and account for 75% of cases. Pigment stones are relatively more common in Far Eastern countries but they account for 20% of stones in the West. Calcium stones made of calcium carbonate and palmitate are rare (porcelain gallbladder).

Pathogenesis of gallstones

Cholesterol stones

The pathogenesis of cholesterol stones is different from that of the pigment variety. As cholesterol is water-insoluble, in bile it is held in solution by being surrounded by bile salts which are water-soluble. These complexes are known as micelles and their formation, which also requires the presence of phospholipids, is essential for the solubility of cholesterol in bile. If for any reason there is too much cholesterol or too little bile salts or phospholipids, the bile becomes unstable or lithogenic and cholesterol then precipitates out as crystals which grow to form cholesterol gallstones. The pathogenesis of cholesterol gallstones is therefore consequent upon a disordered hepatic steroid metabolism which results in a relative deficiency of bile salts in relation to the amount of cholesterol produced and secreted by the hepatocytes.

Bilirubinate stones

The pathogenesis of bilirubinate pigment stones is less clear. Some are associated with chronic haemolysis and excess production of bilirubin and others are related to infections of the biliary tract by certain bacteria which contain an enzyme, β-glucuronidase. This splits the conjugated bilirubin in the bile when the carboxyl group of the bilirubin moiety combines with calcium to form a precipitate of calcium bilirubinate. These pigment stones contain large amounts of bacteria within their various crevices.

Table 13.28 Risk factors for gallstone disease.

Female sex
Obesity
Old age
Genetic and ethnic factors
Diet: fibre-depleted and high in animal fat
Multiple pregnancies
Drugs: clofibrate, thiazide diuretics, oral contraception
Diabetes mellitus
Ileal disease and resection
Haemolytic states
Cirrhosis
Infections of the biliary tract
Parasitic infestations
Cystic fibrosis

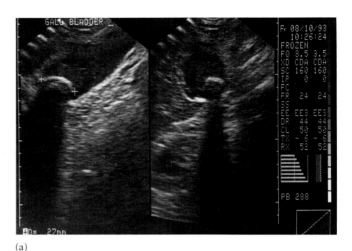

(a)

The risk factors for both types of gallstones are shown in Table 13.28.

Gallstones are best diagnosed by ultrasound examination, which is 90–100% accurate for stones in the gallbladder (Fig. 13.65(a)). Only 15% of gallstones are radiopaque and therefore a plain X-ray of the abdomen misses the vast majority. Other radiological investigations which may be used on occasion are oral cholecystography (Fig. 13.65(b)) and intravenous cholangiography.

Clinical features

Gallstones are two to three times commoner in females than males and their incidence increases with age and obesity. The majority of gallstones are asymptomatic when they are discovered during the course of investigation for some other disorder. Symptomatic gallstone disease may present with chronic symptoms (chronic cholecystitis), with episodes of acute colicky pain (biliary colic) or with complications (acute cholecystitis, jaundice, acute septic cholangitis and acute pancreatitis). Fistula formation between the gallbladder and the duodenum by a large stone which ulcerates through the contiguous organs after they become adherent to each other is rare. The large stone, once it reaches the bowel, may become impacted in the ileum causing intraluminal low small-bowel obstruction (gallstone ileus). The full spectrum of gallstone disease is shown in Table 13.29.

The symptoms of *chronic calculous cholecystitis* are vague and simulate those of other common gastrointestinal conditions such as irritable bowel disease, reflux oesophagitis, colonic cancer and diverticular disease. The pain is situated in the epigastric and right hypochondrial regions and is accompanied by distension, flatulence and intolerance to fatty food. Heartburn is frequently present. It is often difficult for the clinician to be sure whether the patient's

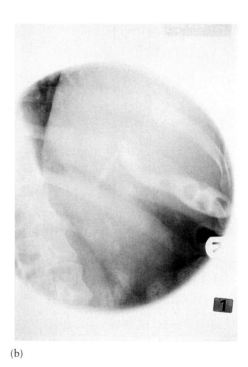

(b)

Figure 13.65 Gallstones may be detected by (a) ultrasonography or (b) oral cholecystography.

symptoms are due to the gallstones or other common gastrointestinal complaints or ischaemic heart disease and certainly these conditions must be excluded before surgical treatment for the gallstones is undertaken.

Acute biliary colic is a severe attack of pain in the right hypochondrium which radiates round the right costal margin to the scapular region (not the shoulder) and may last several hours. The patient rolls about in pain and expe-

Table 13.29 Spectrum of gallstone disease.

Asymptomatic
Chronic cholecystitis
Acute biliary colic
Acute obstructive cholecystitis
Obstructive jaundice
Acute cholangitis
Acute gallstone pancreatitis
Bilioenteric fistula and gallstone ileus

riences sweating, nausea and vomiting. Many attacks of biliary colic seem to occur at night. The attack, which is caused by a stone temporarily blocking the cystic duct or Hartmann's pouch, may subside completely with recurrence weeks or months later, or it may be followed a few days later by the development of jaundice. This is due to migration of the stone into the bile duct with impaction usually at the lower end.

In *acute obstructive cholecystitis*, the stone becomes firmly impacted in the neck of the gallbladder and leads to acute inflammation of the organ. This inflammation is chemical in the first instance but secondary bacterial inflammation ensues in some patients. The gallbladder wall becomes oedematous and thickened and its lumen distended with inflammatory exudate. The rise in the intraluminal pressure caused by the inflammatory exudate eventually lifts the walls of the gallbladder from the impacted stone which then falls into the gallbladder lumen. This effectively results in decompression of the inflamed gallbladder which then drains through the cystic duct with resolution of the inflammation. Although usual, this sequence is not invariable and in some patients the obstruction persists, when the inflammation becomes more severe with the development of gangrenous patches in the gallbladder wall, usually at the fundus. These may perforate and lead to infected biliary peritonitis. Alternatively, the gallbladder becomes a large sac full of pus (*empyema of the gallbladder*). Much less commonly, the obstruction of the neck of the gallbladder by a stone is not followed by inflammation. Instead, the gallbladder becomes grossly distended with mucus secretion from the glands of the gallbladder mucosa. This is known as *mucocele* of the gallbladder and presents with pain and a mobile lump in the right hypochondrium, usually in an elderly female.

The manifestation of acute obstructive cholecystitis includes constant pain in the right hypochondrium which is aggravated by movement and is accompanied by pyrexia and nausea. Jaundice is often present and may be due to oedema of the bile duct or to the presence of ductal stones. On examination, there is tenderness in the right hypochon-drium with a positive Murphy's sign. This consists of midinspiratory apnoea by the patient when the clinician applies gentle pressure on the right hypochondrium and asks the patient to take a deep breath. Patients with an empyema have a tender mass in the right hypochondrium. They are usually ill elderly patients. A plain erect X-ray of the abdomen is performed to exclude a perforated ulcer. A leukocytosis is invariably present but the serum amylase is not elevated or marginally so.

The most serious presentation of gallstone disease is *acute septic cholangitis* which consists of a bacterial infection of the biliary tract in association with ductal calculi. The patient is toxic and has a *high fever* with *rigors* and obvious *jaundice* (Charcot's triad). The rigors are the result of bacteraemia which is invariable in these patients and is most commonly due to Gram-negative aerobic bacteria such as *Escherichia coli*.

Treatment of gallstone disease

Asymptomatic gallstones do not require any treatment. Elective cholecystectomy is needed for patients with proven chronic cholecystitis and especially those with episodes of biliary colic. Nowadays the operation is performed laparoscopically, which is preferable to the open operation as it is attended by a short hospital stay and rapid recovery within 10 days of the operation (Fig. 13.66). During the operation, an operative cholangiogram is performed to exclude common duct stones. If present, these are removed either by the laparoscopic or open surgical approach. Patients with empyema are best managed with insertion of a percutaneous tube into the gallbladder under ultrasound guidance (percutaneous cholecystostomy). This rapidly results in improvement of the patient's condition. If considered fit, these patients will have an elective cholecystectomy. Patients with biliary peritonitis require emergency laparotomy.

In addition to antibiotics and intravenous fluid therapy, patients with acute septic cholangitis are treated as a matter of urgency with endoscopic sphincterotomy and extraction of the ductal calculi. Unless frail and elderly, these patients also require an interval cholecystectomy.

Acalculous gallbladder disease

This term covers a group of benign pathological conditions of the gallbladder not associated with gallstones. They include cholesterolosis (strawberry gallbladder) and adeno-myomatosis of the gallbladder (cholecystitis glandularis proliferans) which may cause chronic ill-defined abdominal pain. Much more important is acute acalculous cholecyst-itis which may develop in seriously ill patients usually

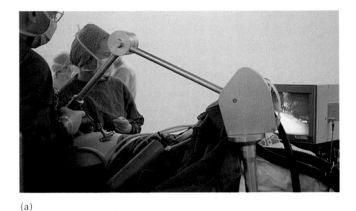

(a)

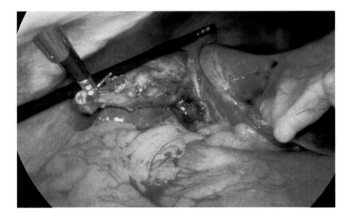

(b)

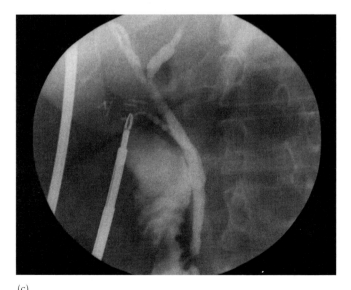

(c)

Figure 13.66 (a) Videolaparoscopic set-up; (b) Laparoscopic cholecystectomy and (c) peroperative cholangiogram.

requiring intensive care, mechanical ventilation, prolonged opiate analgesia and parenteral nutrition, e.g. severe burns, multiple trauma, sepsis, etc. The exact pathogenesis of the acute inflammation of the gallbladder is not known but the condition seems to originate on a background of stasis in the organ. It causes acute abdominal pain and tenderness and is treated by emergency cholecystectomy.

Tumours of the biliary tract

Tumours of the biliary tract are nearly always malignant and affect the gallbladder and the biliary tree.

Carcinoma of the gallbladder

Carcinoma of the gallbladder is a disease of the elderly and is associated with long-standing gallstones. The tumour is either an adenocarcinoma or a squamous cell carcinoma, the latter developing from metaplastic squamous epithelium consequent on chronic irritation by long-standing gallstones. Carcinoma of the gallbladder most commonly presents as acute cholecystitis, when it is usually advanced and incurable. Some gallbladder cancers are only discovered during routine pathological examination of the specimen following cholecystectomy of gallstones.

Cholangiocarcinoma

Tumours of the bile ducts are called cholangiocarcinomas; most commonly they form stenosing infiltrative lesions. The age range at presentation is wide, varying from 30 to 80 years, although they are more frequent in the elderly. They are known risk factors which include ulcerative colitis, sclerosing cholangitis, cystic disease of the biliary tract, parasitic infestations and chronic typhoid carriers. The tumours may arise from the intrahepatic bile ducts, when they are often multifocal, or from the large extrahepatic bile ducts: at the junction of the right and left hepatic ducts (hilar tumours of Klatskin), at the junction of the cystic duct with the common bile duct or from the ampulla. These last are classified with the periampullary tumours of the pancreas.

With the exception of the periampullary tumours, the vast majority of cholangiocarcinomas present at an advanced incurable stage with progressive painless jaundice, hepatomegaly and weight loss. Treatment is therefore usually palliative, either by insertion of a transhepatic stent (endoprosthesis), through the malignant stricture from above or via an endoscope from below. Alternatively a surgical bypass is performed. Following palliation of jaundice by these measures, radiotherapy can impart some benefit. Early lesions are treated by resection which often includes removal of one or other lobes of the liver

Gallstone disease at a glance

DEFINITION

Gallstones are round, oval or faceted concretions found in the biliary tract. They contain, singly or in combination, cholesterol, calcium carbonate or calcium bilirubinate

EPIDEMIOLOGY

M/F–1 : 2 Age 40s onwards. High incidence of mixed stones in western world. Pigment stones commoner in the East

PATHOGENESIS

- Cholesterol stones: imbalance in bile between cholesterol, bile salts and phospholipids producing lithogenic bile
- Bilirubinate stones: chronic haemolysis, infection with β-glucuronidase-producing bacteria

PATHOLOGY

- Gallstones passing through the biliary system may cause biliary colic or pancreatitis
- Stone obstruction at the gallbladder neck with superimposed infection leads to cholecystitis
- Obstruction of the CBD with superimposed infection leads to septic cholangitis
- Migration of a large stone into the gut may cause intestinal obstruction (gallstone ileus)

CLINICAL FEATURES

- May be asymptomatic
- Biliary colic: severe colicky upper abdominal pain radiating around the right costal margin ± vomiting

- Chronic cholecystitis: vague right upper abdominal pain, distension, flatulence, fatty food intolerance
- Acute obstructive cholecystitis: constant right hypochondrial pain, pyrexia, nausea ± jaundice. Tender in RUQ with positive Murphy's sign. Leukocytosis. Unresolved, may lead to an empyema of the gallbladder
- Cholangitis: high fever, rigors, jaundice (Charcot's triad)

INVESTIGATIONS

- 90% of gallstones will be detected on ultrasound examination
- Rarely are other investigations such as oral cholecystography, intravenous cholangiography or HIDA scanning required
- Plain X-ray of the abdomen shows only 10% gallstones
- FBC, U&E, LFTs

MANAGEMENT

Asymptomatic	No treatment required unless diabetic
Biliary colic	Elective cholecystectomy, now usually performed laparoscopically
Chronic cholecystitis	
Acute cholecystitis	Intravenous fluids, antibiotics, cholecystectomy
Empyema	Percutaneous drainage of the gallbladder and interval cholecystectomy usually at same hospital admission
Septic cholangitis	IV fluids, antibiotics, ductal drainage (now usually by ERCP, sphincterotomy and extraction of stones)

COMPLICATIONS OF CHOLECYSTECTOMY

- Leakage of bile from cystic duct or gallbladder bed
- Jaundice due to retained ductal stones or injury to the bile duct. Retained stones can be treated by ERCP or if a T-tube is in place by extraction with a Dormia basket down the T-tube track (Burhenne manoeuvre)

RUQ, right upper quadrant; HIDA, Technetium-labelled immunodiacetic acid compound; LFT, liver function test.

---

because of the extension of the tumour into the hepatic parenchyma.

Benign stricture of the biliary tract

Benign strictures of the biliary tract are the result of *bile duct injuries* usually sustained during cholecystectomy. The stricture gives rise to obstructive jaundice with recurrent attacks of cholangitis and, unless treated, will lead to the development of secondary biliary cirrhosis and portal hypertension. Treatment is surgical and involves anastomosis of the common hepatic duct to a loop of jejunum proximal to the stricture.

Sclerosing cholangitis is an obscure, possibly autoimmune, condition which is characterized by progressive fibrous obliteration of the entire biliary tract. It causes obstructive jaundice, pain in the right hypochondrium and

episodes of cholangitis. At least half the patients have long-standing ulcerative colitis. It often progresses to cirrhosis and may lead to the development of multifocal intrahepatic cholangiocarcinoma. There is no effective medical treatment and, when advanced, sclerosing cholangitis is treated by liver transplantation.

The pancreas

The important surgical disorders of the pancreas are acute and chronic pancreatitis and pancreatic tumours.

Acute pancreatitis

Pancreatitis is defined as an inflammatory condition of the

exocrine pancreas that results from injury to acinar cells. Acute inflammation of the pancreas is a common emergency. The vast majority of cases are mild to moderate with full recovery and a low mortality. However, some 15–20% of patients develop a severe necrotizing disease which is a serious illness carrying a mortality of 30–50%. The important aetiological factors are gallstones and alcoholism, which together account for over 95% of cases (Table 13.30).

Gallstone-associated acute pancreatitis is caused by the migration of small ductal calculi through the ampulla of Vater. The exact mechanism of alcoholic-induced acute pancreatitis is not known.

Clinical features

Mild to moderate pancreatitis

The pancreatic inflammation varies from oedema to actual inflammation without necrosis. The patient complains of upper abdominal pain which is constant and severe. In addition there is nausea and vomiting and a pyrexia with tachycardia. The physical signs include upper abdominal tenderness and diminished or absent bowel sounds. Jaundice may be present. Systemic signs (respiratory difficulty and hypotension) are absent. The serum amylase is elevated above 1000 IU and the plain X-ray of the abdomen may show a sentinel loop of dilated upper jejunum but there is no free gas under the diaphragm.

Severe necrotizing pancreatitis

The pancreas undergoes varying degrees of necrosis and this extends to the peripancreatic fat. The patient complains of severe abdominal pain and is collapsed with a low blood pressure and low urine output. Evidence of respiratory impairment is often present. The abdomen is silent and is usually distended from paralytic ileus. In some patients yellowish-brown staining of the flanks develops during the second to third day of the illness. This is due to tracking of the blood-stained peritoneal exudate through the lumber triangle (Grey Turner sign; see Fig. 13.41).

Management of acute pancreatitis

Following confirmation of the diagnosis, an intravenous line is set up and analgesia is commenced. The severity of the disease is then assessed using clinical criteria and laboratory parameters (Table 13.31). Age over 55 years used to be considered one of the bad prognostic variables, but this is not reliable enough in the assessment of disease severity. Patients with mild to moderate disease are simply monitored for progress clinically and by pulse, blood pressure and temperature charts. There is no evidence that nasogastric tube or antibiotics impart any benefit to these patients. The aetiology of the pancreatitis is established from the history and by an abdominal ultrasound for the detection of gallstones. Cholecystectomy (laparoscopic or open) is performed either during the same hospital admission or as an interval procedure in patients with gallstone-associated disease, as otherwise these patients will experience further attacks.

Patients with severe pancreatitis require resuscitation with intravenous colloids and blood, nasogastric suction for the ileus, oxygen therapy if they are hypoxic and mechanical ventilation if they develop adult respiratory distress syndrome. These patients are best treated in the intensive

Table 13.30 Aetiology of acute pancreatitis.

Duct obstruction
Gallstone migration
Tumours
Cystic fibrosis
Pancreas divisum
Acinar cell injury
Alcohol
Viruses, e.g. mumps
Drugs, e.g. thiazide diuretics
Trauma
Hypercalcaemia (hyperparathyroidism)
Hyperlipidaemia
Hereditary

Table 13.31 Grading of severity of acute pancreatitis.

*Clinical**
Hypotension
Respiratory difficulties
Laboratory†
WBC $> 16 \times 10^9/l$
$PaO_2 < 7.98$ kPa (60 mmHg)
Blood glucose > 11.2 mmol/l
Serum LDH > 350 IU/l
SGOT > 250 IU/l
PCV fall $> 10\%$
Blood urea > 1.8 mmol/l
Serum calcium < 2.0 mmol/l

*Always indicates severe disease.
†Severe disease is present if three or more of these parameters are present.
WBC, White blood cells; LDH, lactate dehydrogenase; SGOT, serum glutamic oxaloacetic transaminase; PCV, packed cell volume.

care unit because they are unstable and require constant monitoring of cardiovascular, respiratory and renal parameters. A contrast-enhanced CT scan is performed to determine the state of the pancreas and, in particular, if the extent of pancreatic necrosis is substantial, a laparotomy is needed to remove the pancreatic slough and drain the pancreatic bed. Often this is followed by irrigation of the region with crystalloid solutions through the drains during the first 3–5 days after surgery. Nutrition of patients with severe necrotizing pancreatitis is maintained by the parenteral route. Patients who have associated gallstone disease will require cholecystectomy but this is performed several weeks later after full recovery from the acute illness.

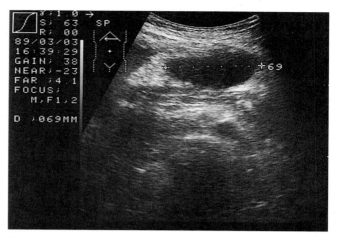

(b)

Table 13.32 Complications of acute pancreatitis.

Pseudocyst formation (moderate disease)
Pancreatic abscess (severe disease)
Intra-abdominal sepsis (severe disease)
Necrosis of the transverse colon (severe disease)
ARDS (severe disease)
Renal failure (severe disease)
Pancreatic haemorrhage (severe disease)

ARDS, Adult respiratory distress syndrome.

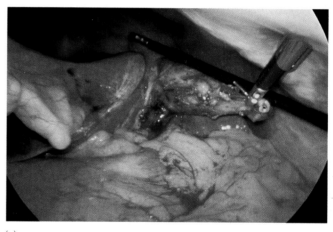

(c)

Figure 13.67 Pancreatic pseudocyst. (a) Clinical photograph; (b) ultrasound scan; (c) operative photograph.

Complications of acute pancreatitis

These are outlined in Table 13.32.

Pseudocyst formation may complicate mild to moderate disease (Fig. 13.67). All the other complications are encountered in patients suffering from severe necrotizing pancreatitis. A pseudocyst is essentially a closed collection of fluid in the lesser sac behind the pancreas. It usually presents with abdominal swelling and gastric compression several months later. It is treated either by percutaneous external drainage or by surgical internal drainage of the cyst into the back wall of the stomach (cystogastrostomy). All the other complications are serious and contribute to the high mortality of severe necrotizing acute pancreatitis.

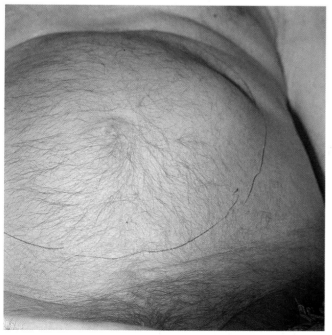

(a)

Chronic pancreatitis

This disorder is on the increase and in western countries is caused by chronic alcohol abuse. The alcoholism induces repeated attacks of relapsing acute pancreatitis, leading to the chronic disease when gradual fibrous replacement of the pancreatic parenchyma and pancreatic calcification occurs. The process leads to exocrine insufficiency with maldigestion of food, especially fat (steatorrhoea) and eventually of the endocrine component with the development of diabetes mellitus. The pancreatic duct is usually narrowed and strictured in several places but may become dilated and sacculated, although this is less common in alcohol-induced pancreatic disease as opposed to the malnutrition-induced chronic pancreatitis encountered in underprivileged countries.

The most important clinical feature of chronic pancreatitis is chronic intractable pain which radiates to the back and which requires large doses of opiate analgesia for its relief. Other surgical complications include obstructive jaundice and duodenal stenosis, both caused by fibrosis in the head of the pancreas. The peripancreatic fibrosis may lead to occlusion of the splenic vein behind the pancreas causing splenomegaly and the development of gastric varices in the distribution of the short gastric vessels (left-sided or sectorial portal hypertension). These may rupture when presentation is with massive upper gastrointestinal haemorrhage. Treatment is by splenectomy.

The only effective treatment is surgical. Resection of the pancreas is most often needed for chronic pain in patients with strictured pancreatic duct. A side-to-side anastomosis between the pancreatic duct and a loop of jejunum is performed in patients with a pancreatic duct which is dilated behind a proximal structure (pancreaticojejunostomy).

Pancreatitis at a glance

DEFINITION

Pancreatitis is an inflammatory condition of the exocrine pancreas that results from injury to the acinar cells. It may be acute or chronic

AETIOLOGY

Gallstones and alcohol abuse account for 95% of cases of acute pancreatitis

PATHOLOGY

- Acinar cell injury allows pancreatic digestive enzymes to be released into the blood stream and peritoneal cavity. The severity of injury varies from mild oedema to a severe haemorrhagic inflammation and necrosis
- An accumulation of pancreatic fluid in the lesser sac is a pseudocyst, i.e. does not have an epithelial lining
- Recurrent episodes of acute inflammation lead to progressive destruction of acinar cells with healing by fibrosis (chronic pancreatitis)

CLINICAL FEATURES

- Mild/moderate pancreatitis: constant upper abdominal pain radiating to back, nausea, vomiting, pyrexia, tachycardia $\pm$ jaundice
- Severe/necrotizing pancreatitis: severe upper abdominal pain, signs of hypovolaemic shock, respiratory and renal impairment, silent abdomen, Grey Turner and Cullen's signs

MANAGEMENT

- Confirm diagnosis: serum amylase >1000 IU

- Assess disease severity (Imrie/Ranson criteria)
(a) Hypotension	(g) Serum LDH >350 IU/l
(b) Age >55	(h) SGOT >250 IU/l
(c) Respiratory difficulty	(i) PCV fall >10%
(d) WBC >16 000/mm³	(j) Blood urea >1.8 mmol/l
(e) PaO_2 <7.98 kPa	(k) Serum calcium <2.0 mmol/l
(f) Blood glucose >11.2 mmol/l	
- Mild/moderate disease: IV fluids, analgesia, monitor progress with pulse, BP, temperature. No need for NG tube or antibiotics. Establish the cause: gallstones, Rx by cholecystectomy; alcohol, Rx by avoiding further exposure
- Severe pancreatitis: full resuscitation in ICU with invasive monitoring. Patient may need laparotomy for debridement of necrotic pancreas

COMPLICATIONS OF ACUTE PANCREATITIS

- Pseudocyst formation: may need to be drained internally or externally
- Pancreatic abscess: usually necrotic pancreas present
- Intra-abdominal sepsis
- Necrosis of the transverse colon
- Respiratory (ARDS) or renal (ATN) failure
- Pancreatic haemorrhage
- Chronic pancreatitis

CHRONIC PANCREATITIS

- Usually caused by chronic alcohol abuse
- Presents with intractable abdominal pain and evidence of exocrine pancreatic failure (steatorrhoea) and eventually diabetes as well
- Medical Rx is with analgesia and exocrine pancreatic enzyme replacement. Surgical Rx is by drainage of dilated pancreatic ducts or excision of the pancreas in some cases

WBC, White blood cells; LDH, lactate dehydrogenase; Rx, treatment; SGOT, serum glutamic oxaloacetic transaminase; PVC, packed cell volume; BP, blood pressure; NG, nasogastric; ICU, intensive care unit; ARDS, adult respiratory distress syndrome; ATN, acute tubular necrosis.

Coeliac axis block is ineffective in relieving the intractable pain in these patients. Vomiting due to duodenal stenosis and jaundice resulting from large bile duct obstruction require surgical bypass — gastrojejunostomy and choledochojejunostomy respectively.

Tumours of the pancreas

The vast majority of tumours of the pancreas affect the exocrine component and are pancreatic ductal carcinomas which carry a dismal prognosis. Also included in the term 'pancreatic cancer' are the periampullary tumours (Fig. 13.68) which are cancers that arise around the ampulla of Vater from the terminal bile duct, the duodenal mucosa or the ampulla itself. These periampullary tumours present early with jaundice and carry a much better prognosis following surgical treatment. The other tumours of the pancreas are of endocrine origin (Table 13.33). These give rise to a variety of syndromes which result from the persistent autonomous secretion of specific peptides.

Pancreatic ductal adenocarcinoma

The incidence of pancreatic ductal carcinoma has increased considerably during the last two decades. Aetiological factors include smoking, diabetes and chronic pancreatitis. The disease usually occurs in patients over 50 years of either sex but may afflict young adults. It may originate in the head or body and tail of the organ. It infiltrates surrounding structures and metastasizes to the peritoneal lining and regional lymph nodes and via the blood stream to the liver and lungs. Pain is an important feature of pancreatic cancer and is caused by infiltration of the retroperitoneal structures. In addition, anorexia and weight loss are marked. Involvement of the bile duct, which occurs earlier in patients with cancer of the head than in those with tumours of the body and tail, results in progressive jaundice. As the occlusion is distal to the insertion of the cystic duct, the gallbladder is enlarged and palpable (Courvoisier's sign). Occlusion of the duodenum results in persistent vomiting. Spread to the liver, which in itself may be the cause of the jaundice, is characterized by nodular hepatomegaly and peritoneal dissemination results in malignant ascites. The diagnosis of pancreatic ductal adenocarcinoma is made by ultrasound and CT examination, laparoscopy and by ERCP.

Periampullary cancer

Periampullary tumours present early with painless progressive obstructive jaundice, anorexia and some weight loss. These patients also complain of itching due to the retention of bile salts. On examination there is a smooth hepato-

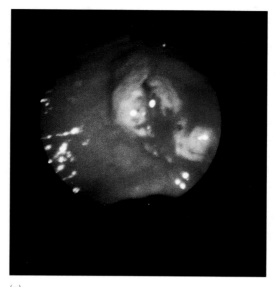

(a)

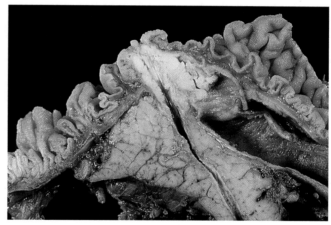

(b)

Figure 13.68 (a) Endoscopic view and (b) pathological specimen of periampullary carcinoma.

Table 13.33 Some endocrine APUD tumours of the pancreas.

Tumour type	Hormone secreted	Effects
Insulinoma	Insulin	Hypoglycaemia
Gastrinoma	Gastrin	Zollinger–Ellison syndrome (intractable peptic ulceration)
Glucagonoma	Glucagon	Diabetes, necrotic migratory erythema, weight loss, weakness and stomatitis
Somatostatinoma	Somatostatin	Diabetes, malabsorption and gallstones

megaly and an enlarged gallbladder. The diagnosis is confirmed by ultrasound and by ERCP when the lesion is biopsied.

Treatment of pancreatic cancer

Pancreatic ductal adenocarcinoma is usually incurable at the time of diagnosis. The exceptions to this are small tumours of the head of the pancreas which have not metastasized to the lymph nodes. Resection by pancreaticoduodenectomy may result in long-term survival in these patients. However, 90% of patients with pancreatic ductal adenocarcinoma are dead within 1 year of diagnosis. Palliative treatment is needed in the majority of patients. Pain is best relieved by coeliac axis block. The jaundice resolves following insertion of stents through the tumour (endoscopic or through the liver) and duodenal obstruction is managed by gastrojejunostomy.

By contrast, the majority of periampullary cancers are operable and, following resection, the 5-year survival averages 50%.

Pancreatic tumours at a glance

DEFINITIONS

Pancreatic ductal carcinoma is a malignant lesion of the head or body of the pancreas. *Periampullary carcinomas* arise around the ampulla of Vater and include tumours arising from the pancreas, the duodenum, the distal bile duct and the ampulla itself. *Endocrine pancreatic tumours* cause a variety of syndromes secondary to the secretion of active peptides

EPIDEMIOLOGY

M:F = 2:1 Age 50–70 years. Incidence of pancreatic carcinoma is increasing in the western world

AETIOLOGY

Predisposing factors
- Smoking
- Diabetes
- Chronic pancreatitis

PATHOLOGY

Site
- 60% involve head of pancreas, 25% body, 15% tail

Macroscopic
- Growth is hard and infiltrating

Histology
- Adenocarcinoma

Spread
- Lymphatics to peritoneum and regional nodes, via blood stream to liver and lung. Metastases often present at time of diagnosis

CLINICAL FEATURES

- Back pain, anorexia, weight loss
- Progressive jaundice (Courvoisier's law: a palpable gallbladder in the presence of jaundice is unlikely to be due to gallstones)
- Duodenal obstruction causing vomiting
- Malignant ascites

INVESTIGATIONS

- Ultrasound — may see mass in head of pancreas and distended biliary tree
- CT scanning — demonstrate tumour mass
- ERCP — very accurate in making diagnosis; obtain specimen for cytology and stent may be placed to relieve jaundice
- Barium meal — widening of the duodenal loop with medial filling defect, the reversed '3' sign (only seen in advanced disease)

MANAGEMENT

Palliation
- Pancreatic adenocarcinoma is usually incurable at time of diagnosis
- Jaundice is relieved by placing a stent through the tumour either transhepatically or via ERCP
- Duodenal obstruction is relieved by gastrojejunostomy
- Pain may be helped with a coeliac axis block

Curative Rx
- Rarely, surgical (Whipple) resection of small tumours of the head of the pancreas is curative if lymph nodes are not involved

Prognosis
- 90% of patients with pancreatic adenocarcinoma are dead within 12 months
- It is important to obtain histology from tumours around the head of the pancreas as the prognosis from *non-pancreatic* periampullary cancers is considerably better (50% 5-year survival) following resection

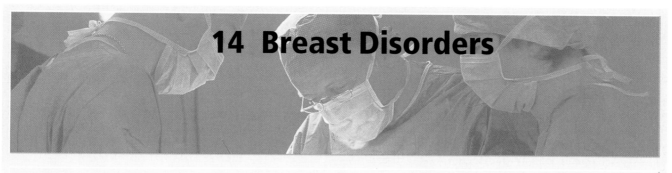

14 Breast Disorders

Breast structure and physiology

The breast is a modified sweat gland enclosed between superficial and deep fascial layers and resting on the pectoralis major muscle between the second and sixth ribs. Cooper's suspensory ligaments support it between the skin and deep fascia, and its blood supply is derived from the intercostal vessels and the lateral thoracic artery. Lymphatic drainage from the breast is mainly to the axilla, but also to smaller lymph nodes along the internal mammary artery. Venous drainage is to the internal mammary vein and the vertebral venous system via the intercostals.

The breast is composed of lobules, with an acinar arrangement, that leads into a ductal system terminating in approximately 20 main lactiferous ducts converging on the nipple. The breast changes during each hormonal cycle in anticipation of pregnancy: under the influence of oestrogen and progesterone, new acini are formed and fluid retention causes oedema in the supporting connective tissues. This is followed by involutionary changes at the end of the cycle — unless pregnancy supervenes.

Evaluation of the patient

Clinical assessment

General history

There are a few general points which should be obtained from all women presenting with breast disease.
• *Age* is important, as malignancy is very rare under the age of 20 and age may affect treatment: a very elderly patient with breast cancer may just receive tamoxifen for treatment.

• *Family history* is important, as the chance of breast cancer developing in a first-degree relative of a patient with breast cancer is greater than that of the general population.
• *Menstrual history*: patients in whom the menarche occurred before 12 years or the menopause after 55 years are at greater risk of breast malignancy than the general population.
• *Age at time of first pregnancy* is relevant as women who have a full-term pregnancy at an early age have a decreased risk of cancer while the risk is increased in nulliparous women and those who become pregnant for the first time after the age of 35 years.
• *Breast-feeding*: infections and breast abscesses are frequent in lactating mothers.
• *Prior history of breast disease*: a history of benign or malignant breast disease is more common in women presenting with breast cancer.

Specific symptoms

• *Breast lump*: The most common symptom of both benign and malignant disease is a palpable mass, which the patient notices either accidentally or because of pain. A palpable mass in the breast may be due to a benign or malignant tumour, a localized area of fibrocystic disease or fat necrosis.
• *Pain* which is often unilateral, is probably the next most common symptom of breast disease. It is frequently confined to the upper outer quadrant of the breast and the axillary tail. Pain may be periodic in nature, being most severe during the second half of the menstrual cycle. Pain — or mastodynia — is common in fibrocystic disease of the breast and is frequently localized to one area; there is often a premenstrual exacerbation of the pain. Pain and tenderness are also associated with mammary duct ectasia and with acute infection, due to streptococcal or staphylococcal infection arising in a cracked nipple. This is common during lactation and may lead to abscess formation, requiring

dependent drainage. However, it may be difficult to drain multilocular abscesses adequately.

• *Nipple discharge* is a less common symptom of breast disease (Table 14.1). The discharge may be serous (green or yellow), opaque (white) or blood-stained (red). A yellow serous discharge is usually due to fibrocystic disease. A green serous discharge may be due to fibroadenosis or mammary duct ectasia. An opaque white discharge indicates lactorrhoea which occurs postpartum and may also be associated with the use of oral contraceptives. Lactorrhoea may also occur in newborn infants from high levels of maternal hormone (witch's milk). A red discharge indicates blood-staining and is associated with duct papilloma and, rarely, with carcinoma.

Table 14.1 The common causes and management of nipple discharge.

Type of discharge	Causes	Management
Serous		
Yellow	Fibrocystic disease	Observe/local excision
Green	Fibrocystic disease	
	Mammary duct ectasia	Subareolar excision of the involved ducts
Opaque (white)	Lactorrhoea	Observe
Blood-stained (red)	Duct papilloma	Excise by microdochectomy
	Carcinoma	Treat as for carcinoma

Physical examination

A detailed account of examination of the breast is given in Chapter 1 and only the salient points are given here.

Inspection

• Inspect the breast with the patient in a sitting position. Look for:
    (a) asymmetry or unilateral elevation of the nipple;
    (b) retraction of the nipple;
    (c) dimpling of the skin, which is often more prominent when the arms are raised above the head;
    (d) *peau d'orange* appearance; and
    (e) eczema of the nipple or skin ulceration.

Palpation

• Palpate the breast with the flat of the hand while the patient lies supine.
• Examine each quadrant separately, including the axillary tail.
• Examine each axilla, supporting the patient's arm to relax her muscles.
• Be systematic in examining the axilla: medial wall, apex, anterior wall, posterior wall and lateral aspect (Fig. 14.1).
• Examination of the supraclavicular fossae should be done from behind.

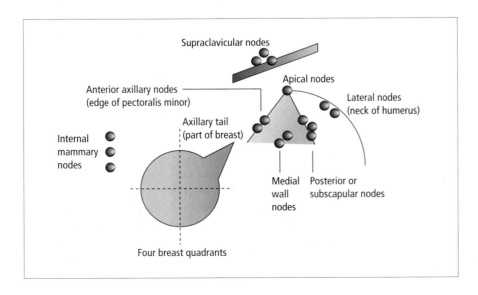

Figure 14.1 The quadrants of the breast and the regional lymph nodes which drain the breast: axillary, supraclavicular and internal mammary.

Determination of breast lump fixation

If a mass is identified it is necessary to look for fixation to the overlying skin. Even if the overlying skin is not directly involved, it may be dimpled due to contraction of Cooper's ligaments. Fixation of a deep-seated mass to the pectoral fascia or muscle is determined by asking the patient to place her hands on her hips and to press medially: this fixes the pectoral muscles and if the mass remains mobile it is not fixed to the pectoral fascia.

Examination of other systems

The chest and abdomen should also be examined — the chest for rib tenderness and pleural effusions, and the abdomen for hepatomegaly or ascites.

Investigations

Mammography

A mammogram is a soft-tissue radiograph of the breast and is the non-invasive method of choice for identifying breast carcinoma. Views are taken in two planes and the technique may identify non-palpable carcinomas. The mammographic signs of malignancy are (Fig. 14.2):
• the presence of a mass — usually, but not exclusively, with irregular margins;
• the presence of microcalcification — fine, elongated and punctated;
• hypervascularity, thickening of the skin and skin retraction.

The sensitivity (i.e. the ability of the test to detect all malignant lesions) and specificity (i.e. all lesions detected are malignant) of mammography are very high — in the order of 90%. The procedure is very safe and exposes the patient to a very low dose of radiation. Fears that repeated mammograms may be carcinogenic have not been substantiated. Mammography is used frequently:
• in breast-screening programmes;
• to assist in the diagnosis of a doubtful lesion;
• to examine the opposite breast when there is a risk of bilateral cancer;
• to examine patients with a strong family history of breast cancer; and
• for assessment of patients with large breasts.

Ultrasonography

Ultrasound can be used to differentiate between solid and cystic breast lesions and can be a useful adjunct to mammography (Fig. 14.3).

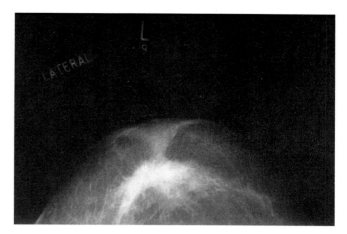

Figure 14.2 Mammogram of the left breast showing a 4 × 4 cm mass deep to the nipple, demonstrating the features of carcinoma: the presence of a mass with irregular margins, microcalcification, thickening of the skin and skin distortion.

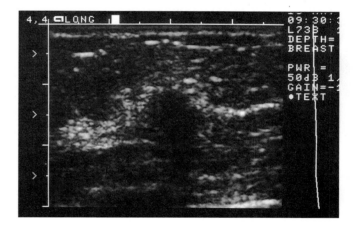

Figure 14.3 Ultrasound of left breast showing a centrally placed irregular mass. Reduced heterogeneous echogenicity, an irregular halo and posterior shadowing are all features of malignancy.

Breast biopsy

Histology is the final proof of malignancy and should always be obtained before definite radical treatment is undertaken.
• *Fine-needle aspiration biopsy* may confirm the presence of malignancy in many cases but a negative aspirate should not be accepted as definitive. Fine-needle aspiration is performed by inserting a needle into the breast lump. Suction is applied to the syringe as the needle is withdrawn, and the aspirate is fixed and stained. An experienced pathologist can make a reliable diagnosis based on the cells contained in the aspirate.

• Larger solid lumps in the breast can be biopsied using a *drill* or a *Tru-cut needle* — the latter is probably preferable. Local anaesthesia is necessary, and the diagnostic accuracy is high.

• An *open biopsy* may have to be performed in some patients. Lesions detected by mammography are often impalpable and have to be localized by inserting a needle under double-view mammographic control. A coloured/radiographic dye or a small wire is left in place which the surgeon excises with a rim of tissue. An X-ray of the specimen is obtained, thus ensuring that the lesion has been biopsied.

Benign breast disorders

Developmental abnormalities

Aplasia, hypoplasia and hypertrophy

The breast may fail to develop (amazia) or be underdeveloped (Fig. 14.4). This may be associated with an absence of pectoral muscles and thoracic cage abnormalities. Hypertrophy of the breast may also occur, with large deposits of fat in the breast. It may be unilateral or bilateral, and the gross enlargement may cause severe discomfort and disability (Fig. 14.5). Occasionally reduction mamoplasty is required to reduce the size of hypertrophied breasts.

Accessory breast tissue

The milk line in different species of animals extends from the axilla to the groin. Normally the embryonic milk line disappears in humans except for that leading to breast tissue over the pectoral muscles. However, accessory breast tissue may persist and accessory nipples may be present.

Breast abscess

Breast infections usually present late in pregnancy or during lactation. They are usually caused by nipple trauma and the organism is invariably *Staphylococcus aureus*. In the early state the typical features of a cellulitis are present with swelling, redness, heat and pain in the breast. If antibiotics (usually flucloxacillin) are given quickly at this stage the infection can be treated successfully. If an abscess develops, incision, drainage and breaking-down of loculations are required. Engorgement of the breast may be treated by expressing milk or by use of a breast pump. There is no need to suppress lactation and breast-feeding should be continued.

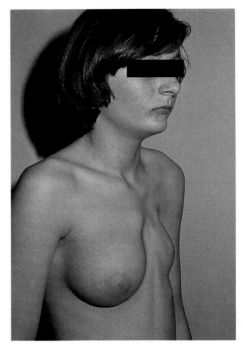

Figure 14.4 Underdeveloped left breast.

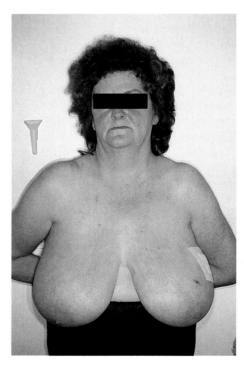

Figure 14.5 Idiopathic benign breast hypertrophy. The breasts have enlarged enormously, have become tender and are disfiguring.

Fibrocystic disease

The cyclical hormonal changes of active reproductive life stimulate proliferative and involutionary changes in the breast tissue. Proliferation of fibrous tissue (*fibrosis*) and hyperplasia of epithelial elements (*adenosis*) occur in varying proportions. Later degenerative changes give rise to *cysts* of varying sizes. Hence the two commonly used names for this condition are *fibrocystic disease* and *fibroadenosis*. Several other names have been used to describe this condition in the past (chronic mastitis, cystic mammary dysplasia, cystic hyperplasia), but we will confine ourselves to fibrocystic disease.

Clinical features

Fibrocystic disease is a common problem in women during the years of ovarian activity but is most often seen between the ages of 25 and 45. Pain and tenderness are common symptoms, most noticeable during the second half of the menstrual cycle and becoming much worse just before menstruation. Many patients present with one or more lumps (often cysts) in the breast which may also be tender. The upper outer quadrant and axillary tail are most often affected. Cysts are usually smooth, spherical and hard but often fibrocystic disease is indicated by a patch of irregular thickening of breast tissue. Nipple discharge is rare.

Treatment

Treatment is directed at pain relief, patient reassurance, cyst aspiration and excision of persistent localized masses after cyst aspiration (Fig. 14.6). The patient's greatest concern is that she may have cancer and once this has been excluded further therapy is often unnecessary. However, a number of patients have marked pain and tenderness which require treatment. Abstinence from xanthine-containing substances (chocolate, cola, coffee, tea) may relieve tenderness and two drugs have been used with good effect: *danazol*, which inhibits pituitary gonadotrophins, and *tamoxifen*, which blocks the effect of oestrogen by combining with oestrogen receptors.

Fibroadenoma

Fibroadenoma is a benign tumour manifesting as one or more round, hard, very mobile and usually painless lumps. It is the most common breast tumour in young women usually under 30 years of age and growth may be accelerated during pregnancy. It is usually detected when it is 2 or 3 cm in size. Histologically a fibroadenoma consists of epithelial elements and connective tissue in varying proportions. The treatment of fibroadenoma is surgical enucleation (Fig. 14.6).

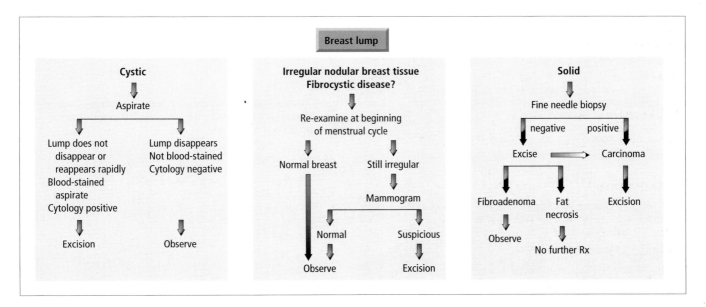

Figure 14.6 Algorithm for the management of a patient presenting with a breast lump.

Cystosarcoma phyllodes

Cystosarcoma phyllodes is a tumour resembling a large fibroadenoma and may attain very large dimensions. Most of the tumours are benign, but about 10% can metastasize. They contain epithelial and connective tissue elements and are not encapsulated. In malignant cases the metastases tend to be blood-borne rather than lymphatic. Removal of cystosarcoma phyllodes should include a generous margin of surrounding breast tissue because of the lack of encapsulation. Simple mastectomy is indicated for large tumours.

Mammary duct ectasia

Mammary duct ectasia occurs in older patients and is most common in the subareolar portion of the breast. Dilated collecting ducts are filled with cellular debris, which escapes to the periductal tissue where it provokes a severe inflammatory-type reaction with pain and tenderness. Clinically, patients present with a green nipple discharge and a lump in the subareolar area. The lump is associated with nipple retraction and skin fixation, and resembles a cancer. Treatment is by subareolar excision of the involved ducts.

Fat necrosis

Despite a history of trauma in half the cases and frequent presence of an ecchymosis, the histological picture of fat necrosis resembles that of mammary duct ectasia with a heavy periductal cellular infiltrate. Clinically the lump is hard and there is dimpling of the overlying skin; differentiation from a carcinoma is impossible on physical examination. Treatment is by surgical excision.

Duct papilloma

Duct papillomas arise within the major breast ducts, are usually benign and, in most cases, are no more than 1–2 mm in diameter — generally too small to be palpable. They give rise to serous or bloody discharge from the nipple. Treatment is by excision of the affected duct by microdochectomy and is curative.

Benign breast disease at a glance

FIBROCYSTIC DISEASE

Definition

Fibrocystic disease is a condition caused by cyclical proliferation and involution of breast tissue producing *fibrosis*, epithelial hyperplasia (*adenosis*) and *cyst* formation

Clinical

- Age 25–45 years
- Breast pain, tenderness and breast lump(s) during the second half of the menstrual cycle

Management

- Patient reassurance, cyst aspiration, excision of persistent localized masses after aspiration
- Avoid xanthine-containing substances
- Drugs:
  (a) Danazol inhibits pituitary gonadotrophins
  (b) Tamoxifen blocks the effects of oestrogen

FIBROADENOMA

Benign breast tumour manifesting as one or more hard mobile painless lumps, usually in women under 30 years of age. Treatment is by excision

BREAST ABSCESS

Infection of the pregnant or lactating breast with *Staphylococcus aureus*. Patient presents with redness, swelling, heat and pain in the breast.

Treatment is with antibiotics (flucloxacillin) initially but if an abscess develops, incision and drainage will be required. Lactation need not suppressed while the abscess is being treated.

MAMMARY DUCT ECTASIA

Dilated subareolar ducts are filled with cellular debris which causes a periductal inflammatory response. The usual presentation is a green nipple discharge and a subareolar lump. Treatment is by subareolar excision of the involved ducts

DUCT PAPILLOMA

Small papillomas arise in the major breast ducts. They cause a bloody or serous nipple discharge. Treatment is by excision of the affected duct by microdochectomy

FAT NECROSIS

- History of trauma to the breast in 50% of cases
- Often associated ecchymoses
- Histology — periductal cellular infiltrate
- Treatment is by surgical excision

Malignant breast disease

Breast cancer

Epidemiology and aetiology

• Breast cancer is most common in western countries and, in mixed-race populations, it is more common in white women than in black women
• Women in social classes I and II with a strong family history of breast cancer have the highest risk of developing the disease: such a family history would include several members of the same or the preceding generation with breast cancer and does not include isolated incidence within the family
• Early menarche and late menopause may be predisposing factors, particularly in nulliparous women
• There may be an increased risk among women who have benign breast disease
• Multiple and early pregnancies may confer some protection
• There is no evidence that trauma or the use of oral contraceptives or oestrogen replacement therapy has any role in the aetiology

Clinical presentation of breast cancer

Clinically, a carcinoma of the breast is *early* if at the time of diagnosis it is confined to the breast and there is no evidence of distant metastases, whereas *late* breast cancer describes a tumour that has spread to the regional lymph glands or to distant sites such as the liver or bone. Even the smallest of malignant breast tumours may have given rise to distant metastases.

The most common presentation is as a palpable lump, often first felt by the patient herself. More than 90% are painless, but pain does not exclude the possibility of tumour. If the tumour is centrally located the nipple may be involved, causing retraction of the nipple or producing a blood-stained or serous discharge. In *Paget's disease of the nipple* an eczema of the nipple develops over a centrally located tumour.

A variety of signs may be manifest:
• skin dimpling may be evident due to involvement of Cooper's ligaments;
• *peau d'orange* is seen when cutaneous lymphatics are blocked by tumour cells and cutaneous oedema occurs; and
• palpable axillary lymph glands are not an indication of regional spread *per se* — only about 50% of palpable axillary nodes contain tumour metastases.

Pathology of breast cancer

Histologically, breast cancer is a duct carcinoma arising, in most cases, from the terminal duct lobular unit. Breast carcinomas can be divided pathologically into two broad groups: non-invasive and invasive carcinomas (Table 14.2).

Table 14.2 Pathological classification of breast carcinoma.

Type	Frequency (%)
Non-invasive	
Intraductal (including comedocarcinoma*)	1
Lobular carcinoma-*in-situ*	Rare
Intraductal papillary carcinoma	Rare
Invasive	
Invasive ductal carcinoma (nos)	78
Paget's disease	2
Invasive lobular carcinoma (multicentric)	10
Medullary carcinoma (lymphocytic infiltrate)	6
Mucoid carcinoma (extracellular mucin)	2
Tubular carcinoma (well-differentiated)	Rare
Invasive papillary (well-differentiated)	Rare

*In comedocarcinoma the ducts are filled with cellular debris.
nos, not otherwise specified

The vast majority of breast cancers are invasive and are *ductal* carcinomas not otherwise specified (nos). Most invasive ductal carcinomas have a *scirrhous* pattern with dense fibrous tissue and tumour infiltration of the surrounding breast tissue. Lobular carcinoma has a better prognosis than ductal carcinoma, but as it is multicentric it tends to be bilateral. The apparently tumour-free opposite breast should be examined carefully for a second tumour and follow-up with repeated mammograms may be indicated; it may even be reasonable to consider mastectomy. Other forms of invasive carcinoma are:
• *medullary* characterized by a lymphocytic infiltration;
• *mucoid*, in which are seen large amounts of extracellular mucin;
• *tubular* which is well-differentiated; and
• *papillary*, characterized by a well-differentiated papillary structure.

These variants of invasive cancer generally have a better prognosis than invasive ductal carcinoma.

Paget's disease of the nipple is an uncommon manifestation of invasive ductal carcinoma. Tumour cells invade the nipple, resulting in an eczema-like appearance. Paget cells are large, clear, vacuolated cells with dark nuclei.

Inflammatory carcinoma is likewise a variant of invasive ductal carcinoma and is uncommon. The breast is enlarged, oedematous and indurated, and is hot and painful to palpation. This type of tumour is aggressive and there is early and wide invasion of lymphatic and blood vessels. Its prognosis is poor.

Staging of breast cancer

The commonest site for a primary breast cancer is the upper outer quadrant of the breast followed by the subareolar area. Cancers spread by the lymphatics usually to the axillary nodes (even when the primary is medially placed in the breast) and disseminate to produce metastases in lung, bone, liver, brain, adrenal and ovary. An assessment of the extent of disease , i.e. staging, is important as it:
• gives an indication of probable prognosis;
• provides guidelines for treatment;
• allows comparison of data from different centres.

Accurate clinical staging is handicapped by difficulty in palpating lymph nodes in the axilla and determining if those palpated are involved by tumour. False-positive and false-negative observations may be as high as 40%. However, a relatively simple clinical staging system is:

Stage I: Primary tumour < 2 cm, no palpable axillary nodes;
Stage II: Primary tumour < 2 cm, with palpable axillary nodes;
           Primary tumour 2–5 cm, with or without palpable axillary nodes;
Stage III: Primary tumour > 5 cm, with or without fixed axillary nodes;
Stage IV: Distant metastases or extensive local involvement, e.g. skin or chest wall.

More accurate staging may be carried out retrospectively after surgery, when the axillary glands can be examined histologically and the internationally accepted TNM classifications (there are both clinical and pathological classifications) are currently used.

Investigation of breast cancer

Mammography and *breast biopsy* (see above) are indicated in patients suspected of having breast cancer. The following investigations are indicated in a patient in whom the diagnosis has been established.

Imaging

Chest radiography is always necessary, and isotope bone scans with radiography of 'hot' spots is indicated if bony metastases are suspected. An ultrasound liver scan is also performed routine, irrespective of the findings of the liver function tests.

Biochemistry

A raised serum alkaline phosphatase and/or γ-glutamyl transpeptidase may indicate liver metastases, while an abnormal serum calcium or alkaline phosphatase level may suggest bony metastases.

Hormone receptor status

Normal breast tissue cells respond to hormones such as oestrogen and progesterone through protein receptor sites, which bind these hormones. Breast cancer cells may also have these receptor sites which have an ability to bind sex hormones: their binding capacity is an indication of the extent to which the tumour can be subjected to and influenced by hormone manipulation, and may be important for therapy. Tissue for hormone receptor assay is obtained at operation and is immediately frozen in liquid nitrogen or dry ice. Patients whose cancer cells have oestrogen receptors (ER+) have a better prognosis than those whose cells do not have oestrogen receptors (ER–).

Management of breast cancer

Management of a patient with breast cancer can be considered as a series of strategies:
• to establish the diagnosis;
• to obtain as much information as possible for prognosis (staging, histological type, ER status);
• to treat and prevent recurrence of locoregional disease;
• to treat recurrent and metastatic disease;
• to consider breast reconstruction.

Today several options, including breast conservation and total mastectomy, radiotherapy, chemotherapy and hormonal manipulation, are available to achieve these goals and a full discussion of the benefits and risks of the various therapies should be had with the patient before embarking on treatment. Patients present in one of two groups: early breast cancer (stages I and II) and advanced breast cancer (stages III and IV).

Early breast cancer

Surgery • *Total mastectomy* (i.e. removal of the breast containing the tumour) with axillary dissection to remove the lymph nodes is currently the standard operation for locally confined breast cancer where the primary is 3.0 cm or more. The extent of the axillary dissection varies with different surgeons and may consist of a full clearance of axillary contents downwards from the axillary vein or a less extensive lower axillary clearance.

• *Radical mastectomy* (i.e. removal of the pectoral muscles, breast and underlying fascia, and the contents of the axilla) is no longer considered to be an appropriate operation because it is excessively mutilating and unlikely to confer additional benefit over total mastectomy.)

• *Lumpectomy or segmental resection* with radiotherapy to the residual breast involves a limited clearance around the tumour with breast conservation. The axilla is also dissected for nodal staging. Breast conservation is usually preferred for tumours up to 3 cm.

Radiation is given if there is tumour in the axillary nodes, and it may be advisable to irradiate the internal mammary chain of glands as well, particularly if the primary tumour is located centrally or medially in the breast.

Chemotherapy and hormonal manipulation Adjuvant chemotherapy using cyclophosphamide, methotrexate and 5-fluorouracil (CMF) is used for premenopausal women with positive axillary nodes. The same regimen (CMF) is used for postmenopausal patients with ER– tumours and positive axillary nodes, while the antioestrogen drug tamoxifen is used for postmenopausal patients with ER+ tumours and positive axillary nodes.

Prognosis The prognosis for early-treated breast cancer is quite good, with an 80% 10-year survival rate.

Advanced breast cancer

Surgery Surgery is certainly not going to cure a patient with advanced breast cancer. However, toilet mastectomy may be indicated for patients with breast cancer ulcerating through the skin (Fig. 14.7), though sometimes the response to tamoxifen in this situation may be quite dramatic.

Radiotherapy Radiotherapy is often used in patients with advanced breast cancer and may reduce the tumour size to enable mastectomy. It is especially indicated in inflammatory breast cancer. External-beam irradiation is also helpful for pain from bony metastases.

Chemotherapy and hormonal manipulation Chemotherapy (20–30 different drugs have been used with varying response rates) and hormonal manipulation, using tamoxifen or oopherectomy, may be of value for visceral and other distant metastases. Suppression of corticosteroid production by administration of aminoglutethamide (an

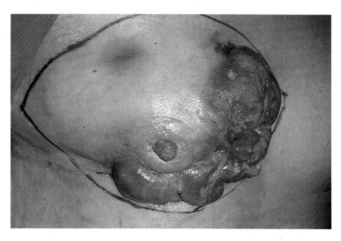

Figure 14.7 Advanced carcinoma of the breast. There is a large ulcerated and fungating carcinoma of the left breast. This patient clearly requires a toilet mastectomy.

anticonvulsant which suppresses corticosteroid synthesis) induces regression in up to 30% of patients but these treatments have now been superseded by tamoxifen. Aminoglutethamide, however, may be useful in the management of bony metastases, but it is associated with significant side-effects, including lethargy, ataxia, blurred vision and skin rashes.

Prognosis The prognosis for patients with advanced breast cancer is poor. Only 30–40% of patients respond to therapy and then the response only lasts for about a year. The mean survival of the responders is 2 years, by which time most of the non-responders will have died.

Breast reconstruction

The results of breast reconstruction after mastectomy have improved considerably in recent years and patients undergoing mastectomy for potential cure should be counselled regarding reconstruction. The criteria for selection and timing of reconstruction are not clearly defined and several different methods of reconstruction are available (Fig. 14.8).

Screening for breast cancer

In biological terms a clinically detectable carcinoma of the breast is a late manifestation of the disease. Earlier diagnosis of an impalpable lesion by radiology is likely to be attended by a reduction in the mortality rate. Screening programmes employing mammography have been introduced in various countries around the world and the results

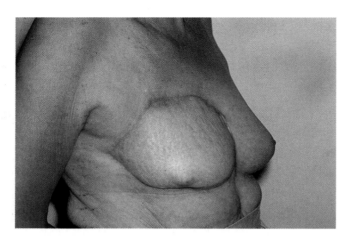

Figure 14.8 Breast reconstruction following mastectomy. In this patient after resection of the tumour, the contralateral rectus muscle and overlying skin were mobilized and tunnelled subcutaneously to reach the right chest defect. The abdominal defect was closed using polypropylene mesh.

Table 14.3 Requirements for a successful screening programme.

Selectivity	Screening should be confined to high-risk groups
Sensitivity	The test used must be able to detect most of the malignancies (or disease) present in the screened population
Specificity	The majority of the lesions deteced by the test should be malignancies (or the disease being screened for)
Simplicity	The test should be relatively simple to perform
Safety	The risk to the patient from the test should be negligible
Savings	The test should be cheap and cost–benefit analysis should demonstrate that significant savings result from detection and treatment of the disease
Sensible	There must be an effective treatment available for the disease
Suitability	The screening programme must be acceptable to most of the people invited to be screened so that compliance is high

of these programmes suggest that there is a reduction in mortality from breast cancer in the study group, i.e. those women undergoing mammography, when compared with the control group who did not undergo mammography. The mortality reduction is statistically significant in women over the age of 50 years.

For such screening programmes to be successful there must be a high compliance rate amongst those invited to participate. Identification of a suspicious lesion at mammography must be followed by careful assessment with fine-needle aspiration cytology or biopsy. Formerly, anxiety was expressed at the risk of repeated doses of irradiation in a screening programme but it is now accepted that the radiation dose is minimal and without risk. Cost-effectiveness is an important consideration in screening programmes and the cost of the undertaking must be set against the number of possible lives saved (Table 14.3). If benefits are minimal and resources limited, a more rewarding preventive programme with a higher yield may take precedence.

Disorders of the male breast

Gynaecomastia

Enlargement of the adolescent male breast, either unilaterally or bilaterally, may occur in response to the changing hormone environment after puberty. If often regresses spontaneously, but frequently it is necessary to remove the redundant breast tissue because of the patient's embarrassment. Gynaecomastia is also associated with testicular atrophy in Klinefelter's syndrome and with advanced liver disease. It may also be drug induced (oestrogens, cimetidine, epanutin etc.).

Male breast cancer

Male breast cancer is rare. The tumour is often hormone-dependent, being seen in patients with high oestrogen levels, e.g. Klinefelter's syndrome, oestrogen therapy for prostate cancer. Gynaecomastia, however, is not associated with the development of male breast cancer. It is not always highly invasive locally, but has a high incidence of lymph node involvement as it is usually diagnosed in a more advanced state than in females. The prognosis is poor.

The standard treatment for breast cancer in men is a mastectomy. Eighty per cent of male breast tumours are ER+ and should respond to tamoxifen.

Breast cancer at a glance

DEFINITION

Malignant lesion of (predominantly) the female breast

EPIDEMIOLOGY

M/F = 1:100   Any age (usually >30 years)   High incidence in western world and in whites more than blacks

AETIOLOGY

Predisposing factors are:
- Strong family history of breast cancer
- Early menarche and late menopause, especially in nulliparous women
- Benign breast disease
- Social class I and II

PATHOLOGY

Histology
- Ductal carcinoma. Commonest type is *invasive ductal* or *nos* carcinoma. *Paget's disease* is ductal carcinoma involving the nipple

Spread
- Lymphatics, vascular invasion, direct extension; spreads to lung, liver, bone, brain, adrenal, ovary

Staging
- TNM classification, important for treatment and prognosis

CLINICAL FEATURES

- Palpable breast lump, usually painless
- Nipple retraction and skin dimpling
- Nipple eczema in Paget's disease
- *Peau d'orange* (cutaneous oedema secondary to lymphatic obstruction)
- Palpable axillary nodes

INVESTIGATIONS

- Mammography — infiltrating radiopaque mass and microcalcification indicate malignancy
- Ultrasound — differentiates cystic from solid lesions
- Breast biopsy — fine-needle aspiration of suspicious lump usually confirms the diagnosis. Excision biopsy occasionally required
- Imaging: CXR, isotope bone scan and radiography of hot spots, ultrasound scan of liver
- FBC, serum alkaline phosphatase, γ-glutamyl transpeptidase, serum calcium indicate liver or bone metastases
- Breast tissue for hormone receptor status (ER+/−) important for treatment and prognosis

MANAGEMENT

Early breast cancer (i.e. no evidence of distant spread at time of diagnosis)

Surgery	• Total mastectomy/breast conservation i.e. lumpectomy and radiotherapy to the residual breast. With all of these resections the axilla should be dissected to assess the node status histologically
Radiotherapy	• Radiation is given if the axillary nodes are involved
Chemotherapy/ hormonal therapy	• Adjuvant chemotherapy (cyclophosphamide, methotrexate, 5-FU) is given to premenopausal women with positive nodes and to postmenopausal women who are ER− . Tamoxifen is given to postmenopausal women who are ER+
Prognosis	• 80% 10-year survival rate

Advanced breast cancer (i.e. spread to regional nodes or distant sites at time of diagnosis)

Surgery	• Only for toilet mastectomy
Radiotherapy	• To deal with primary especially if inflammatory, to relieve pain from bony metastases
Chemotherapy	• Tamoxifen, aminogluthetamide
Prognosis	• Poor: only 30–40% respond to treatment with mean survival of 2 years, by which time the non-responders have died

CXR, Chest X-ray; FBC, full blood count; 5-FU, 5-fluorouracil; nos, not otherwise specified.

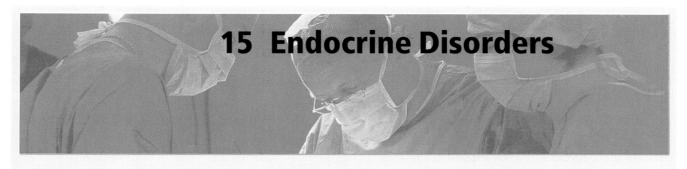

15 Endocrine Disorders

The extirpation of the thyroid gland for goitre typifies, perhaps better than any operation, the supreme triumph of the surgeon's art. (William S. Halsted 1852–1922)

The thyroid gland

Clinical assessment

The surgical anatomy of the thyroid and parathyroid glands is given in Fig. 15.1. Patients with disorders of the thyroid gland present with either systemic or local manifestations. The systemic manifestations result from either overactivity (hyperthyroidism or thyrotoxicosis) or underactivity (hypothyroidism) of the thyroid gland and involve many systems. The local features include generalized enlargement of the thyroid gland (goitre) and the development of a neck swelling.

Symptoms

The main symptoms and signs of thyroid disease are caused by an excess or paucity of circulating thyroid hormone

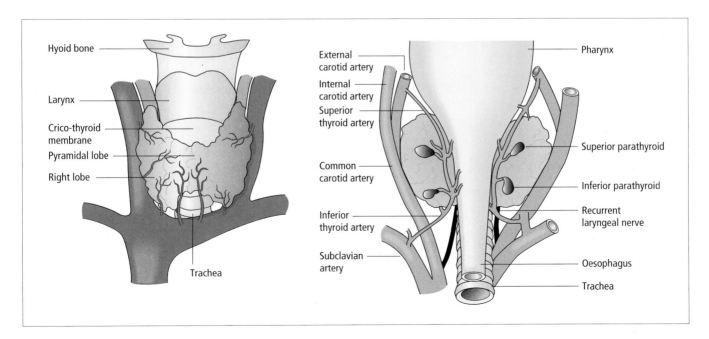

Figure 15.1 Surgical anatomy of thyroid and parathyroid glands.

Table 15.1 Clinical features of hyperthyroidism (thyrotoxicosis) and hypothyroidism (myxoedema).

Hyperthyroidism/thyrotoxicosis	Hypothyroidism/myxoedema
Symptoms	
Preference for cold weather	Intolerance to cold
Excessive sweating	Decreased sweating
Increased appetite	Hoarseness
Weight loss	Weight increase
Anxiety	Slow cerebration
Tiredness	Tiredness and decreased energy
Diarrhoea	Constipation
Palpitations	Muscular pains
Oligomenorrhoea	
Signs	
Goitre	Pallor or slightly yellow skin
Exophthalmos	Periorbital puffiness
Lid retraction	Loss of outer third of eyebrows
Lid lag	Dry, thickened skin and hair
Warm moist palms	Dementia (myxoedema madness)
Tremor	Slow-recovery phase ankle jerk
Onycholysis	Nerve deafness, coma
Atrial fibrillation	Slow pulse
Pretibial myxoedema	Large tongue
	Peripheral oedema

resulting in hyper- or hypothyroidism (Table 15.1). Hyperthyroidism may or may not be associated with a goitre which may be diffuse enlargement of the gland (Graves' disease) or a multinodular goitre (Plummer's disease).

Physical examination

Examination of the thyroid gland has been discussed in Chapter 1 but the key features are summarized in Table 15.2. A thyroid swelling moves with swallowing.

Investigations

The aims of investigations of the thyroid are:
• to determine accurately the size, shape and location of the gland;
• to assess the effects on surrounding structures;
• to measure its functional activity and autoimmune status; and
• to obtain tissue diagnosis of suspicious lesions.

To determine accurately the size, shape and location of the gland and to assess the effects on surrounding structures:

(a) *Ultrasound* examination is a safe non-invasive test that provides information on the general shape and outline of the gland and can also determine displacement of the trachea. More importantly, ultrasound can establish whether a discrete lump is cystic or solid.

(b) *Plain radiographs of the chest and thoracic inlet* may also demonstrate tracheal displacement and compression, or retrosternal extension of a goitre.

To measure its functional activity and autoimmune status:

(a) *Serum tests*: Serum thyroxine (T_4) levels will usually establish whether the gland is overactive or not. If there is clinical evidence of hyperactivity and T_4 is normal, tri-iodothyronine (T_3) levels should be done. Thyroid-stimulating hormone (TSH) levels are elevated in patients with hypothyroidism and the presence of long-acting thyroid-stimulating factor (LATS) is diagnostic of Graves' disease. (LATS is in fact an immunoglobulin-G mimicking TSH through its reaction with TSH receptors on the thyroid, but it has a much longer half-life in the circulation than TSH.) Thyroid antibodies such as antithyroglobulin or antimitochondrial antibodies are elevated in Hashimoto's disease.

Table 15.2 Examination of the thyroid gland.

Inspection	Palpation	Percussion	Auscultation
From the front	*From behind*	Percuss the manubrium from one side to the other for dullness, indicating a retrosternal extension	A bruit may be heard over each lobe in thyrotoxicosis
Look for generalized swelling of the gland	Size, shape, consistency (smooth/nodular), tenderness, mobility, thrill, lymph nodes		
Does it move on swallowing?			
Distended neck veins may indicate retrosternal extension*	*From the front*		
	Tracheal displacement		

*Pemberton's sign: when the patient lifts both arms as high as possible, venous congestion of the face and neck occurs after a few minutes if a retrosternal goitre is present.

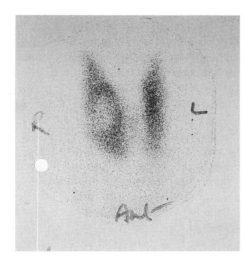

Figure 15.2 Isotope scan of thyroid gland showing a cold nodule in the right lobe.

(b) *Isotope scan*: Technetium 99m pertechnetate is the most frequently used isotope in thyroid assessment. The injected isotope is taken up by the thyroid gland. It is distributed uniformly in a normal thyroid. In a multinodular goitre the activity is unevenly distributed. Areas without activity corresponding to isolated single nodules in the thyroid are indicative of cyst or tumour (Fig. 15.2). A highly active nodule suggests a toxic nodule with secondary hyperthyroidism. Generalized high activity is found in Graves' disease.

To obtain tissue diagnosis of suspicious lesions:
(a) *Fine-needle aspiration cytology* may be diagnostically useful in solid, cold nodules. It may give rise to false negatives with well-differentiated tumours.
(b) *Excision biopsy* with frozen section is an alternative, but many pathologists express reservations about providing a definitive diagnosis with frozen section material only.

An algorithm for the management of a thyroid swelling is given in Fig. 15.3.

Neck swellings

The common causes of neck swelling are given in Table 15.3. Only thyroglossal cyst and goitre will be discussed here.

Thyroglossal cyst

This fluctuant swelling occurs in the middle of the neck, usually below the hyoid bone, but may occur anywhere

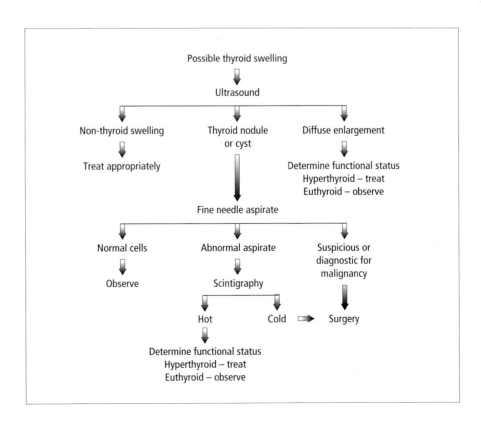

Figure 15.3 Algorithm for the management of a thyroid nodule.

Table 15.3 Causes of neck swelling.

Midline
Thyroglossal cyst (moves on protruding tongue) (relatively rare)
Goitre (moves on swallowing) (common)
Submental lymph nodes (common)

Lateral
Cervical lymphadenopathy (commonest cause overall)
Enlarged submandibular or parotid glands (not uncommon)
Branchial cyst
Cystic hygroma   rare
Pharyngeal pouch
Subclavian artery aneurysm

along the embryonic line of descent of the thyroid gland from the foramen caecum (Fig. 15.4). The track may lie in front or behind the hyoid bone and runs downwards from the foramen caecum at the junction of the anterior two-thirds and posterior third of the tongue to the suprasternal notch. The cyst is due to persistence of the epithelial lining of some part of the thyroglossal duct which normally atrophies.

Infection of a thyroglossal cyst, incision of the cyst or incomplete excision may result in a *thyroglossal fistula*, which discharges clear fluid or pus intermittently.

Clinical features

The swelling is located in the midline of the neck, usually below the hyoid bone. Because of its anatomical connection it moves upwards on swallowing and on protrusion of the tongue (Fig. 15.5.)

Treatment

Treatment may be required because of the size of the cyst or symptoms such as tenderness. The cyst should be excised and the fibrous track dissected out until it reaches the foramen caecum. It is necessary to excise the mid-portion of the hyoid bone in order to excise completely this portion of the thyroglossal duct.

Goitre

The word *goitre* comes from the Latin word *guttur*, meaning throat.

Goitre is the common clinical term used for a variety of thyroid swellings (Fig. 15.6). Many patients with goitre are euthyroid. A toxic goitre is a thyroid enlargement with either primary (Graves' disease) or secondary (Plummer's disease) hyperthyroidism. The causes of goitre are summarized in Table 15.4.

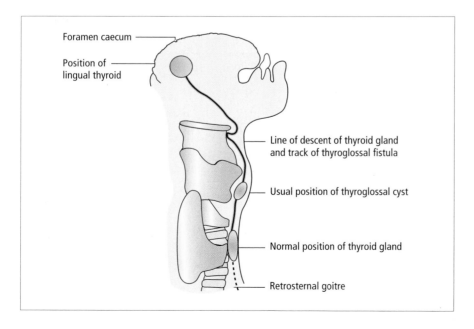

Foramen caecum

Position of lingual thyroid

Line of descent of thyroid gland and track of thyroglossal fistula

Usual position of thyroglossal cyst

Normal position of thyroid gland

Retrosternal goitre

Figure 15.4 The embryonic descent of the thyroid gland from the foramen caecum to the suprasternal notch may be interrupted at several points, resulting in ectopic thyroid tissue, thyroglossal cysts or thyroglossal fistula.

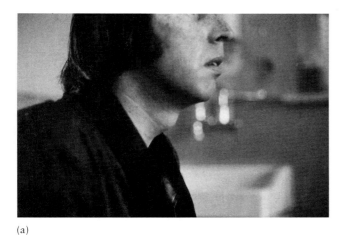

(a)

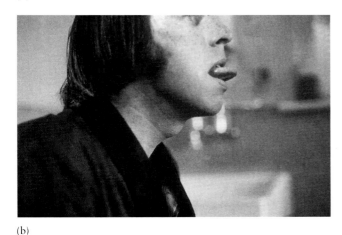

(b)

Figure 15.5 (a) Thyroglossal cyst; (b) the cyst moves upwards on protrusion of the tongue.

Physiological goitre

Because of the increased demands for thyroid hormone at puberty and during pregnancy, a mild diffuse enlargement of the thyroid takes place. The patient remains euthyroid but the enlargement of the gland may persist after the stimulus for increased thyroid hormone production has subsided. Treatment is not usually required.

Iodine-deficient (endemic) goitre

In areas far from salt water and seafood, a rich source of iodides, the soil is deficient in iodine and without iodine supplements, e.g. addition of iodine to salt, there is inadequate iodine uptake for conversion to T_4 resulting in low T_4 levels. The thyroid gland is subjected to continuous stimulation from TSH and enlarges progressively until it reaches enormous proportions in some cases. The huge enlargement

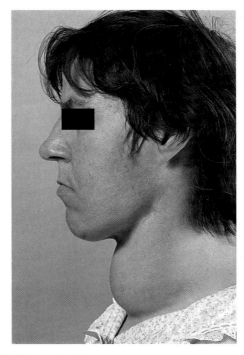

Figure 15.6 Large goitre in young woman.

Table 15.4 Causes of goitre.

Physiological (puberty and pregnancy)
Iodine deficiency (endemic, simple)
Primary hyperthyroidism (Graves' or Basedow's disease, exophthalmic goitre)
Adenomatous or nodular
Thyroid malignancies 　Papillary 　Follicular 　Anaplastic 　Medullary
Thyroiditis 　Autoimmune (Hashimoto's) 　Subacute (de Quervain's) 　Riedel's (struma)
Ingestion of goitrogens, e.g. excess iodides, drugs (para-aminosalicylic acid, phenylbutazone)
Pendred's syndrome (autosomal recessive condition characterized by goitre, hypothyroidism and nerve deafness)

may be either diffuse or nodular, and the goitre is usually asymptomatic.

Primary hyperthyroidism (Graves' disease — Basedow's disease — exophthalmic goitre)

Hyperthyroidism or thyrotoxicosis in Graves' disease is associated with diffuse thyroid enlargement. The gland is extremely hyperactive, producing excessive amounts of thyroid hormone. It has an increased blood supply, manifested by a thrill or palpation and a bruit on auscultation. These manifestations of overactivity are due to a circulating immunoglobulin known as LATS (see above).

Examination of the thyroid gland reveals a smooth moderate enlargement with sometimes a palpable thrill and an audible bruit. A varying degree of exophthalmos may be present with lid retraction, lid lag and proptosis. The metabolic effects are manifested by weight loss, sweating, nervousness, increased appetite, heat intolerance, diarrhoea, a fine tremor in the fingers and pretibial myxoedema. Cardiac manifestations are tachycardia and atrial fibrillation (Table 15.1).

Adenomatous or nodular goitre

This is a benign hyperplasia of the thyroid gland which may be diffuse or multinodular. Adenomatous and colloid nodules are scattered throughout the gland. Cystic degeneration may occur. Sometimes the enlargement is confined to a single adenomatous nodule. It is much more commonly seen in females than in males. In goitres with cystic degeneration there may be acute painful enlargement of the gland due to haemorrhage into a cyst. This may cause pressure symptoms in retrosternal goitres. If the patient remains euthyroid, the indications for resection are cosmesis, retrosternal projection causing pressure symptoms on the trachea and venous congestion, and haemorrhage into a cyst.

Secondary hyperthyroidism (Plummer's disease)

Excess thyroid hormone may be secreted by an adenomatous goitre or single adenomatous nodule. This usually occurs in middle-aged patients in whom the goitre has been present for some time, in contrast to Graves' disease where the goitre and the signs of toxicity appear simultaneously in young patients. In patients with secondary toxic goitre the cardiac signs are much more prominent than the metabolic features.

Thyroid malignancies

Thyroid malignancies (see below) usually present with a nodule in the thyroid gland.

Thyroiditis

Hashimoto's thyroidits, de Quervain's thyroiditis and Riedel's struma (see below) may all cause a goitre.

Management of thyrotoxicosis

Medical

Antithyroid drugs

The use of antithyroid drugs which inhibit the synthesis of thyroid hormone will control the disease in most patients and is curative in >50%. *Carbimazole* is effective in reducing T_4 levels to normal within 4–6 weeks. If tachycardia is excessive, *propranolol* may be used to control the heart rate more quickly. Patients should remain on maintenance dosage of carbimazole for up to 2 years, after which the majority will remain euthyroid. Some will relapse and require further courses of treatment or may be referred for surgery or radioactive iodine. Side-effects of carbimazole are joint pains, headache, nausea and skin rashes but the most serious effect is leukopenia. The white cell count should be regularly checked and patients should be warned to report a sore throat to their doctor immediately.

Radioactive iodine

Radioactive iodine is taken up by the thyroid gland and in appropriate dosage will destroy most of the active thyroid tissue. The effects of the radiation are variable but tend to be progressive, so that hypothyroidism is an almost inevitable sequel to treatment. Nevertheless, radioactive iodine may be the ideal treatment where medical therapy has failed and the patient is unfit for or refuses surgery. The risk of inducing malignancy is low but irradiation is preferably reserved for middle-aged and elderly patients and is absolutely contraindicated in pregnancy.

Surgical

Surgery for hyperthyroidism consists of removing most of the thyroid gland. The first removal of a thyroid gland was probably performed by Abul Casem Khalaf Ebn Abbas (Albucasis) in Baghdad in the 10th century AD. The fate of the patient is not known.

The indications for surgery are:

- failure of medical treatment;
- drug sensitivity in the younger patient; and
- large goitres with pressure symptoms (usually multinodular).

The advantages of surgery are:
• an immediate response is achieved in thyrotoxicosis;
• satisfactory cosmetic effect if the goitre has been large and prominent; and
• restoration of normal function in the remainder of the gland when a toxic nodule is removed.

Disadvantages include:
• possible damage to the recurrent laryngeal nerves;
• the risk of postoperative haemorrhage; and
• cardiac arrhythmias and the risk of precipitating a thyroid crisis or storm.

Thyroid crisis may occur following release of large quantities of T_4 into the circulation during surgical manipulation of the gland. The risk can be minimized or abolished by appropriate preoperative preparation.

Preoperative preparation

Signs and symptoms of thyrotoxicosis should be controlled before embarking on surgery. Up to 6 weeks may be required to achieve this. The effectiveness of the antithyroid therapy (carbimazole) is reflected in a falling pulse rate, particularly the sleeping pulse, and a reduction in the hyperkinetic state. β-Adrenergic blockers such as propranolol may also be used to achieve this effect. Antithyroid drugs are thought to increase the vascularity of the thyroid and some surgeons give Lugol's iodine for 10 days after the toxic symptoms have been controlled and before surgery. The recurrent laryngeal nerves must be examined preoperatively in case of subsequent damage at operation. Prior to surgery indirect laryngoscopy should be performed to ensure that both vocal cords are moving normally.

Technique of subtotal thyroidectomy

Subtotal thyroidectomy is the operation indicated in Graves' disease. A transverse incision is made in the neck, incising skin and platysma. The skin flaps are reflected to the notch in the thyroid cartilage superiorly and the suprasternal notch inferiorly. The deep cervical fascia is divided in the midline. The strap muscles are mobilized and retracted or divided at the upper ends to maintain their nerve supply. Each lobe of the thyroid is dissected separately. The middle thyroid vein is divided. The upper pole vessels are divided individually. The recurrent laryngeal nerve is identified in the groove between trachea and oesophagus and the inferior thyroid artery ligated in continuity well lateral to it. Division of the inferior thyroid veins now allows full mobility of the thyroid lobe.

In a toxic goitre all but 10 g of the gland is removed on either side. The posterior aspect of each lobe is retained with the parathyroid glands and the raw surface sutured to the side of the trachea. The isthmus of the thyroid must also be removed, otherwise an unsightly midline enlargement may occur.

Complications

• *Haemorrhage*: Postoperatively the immediate problem may be haemorrhage, which occurs in the first 24 h after surgery and requires emergency reopening of the wound. The compression caused by the bleeding may include laryngeal oedema giving rise to stridor and dyspnoea. Treatment is by tracheal intubation with subsequent evacuation of the haematoma.

• *Nerve injury*:
(a) *Recurrent laryngeal nerve* damage occurs in about 0.2% of thyroidectomies. During surgery the recurrent laryngeal nerves should be identified and protected. Damage to the recurrent laryngeal nerve is manifested by hoarseness. It may be temporary due to neuropraxia. Teflon injection of the cord will improve the voice if the condition is permanent. Bilateral recurrent laryngeal nerve injury is a devastating complication. The patient is unable to speak and any exertion causes airway obstruction. Immediate treatment is by tracheostomy and subsequently arytenoidectomy may be performed to hold the airway open.
(b) *Superior laryngeal nerve* (external branch) damage is characterized by a loss of pitch and inability to make explosive sounds. However, it is usually transient.

• *Hypoparathyroidism*: Hypoparathyroidism occurs in about 8% of patients following thyroidectomy. The serum calcium should be checked postoperatively. If the parathyroids have been damaged, tingling sensations and carpopedal spasm are experienced at an early stage. Hypoparathyroidism usually presents within a week of surgery. Symptoms may be relieved by immediate injection of calcium gluconate and prevented by giving oral calcium 2–3 g/day. Vitamin D (calciferol 25 000–100 000 units/day) is indicated if hypocalcaemia persists in spite of calcium supplementation.

• *Hypothyroidism*: If too much thyroid glandular tissue has been removed, the patient may eventually develop hypothyroidism and this occurs in about 15% of patients. The symptoms, which include weight gain, intolerance to cold, mental deterioration and depression, are of slow onset and are not easily recognized (Table 15.1). Treatment is by maintenance dosage of T_4. If too much thyroid tissue was left behind recurrence of hyperthyroid symptoms may occur.

• *Thyrotoxic crisis*: A 'thyroid storm' is very rare nowadays due to appropriate preoperative control of toxicity. It occurs following surgery on thyrotoxic patients but other events, e.g. pneumonia, can precipitate a crisis in hyperthyroid patients. Clinically a thyroid crisis presents with pyrexia, agitation and confusion, extreme tachycardia or atrial fibrillation and profuse sweating. Treatment is aimed at rapid control of thyrotoxicosis by administration of antithyroid drugs (propylthiouracil or methimazole and iodine) and blocking the peripheral actions of the hormone by administering β-adrenergic blockade and hydrocortisone. Supportive therapy, including intravenous fluids, cooling for hyperthermia (aspirin should not be used), diuretics and digoxin for heart failure should also be instituted. Treatment is usually effective but there is a significant mortality.

Malignant exophthalmos

Control of thyrotoxicosis has no effect on exophthalmos. Malignant exophthalmos is fortunately rare. It is characterized by increased lacrimation, venous congestion and chemosis. Orbital tissue oedema occurs with ophthalmoplegia, corneal ulceration and loss of sight due to optic nerve involvement. Treatment consists of steroids and eye protection, including when necessary tarsorrhaphy to appose the lids and prevent corneal ulceration. Occasionally, surgical decompression of the orbit via a transfrontal approach may be necessary.

Tumours of the thyroid gland

Most tumours of the thyroid gland are epithelial in origin and are thus carcinomas. They are classified histologically as papillary, follicular and anaplastic carcinomas, but mixed papillary and follicular patterns are not unusual. Medullary thyroid carcinoma arises from parafollicular (C-cell) elements. Very occasionally the thyroid is the site of a metastasis or lymphoma.

Goitre at a glance

DEFINITION

- A goitre is an enlargement of the thyroid gland from any cause

CAUSES

- *Physiological* — gland increases in size as a result of increased demand for thyroid hormone at puberty and during pregnancy
- *Iodine-deficient (endemic)* — deficiency of iodine results in decreased T_4 levels and increased TSH stimulation, leading to a diffuse goitre
- *Primary hyperthyroidism* (Graves' disease) — goitre and thyrotoxicosis due to circulating immunoglobulin LATS
- *Adenomatous* (nodular) goitre — benign hyperplasia of the thyroid gland
- *Thyroiditis*
  (a) Autoimmune (Hashimoto's)
  (b) Subacute (de Quervain's)
  (c) Riedel's (struma)
- *Thyroid malignancies*

CLINICAL FEATURES

Hyperthyroidism

Symptoms
- Preference for cold
- Excessive sweating
- Increased appetite
- Weight loss, diarrhoea
- Anxiety and tiredness
- Palpitations
- Oligomenorrhoea

Signs
- Goitre
- Exophthalmos
- Lid lag and retraction
- Warm, moist palms
- Tremor
- Atrial fibrillation
- Pretibial myxoedema

Hypothyroidism

- Cold intolerance
- Decreased sweating

- Pale/yellow skin
- Periorbital puffiness

- Hoarseness
- Weight increase
- Slow cerebration
- Tiredness
- Constipation
- Muscle pains

- Loss of outer third of eyebrow
- Dry, thickened skin and hair
- Dementia, nerve deafness
- Slow pulse
- Large tongue
- Peripheral oedema

INVESTIGATION

- Ultrasound — for position of gland and to differentiate cystic from solid lesions
- Plain X-ray of thoracic outlet and chest — retrosternal goitre
- Serum tests — T_4, T_3, TSH, thyroid antibodies
- Isotope scan — identifies hot or cold nodules
- Fine-needle aspiration

MANAGEMENT

- *Physiological* — reassurance
- *Iodine-deficient (endemic)* — supplemental iodine in the diet
- *Primary hyperthyroidism* (Graves' disease)
  (a) Medical: Antithyroid drugs (carbimazole (side-effect leukopenia), propranolol); radioactive iodine (hypothyroidism is inevitable with this prescription)
  (b) Surgical: Subtotal thyroidectomy (difficult to judge how much gland should be taken, risk of nerve injury, haemorrhage and hypoparathyroidism)
- *Adenomatous* (nodular) goitre — thyroidectomy
- *Thyroiditis*
  Autoimmune (Hashimoto's) — thyroid replacement therapy
  Subacute (de Quervain's) — simple analgesia, sometimes steroids
  Riedel's (struma) — resection only for compression symptoms
- *Thyroid malignancies* — see following text

Papillary carcinoma

Papillary carcinoma is the commonest type of thyroid cancer, accounting for 60% or more of cases. This is a slow-growing tumour with a papillary structure metastasizing mainly to regional lymph nodes and found in children and young adults. There is a preponderance of female patients. The tumour is multifocal in origin and glandular metastases may be the first manifestation of the disease. More usually the presentation is of a solitary nodule in the thyroid. The patient is euthyroid and an isotope scan will identify a cold or inactive nodule, and may occasionally identify other impalpable nodules.

The standard treatment is by total thyroidectomy and removal of involved lymph nodes (although some surgeons prefer to remove only one lobe if the primary is small and there are no metastases). All patients should receive L-thyroxine to suppress TSH postoperatively as TSH stimulates the growth of both papillary and follicular carcinoma. TSH suppression is most effective in well-differentiated tumours which are most likely to be hormone-dependent but a response may also be obtained in poorly differentiated tumours. The prognosis for papillary thyroid cancer is excellent, even in the presence of lymph node metastases.

Follicular carcinoma

Follicular carcinoma comprises about 20% of all malignant thyroid lesions. This is a well-differentiated tumour which occurs in an older age group than papillary carcinoma. It is seen most frequently in middle age. The tumour is slow-growing but eventually produces distant haematogenous metastases in lungs, bone, etc. Treatment depends on the stage at which the disease is identified. If there is no evidence of distant metastases, thyroid lobectomy is adequate since the tumour is rarely multifocal. However, if distant metastases are present, total thyroidectomy is indicated, after which the distant metastases can be treated by radioactive iodine (^{131}I). Prognosis depends on the degree of vascular invasion in the primary tumour. If extensively present, the outlook falls from more than 90% 10-year survival to around 30%.

Anaplastic carcinoma

These undifferentiated tumours occur most commonly in elderly females. They represent 10% of all thyroid cancers and are very aggressive. They grow rapidly, giving rise to pressure symptoms on the trachea and oesophagus. Laryngeal nerve paralysis is common. They usually infiltrate widely outside the thyroid and, although surgical intervention may be required to relieve pressure symptoms, complete resection of the tumour is usually not possible. Radiotherapy and chemotherapy are relatively ineffective. Metastases occur in the regional lymph nodes, lungs and bone. Prognosis is dismal and the tumour usually proves fatal within 12 months of diagnosis.

Medullary carcinoma

Medullary carcinoma of the thyroid is an uncommon, slow-growing tumour of the parafollicular cells of the thyroid, accounting for less than 5% of all thyroid cancers. Parafollicular cells are derived from the embryonic neural crest and are part of the amine precursor uptake and decarboxylation (APUD) system, demonstrating an ability to synthesize amines and polypeptides. The cells secrete *calcitonin*, which may act as a tumour marker. Metastases from medullary tumours are found in lymph glands, lungs, liver and bone.

Medullary carcinoma is more common in women and is most frequently seen in the sixth decade. Both sporadic and familial forms occur. Familial tumours may be part of the multiple endocrine neoplasia (MEN) syndromes. These are MEN type IIA (medullary thyroid carcinoma, phaeochromocytoma and hyperparathyroidism) and MEN type IIB (medullary thyroid carcinoma, phaeochromocytoma, multiple mucosal neuromas, Marfanoid habitus and typical facies). Treatment of medullary thyroid carcinoma should be undertaken only after a phaeochromocytoma has been sought (24-h urinary vanillylmandelic acid (VMA) and computed tomographic (CT) scan) and treated or excluded. Treatment consists of total thyroidectomy and excision of regional lymph glands. Prognosis is slightly worse than follicular carcinoma, with an overall 5-year survival of about 50%. However, operative treatment in the absence of metastases is usually curative. Other family members should be screened for phaeochromocytoma.

Lymphoma

Lymphomas of the thyroid gland are uncommon. They are associated with Hashimoto's disease. They tend to occur in the fifth decade and are responsive to radiotherapy.

Thyroiditis

Autoimmune (Hashimoto's) thyroiditis

Hashimoto's thyroiditis is the commonest form of thyroiditis. It is familial, being found in families who have a high incidence of thyroid autoantibodies, thyroiditis and other autoimmune diseases. High levels of thyroid antibodies against thyroglobulin or thyroid cell microsomes are

Thyroid malignancies at a glance

DEFINITION

Malignant lesions of the thyroid gland

EPIDEMIOLOGY

M/F = 1 : 2 Age depends on histology (papillary, young adults; follicular, middle age; anaplastic, elderly; medullary, any age)

AETIOLOGY

Predisposing factors are:
- Pre-existing goitre
- Radiation of the neck in childhood

PATHOLOGY

Histology

Type	(% of total)	Cell of origin	Differentiation	Spread
• Papillary	(60%)	Epithelial	Well	Lymphatic
• Follicular	(25%)	Epithelial	Well	Haematogenous
• Anaplastic	(10%)	Epithelial	Poor	Direct, lymphatic and haematogenous
• Medullary	(5%)	Parafollicular	Moderate	Lymphatic and haematogenous

CLINICAL FEATURES

- Papillary: Solitary thyroid nodule
- Follicular: Slow-growing thyroid mass, symptoms from distant metastases
- Anaplastic: Rapidly growing thyroid mass causing tracheal and oesophageal compression
- Medullary: Thyroid lump, may have MEN IIA (medullary thyroid carcinoma, phaeochromocytoma, hyperparathyroidism) or IIB (medullary thyroid carcinoma, phaeochromocytoma, multiple mucosal neuromas, Marfanoid habitus) syndrome

INVESTIGATIONS

- Ultrasound of the thyroid gland
- Isotope scan — a 'cold' nodule is suspicious for malignancy
- Fine-needle aspiration — gives histological diagnosis
- Bone scan and radiographs of bones for secondary deposits
- Calcitonin levels as a marker for medullary carcinoma

MANAGEMENT

Papillary

Surgery	Total thyroidectomy and removal of involved lymph nodes
Adjunctive Rx	L-thyroxine postoperatively to suppress TSH production which stimulates papillary tumour growth
Prognosis	Excellent

Follicular

Surgery	Thyroid lobectomy or total thyroidectomy if metastases are present
Adjunctive Rx	Radioactive iodine (I^{131}) for distant metastases and L-thyroxine for replacement therapy and to suppress TSH
Prognosis	No metastases: 90% 10-year survival
	Metastases: 30% 10-year survival

Anaplastic

Surgery	Only to relieve pressure symptoms
Adjunctive Rx:	Neither radiotherapy nor chemotherapy is effective
Prognosis	Dismal: most patients will be dead within 12 months of diagnosis

Medullary

Exclude phaeochromocytoma before treating

Surgery	Total thyroidectomy and excision of regional lymph nodes
Prognosis	Overall 50% 5-year survival

present in patients with Hashimoto's thyroiditis. It usually presents in young adult females as a diffuse thyroid enlargement. The thyroid may be tender initially and there may be signs of mild hyperthyroidism in some patients. In the early stages of the disease most patients continue to be euthyroid but, gradually, hypothyroidism develops with destruction of thyroid tissue and increasing atrophy and fibrosis. Treatment is by thyroid replacement therapy, which is needed to maintain the euthyroid state.

Subacute (de Quervain's) thyroiditis

This is an uncommon condition in which the thyroid gland undergoes diffuse painful enlargement. The cause is uncertain, but is thought to be viral in origin. The onset is sudden and thyroid enlargement is often accompanied by fever, general malaise and weight loss. The gland is tender throughout and some patients develop a transient moderate hyperthyroidism. The erythrocyte sedimentation rate is elevated in the early stages of the disease. The condition may last weeks or months and may recur. Treatment consists of simple analgesia but occasionally steroids are required for symptom relief.

Riedel's (struma) thyroiditis

This very rare condition gives rise to a very hard irregular swelling of the thyroid gland with progressive fibrosis. It resembles a tumour and may produce compression symptoms. Despite the dense fibrosis, the patient may continue to be euthyroid. Resection is not normally undertaken but may be necessary if the fibrotic gland shows signs of compression.

The parathyroid glands

Introduction

Anatomy

The parathyroid glands are located on the posterior surface of the thyroid gland. There are normally four parathyroid glands, one at each upper pole and one at each lower pole of the thyroid gland (Fig. 15.1). Each gland is about 15 mm long and 3 or 4 mm wide. In 1% of patients more than four glands may be present. Aberrant location of the lower parathyroids is not uncommon and such ectopic glands may be lateral or inferior to the thyroid or may be situated retrosternally.

Physiology

The parathyroid gland secretes parathyroid hormone whose function is to regulate plasma calcium levels and influence calcium metabolism in the skeleton, kidneys and the gastrointestinal tract (Fig. 15.7). Parathyroid hormone:
• stimulates osteoclastic activity in bone with release of calcium, which passes into the circulation;
• enhances renal tubular reabsorption of calcium and inhibits reabsorption of phosphate; and
• facilitates, in conjunction with vitamin D, the absorption of calcium from the small intestine.

Calcium levels in the blood are maintained within very narrow limits (2.25–2.6 mmol/l) by the opposing actions of parathormone and calcitonin. This is a negative feedback mechanism through which rising blood calcium levels inhibit secretion of parathormone from the chief cells of the parathyroid gland. The presence of excessive amounts of parathyroid hormone causes hypercalcaemia. Some causes of hypercalcaemia are listed in Table 15.5 (see also Box 6.2 in Chapter 6).

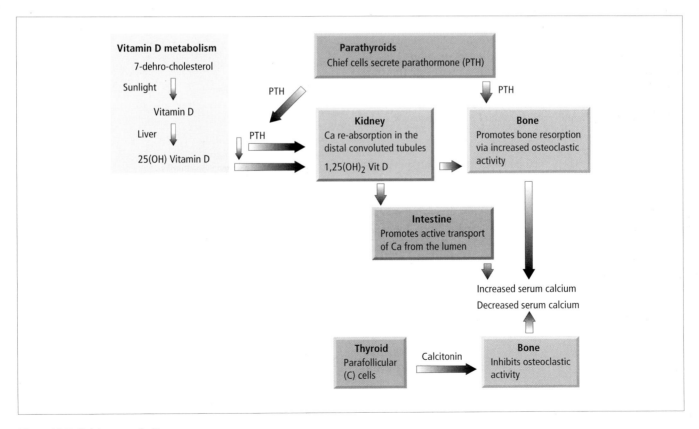

Figure 15.7 Calcium metabolism.

Table 15.5 Causes of hypercalcaemia.

Hyperparathyroidism
Bone metastases
Multiple myeloma
Paget's disease of bone
Sarcoidosis
Hypervitaminosis D
Milk alkali syndrome
Drugs (thiazides)
Hyperthyroidism

Disorders of the parathyroid glands: hyperparathyroidism

Pathology

Primary hyperparathyroidism

Primary hyperparathyroidism is due either to a tumour of the parathyroid (adenoma) or to hyperplasia of the parathyroid glands.

Parathyroid adenoma Single adenomas are the most common tumours producing hyperparathyroidism. However, multiple adenomas are present in 20% of patients. They consist of a mixture of chief cells and oxyphil cells and water-clear cells and tend to be encapsulated. The tumours secrete abnormally high amounts of parathormone with a corresponding suppression of secretion in the other parathyroids. Tumours are not usually large enough to be palpable. Malignant change is very rare.

Primary hyperplasia In primary parathyroid hyperplasia there is a general increase in the size of the parathyroids with an increase in the number of cells in each gland. Hypersecretion of parathormone occurs and the plasma calcium rises. The condition is more common in middle age and is seen more frequently in females than in males.

Secondary hyperparathyroidism

Secondary hyperparathyroidism is characterized by hyperplasia of the glands secondary to chronic renal failure. Increased parathormone production occurs in response to a low serum calcium due to decreased absorption of calcium from the gut in such patients. The impairment of calcium absorption is due to failure of the diseased renal parenchyma to convert 25 hydroxycholecalciferol to 1–25 dehydroxycholecalciferol. This stimulus to increased parathormone production is further enhanced by phosphate retention and hyperphosphataemia in the failing kidney. Serum calcium may be normal or low.

Tertiary hyperparathyroidism

In most cases, patients who undergo renal transplantation have their ability to absorb calcium restored, the serum calcium becomes normal and the parathyroid hyperplasia regresses. In some patients, however, the constant and persistent stimulus to the parathyroids renders this secretion autonomous and no longer responsive to the negative feedback stimulus of a rising serum calcium.

MEN syndromes and ectopic parathormone production

Hyperparathyroidism may be part of MEN syndromes. These are listed in Table 15.6. These endocrine abnormalities may occur sequentially rather than synchronously.

Table 15.6 The different types of multiple endocrine neoplasia (MEN).

MEN I
Islet cell tumour of pancreas
Pituitary tumour
Parathyroid hyperplasia

MEN IIA
Phaeochromocytoma
Medullary carcinoma of thyroid
Parathyroid adenoma

MEN IIB
Phaeochromocytoma
Medullary carcinoma of thyroid
Mucosal neuromas and ganglioneuromas

Oat cell tumours of the lung may secrete sufficient quantities of a parathormone-like substance to cause an increase in the serum calcium. The substance or substances involved are thought to alter the calcium levels by causing bone resorption. Prostaglandins, epidermal growth factors and other substances have been implicated.

Symptoms and signs

• *Stones, bones, abdominal groans and psychic moans!*
• Renal calculi and/or renal calcification is the most common consequence of the hypercalcaemia associated with hyperparathyroidism.

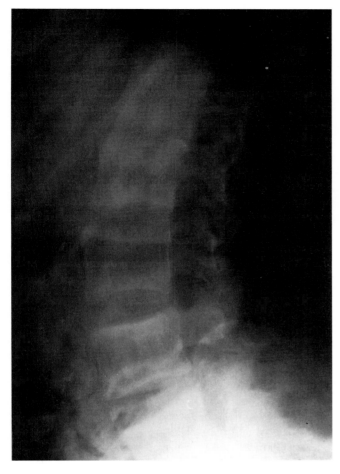

Figure 15.8 Typical appearance of the spine in a patient with hyperparathyroidism. There is resorption of bone from the vertebral bodies, producing the classic 'rugger jersey' appearance.

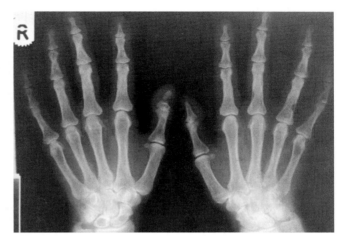

Figure 15.9 Subperiosteal erosions, scalloping of the middle phalanges and tufting of the terminal phalanges are typical X-ray features found in patients with hyperparathyroidism. Multiple cysts of the long bones (brown tumours) are also seen.

• Bone pain, sometimes manifesting itself as severe backache, is the result of decalcification of bone (Fig. 15.8).
• Severe bony deformity may be produced in young patients with secondary hyperparathyroidism and renal rickets.
• Pathological fractures may occur, especially when there is generalized cystic degeneration in the bones. The bone lesions are called either *brown tumours*, because the fibrous tissue is pigmented with haemosiderin, or *osteitis fibrosa cystica* (von Recklinghausen's disease of bone), which describes the radiological appearances of the cystic bone (Fig. 15.9). Early signs may show nothing more than subperiosteal erosions. Degeneration in a single bone may be mistaken for osteoclastoma.
• Hypercalcaemia has a direct depressive effect on nerve conduction and this is manifested clinically by muscular weakness, anorexia and intestinal atony.
• Psychiatric disorders may occur.

• Polyuria is not uncommon.
• Peptic ulcer and both acute and chronic pancreatitis are common.

Diagnosis

The history may be suggestive and radiological results may offer objective evidence but the definitive diagnosis depends on the biochemical profile. A fasting sample of blood is taken without a tourniquet with the patient at rest to measure the serum calcium. Any elevation should be confirmed on two further occasions. A raised parathormone level is also present and may continue to rise over a period of observation. Occasionally the veins draining the parathyroids are catheterized selectively and blood samples obtained for parathormone assay. This technique is sometimes useful in identifying a hyperactive gland.

Cortisone suppression test

The administration of cortisone (150 mg/day for 10 days) will restore serum calcium levels to normal in patients with sarcoidosis, thyrotoxicosis or hypervitaminosis D. It will also correct the hypercalcaemia due to the bone destruction accompanying metastatic deposits. Excessive absorption of calcium can be counteracted by giving sodium phytate, which will restore calcium levels to normal.

Imaging the parathyroids

Several techniques are available for imaging the parathyroids. These include high-resolution ultrasound, CT and magnetic resonance (MR) scanning. Dual isotope imaging using two tracers, thallium 201 to outline both thyroid and parathyroids and sodium (^{99m}Tc) pertechnetate or iodine as a subtraction marker for the thyroid, also gives useful information. Invasive procedures such as selective vein catheterization and digital subtraction arteriography are also useful in localizing parathyroids in patients in whom surgical exploration has been unsuccessful.

Treatment

Primary hyperparathyroidism is treated surgically. Tertiary hyperparathyroidism where the hyperplastic glands have become autonomous must also be treated surgically. Secondary hyperactivity can often be treated satisfactorily by vitamin D and/or calcium.

Surgery

The surgical approach is similar to that for thyroidectomy. An adenoma is present if one parathyroid gland is significantly larger than the others. However, all glands must be identified. Repeated frozen-section examination of biopsy material may be needed during the operation. If an adenoma is not identified, enough parathyroid tissue must be removed from the hyperplastic glands to restore normality but at the same time parathyroid function should be preserved. Preservation of at least 50 mg of parathyroid tissue with its blood supply is recommended.

Failure to find an adenoma or hyperplasia means that all investigations must be repeated after operation and, if positive, re-exploration must take place about 3 months after the original operation. Even though the 'second look' very often identifies an adenoma in the upper mediastinum, the cervical approach usually provides adequate access without the need for a sternum-splitting procedure.

Hypoparathyroidism

Parathyroid deficiency occurs after thyroid surgery, when the parathyroid may have been inadvertently injured or after parathyroid surgery. Transient hypoparathyroidism may occur after removal of a parathyroid adenoma until the remaining suppressed glands begin to function normally.

The fall in serum calcium increases neuromuscular excitability, giving rise to paraesthesiae around the mouth, muscular cramps and tetany. If hypoparathyroidism is suspected, Chvostek's sign and Trousseau's sign may be elicited.

Chvostek's sign

When the sign is positive, tapping over the facial nerve in front of the ear induces contractions in the facial muscles.

Trousseau's sign

This is elicited by inflating a sphygmomanometer cuff to above systolic blood pressure. After a few minutes carpal spasm occurs, producing the classic *main d'accoucheur* with apposed thumb, extended fingers flexed at the metacarpophalangeal joints and wrist flexed.

Calcium deficiency also increases electrocardiogram changes and there is prolongation of the QT interval. Parathormone levels and calcium levels will both be low. Calcium gluconate will abolish symptoms rapidly when given intravenously. Long-term treatment involves the oral administration of calcium and vitamin D.

The pituitary gland

Introduction

The pituitary gland (hypophysis), which lies in the pituitary fossa at the base of the skull, can be divided anatomically into anterior (adenohypophysis) and posterior lobes (neurohypophysis). The gland is intimately related to the optic chiasma (Fig. 15.10a). The anterior lobe produces at least seven hormones while the posterior produces two (Table 15.7). The production of most of these hormones is controlled by hypothalamic factors and feedback mechanisms from their target organs. Diseases of the pituitary are rare and are characterized by the syndromes resulting from excessive production (usually from a tumour) or lack of production (hypopituitarism) of hormones and by pressure effects on adjacent structures (especially the optic chiasma). Classically, pituitary tumours cause bitemporal hemianopia (Fig. 15.10b) and patients suspected of having pituitary tumours should have their visual fields plotted (perimetry). Headaches are also characteristic.

The pituitary gland can be imaged by plain radiography, CT or MR scanning and the various hormones can be assayed to measure serum levels.

Disorders of the pituitary gland (see Table 15.8)

Panhypopituitarism (Simmond's disease)

Any process that destroys pituitary tissue may cause hypopituitarism, e.g. pressure from a tumour, infection, ischaemia. A specific cause of hypopituitarism is postpartum shock-induced infarction of the anterior pituitary gland (Sheehan's syndrome) which is now, thankfully, rare. The clinical features depend on which hormones are affected but often all are decreased or absent. Thus the patient may be pale (melanocyte-stimulating hormone; MSH), hypothyroid (TSH), fail to lactate (prolactin; PL), have chronic

Parathyroid disease at a glance

HYPERPARATHYROIDISM

Definition
Hyperparathyroidism is a condition characterized by hypercalcaemia caused by excess production of parathyroid hormone

Causes
- *Primary* hyperparathyroidism is due to a parathyroid adenoma or parathyroid hyperplasia
- *Secondary* hyperparathyroidism is hyperplasia of the gland in response to *hypo*calcaemia (e.g. in chronic renal failure there is failure of conversion of 25-hydroxycholecalciferol to 1-25 dehydroxycholecalciferol, resulting in impaired calcium absorption)
- In *tertiary* hyperparathyroidism autonomous secretion of parathormone occurs when the secondary stimulus has been removed (e.g. after renal transplantation)
- *MEN syndromes* and *ectopic* parathormone production (e.g. oat cell carcinoma of the lung)

Pathology
Parathormone mobilizes calcium from bone, enhances renal tubular absorption and, with vitamin D, intestinal absorption of calcium. The net result is *hypercalcaemia*

Clinical features
- Renal calculi or renal calcification, polyuria
- Bone pain, bone deformity, osteitis fibrosa cystica, pathological fractures
- Muscle weakness, anorexia, intestinal atony, psychosis
- Peptic ulceration and pancreatitis

Diagnosis
- Serum calcium (specimen taken on three occasions with patient fasting, at rest and without a tourniquet). Normal range 2.2–2.6 mmol/l. Calcium is bound to albumin and the level has to be corrected when albumin levels are abnormal
- Parathormone level
- Imaging:
  (a) High-resolution ultrasound
  (b) CT and MR scanning
  (c) Dual isotope imaging (thallium 201 and Na^{99m} Tc pertechnetate)
- Selective vein catheterization and digital subtraction angiography in patients in whom exploration has been unsuccessful

Treatment
- Primary and tertiary hyperparathyroidism are treated surgically. Excise adenoma if present; remove $3\frac{1}{2}$ glands for hyperplasia
- Secondary hyperplasia — vitamin D and/or calcium

HYPOPARATHYROIDISM

Definition
A rare condition characterized by hypocalcaemia due to reduced production of parathormone

Causes
- Postthyroid or parathyroid surgery
- Idiopathic
- Pseudohypoparathyroidism (reduced sensitivity to parathormone)

Pathology
- Reduced calcium increases neuromuscular excitability

Clinical features
- Perioral paraesthesia, cramps, tetany
- *Chvostek's sign:* tapping over facial nerve induces facial muscle contractions
- *Trousseau's sign:* inflating blood pressure cuff to above systolic pressure induces typical *main d'accoucheur* carpal spasm
- Prolonged QT interval on ECG

Diagnosis
- Calcium and parathormone levels decreased

Treatment
- Calcium and vitamin D

Table 15.7 The hormones of the pituitary gland and some disease states associated with them.

Pituitary hormones	Pathology	Clinical features
Anterior		
Prolactin (PL)	Prolactinoma	*Female*: galactorrhoea, amenorrhoea, infertility
		Male: impotence, galactorrhoea, gynaecomastia
Growth hormone (GH)	GH tumours	Acromegaly
Adrenocorticotrophic hormone (ACTH)	ACTH tumours	Cushing's disease
Follicle-stimulating hormone (FSH)		
Luteinizing hormone (LH)	'Gonadotrophinoma'	Panhypopituitarism and retained libido
Thyroid-stimulating hormone (TSH)	TSHoma	Mild thyrotoxicosis
Melanocyte-stimulating hormone (MSH)		
Posterior		
Antidiuretic hormone (ADH; vasopressin)	Absence of ADH	Diabetes insipidus
Oxytocin		

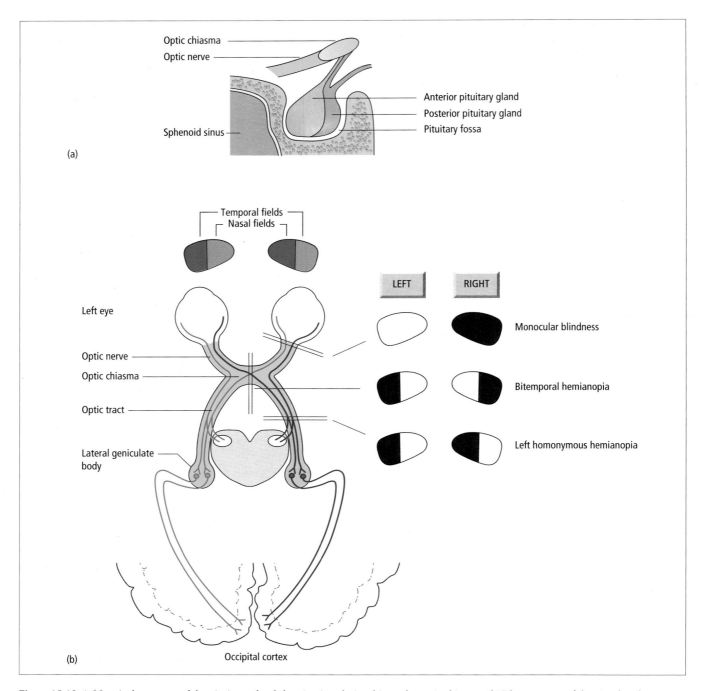

Figure 15.10 (a) Surgical anatomy of the pituitary gland showing its relationship to the optic chiasma. (b) The anatomy of the visual pathway showing how lesions at different points along the pathway produce different eye signs. Classically, pituitary lesions which affect the optic chiasma cause bitemporal hemianopia.

adrenal insufficiency (adrenocorticotrophic hormone; ACTH) and ovarian failure with amenorrhoea (follicle-stimulating hormone (FSH), luteinizing hormone (LH)). Diagnosis is by serum assay of the pituitary and target organ hormones and by dynamic tests of hypothalamic–pituitary function. Treatment is by replacement therapy: cyclical oestrogen–progesterone, hydrocortisone and T_4.

Tumours of the pituitary gland

All tumours of the pituitary gland are uncommon, accounting for only 8% of all intracranial tumours. They are usually adenomas, may be endocrinologically active or inactive and cause symptoms by pressure effects. The commonest pituitary tumours are:
- Endocrinologically active (75%):
  (a) Prolactinomas (35%) — cell type: acidophil;
  (b) GH-secreting tumours (20%) — cell type: acidophil;
  (c) Mixed PL and GH (10%) — cell type: acidophil;
  (d) ACTH-secreting tumours (10%) — cell type: basophil (causes Cushing's disease);
- Endocrinologically inactive (25%) — chromophobe;
- Craniopharyngioma — Rathke's pouch.

Diagnosis is made by a combination of clinical suspicion (e.g. presentation of bitemporal hemianopia), hormone assay and imaging by CT or MR scanning of the pituitary gland. A variety of treatments is available, including bromocriptine, yttrium 90 implantation and surgery. Surgery is now less commonly performed for pituitary tumours because *prolactin-secreting tumours can be controlled with bromocriptine*. The transphenoidal route is the fashionable approach to the gland, but if the optic nerves are compressed the transcranial route is still used.

Acromegaly

Excess growth hormone causes acromegaly in adults and giantism in children by its action on the long bones before the epiphyses have fused. The usual cause is an acidophilic adenoma of the pituitary. The clinical picture results from the action of growth hormone on skin, tongue, viscera and bones. Patients may also be diabetic because of the anti-insulin effects of growth hormone (Fig. 15.11).

The clinical features of acromegaly are:
- thickened skin (hypertrophy of sebaceous and sweat glands);
- acromegalic facies: increased size of skull, prognathism;
- enlarged tongue;
- goitre;
- osteoporosis causing kyphosis;

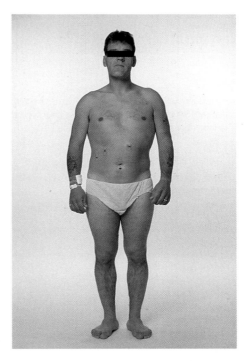

Figure 15.11 A patient with acromegaly. Note the recent scars from laparoscopic cholecystectomy.

- barrel chest;
- cardiomegaly (hypertension);
- hepatomegaly;
- enlarged (spade-like) hands and feet, carpal tunnel syndrome;
- degenerative arthritis;
- male sexual dysfunction; and
- menstrual irregularities in women.

Treatment is by ablation of the growth hormone-producing tissue, i.e. hypophysectomy. This has been largely replaced by somatostatin therapy.

Diabetes insipidus

Diabetes insipidus is a rare condition with many causes, including trauma (accidental or surgical) to the neurohypophysis, localized haemorrhage or ischaemia, and tumours. The production of antidiuretic hormone (ADH) by the posterior pituitary is thus prevented. ADH normally promotes water resorption in the distal tubules and collecting ducts of the kidney and its absence results in huge daily water losses (5–20 l), characterized by polyuria and polydipsia, i.e. diabetes insipidus. A very low urinary specific gravity which fails to increase with water deprivation confirms the diagnosis. Treatment is with the vasopressin analogue *desmopressin* administered as a nasal spray.

Pituitary disorders at a glance

DEFINITION

Pituitary disorders are characterized by either a *failure of secretion* of pituitary hormones or *tumours*, which cause local pressure effects or specific syndromes due to hormone overproduction

CAUSES

- Failure of secretion, panhypopituitarism (Simmond's disease)
  (a) Pressure from a tumour, infection, ischaemia
  (b) Postpartum-induced infarction of the anterior pituitary (Sheehan's syndrome)
- Failure of antidiuretic hormone production from the posterior pituitary gland leads to diabetes insipidus
  (a) Trauma, local haemorrhage, ischaemia, tumours
- **Tumours (% of total)**   **Cell type**
  Endocrinologically active (75%)
    Prolactinomas (35%)   Acidophil
    Growth hormone (GH)-secreting tumours (20%)   Acidophil
    Mixed PL and GH (10%)   Acidophil
    ACTH-secreting tumours (10%)   Basophil
  Endocrinologically inactive (25%)   Chromophobe
  Craniopharyngioma   Rathke's pouch

CLINICAL FEATURES

- Panhypopituitarism: pallor (MSH), hypothyroid (TSH), failure of lactation (PL), chronic adrenal insufficiency (ACTH), ovarian failure and amenorrhoea (FSH, LH)
- Diabetes insipidus: polyuria (5–20 litres/day), polydipsia
- Tumours

Pressure effects: headache, bitemporal hemianopia
Specific syndromes:
(a) *Acromegaly* (excess GH): Thickened skin, increased skull size, prognathism, enlarged tongue, goitre, osteoporosis, organomegaly, spade-like hands and feet
(b) *Cushing's disease* (excess ACTH): Malaise, muscle weakness, weight gain, bruising, moon facies, buffalo hump, hirsutism, amenorrhoea, impotence, polyuria, diabetes, emotional instability

INVESTIGATIONS

- Panhypopituitarism
  (a) Serum assay of pituitary and target gland hormones
  (b) Dynamic tests of pituitary function
- Diabetes insipidus: very low urinary specific gravity which does not increase with water deprivation
- Tumours
  (a) Visual field measurements
  (b) Hormone assay
  (c) CT or MR scanning

MANAGEMENT

- Panhypopituitarism: replacement therapy: cyclical oestrogen–progesterone, hydrocortisone, thyroxine
- Diabetes insipidus: vasopressin analogue, *desmopressin*, administered as nasal spray
- Tumours: bromocriptine suppresses PL release from prolactinomas, yttrium 90 implant for pituitary ablation, surgery (hypophysectomy via nasal or transcranial route), somatostatin for acromegaly.

The adrenal glands

Introduction

The adrenal glands are located at the upper poles of the right and left kidneys and are adjacent to the inferior vena cava and the aorta (Fig. 15.12). The arterial supply is derived from small branches of the aorta, renal arteries and phrenic arteries. The venous drainage is of more importance surgically because of the large calibre of the vessels with consequent potential for serious bleeding. The right adrenal vein drains directly into the inferior vena cava and the left drains into the left renal vein.

The adrenal glands are composite glands with a cortex made up of three different functional zones and a medulla whose functional role is quite separate and distinct. The cortex is derived from the embryonic mesoderm while the medulla arises from the ectoderm of the neural crest. The adrenal cortex has three zones, which are from without inwards:

- zona glomerulosa — produces aldosterone;
- zona fasciculata — produces cortisol;
- zona reticularis — produces adrenal androgen and oestrogen.

The adrenal medulla is part of the APUD system, indicating an ability to synthesize amines and polypeptides. Adrenaline and noradrenaline are the two hormones produced by the adrenal medulla.

Disorders of the adrenal cortex

Cushing's syndrome

Aetiology

Cushing's syndrome is the result of excess corticosteroid. The causes of Cushing's syndrome are:

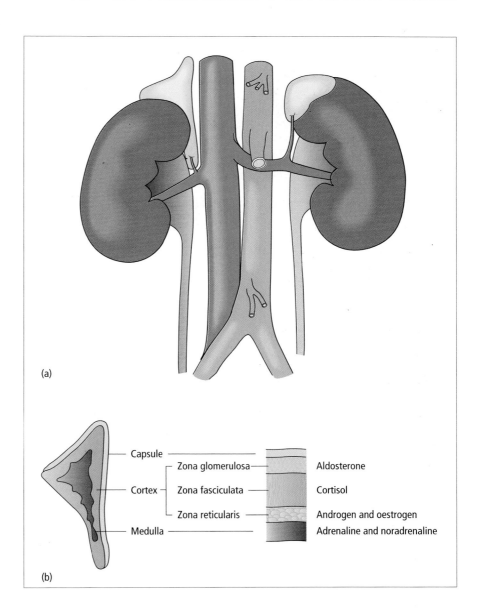

(a)

(b)

Capsule

Cortex — Zona glomerulosa —————— Aldosterone

Zona fasciculata —————— Cortisol

Zona reticularis —————— Androgen and oestrogen

Medulla —————————— Adrenaline and noradrenaline

Figure 15.12 (a) Surgical anatomy of the adrenal glands showing their position in relation to the kidneys and (b) the various zones of the gland.

• prolonged or excessive steroid therapy (probably the commonest cause);
• an ACTH-producing tumour of the pituitary gland or Cushing's disease (see above);
• adenoma or carcinoma of the adrenal cortex or adrenal cortical hyperplasia; and
• ectopic ACTH production from a tumour outside the adrenal–pituitary axis, e.g. oat cell bronchial carcinoma.

Clinical features and diagnosis

Patients with Cushing's syndrome complain of malaise, muscular weakness, bruising and weight gain. The physical signs are characteristic with moon facies (Fig. 15.13), cutaneous striae, dorsal fat pad (buffalo hump), supraclavicular fat pads, hirsutism and acne, muscle wasting and bruising. Female patients experience amenorrhoea and males may become impotent; headache is common and polyuria and diabetes occur. Patients develop hypertension but this tends to be moderate. Emotional instability is common.

Elevation of plasma cortisol and loss of the normal diurnal variation in cortisol level is helpful but there are many false-negative and false-positive results.
• Urinary cortisol levels are elevated in Cushing's syndrome and there are few misleading results.

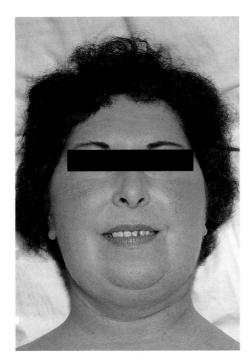

Figure 15.13 Typical moon facies of a patient with Cushing's syndrome.

• The dexamethasone suppression test is used to distinguish between pituitary and adrenal disease. Daily dosage of 8 mg of dexamethasone for 48 h will cause a 50% or more reduction in plasma and urinary cortisol levels in patients whose symptoms are due to an adrenal tumour or ectopic ACTH secretion.

• Assay of immunoreactive ACTH is useful in distinguishing between an adrenal origin for the syndrome (ACTH levels are very low), a pituitary origin (moderate elevation) or non-endocrine tumour (plasma ACTH levels are very high).

• Tomography of the sella turcica and visual field measurements are done if a pituitary tumour is suspected. Localization of suspected adrenal tumour is by ultrasound and CT scan.

Treatment

Treatment of Cushing's syndrome depends on the cause.

• If a *pituitary adenoma* is responsible for Cushing's syndrome, then treatment is by pituitary ablation (see above). This may be achieved by transsphenoidal hypophysectomy, microdissection of a pituitary adenoma, cryosurgery or irradiation of the pituitary. Irradiation may be by external-beam irradiation or the implantation of radioactive yttrium

or gold. (In the past, bilateral adrenalectomy was the major form of treatment for Cushing's disease (i.e pituitary adenoma) but it was associated with a 5–10% mortality and considerable morbidity; it made the patient dependent on steroid replacement therapy and induced Nelson's syndrome (rapid enlargement of a pituitary microadenoma into a fast-growing aggressive pituitary tumour with encroachment on the optic chiasma) in 10% of patients.)

• *Adrenal adenoma* is treated by unilateral adrenalectomy with excellent results.

• *Adrenal carcinoma* has a poor prognosis (median survival 4 years) as metastases are usually present by the time the diagnosis is made. Surgery is indicated to debulk the tumour and thereby reduce corticosteroid production. The tumours are not radiosensitive and chemotherapy has little to offer, although *mitotane*, a mitochondrial poison, is used to reduce cortisol secretion in patients with metastases.

• The management of an *ectopic ACTH-secreting* tumour is resection of the tumour when possible, e.g. carcinoid tumour. However, it is often due to an inoperable carcinoma of the bronchus (see Chapter 19) and in this situation inhibitors of adrenal enzyme synthesis (e.g. metyrapone and ketoconazole) are the treatments of choice.

Primary hyperaldosteronism (Conn's syndrome)

Introduction

Primary hyperaldosteronism is responsible for the elevated blood pressure in 1% of hypertensives. The condition is due to a benign adrenocortical adenoma or, more rarely, bilateral cortical hyperplasia. Very rarely, a carcinoma of the adrenal gland may be responsible. The hyperplasia occurs in the zona glomerulosa of the cortex, although the adenoma contains cells resembling both glomerulosa and reticularis-type cells. The condition must be distinguished from secondary hyperaldosteronism with high renin levels, sodium depletion and renal disease. Hypokalaemia accompanies the hypertension and patients may have hypokalaemic alkalosis. The plasma sodium may be normal or elevated and renin levels are low.

Clinical features and diagnosis

Patients present with hypertension and complain of muscle weakness and tetany. They are affected by thirst, nocturia and polyuria. These are all features of the hypokalaemic alkalosis.

The presence of hypertension with low potassium and normal or high sodium suggests Conn's syndrome, especially if renin levels are low. These biochemical parameters can be affected by a number of drugs, including carbenoxolone, oral contraceptives, methyldopa or β-adrenergic blockade. Biochemical confirmation, therefore, must await a 4-week period of normal sodium and potassium intake, without the drugs listed above. Plasma levels of aldosterone and renin may be measured directly.

Direct sampling of adrenal vein blood to assess aldosterone levels may be necessary to localize a tumour. Aldosterone levels from the side with a tumour are three times higher than normal. More indirect methods of identifying tumour are arteriography, venography, scintigraphy, ultrasonography and CT scan.

Treatment

• *Adenoma*: Adrenalectomy is the definitive treatment for an adrenal adenoma and the result is usually very satisfactory.
• *Carcinoma*: Surgical removal is also indicated for a carcinoma but the prognosis is poor.
• *Bilateral hyperplasia*: There is controversy about the most appropriate treatment for patients with bilateral hyperplasia. Initially, spironolactone or amiloride is used and if the response is satisfactory and side-effects are tolerable, this treatment should be continued. If not, resection should be undertaken with either subtotal adrenalectomy or total adrenalectomy with replacement therapy. If adrenalectomy is to be undertaken, preoperative treatment with spironolactone or amiloride should be given in order to control the blood pressure and correct electrolyte abnormalities.

Adrenogenital syndrome

In this congenital condition there is a partial or complete absence of enzymes involved in the synthesis of cortisol and aldosterone. As a result, excess ACTH production gives rise to adrenal cortical hyperplasia. This may or may not boost the production of cortisol but will cause excess androgen production.

The clinical conditions produced are virilization in female children and precocious puberty or feminization in boys. Glucocorticoid and mineralocorticoid deficiency may be present and the salt-losing syndrome is potentially fatal. Hypertension may occur and patients are of low stature because of early epiphyseal closure.

Pseudohermaphroditism may give rise to clitoral enlargement and fused labia in girls, cleft scrotum and hypospadias in boys; penile enlargement may also occur in male children. Both sexes undergo premature puberty. Treatment with cortisol will suppress the ACTH-stimulated secretion of androgens and supply corticosteroids. Surgery may be required for correction of abnormalities of the external genitalia. Steroids should be given preoperatively. Fluid,

electrolytes and steroids are needed in the salt-losing syndrome.

Adrenal insufficiency (Addison's disease)

• *Acute adrenal insufficiency* may be precipitated *de novo* or may be due to the stress of a surgical operation or an infection in patients suffering from chronic adrenal insufficiency. The latter is the most common. Primary adrenal failure arising *de novo* may be due to bilateral adrenal haemorrhage in association with severe sepsis (Waterhouse–Friderichsen syndrome). This is particularly prone to occur in children with meningococcal septicaemia. Haemorrhage related to anticoagulation is a rare cause, as is adrenal vein thrombosis. Bilateral adrenalectomy without replacement therapy may occur inadvertently when one adrenal is removed when the other is already destroyed by tumour or other disease.
• Formerly the *chronic adrenal insufficiency* of Addison's disease was largely due to tuberculosis. Currently autoimmune disease of the adrenal accounts for 70% of cases with about 25% being due to tuberculosis. Metastatic deposits, amyloidosis and damage from drugs account for many of the remainder.
• *Secondary adrenal failure* is caused by pituitary insufficiency either due to tumour or infarction as in Sheehan's syndrome (see above). It may also be due to granulomatous disease or to prolonged treatment with corticosteroids which suppress the production of ACTH.

Clinical features and diagnosis

Lethargy, weakness, nausea and vomiting, anorexia and weight loss are all chronic symptoms. Pigmentation may occur, particularly in pressure areas. Dizziness, hypotension and fainting are frequent. An acute Addisonian crisis may present like an acute abdominal emergency with rigidity, vomiting, hypotension and collapse. If it is mistaken for a surgical condition and operation is undertaken the result is fatal.

Low plasma sodium levels are frequently seen. Low plasma cortisol levels with high ACTH levels suggest primary adrenal insufficiency. Low plasma cortisol levels and low ACTH levels suggest secondary adrenal failure. The tetracosactrin (Synacthen) tests are used to differentiate between primary and secondary adrenal insufficiency.

Treatment

Maintenance therapy with cortisol 20 mg in the morning and 10 mg at night and fludrocortisone 0.1 mg daily is usually sufficient. This replacement therapy is permanent and should be increased in stressful situations. All surgical procedures, however minor, require substantially increased dosage of steroids preoperatively, during operation and postoperatively. In acute adrenal crises intravenous hydrocortisone, intravenous saline and glucose are required.

Disorders of the adrenal medulla

Phaeochromocytoma

Phaeochromocytomas are rare tumours composed of chromaffin cells derived from sympathetic nervous tissue.

Nine-tenths of these tumours occur in the adrenal medulla. The remainder may arise anywhere in the sympathetic chain from neck to pelvis. Phaeochromocytoma is of clinical importance because it induces hypertension which, if not treated, invariably causes death due to stroke, myocardial infarction, cardiac arrhythmias or congestive cardiac failure. Functioning phaeochromocytomas produce excessive amounts of catecholamines. While adrenal medullary tumours produce both adrenaline and noradrenaline, extramedullary tumours (called paragangliomas) produce noradrenaline only.

Table 15.8 Eponyms associated with endocrine dysfunction.

Name	Dates	Pathology	Eponym
Thyroid			
Robert Graves, Dublin	1796–1853	Autoimmune thyrotoxicosis	Graves' disease
Carl von Basedow, Merseburg	1799–1854	Autoimmune thyrotoxicosis	Basedow's disease
Henry Plummer, Rochester	1874–1937	Thyrotoxicosis with multinodular goitre	Plummer's disease
Hakaru Hashimoto, Mie	1881–1934	Autoimmune thyroiditis	Hashimoto's thyroiditis
Fritz de Quervain, Berne	1868–1940	Subacute thyroiditis	de Quervain's thyroiditis
Bernhard Riedel, Jena	1846–1916	Thyroiditis	Riedel's struma
Hugh Pemberton, England	1891–1956	Venous congestion of face and neck on arm elevation	Pemberton's sign
Vaughan Pendred, Surrey	1896–1946	Congenital goitre, hypothyroidism and nerve deafness	Pendred's syndrome
Parathyroid			
Friedrich von Recklinghausen, Strasbourg	1833–1910	Cystic bone disease in hyperparathyroidism	von Recklinghausen's disease of bone
Frantisek Chvostek, Vienna	1835–1884	Tapping over the facial nerve induces facial muscle contractions	Chvostek's sign
Armand Trousseau, Paris	1801–1867	Ischaemia induces carpal spasm	*Trousseau's sign*
Pituitary			
Morris Simmonds, Hamburg	1855–1925	Panhypopituitarism	Simmond's disease
Harold Sheehan, Liverpool	b.1900	Hypopituitarism following postpartum haemorrhage	Sheehan's syndrome
Harvey Cushing, Boston	1869–1939	Excess glucocorticoid production secondary to ACTH-producing pituitary adenoma	Cushing's disease
Warren Nelson, USA	1906–1964	Rapid enlargement of a pituitary adenoma following bilateral adrenalectomy	Nelson's syndrome
Adrenal			
Harvey Cushing, Boston	1869–1939	Excess glucocorticoid production for any reason	Cushing's syndrome
Jerome Conn, Ann Arbor	b.1907	Primary hyperaldosteronism	Conn's syndrome
Thomas Addison, London	1793–1860	Adrenal insufficiency	*Addison's disease*
Rupert Waterhouse, Bath Carl Friderichsen, Copenhagen	1873–1958 b.1886	Acute adrenal insufficiency due to adrenal cortical haemorrhage	Waterhouse–Friderichsen syndrome

The majority of tumours are benign but about 5% are malignant and these tend to be bilateral. The tumour may have a familial tendency. Because of its neuroectodermal origin it may be associated with other lesions of neuroectodermal origin such as acoustic neuroma, meningioma, glioma and neurofibromatosis. Its association as a familial bilateral tumour with medullary carcinoma of the thyroid and parathyroid adenoma has been mentioned earlier in this chapter.

Clinical features and diagnosis

Hypertension, either paroxysmal or sustained, is present. The paroxysmal attacks are accompanied by palpitation, tremor, flushing or pallor and sweating. The patient experiences acute anxiety. Other symptoms include headache, nausea, vomiting, chest pain, diarrhoea and weight loss.

Twenty-four-hour urinary estimations of dopamine, adrenaline, noradrenaline and VMA are carried out. The

Adrenal disorders at a glance

DEFINITION

Adrenal gland disorders are characterized by clinical syndromes resulting from either a *failure of secretion* or *excessive secretion* of adrenal cortical or medullary hormones

CAUSES

- Failure of secretion of adrenocortical hormones
  - (a) *Adrenal insufficiency, Addison's disease*: bilateral adrenal haemorrhage in sepsis (Waterhouse–Friderichsen syndrome), autoimmune disease, TB, pituitary insufficiency, metastatic deposits
- Excessive secretion
  - (a) *Cushing's syndrome* — excess corticosteroid: steroid therapy, ACTH-producing pituitary tumour, adenoma or carcinoma of the adrenal cortex, ectopic ACTH production, e.g. oat cell carcinoma of lung
  - (b) *Conn's syndrome, primary hyperaldosteronism* — excess aldosterone: adenoma or carcinoma of adrenal cortex, bilateral cortical hyperplasia
  - (c) *Adrenogenital syndrome* — excess androgen: abnormal cortisol synthesis causes excess ACTH production which boosts androgen production, adrenal cortical tumour
  - (d) *Phaeochromocytoma* — excess catecholamines: adrenal medullary tumours, 95% are benign

CLINICAL FEATURES

Adrenal insufficiency, Addison's disease
Lethargy, weakness, nausea, vomiting, weight loss, skin pigmentation, dizziness, hypotension. Addisonian crisis: an acute collapse which may mimic an abdominal emergency

Cushing's syndrome
Malaise, muscle weakness, weight gain, bruising, moon facies, buffalo hump, hirsutism, amenorrhoea, impotence, polyuria, diabetes, emotional instability

Conn's syndrome, primary hyperaldosteronism
Muscle weakness, tetany, polyuria, polydipsia, hypertension

Adrenogenital syndrome
Virilization in female children, pseudohermaphroditism, precocious puberty

Phaeochromocytoma
Paroxysmal hypertension, palpitations, tremor, flushing or pallor, sweating, anxiety

INVESTIGATIONS

Adrenal insufficiency, Addison's disease
Low sodium, low plasma cortisol, Synacthen test to differentiate primary (adrenal) from secondary (pituitary) insufficiency

Cushing's syndrome
Elevated plasma cortisol and loss of diurnal variation; dexamethasone suppression test to distinguish adrenal from pituitary disease

Conn's syndrome, primary hyperaldosteronism
Low K^+, normal or high Na^+, raised aldosterone and normal renin levels

Adrenogenital syndrome
Elevated urinary 17-ketosteroids

Phaeochromocytoma
24-hour urinary VMA, dopamine, adrenaline and noradrenaline

- Imaging of the adrenal gland is achieved with US and CT scanning Arteriography and venous sampling may also be required

MANAGEMENT

Adrenal insufficiency
Replacement therapy. Cortisol 20 mg mane, 10 mg nocte, fludrocortisone 0.1 mg daily. Increase dose at times of stress

Cushing's syndrome
Adrenalectomy for adenoma and to debulk carcinoma. Mitotane reduces steroid production in metastases

Conn's syndrome
Adrenalectomy for adenoma and carcinoma. Spironolactone or amiloride for hyperplasia. If poor response, subtotal adrenalectomy or total adrenalectomy with replacement therapy

Adrenogenital syndrome
Cortisol to suppress ACTH and provide corticosteroids. Surgery to correct abnormalities of external genitalia

Phaeochromocytoma
Surgery under α- and β-adrenergic blockade

urinary collections are more reliable when taken during symptomatic episodes or when blood pressure is elevated. CT scanning, ultrasonography and ^{131}MIBG isotope scanning are the best means to localize the tumour.

Treatment

α- and β-adrenoceptor blockade with the drugs *phenoxybenzamine* (α-blocker) and *propranolol* (β-blocker) is used to control the blood pressure and prevent arrhythmias during investigations such as angiography and while waiting for surgery. Anaesthetic agents should be chosen with care. Nitrous oxide, isoflurane and enflurane are suitable; halothane is not. *Phentolamine* (short-acting α-blocker) and propranolol are used throughout surgery with careful monitoring of pulse and blood pressure. The tumour should be handled as little as possible to minimize catecholamine release. When the tumour is removed, large volumes of plasma and plasma substitutes are needed to maintain the blood pressure. Operative mortality has improved dramatically from about 20% in the early 1950s to less than 2% now. The prognosis for benign phaeochromocytoma is excellent, with 96% 5-year survival after resection. This falls to 44% for malignant lesions.

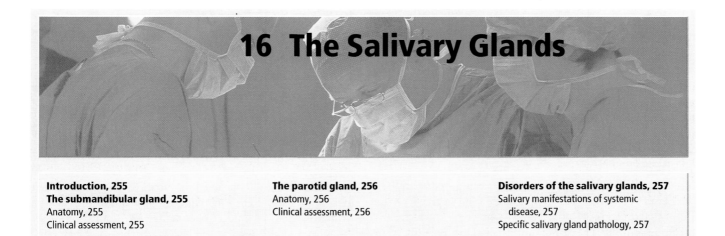

16 The Salivary Glands

Introduction

The salivary tissues comprise the paired parotid, sub-mandibular and sublingual glands as well as tiny accessory salivary glands scattered over the buccal membrane. The normal function of the salivary glands is to produce saliva. Approximately 1500 ml of saliva is produced each day. Saliva has several important physiological functions.
- It facilitates swallowing.
- It keeps the mouth moist and aids speech.
- It serves as a solvent for molecules which stimulate the taste buds.
- It cleanses the mouth, gums and teeth.
- It contains an enzyme, ptyalin, which breaks down starch.

The glands most often involved by a pathological process are the submandibular and the parotid glands. Rarely do the sublingual glands or the accessory glands cause trouble.

The submandibular gland

Anatomy

The submandibular gland, which is about the size of a walnut, lies beneath and in front of the angle of the jaw. The gland envelops the posterior margin of the myelohyoid muscle which separates it into a superficial and a deep part. The sub-mandibular duct (Wharton's duct) passes forwards for 5 cm from the deep part of the gland to the floor of the mouth where it has its orifice just lateral to the frenulum of the tongue (Fig. 16.1). Most of the problems with the submandibular gland arise because the duct becomes obstructed.

Clinical assessment

Symptoms

The symptom of submandibular pathology is a history of swelling beneath and in front of the angle of the jaw, usually

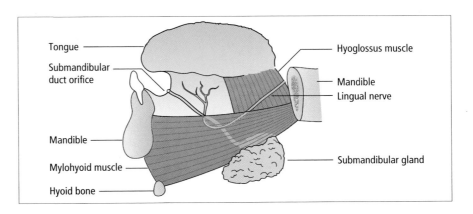

Figure 16.1 Surgical anatomy of the submandibular gland.

associated with pain. A history that the pain and swelling are induced or exacerbated by eating is indicative of sub-mandibular duct obstruction.

Physical examination

Normally the submandibular gland is not palpable. When the gland is enlarged it is palpable 2–3 cm in front of the sternomastoid muscle just beneath the horizontal ramus of the mandible. The submandibular gland is rubbery in consistence and should not be confused with enlarged cervical lymph nodes. Inspection of the orifice of the duct is mandatory when examining the submandibular gland. The orifices of both ducts should be inspected with the aid of a torch. The patient opens the mouth and lifts the tongue to the roof of the mouth, thus displaying the orifices of the two ducts on either side of the frenulum of the tongue. The presence of inflammation or a bead of pus at the orifice should be noted and sometimes a bulge indicating the presence of a stone in the duct may be seen in the floor of the mouth. Finally, bimanual palpation of the gland and duct should be performed. Submandibular swellings should be palpable between the index finger of one hand inside the mouth and the fingers of the other hand over the outer surface of the lump in the neck. Finally the duct should be palpated for the presence of a stone.

Investigations

Generally a plain radiograph of the jaw area is all that is required to demonstrate a calculus, which is invariably radiopaque, in the submandibular duct.

The parotid gland

Anatomy

The parotid gland is an irregular structure which lies *below* the external auditory meatus between the vertical ramus of the mandible and the mastoid process. Swellings of the parotid are seen in this area and not in front of the ear — a common mistake made by students. The confusion arises because a small portion of the gland (the accessory part) projects forwards on to the masseter muscle but the bulk of the gland lies deep in the space between the mandible and the mastoid. The 5 cm long parotid duct passes forwards from the gland across the masseter muscle (where it may be palpated) to gain entry to the mouth via a small papilla on the buccal membrane opposite the crown of the second upper molar tooth. An important anatomical feature of the parotid gland is that the facial nerve passes through the gland and divides into its branches as it does so (Fig. 16.2).

Clinical assessment

Symptoms

The symptoms of parotid disease are a history of swelling of the gland which may or may not be associated with pain, depending on the underlying pathology.

Physical examination

Examination of the parotid consists of inspection and palpation of the swelling. If the patient has parotitis then

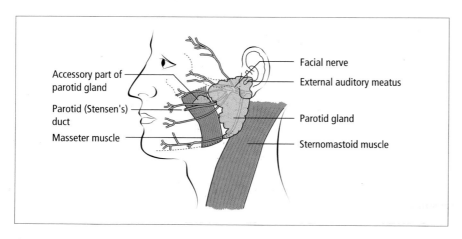

Figure 16.2 Surgical anatomy of the parotid gland.

the signs of inflammation will be present. Tumours present as painless swellings. The anterior part of the parotid duct can be palpated as it crosses the anterior border of the masseter muscle one finger-breadth below the inferior border of the zygomatic bone. Rarely, a calculus may be palpated in this part of the duct. The orifice of the duct in the mouth (opposite the second upper molar) should also be inspected by retracting the cheek with a spatula. Pressure applied to the body of the gland may cause a bead of pus to appear at the orifice in patients with parotitis.

Investigations

Baseline haematological and biochemical investigations are indicated if salivary pathology is part of a systemic disease, such as Sjögren's syndrome, sarcoidosis or leukaemia, and more specific investigations may be required depending on the nature of the systemic problem. Imaging of the parotid (and occasionally the submandibular) ducts can be performed by *sialography*, i.e. introducing a small catheter into the orifice of the duct and injecting a small volume of contrast. In this way obstructions, dilations and narrowings of the duct may be demonstrated. It is particularly useful in the diagnosis of sialectasis (see below).

Disorders of the salivary glands

Salivary manifestations of systemic disease

Xerostomia

Xerostomia is defined as decreased salivary flow and it may result from many causes. These include mumps, Sjögren's syndrome, sarcoidosis, radiation-induced atrophy (e.g. following radiation therapy to oral cancer) and drugs (antihistamines, phenothiazines, atropine).

Sialorrhoea

Sialorrhoea is defined as increased salivary flow and is associated with many conditions: aphthous stomatitis, rabies, mental retardation, unrelieved oesophageal obstruction.

Specific salivary gland pathology

Salivary calculi

Sialolithiasis is common in the submandibular gland and Wharton's duct and more rarely in the parotid gland. The aetiology of salivary stones is unknown but some have been found in association with a foreign body and toothpaste has been offered as an aetiological factor in this situation. The stones are composed of mucus, cellular debris and calcium and magnesium phosphates. The most important consequence of stone formation is obstruction of the salivary duct which may lead to inflammation characterized by swelling of the gland. Calculi in the submandibular duct may be removed via an incision into the duct in the floor of the mouth while stones in the substance of the submandibular gland are removed by gland excision. Anteriorly placed parotid duct stones may also be removed *per oram* while symptomatic stones in the gland require formal exploration.

Inflammation

Mumps

Mumps (endemic parotitis) is an infectious viral disease with an incubation period of 17–21 days. It usually affects the parotid glands bilaterally, but the submandibular and sublingual glands may also be affected. Viral-induced pancreatitis and orchitis are not uncommon in adolescents. The disease is self-limiting without serious sequelae in most patients. Rarely, however, bilateral orchitis can lead to sterility or failure of testosterone production.

Acute suppurative (postoperative) parotitis

Suppurative parotitis is caused by ascending infection from the oral cavity with reduced salivary flow. *Staphylococcus aureus* is the usual causative agent. This condition is usually seen in debilitated or postoperative (hence the name) patients in whom there is dehydration, dental sepsis and poor oral hygiene. Clinically one or both glands may be enlarged and painful and there may be a purulent discharge from the duct. Prophylaxis is achieved by removing the aetiological factors and maintaining good hydration and mouth care preoperatively. Established cases required antibiotics and surgical drainage if an abscess develops.

Chronic parotitis

Chronic inflammation of the parotid gland is often associated with obstruction and infection of the gland leading to *sialectasia*, i.e. dilatation of the duct system analogous to bronchiectasis. Sialography (see above) demonstrates these changes in the duct system. Treatment is by removing any duct obstruction (calculi or strictures) and promoting salivary flow. Occasionally gland excision is required.

Sjögren's syndrome

Sjögren's syndrome is an autoimmune chronic inflammatory disease. It is characterized by keratoconjunctivitis sicca (dry eyes; *siccus* is Latin, meaning dry), xerostomia, parotid swelling and rheumatoid arthritis. Sjögren's syndrome may be accompanied by other autoimmune disorders, e.g. scleroderma, systemic lupus erythematosus, primary biliary cirrhosis, etc. and is found mostly in postmenopausal women. *Mikulicz's disease* is a symmetrical enlargement of the salivary and lacrimal glands caused by the benign inflammatory infiltrate characteristic of Sjögren's syndrome. Treatment is difficult and is mostly symptomatic. Good oral hygiene is to be encouraged. Closure of the lacrimal punctum and regular instillation of 1% methylcellulose (artificial) tears helps to relieve the ocular symptoms. The prognosis is that of the associated disease.

Tumours of the salivary glands

Tumours of the salivary glands occur quite frequently and are classified on the basis of their clinical and pathological features (Table 16.1). Only the common tumours will be discussed.

Pleomorphic adenoma

This is the most common tumour of the salivary glands, occurring more frequently in the parotid gland than in the

Table 16.1 Pathological classification of salivary tumours.

	Percentage of tumours in	
	Major glands	**Minor glands**
Adenomas		
Pleomorphic adenoma	70	50
Monomorphic adenoma	5–10	5–10
Adenolymphoma (Warthin's tumour)		
Oncocytoma (oxyphilic adenoma)		
Carcinomas		
Mucoepidermoid	5–10	10
Adenoid cystic	5	20
Carcinoma in pleomorphic adenoma	Rare	Rare
Adenocarcinoma	Rare	Rare
Undifferentiated carcinoma	Rare	Rare

submandibular gland and usually in the superficial portion of the parotid (Fig. 16.3). It presents in middle age as a slow-growing, painless smooth mass in the parotid. Histologically, pleomorphic adenomas consist of epithelial cells mixed with myxoid, mucoid and chondroid elements and the tumour is surrounded by a fibrous capsule. The tumour also has projections which protrude beyond the fibrous capsule into the surrounding parotid gland. Failure to remove these projections at surgery may result in tumour recurrence. Treatment of a parotid tumour is resection, en-

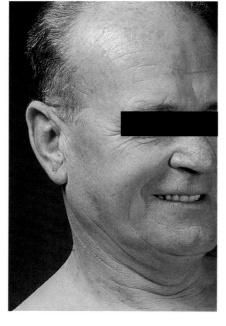

(a)

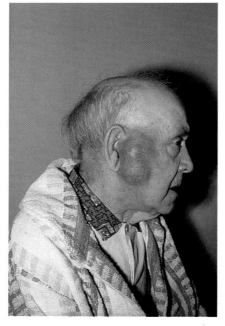

(b)

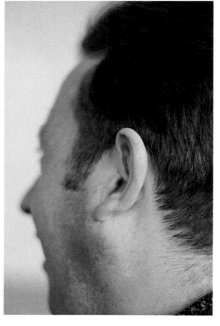

(c)

Figure 16.3 (a) Early and (b) late presentation of parotid tumours. (c) Typical site of parotid tumour between angle of mandible and mastoid process. Note the way the tumour distorts the ear lobe.

suring that a rim of normal parotid gland is taken around the fibrous tumour capsule. Great care must be taken not to damage the facial nerve. If a salivary tumour involves a gland other than the parotid, complete excision of that gland is indicated. Complete removal of the tumour carries an excellent prognosis.

Adenolymphoma (Warthin's tumour)

These account for about 10% of parotid tumours. They present as soft cystic masses in men over 50 years of age. It is the only salivary tumour that is more common in men than in women. Histologically they are composed of cystic glandular spaces with papillary projections, surrounded by lymphoid tissue. Treatment is by surgical excision and the prognosis is very good.

Carcinomas

Several histological types are recognized (Table 16.1) but these tumours usually present as a hard, rapidly growing, infiltrating parotid mass in a middle-aged or elderly patient. The mass may be painful and the facial nerve may be involved. Spread is to local lymph nodes and, if left untreated, ulceration of the tumour through the skin will occur.

Treatment consists of radical parotidectomy with sacrifice of the facial nerve (Fig. 16.4), block dissection of the regional lymph nodes and radiotherapy. Carcinomas of the submandibular glands are similarly treated by radical resection. Prognosis is poor for this tumour.

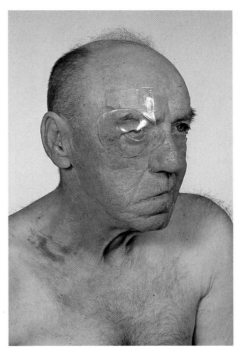

Figure 16.4 Facial nerve palsy following surgery for a carcinoma of the parotid gland.

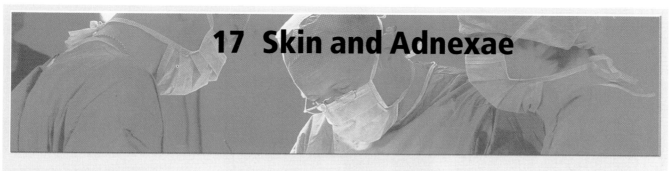

17 Skin and Adnexae

I stuff my skin, so full within,
Of jolly good ale and old.
William Stevenson (1530–75)

The skin

Cysts

Sebaceous cyst

Sebaceous cysts are more correctly called *epidermal inclusion cysts* as they are composed of thin layers of epidermis and contain epidermal debris. They are retention cysts produced by obstruction to the mouth of a sebaceous gland. They commonly occur on the face, neck, scalp, scrotum and vulva (Fig. 17.1). They cannot occur on gland-free areas such as the palm of the hand or the sole of the foot. Clinically they are smooth, soft or firm and are attached to the skin. A pathognomonic *punctum* is often visible in the overlying skin. They contain soft, cheesy material and occasionally become infected. Sebaceous cysts may be complicated by infection, ulceration (Cock's peculiar tumour), calcification and horn formation. For these and cosmetic reasons they are best treated by surgical excision, which is performed under local anaesthetic.

Hyperplasia of the sebaceous glands at the tip of the nose leads to the development of a protruberant mass called a rhinophyma. This is treated by shaving the mass down to a reasonable size. Skin regeneration occurs rapidly.

Dermoid cyst

Congenital dermoid cysts lie deep to the skin, and are not attached to it. They arise from epidermal cells separated from the skin during fusion of the embryological lines in the face and are found at the junctions of lines of fusion of facial skin. External angular (Fig. 17.2a) and midline (Fig. 17.2b) angular dermoids are the most common examples seen. They usually present as a pea-sized swelling under the skin but fixed to the underlying bone. Occasionally a dermoid (usually a midline dermoid) may extend through bone to communicate with a cyst in the anterior fossa of the skull. Skull X-ray or computed tomographic (CT) scan may be necessary to exclude this.

An *implantation dermoid* is a cystic lesion which develops following a puncture injury in which epithelial cells are implanted into the subcutaneous tissue. They are often found on the fingers. Excision is the treatment for these cysts (Fig. 17.3).

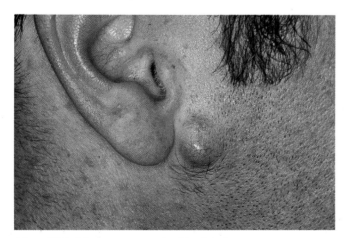

Figure 17.1 Sebaceous cyst on the side of the face.

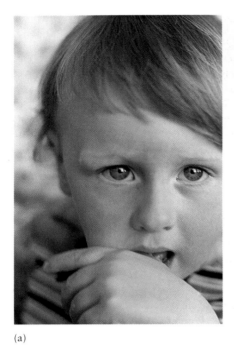

(a)

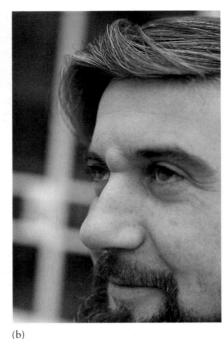

(b)

Figure 17.2 (a) External and (b) internal angular dermoids.

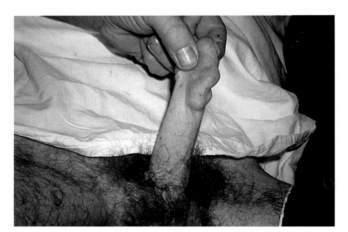

Figure 17.3 Implantation dermoid of the penis following a 'zipper' injury.

Ganglion

A ganglion is a unilocular synovial fluid-filled cyst arising from synovial tissue in relation to joints or tendons. A ganglion is not a pouch from the joint space but arises from other synovial tissues near the wrist, ankle or digits. The most frequent location for a ganglion is the dorsum of the wrist and patients usually present with a hard lump which

may or may not cause discomfort. On examination they are 1–2 cm in diameter, they are smooth, firm and slightly fluctuant and not attached to the overlying skin. Treatment is by formal surgical excision.

Vascular lesions of the skin

Vascular malformations can be categorized as arterial, venous, capillary, lymphatic or mixed. Vascular malformations are the commonest of all malformations and occur in 10% of the normal population, being somewhat higher in premature infants.

Strawberry naevus

A strawberry mark or naevus (capillary–cavernous angioma) characteristically appears as small red marks at a week to 10 days after birth and rapidly enlarges over a few weeks to several centimetres in diameter. They are raised, fleshy, compressible vascular lesions (Fig. 17.4). These regress spontaneously over 5 years, leaving either no mark at all or occasionally a small whitish scar which may need excision. Treatment of strawberry naevi is therefore conservative.

Lesions involving the eyelids may impair vision and lead to sympathetic ophthalmoplegia. Treatment of such lesions must be by early surgery (Fig. 17.5).

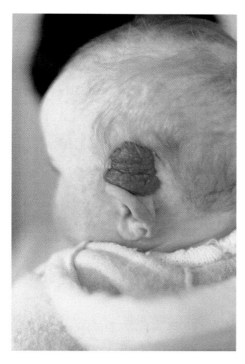

Figure 17.4 Strawberry naevus adjacent to the left ear. In the vast majority of patients these lesions are treated conservatively and eventually disappear or leave only a small blemish.

Capillary haemangioma (portwine stain)

Capillary haemangiomas may occur at any site. However, they often conform to sensory dermatomes, especially when seen on the face (Fig. 17.6). Ipsilateral meningeal involvement may occur in conjunction with hemifacial haemangiomas — Sturge–Weber syndrome. Treatment is usually not required for portwine staining as attempts at trying to remove the haemangioma often result in unsightly scarring. The Klippel–Trenaunay syndrome is a triad of varicose veins, limb hypertrophy and portwine staining (see Chapter 18).

Cavernous haemangioma

Cavernous haemangiomas (localized collections of dilated veins) are commonly found on the limbs and trunk. They are usually asymptomatic but may be associated with arteriovenous fistula which may cause either local gigantism because of the increased local blood flow or high-output cardiac failure. After excision they are prone to recurrence.

Lymphangioma

The *linear naevus* is the commonest form of lymphangioma comprising small vesicles, often arranged in a linear fashion

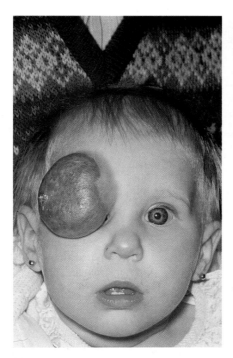

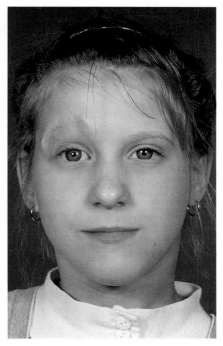

Figure 17.5 (a) In this patient the haemangioma was obstructing vision, and hence surgery was required to prevent amblyopia. (b) Late postoperative appearance in the early teens.

(a)

(b)

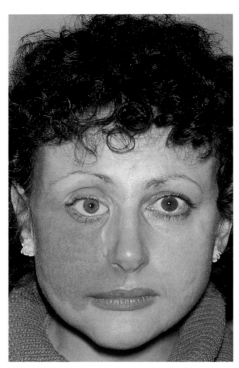

Figure 17.6 Portwine stain affecting the right cheek in the distribution of the maxillary division of the trigeminal nerve.

as a skin naevus. These vesicles contain lymphatic channels with clear fluid within them. The larger and much rarer form of lymphangioma is the highly transilluminable *cystic hygroma*, often found in the neck (see Fig. 1.8).

Glomus body tumour

A *glomangioma* is a tumour of the glomus body, a convoluted arteriovenous formation which is sensitive to temperature and controls local arterial blood flow. Glomus bodies are distributed widely through the skin with a preference for the fingers and toes. Glomangiomas are small (<1 cm) rounded, firm, purple tumours frequently found beneath the nail. Their outstanding feature is that they are exquisitely tender, and for this reason they should be excised.

Spider naevus

Spider naevi are subcutaneous endarterioles and therefore when emptied by compression fill from the centre outwards (centripetally). They appear in the distribution of the superior vena cava and are found in patients with liver disease (see Fig. 13.61).

Campbell de Morgan spots

These are small (1–2 mm) bright red spots which occur in the skin of the trunk in middle-aged and elderly patients. They are localized capillary proliferations. At one time they were thought to indicate deep-seated malignancy but in fact they have no clinical significance.

Benign skin tumours

Benign papilloma (skin tag)

A benign papilloma is an overgrowth of the skin which presents as a sessile or pedunculated polyp. They may occur at any age, but usually in adult life. They are completely harmless but should be removed if cosmetically unacceptable or liable to trauma.

Warts (verruca vulgaris)

Warts are a very common problem. They are caused by viruses and pathologically consist of papillary hyperplasia of the epidermis and excessive keratinization. Warts are common on the fingers and hands and when they occur on the sole of the foot they are called plantar warts or verrucas. Verrucas are commonly transmitted in swimming pools and may occur in epidemics in schools. Warts occurring on the genitalia, in the perineum and perianally are spread by sexual contact. These are caused by human papilloma-viruses and are also referred to as venereal warts or *condylomata acuminata*.

Warts often disappear spontaneously. This phenomenon probably explains the efficacy of the myriad folk cures which have been used to treat warts over the centuries. However, sometimes they require treatment because they are cosmetically unacceptable, cause pain or discomfort. Several treatments exist, including applications of podophyllin and salicylic acid or silver nitrate, curettage or excision with diathermy or cryosurgery. Plantar warts should be curetted if they cause a lot of pain on walking.

Keloid scar

Keloid (Κελοιδ, Greek crab claw) scar formation is a complication of wound healing caused by excessive deposition of extracellular matrix at the wound site. Histologically there is excessive production of collagen, fibroblasts and capillaries in the healing wound. Typically keloids are raised pink deforming lesions along the course of the wound. They commonly occur on the skin of the head and neck and upper trunk (Fig. 17.7). Unfortunately, keloid formation frequently follows piercing of the earlobes for ear-

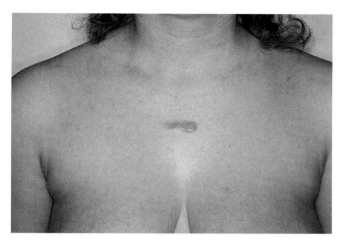

Figure 17.7 Presternal keloid scar.

rings. They are much more frequent in blacks and orientals than in Caucasians. Treatment is difficult. Low-dose radiotherapy and local steroid injections have been effective in some cases.

Pyogenic granuloma

A pyogenic granuloma is a mass of vigorously growing granulation tissue which arises in relation to an area of minor skin trauma. The patient notices a rapidly growing reddish/pink lump on the skin which bleeds easily. They usually occur in areas most likely to be traumatized, e.g. the hands, feet, face and lips. They are not painful. Treatment is by excision and curettage (Fig. 17.8).

Histiocytoma

A histiocytoma is a benign skin nodule caused by infiltration of lipid-filled macrophages (*histiocytes*). They are firm hemispherical nodules of about 1 cm in diameter. They occur singly in adults and are found slightly more often on the limbs. While they are benign, treatment is by excision to confirm the diagnosis.

Keratoacanthoma

Keratoacanthomas are thought to arise from hair follicles. They are frequently misdiagnosed clinically as squamous carcinomas. They commonly occur on the face or hand in older adults (Fig. 17.9). The patient complains of a rapidly growing lump which may measure up to 2 cm in 6 weeks. The centre then ulcerates and the lesion begins to regress and will eventually heal in 2–3 months. Keratoacanthomas are not painful. Treatment should be excision for cosmetic

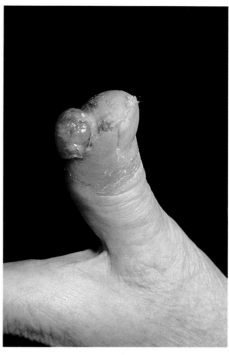

Figure 17.8 Pyogenic granuloma of the thumb following an injury.

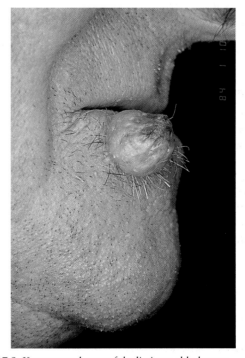

Figure 17.9 Keratoacanthoma of the lip in an elderly man.

reasons and to confirm that the lesion is not a squamous carcinoma.

Keratoses

Keratoses are lesions caused by hypertrophy of the epidermis. They are very common and solar ketatoses may undergo malignant change. Two types are recognized:

Solar keratosis

These are well-demarcated *premalignant* lesions which are caused by solar damage and histologically are areas of hyperkeratosis. They usually occur on the back of the hands or face or the ears (all areas exposed to the sun) and they are commoner in the elderly and outdoor workers and in fair-skinned people living in the tropics and subtropics. Clinically solar keratoses develop as an adherent scale which can be removed with difficulty to reveal a hyperaemic base. Often a small ketatotic horn develops. As they are precancerous, isolated lesions should be removed (by excision or cryotherapy) and the patients advised to avoid exposure to the sun and to use appropriate protection (e.g. hats and sunscreen creams) when exposure is inevitable.

Seborrhoeic keratosis

These are multiple, raised, frequently pigmented lesions which develop on the trunk in middle-aged or elderly people (Fig. 17.10). They are extremely common and their aetiology is unknown. Histologically they consist of cords of stratified squamous epithelium with keratin cysts. They are benign and generally require no treatment.

Bowen's disease

Bowen's disease is squamous cell carcinoma-*in-situ* and is a *premalignant* lesion. This is a rare condition characterized by a red, raised hyperkeratotic plaque with well-defined margins. Exposure to arsenic compounds is an aetiological factor in some patients. Local cytotoxic therapy (e.g. 5-fluorouracil) and cryotherapy has been employed to treat it but local recurrence is frequent after such therapy and surgical excision gives the best results. Bowen's disease involving the glans penis glories in the exotic name *erythroplasia of Queyrat*.

Malignant skin tumours

Aetiological factors

Several aetiological factors for skin malignancies have been identified, the most important of which are summarized in Table 17.1.

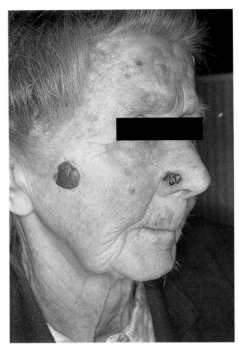

Figure 17.10 Seborrhoeic keratosis on the face. (Note that this lady also has a basal cell carcinoma on the side of the nose.)

Table 17.1 Aetiological factors for skin malignancy.

Factor	Evidence
Exposure to sunlight	Keratinocytes are damaged by ultraviolet light
	90% of cancers occur in exposed sites
	Skin cancer is common in outdoor workers
	Incidence increases in fair-skinned races
	Increased incidence in areas of high annual sunshine (e.g. Australia (*Slip, Slap, Slop!*), southern USA)
Immunosuppression	Increased incidence in patients on immunosuppressive therapy (e.g. after renal transplantation) and in patients with AIDS
Radiation exposure	Increased incidence following radiotherapy and among radiologists
Chemical carcinogens	Hydrocarbons, arsenic, coal tar, oils, soot (chimney sweeps' scrotal carcinoma was described by Percival Pott in 1775)
Inherited disorders	Very high occurrence of skin cancer in *albinism and xeroderma pigmentosum*
Chronic irritation	Carcinoma may develop in scars or in relation to a chronic ulcer (Marjolin's ulcer)

Basal cell carcinoma

A basal cell carcinoma (BCC) is a malignant tumour of the skin arising from basal cells in the epidermis. BCCs are very common tumours, particularly in those exposed to ultraviolet light. They usually appear after the age of 50 and 90% are found on the forehead, face and hair margin. Clinically, BCCs present as small nodules which soon become ulcerated centrally, producing an umbilicated lesion (Fig. 17.11a). A history of a lesion which apparently heals only to recur soon after is not unusual. As the lesion progresses large areas of ulceration with slightly raised pearly coloured edges develop and, untreated, large areas of the face may be eaten away with invasion of bone and cartilage (rodent ulcer; Fig. 17.12). BCCs do not, however, metastasize.

The diagnosis is made clinically but if there is any doubt a biopsy may be obtained prior to definite treatment. Five methods of treatment are available for BCC:
• Curettage and cautery: effective for small lesions, but leaves an open wound.

• Cryotherapy: no tissue for histology and clearance of margins is uncertain.
• Surgical excision: clean closed wound, provides specimen for histology and proof that margins are clear. Larger lesions may require skin grafting (Fig. 17.11b) and more extensive lesions may even require reconstructive surgery (see Chapter 23).
• Radiotherapy: produces excellent results. No tissue for histology and should be avoided near cartilage, which may undergo necrosis. The usual dose is 40–60 Gy given over 2–3 weeks.
• Topical chemotherapy: not as effective as the other methods. The most frequently used agent is 5-fluorouracil (5-FU).

Squamous cell carcinoma

Squamous carcinoma of the skin arises from the keratinocytes in the epidermis. It grows rapidly with anaplasia, local invasion and metastases. Solar keratoses and Bowen's disease are precursors of squamous carcinoma of the skin

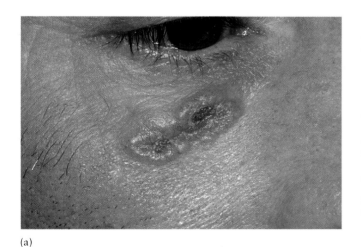

(a)

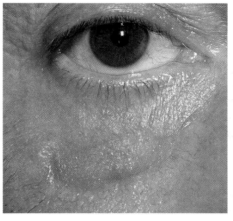

(b)

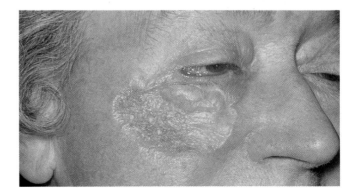

(c)

Figure 17.11 (a) A basal cell carcinoma just below the right eye. Note the rolled edge and pearly colour. (b) Early postoperative result following excision of the lesion and full-thickness skin grafting of the defect (Wolfe graft). (c) A split-skin graft would contract and cause ectropion.

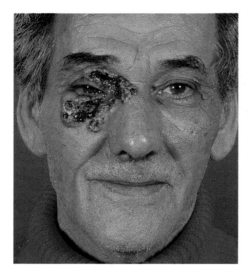

Figure 17.12 A neglected basal cell carcinoma around the left orbit. This patient required extensive reconstructive surgery (see Chapter 23).

(see above). Squamous carcinoma also occurs mostly on the exposed areas of the body (75% on the head, 15% on the hands) and may present with a variety of lesions ranging from a superficial skin ulcer to a fungating lesion or extensive ulceration with heaped-up edges. These are aggressive tumours and will invade the structures deep to the dermis and metastases to regional lymph nodes (Fig. 17.13).

Establishing the diagnosis is the first step in the management of squamous carcinoma. This is done by obtaining a biopsy for histological diagnosis. The main forms of treatment are surgical excision and radiotherapy, but occasionally cryotherapy or currettage and cautery are used for small lesions. In general, results of treatment are very good but patients should be followed for 5 years post-treatment.

Malignant melanoma

See below.

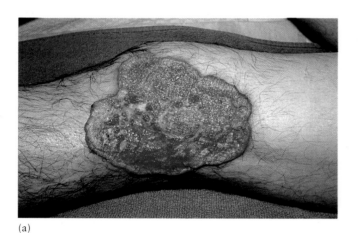

(a)

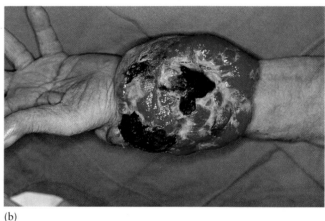

(b)

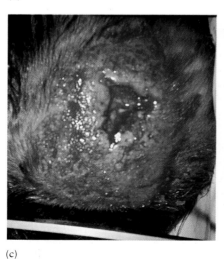

(c)

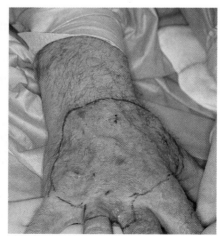

(d)

Figure 17.13 (a) Squamous cell carcinoma of the right leg. Note the extensive ulcer and the heaped-up everted edges. (b) A neglected squamous cell carcinoma of the right wrist. The tumour has grown around the wrist like a bracelet. (c) A squamous cell carcinoma of the scalp which the patient concealed under his hat for years. When he presented, the tumour had penetrated his skull to the dura. (d) Multiple squamous carcinomas on the dorsum of the hand.

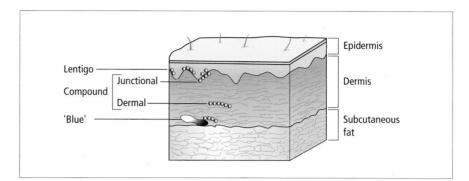

Figure 17.14 Classification of naevi; the sites of melanocyte accumulation in different types of naevi.

Kaposi's sarcoma

Kaposi's sarcoma is a multicentric angiomatous neoplasm affecting the skin characterized by purple-brown tumour nodules that vary from 1 mm to 1 cm in diameter. The tumour occurs most often on the hands and feet. Classically, Kaposi's sarcoma occurred in elderly men and was common in parts of Central Africa. Recently, however, this condition has been recognized as one of the most frequent presentations of acquired immunedeficiency syndrome (AIDS), almost in epidemic proportions. Treatment of individual lesions is by excision, but this is not always possible when large numbers of tumours are present.

Pigmented skin lesions

Naevi

Naevi are benign pigmented lesions of the skin which arise from increased numbers of melanocytes. A number of different types are recognized depending on the site of melanocyte accumulation (Fig. 17.14):

- *Lentigo:* accumulation of melanocytes within the basal layer of the epidermis. Usually found as pigmented lesions on the face and hands of the elderly (Fig. 17.15);
- *Junctional:* proliferation of melanocytes at the dermal–epidermal junction. Clinically present as smooth, flat, and often irregularly pigmented lesions. They arise most commonly at or before puberty;
- *Dermal:* melanocytes entirely within the dermis. These are elevated fleshy to brown-coloured, sometimes pedunculated and may contain hair. They usually occur in adults;
- *Compound:* melanocytes lie both at the dermal–epidermal junction and within the dermis and clinically display features of both junctional and dermal naevi. These may develop into malignant melanomas;
- *Blue:* melanocytes lie deep within the dermis. Clinically they are small, sharply defined dark blue or blue-grey lesions

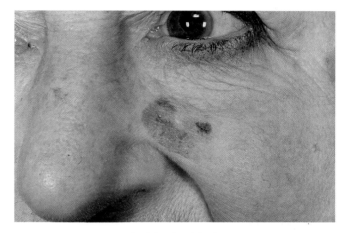

Figure 17.15 Lentigo on the left side of the face.

found anywhere on the body but most commonly on the head and neck. It is the depth of the cells in the dermis that accounts for the blue rather than brown appearance of these lesions.

Management of pigmented lesions

Most pigmented lesions are benign and do not require any treatment. A proportion require treatment for aesthetic reasons and a number are treated because of a suspicion of malignant change. Treatment is by excision and lesions which should be removed are:

- newly discovered pigmented lesions in an adult;
- lesions which have undergone a change in colour, shape or size;
- lesions which bleed;
- lesions subject to chronic irritation;
- lesions on the sole of the foot or palm of the hand;
- any lesion about which the patient is concerned.

The majority of these lesions will turn out to be naevi of various sorts but a few will be malignant melanoma.

Malignant melanoma

Malignant melanoma is a malignant tumour arising from the melanocytes. The incidence of the commonest type of malignant melanoma (superficial spreading type) is increasing more rapidly than any other human cancer and it has been estimated that approximately 1% of all children born today will develop this condition. Since 1979 the incidence of malignant melanoma has been rising at a rate of 6% per annum and it causes about 1000 deaths annually in the UK. Approximately 50% of all melanomas arise in pre-existing naevi and exposure to intense ultraviolet radiation from sunlight is the most important aetiological factor (Table 17.1). Fair-skinned people are affected most often.

Pathology

Pathologically the two commonest form of malignant melanoma are:
- superficial spreading (Fig. 17.16);
- nodular (Fig. 17.17);

while less frequently encountered varieties are:
- lentigo maligna melanoma (Hutchinson's freckle, Fig. 17.18);
- acral lentiginous melanoma.

Two phases of tumour progression occur in malignant melanoma. First, the malignant cells grow in all directions. This is referred to as the *radial growth phase*. It is important to recognize this phase as tumours treated at this stage do not metastasize. After 1–2 years a change occurs in some of the malignant cells which grow as spheroidal nodules and expand more rapidly than the rest of the cells. The direction of this rapid growth is vertical and this phase is called the *vertical growth phase*. The tumour now has the potential to

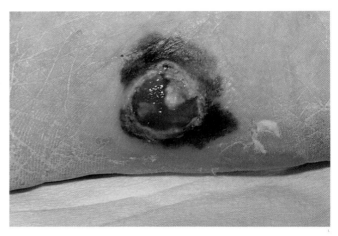

Figure 17.17 Nodular malignant melanoma of the sole of the foot.

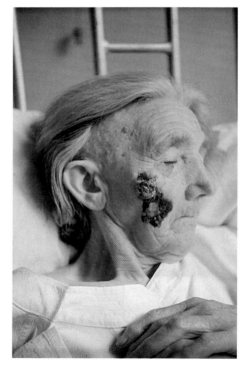

Figure 17.18 Lentigo maligna melanoma (Hutchinson's freckle).

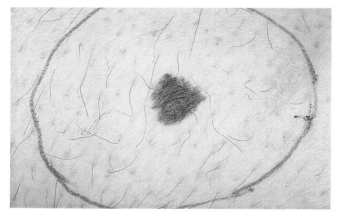

Figure 17.16 Superficial spreading malignant melanoma. This is the commonest type of malignant melanoma.

metastasize. Spread to regional lymph nodes occurs early. Haematogenous spread is to liver, bone and brain.

Staging of malignant melanoma is determined in two ways: Clarke's levels and Breslow tumour thickness. Details of Clarke's levels are given in Fig. 17.19.

In Breslow's method the tumour thickness in millimetres is used to predict outcome (Table 17.2).

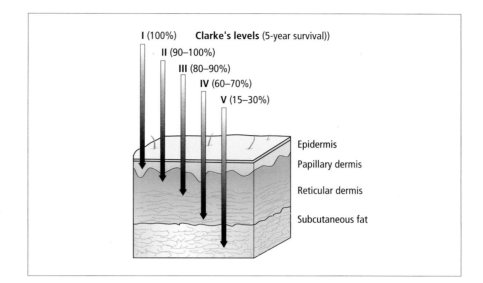

Figure 17.19 Five Clarke's levels are recognized. Epidermal involvement only (level I) is non-invasive and has a 100% 5-year survival rate. In level II disease the papillary dermis only is involved, while level III tumour involves the junction of the papillary and reticular dermis. Level IV disease means that tumour extends to the reticular dermis and the subcutaneous fat is involved in level V disease.

Table 17.2 Breslow method of staging tumour thickness.

Tumour thickness (mm)	5-year survival (%)
< 0.76	98
0.76–1.49	95
1.50–2.49	80
2.50–3.99	75
4.00–7.99	60
>8.00	40

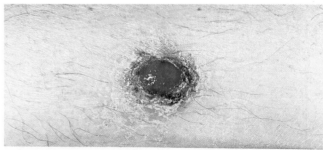

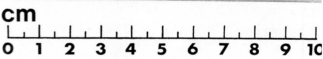

Figure 17.20 Amelanotic melanoma.

Other prognostic factors include:
• Ulceration of the lesion: prognosis is worse if ulceration is present.
• Sex of patient: men do worse than women.
• Anatomical location: extremities do better than the trunk.
• Age of onset of lesion: prognosis is better with lesions which arise before puberty or in the elderly.

Clinical features

Malignant melanomas are found most commonly on the lower limbs, feet, head and neck. They are usually pigmented but a small number lack pigment (amelanotic melanoma; Fig. 17.20). Usually the patient presents with a history of a *change* in a pigmented lesion. Such changes include:
• increasing size;
• increasing pigmentation;
• bleeding;
• pain or itching;

• ulceration; and
• development of satellite lesions.
The appearance of a melanoma varies considerably. Most are brown/black, irregular lesions on the skin, approximately 1 cm in diameter. The colour is not uniform and there may be evidence of bleeding or ulceration. Satellite lesions are like a number of small moons surrounding a planet, represented by the melanoma.

Management of malignant melanoma

Surgical excision is the treatment of choice for almost all melanomas. Definitive surgery may be undertaken *ab initio* or following a biopsy. In the past very wide margins of excision (>5 cm) were recommended but it is now recognized that lateral margins of 2–3 cm are adequate. Usually the subcutaneous tissue is excised with the lesion but it is not necessary to excise fascia or muscle underneath the lesion.

These smaller excisions allow primary closure of the wounds in the majority of patients.

Controversy exists regarding the surgical management of regional lymph nodes. In a patient in whom there is clinical evidence of regional node involvement a lymph node dis-

Skin cancer at a glance

DEFINITION

Malignant lesions of skin — basal cell (BCC) and squamous cell (SCC) carcinomas and malignant melanoma (MM)

EPIDEMIOLOGY

M/F=2:1 for BCC and SCC. Elderly males. Equal sex distribution and all adults for MM. All tumours common in areas of high annual sunshine (e.g. Australia, southern USA)

AETIOLOGY

Predisposing factors
- Exposure to sunlight (especially in fair-skinned races)
- Immunosuppression (high incidence after renal transplant)
- Radiation exposure (radiotherapy, among radiologists)
- Chemical carcinogens (hydrocarbons, arsenic, coal tar)
- Inherited disorders (albinism, xeroderma pigmentosum)
- Chronic irritation (Marjolin's ulcer)
- Naevi (50% of malignant melanomas arise in pre-existing benign pigmented lesions)
- Bowen's disease and erythroplasia of Queyrat

PATHOLOGY

BCC
- Arises from basal cells of epidermis
Aggressive local spread but do *not* metastasize

SCC
- Arises from keratinocytes in the epidermis
Spreads by local invasion and metastases

MM
- Arises from the melanocytes, often in pre-existing naevi
Superficial spreading and nodular types. Radial and vertical growth phases. Lymphatic spread is to regional lymph nodes and haematogenous spread to liver, bone and brain

Staging
Clarke's levels I–V, Breslow's tumour thickness

CLINICAL FEATURES

BCC
- Recurring ulcerated umbilicated skin lesion on forehead or face. Ulcer has a raised pearl-coloured edge. Untreated, large areas of the face may be eroded (rodent ulcer)

SCC
- Lesions (ulcers, fungating lesions with heaped-up edges) on exposed areas of the body

MM
- Pigmented lesions (occasionally not pigmented — amelanotic), 1 cm in diameter on lower limbs, feet, head and neck. Usually present as a change in a pigmented lesion: increasing size or pigmentation/bleeding/pain or itching/ulceration/satellite lesions

INVESTIGATIONS

- Biopsy (usually excisional) of the lesion

MANAGEMENT

BCC
- Curettage/cautery/cryotherapy/topical chemotherapy (5-FU). These treatments are suitable for small lesions
- Surgical excision/radiotherapy (40–60 Gy over 2–3 weeks)

SCC
- Surgical excision/radiotherapy

MM
- Surgical excision with 2–3 cm margin
Nodes involved — node dissection
Immunotherapy, chemotherapy (systemic and local limb perfusion), radiotherapy

PROGNOSIS

- BCC ⎫ Prognosis is usually excellent but patients with SCC
- SCC ⎬ should be followed for 5 years
- MM: Prognosis depends on staging:

Clarke's level	5-year survival	Tumour thickness	5-year survival
I (epidermis)	100%	<0.76 mm	98%
II (papillary dermis)	90–100%	0.76–1.49 mm	95%
III (papillary/reticular dermis)	80–90%	1.50–2.49 mm	80%
IV (reticular dermis)	60–70%	2.50–3.99 mm	75%
V (subcutaneous fat)	15–30%	4.00–7.99 mm	60%
		>8.00 mm	40%

section of that area is appropriate. Some surgeons also advocate node dissections prophylactically with intermediate-stage primary lesions (i.e. Clarke levels III and IV and Breslow's 0.76–3.99 mm thickness).

Other forms of treatment include immunotherapy, chemotherapy (both systemic and local perfusion, e.g. of a limb) and radiotherapy. However, survival rates have not been drastically altered by any of several innovative treatments. Occasionally spontaneous remission of a primary malignant melanoma occurs.

The subcutaneous tissue

Lipoma

Lipomas are multilobular benign tumours of fat usually arising in the superficial subcutaneous tissues of the trunk and limbs but may also be found in the peritoneal cavity and within muscles. Lipomas present as soft, fluctuant, painless subcutaneous lumps measuring anything from 2 to 20 cm in diameter. Most lipomas are excised for cosmetic reasons. Usually an incision in the skin over the lump allows the lipoma to be enucleated. *Liposarcomas* are rare and tend to occur in the body cavities rather than subcutaneously.

Neurofibroma

Benign nerve sheath tumours may be either schwannomas (neurilemmomas) or neurofibromas. *Schwannomas* are benign slowly growing neoplasms of Schwann cells and may arise in any nerve. They are oval, well-demarcated tumours ranging in size from a few millimetres to several centimetres and are often solitary. *Neurofibromas* are also thought to arise from the Schwann cell and should be differentiated from schwannomas because of their potential for sarcomatous degeneration. Neurofibromas present as small, firm, smooth, mobile, subcutaneous masses of variable size.

Neurofibromatosis (also called von Recklinghausen's disease) is an autosomal dominant inherited disorder of the ectoderm characterized by multiple neurofibromas and *café-au-lait* spots. Some members of affected families may only have cutaneous pigmentation while others have a fuller clinical picture, including:
• cutaneous pigmentation: brownish spots or areas invariably present;
• cutaneous fibromas: soft pinkish sessile or pedunculated swellings, usually on the trunk;
• neurofibromas: usually along the course of the superficial cutaneous nerves;

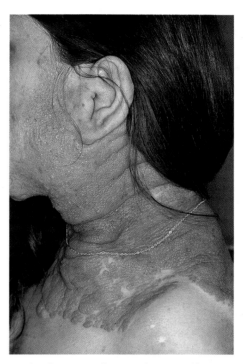

Figure 17.21 Plexiform neurofibroma of the neck.

• plexiform neuroma: diffuse neurofibromatosis of nerve trunks associated with hypertrophy of the skin and subcutaneous tissue (Fig. 17.21; Box 17.1);
• acoustic neuroma: often bilateral. Presents in middle age with tinnitus and progressive deafness.

The Elephant Man

John Merrick was a Londoner whose horrendous deformities, thought to be from neurofibromatosis, resulted in his being called 'The Elephant Man'. His contemporaries and tormentors thought his condition was due to his mother being jostled by an elephant when pregnant. In fact he probably had a very rare condition called Proteus syndrome. In 1886 he came under the care of Sir Frederick Treves and was given a room at the London Hospital, where he lived until his death in 1890 and where his skeleton is preserved. Treves was sergeant surgeon to the King and in that role he performed an appendicectomy on his most famous patient, Edward VII, just prior to the latter's coronation in 1902.

Box 17.1

The nails

The nails in systemic disease

Abnormalities of the nails often indicate the presence of systemic disease and examination of the nails in an important part of the physical examination of a patient. Such abnormalities include the following.

Clubbing

This is swelling of the finger (or toe) tips such that there is a loss of the normal angle between the nail and the skin covering the nail bed or, more simply, the depression at the base of the nail is replaced with a convexity (Fig. 17.22). Clubbing is associated with:
- bronchogenic carcinoma;
- bronchiectasis;
- cyanotic congenital heart disease; and
- cirrhosis of the liver.

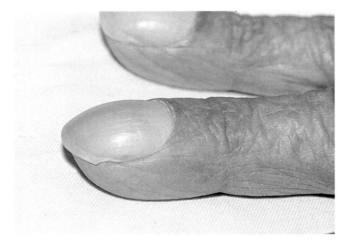

Figure 17.22 Clubbing of the nails of the hands. This patient also had clubbing of his toenails.

Koilonychia (Greek κοιλοσ = concave, ονψχ = nail)

Thin, brittle, concave nails are referred to as koilonychia. This physical sign is associated with iron-deficiency anaemia and may also be found after trauma to the nail and in the skin disease lichen planus.

Leukonychia

White patches or discoloration of the fingernails are referred to as leukonychia. It is sometimes seen with cirrhosis of the liver.

Splinter haemorrhages

These are small linear streaks of blood under and in the long axis of the nail caused by small haemorrhages from the vessels of the nail bed. They are caused by microembolic disease and classically are found in patients with bacterial endocarditis.

Paronychia (whitlow)

Paronychia is an infection of the soft tissue at the margin of the nail. The diagnosis is easily made. The margin of the nail is red, hot, tender and swollen and a small collection of pus may be visible. Treatment usually involves drainage of the collection of pus under local anaesthetic through an incision into the affected part. As with all hand infections, antibiotics and elevation of the hand are also required. Extensive infection may require avulsion of the nail.

(Infection of the pulp space of a fingertip is caled a *felon* and these frequently require surgical drainage via an incision placed at the periphery of the pulp space.)

Onychogryphosis

Onychogryphosis is a deformity of the toenail which usually affects the big toe (Fig. 17.23). It is referred to as a 'ram's horn' deformity because there is exuberant growth of the nail resulting in a nail that looks like a ram's horn. It is usually seen in the elderly but may also occur after trauma. Clipping and filing the nail may keep it under control. Avulsion of the nail does not cure the condition as the new nail will also be onychogryphotic. If a cure is desired then ablation of the nail bed is necessary.

Ingrowing toenail

An ingrowing toenail is a common problem in adolescents and young adults (Fig. 17.24). It most commonly affects the hallux but other toenails may be affected. One should be wary of making this diagnosis in the elderly as a toe problem in this age group is often a manifestation of peripheral vascular disease.

An ingrowing toenail is caused by the lateral edge of the toenail cutting and growing into the adjacent soft tissue of

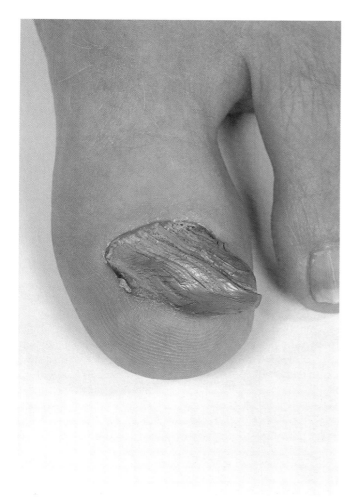

Figure 17.23 Onychogryphosis.

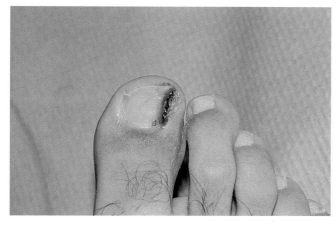

Figure 17.24 Ingrowing toenail.

the nail fold. Superimposed infection (bacterial or fungal) causes inflammation and attempted tissue repair results in exuberant granulation tissue formation. A combination of factors leads to ingrowing toenails:

• tight-fitting shoes (e.g. winkle pickers, beloved of the teddy-boys of a generation ago);
• cutting (or picking!) the nail down into the nail fold rather than transversely;
• sweaty feet and poor hygiene.

Clinically the patient may present with anything ranging from the nail fold riding up on to the nail to a grossly infected, painful nail fold with cellulitis and weeping granulation tissue. One side, or more rarely both sides of a nail may be affected.

Management

If seen in the early stages, an ingrowing toenail may be treated conservatively by:

• regular soaking and washing of the feet;
• carefully drying the feet after washing;
• wearing clean socks and wide-fitting shoes;
• avoiding trauma;
• cutting toenails properly (i.e. transversely);
• the use of a cotton-wool pledget placed under the corner of the nail to help it grow out from the nail fold.

With perseverence these measures are very successful in many cases.

With more severe cases surgery is necessary. The aim of surgery in the acute situation is to remove the ingrowing nail from the nail fold, thus allowing the wound to heal. This can be achieved by:

• avulsion of the whole nail; or
• avulsion of the side of the nail that is ingrowing.

Following avulsion the nail will regrow and if the conservative measures listed above are followed the new nail should grow normally.

If recurrence occurs then more drastic measures are undertaken:

• *Wedge resection* removes about 25% of the width of the nail *and the nail bed* on the affected side. Ablation of the nail bed is achieved by a combination of surgery and phenolization (i.e. a small amount of liquid phenol is left in contact with the nail bed wound for a minute or two). If the nail bed has not been completely ablated, little spikes of nail regenerate and can be a considerable nuisance.

• In *Zadek's operation* the entire nail bed is removed surgically so that the patient is left without a toenail. This is reserved for the severest cases.

Subungual haematoma

Trauma to a fingertip frequently results in a haematoma under the nail. This is an extremely painful condition as there is no room for the haematoma to expand in the confined space under the nail. Drilling a small hole through the nail with a sterile needle produces a small quantity of old blood and instant relief. Frequently, the nail separates after a few days. Occasionally a malignant melanoma presents under a nail (*subungual melanoma*) and may be mistaken for a subungual haematoma. Lesions under the nail should be biopsied.

18 Cardiovascular Disorders

**Tobacco surely was designed
To poison and destroy mankind.**   (Philip Freneau, 1752–1832)

Introduction

Disorders of the circulation are common and can conveniently be considered under four headings: cardiac problems, arterial problems, venous problems and lymphatic problems. Coronary artery disease and peripheral vascular disease are serious problems which are the leading causes of death in the western world today. Venous thromboembolism frequently causes death by pulmonary embolism while other venous disorders, such as varicose veins, are a major cause of morbidity worldwide. Lymphatic disease is uncommon but causes considerable distress in those unfortunate enough to be afflicted by it. In this chapter we will consider the causes, clinical manifestations and management of the common cardiac and vascular problems encountered in clinical practice (and exams!).

Pathophysiology

The primary function of the circulation is the delivery of oxygen and nutrients to maintain the viability of the cell. This is achieved by the heart pumping oxygenated blood through a series of viscoelastic tubes to the periphery.

Inadequate blood supply is the single most important determinant in the pathogenesis of cellular injury in human disease. This inadequacy, which is called *ischaemia*, arises from either a failure of a pumping action of the heart or from local interference with the circulation through disease of blood vessels or a combination of both.

The consequences of circulatory failure depend on the severity of circulatory disruption, the acuteness of the event and the vulnerability of the tissue to ischaemia. A range of cellular injury may occur from rapidly reversible anaerobic metabolism, loss of membrane integrity and cellular swelling to cell death and death of tissue *en masse*. In addition, restoration of normal blood flow after a period of ischaemia results in *reperfusion injury* — further tissue injury locally and systemically when the products of ischaemia are carried into the systemic circulation. Thus, reperfusion may cause cardiac, renal and pulmonary dysfunction.

Interference with arterial blood flow may result from external compression of the artery (trauma), disease in the arterial wall (atherosclerosis), an intraluminal obstruction (thromboembolism) and variations in arterial tone (vasospastic disorders). Each of these events may cause endothelial damage with subsequent activation of the clotting mechanism.

The human body contains one artery and the symptoms and signs of coronary, cerebral, and peripheral arterial disease simply reflect underlying arterial pathology in those areas. The most important disease to affect arteries is atherosclerosis, an acquired condition, the complications of which account for more than half of the entire annual mortality of the USA. The main sites of atherosclerosis in the human body are shown in Fig. 18.1. Atherosclerosis is characterized by the proliferation of intimal smooth-muscle cells and the accumulation of lipid in the intima. Expansion and ulceration of this intimal lesion (plaque) lead to narrowing of the lumen of the artery, thrombosis and occlusion of a distributing artery. The risk factors for atherosclerosis are shown in Table 18.1. The effects of smoking, which is the most important (and most preventable) risk factor, are additive to those of the other risk factors.

Rarer causes of arterial disease are inflammatory conditions such as thromboangiitis obliterans or Buerger's disease. Vasculitis is defined as inflammation and necrosis of blood vessels and may be caused by infectious agents (e.g. syphilis), trauma (e.g. frostbite, radiation) and altered immunology (e.g. temporal arteritis). Whatever the cause of the arterial lesion, the resulting clinical picture depends on the site and speed of onset of arterial occlusion or arterial rupture.

Less severe occlusion, in which blood flow is restricted by a gradual narrowing of the arterial lumen, produces ischaemia on exercise. During exercise the blood supply to the tissues is not adequate for energy demands and the byproducts of anaerobic metabolism (lactic acid and potassium) accumulate and cause pain. Long-recognized symptoms of this process are angina pectoris in the heart and intermittent claudication in the limbs. Sudden occlusion of an artery usually results in death of the tissues supplied by that artery and, if it is an important vessel, e.g. the anterior descending branch of the left coronary artery ('the widowmaker'), death of the individual.

Occasionally an artery is occluded by an embolus, usually a thrombus which has migrated from the heart or a larger proximal vessel. For example, small emboli from plaques at the origin of the internal carotid artery migrate into the brain and cause strokes or, if the neurological deficit is temporary, transient ischaemic attacks (TIAs).

Atherosclerosis (or other factors) may also weaken the wall of an artery so that the artery expands and becomes an aneurysm. The tension on the wall of the aneurysm is directly related to the blood pressure and the diameter of the lumen (law of Laplace); as the lumen increases the tension on the wall increases and, like a balloon, the aneurysm will eventually burst and, if it is an abdominal aortic aneurysm, kill the patient.

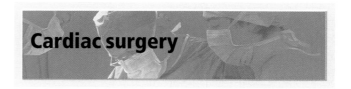

Cardiac surgery

Table 18.1 Risk factors for atherosclerosis*.

Cigarette smoking
Hypertension
Raised serum cholesterol
Diabetes mellitus
Age and sex

*Any factor associated with 100% increase in the incidence of atherosclerosis.

Introduction

The successful use of cardiopulmonary bypass in the 1950s revolutionized cardiac surgery. While the heart was paralysed, the patient's blood could be moved around the circulation and oxygenated. For the first time the heart became amenable to surgical treatment, just like any other organ.

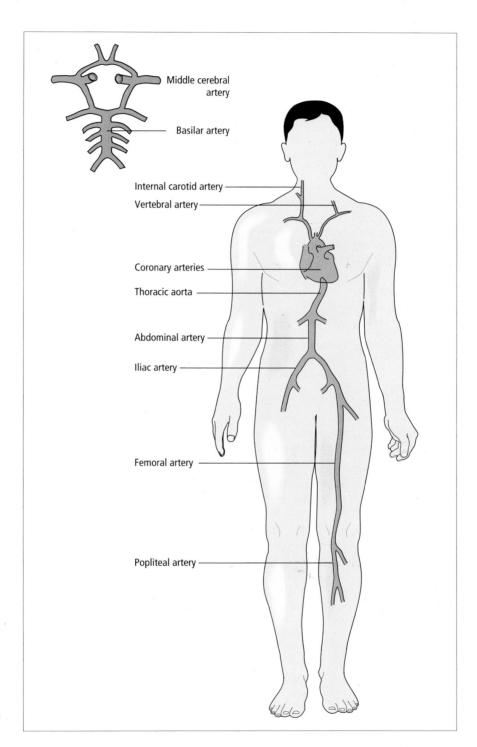

Figure 18.1 Common sites of atherosclerosis in the human body.

Heart surgery has continued to expand, to the extent that now many cardiac operations are regarded as routine and carry negligible risk. In this chapter, the more common aquired cardiac surgical problems and the principles underlying their treatment are presented with special reference to basic pathophysiology.

Table 18.2 Important questions to ask the patient about to undergo cardiac surgery.

General	*Cardiac*
Family history of coronary artery disease	Hypertension (140/90 mmHg or treated)
Smoking, calculated as the number of pack-years (see Chapter 19)	Previous myocardial infarction
Hypercholesterolaemia (>6.5 mmol/l or treated)	Previous cardiac or thoracic surgery
Advancing age	History of rheumatic fever/scarlet fever
Alcoholism	History of bacterial endocarditis
Ankylosing spondylitis, Marfan's syndrome, osteogenesis imperfecta, Ehlers–Danlos syndrome	Known congenital valve abnormality
Endocrine	*Vascular*
Diabetes (diet-controlled, oral therapy or insulin)	Carotid bruit, previous TIA or CVA
Hypothyroidism	Peripheral vascular disease
	Previous DVT or pulmonary embolus
	Varicose veins
Gastrointestinal tract	
History of peptic ulcer, hiatus hernia, gallstones	*Renal*
Diverticular and inflammatory bowel disease	Functioning transplant
Previous abdominal surgery	Acute or chronic renal failure: dialysis
	Cr ⩾200 μmol/l
Respiratory	
Clinical COAD	
Asthma	
History of tuberculosis	

TIA, Transient ischaemic attack; CVA, cerebrovascular accident; DVT, deep venous thrombosis; Cr, creatinine; COAD, chronic obstructive airways disease.

Evaluation of the patient

Despite the development of sophisticated invasive and non-invasive techniques by which the heart and its pathology may be investigated, a highly important means of evaluation, both pre- and postoperatively, remains the clinical history and examination. It should be remembered that investigations demonstrate the patient's haemodynamics at only one point in time, often extending to no more than a few heart beats. A better understanding of the patient's ability to function may be obtained from a careful history and detailed physical examination.

Clinical assessment

General medical history and risk factors

Routine cardiac surgery is now commonplace, and the mortality for operations such as coronary artery bypass grafts is of the order of 1–4%. None the less, it is still a major undertaking and the low mortality is a reflection of improved surgical techniques, technological advances in cardiopulmonary bypass, myocardial preservation techniques, and at least in part, identification of risk factors for morbidity and mortality. These are of paramount importance if complications are to be avoided, and adequate pro-

phylaxis and early institution of therapy are to be carried out (Table 18.2).

Symptoms

The common symptoms of cardiac disease are listed in Table 18.3. For the patient with cardiac disease these symptoms should be specifically sought; assessment should also be made at the same time of the duration of symptoms, and whether they are stable or have recently undergone a deterioration.

Table 18.3 Symptoms of cardiac disease.

Chest pain
Dyspnoea
Syncope
Palpitations
Fatigue
Haemoptysis
Oedema

Chest pain (Table 18.4)

Chest pain is a common feature of cardiac surgical disease. *Angina pectoris* is pain derived from the heart itself when the oxygen demand of the myocardium exceeds supply. The

Table 18.4 New York Heart Association (NYHA) grading of cardiac symptoms.

NYHA 1	No limitation of ordinary physical activity
NYHA 2	Ordinary physical activity causes discomfort
NYHA 3	Moderate to great limitation of ordinary physical activity
NYHA 4	Unable to perform any physical activity without discomfort

In the assessment of a patient whose predominant features are *angina or dyspnoea*, a system of grading by severity of symptom occurrence has been instituted by the New York Heart Association (NYHA). It represents a means by which subsequent improvement or deterioration may be measured.

causes are given below but it is not uncommon for these factors to coexist.

• Commonly, angina results from *coronary artery stenosis* due to atheroma.

• However, angina may also occur when the oxygen supply is insufficient to meet the demands of an *increase in cardiac muscle mass* as a result of aortic stenosis or systemic hypertension. In these cases the increased bulk of the myocardium is due to left ventricular hypertrophy.

• A *low cardiac output* which may occur from ischaemic damage or a cardiomyopathy may also cause angina.

Angina is a strangulating pain felt substernally which may radiate to the arm, jaw or neck. It is commonly exacerbated by exercise and cold weather and relieved by rest and sublingual nitrates. It may also occur at night and wake the patient from sleep, and it may occur after eating. The clinician should always be vigilant as angina often may manifest itself atypically, for example as epigastric pain and thus mimic the pain of a peptic ulcer. An episode of pain lasting longer than a few minutes and associated with nausea or vomiting may signify that the angina has become unstable, or that the patient has sustained a myocardial infarction.

Severe pain felt in the anterior chest with radiation through to the back is characteristic of an acute dissection of the thoracic aorta.

Dyspnoea (Table 18.4)

In the cardiac patient, dyspnoea results from a loss of elasticity of the lungs secondary to passive congestion. This may be due to left ventricular failure or valvular obstruction. In such cases congestion is *passive*, in contrast to *active* congestion seen with increased pulmonary blood flow (from a left to right shunt) in congenital heart disease. Congested lungs become turgid and stiff and increased effort is required to inflate them.

• *Orthopnoea* is defined as breathlessness on lying flat. When a patient adopts a recumbent position there is an in-

crease in venous return to the heart which cannot be adequately dealt with by a failing or obstructed heart. In addition, in the supine position, there is 'splinting' of the diaphragm by the abdominal viscera and the volume of potential lung expansion is reduced. It is useful to enquire how many pillows a patient sleeps with, as this will help reduce the splinting effect.

• *Paroxysmal nocturnal dyspnoea* (*PND*) is breathlessness which wakes the patient from sleep. Typically the patient describes 'gasping for air' and may open a window to try and ease the distress. The mechanism is similar to orthopnoea but because sensory awareness is reduced during sleep, severe interstitial and alveolar oedema can accumulate.

• *Wheezing* may occur in association with the above due to bronchial endothelial oedema (cardiac asthma), and the sputum may be tinged with blood.

Syncope

Syncope of cardiac origin is sudden and of brief duration.

• It occurs on exercise in patients with *aortic stenosis*. It may be due to decrease in cerebral blood flow as peripheral resistance falls secondary to exercise, or to high intraventricular pressures generated within the left ventricle.

• *Pulmonary and mitral stenosis* (when associated with pulmonary hypertension) may also cause syncope on exercise. The fixed low cardiac output which results from these conditions is unable to increase to accommodate the demands of exercise.

• *Arrhythmias and atrioventricular block*, themselves caused by ischaemic heart disease, may also cause syncope. Syncope due to heart block is known as the Stokes–Adams syndrome.

• Rarely, tumour or clot within the left atrium may cause a low cardiac output which secondarily leads to diminished ventricular filling and may present with syncope on exercise.

Palpitations

A palpitation is an increased awareness of the normal heart beat. It may be the result of *extra systoles* or *tachyarrhythmia*; an example of the latter is atrial fibrillation which often occurs in patients with mitral stenosis due to enlargement of the left atrium. Atrial fibrillation may be a further manifestation of ischaemic heart disease. Palpitations may also be due to an increased force of contraction, as occurs in *aortic regurgitation*, due to volume loading of the left ventricle.

Fatigue

Fatigue consists of *tiredness* and *lethargy*. As an indicator of heart disease *per se*, the symptom is of little use. However, commonly in patients with severe heart disease, fatigue is experienced as a result of a poor cardiac output leading to reduced cerebral and peripheral perfusion. β-Blockers used in the treatment of hypertension or angina may also cause fatigue.

Haemoptysis

A variety of underlying pathological processes may cause haemoptysis (see also Chapter 19). Cardiac causes include those listed below.
- *Mitral stenosis* may be due to rupture of congested bronchial capillaries or pulmonary hypertension causing pulmonary congestion.
- *Pulmonary apoplexy* is the effortless sudden coughing of a large volume of bright red blood. It occurs in cases of pulmonary venous hypertension, and the event acts as a physiological venesection.
- The pink blood-stained frothy sputum of *pulmonary oedema* is of sinister significance.
- *Pulmonary infarction*, which may occur as a result of pulmonary embolism, is another cause of haemoptysis. Pulmonary venous or arterial thrombosis as a result of a large left-to-right shunt is a rarer cause.

Oedema

This is the result of salt and water retention consequent upon heart failure. Retained fluid will accumulate in the feet and ankles of ambulant patients, and over the sacrum in bed-ridden patients. It generally worsens during the day and may be absent on initial rising as the fluid is resorbed on lying down. In severe cases, ascites, pleural effusions, leg and thigh oedema may occur.

Physical examination

General examination

A general assessment of the patient is made first. This should include an assessment of whether the patient is well, unwell, ill or very ill and whether the patient is anaemic, jaundiced, obese or cachectic. Examination of a patient's teeth is also important when implanting a new heart valve as poor dental hygiene is a common source of valve infection. The liver should be palpated to see if it is enlarged, tender and, in the case of tricuspid regurgitation, pulsatile. The spine and limbs should be examined for pitting oedema of the sacrum and ankles and the lung bases should be auscultated for crackles after the patient has coughed.

Examination of the cardiovascular system

Clubbing

The common cardiac causes of clubbing are *subacute infective endocarditis* and *cyanotic congenital heart disease*. Clubbing takes many months to develop and is therefore not seen in infants or neonates, or in acute endocarditis. The mechanism remains obscure; clubbing might be due to hepatic impairment, or as part of the condition of *hypertrophic pulmonary osteoarthropathy*. Another possible mechanism is that clubbing is due to a blood-borne factor either produced in or not deactivated by the lungs; this would explain clubbing in right-to-left shunts where a portion of the blood effectively bypasses the pulmonary circulation. Clubbing appears first in the thumb and in the great toe (Fig. 17.22).

Cyanosis

The dusky blue discoloration of the skin and mucous membranes is due to the presence of unoxygenated haemoglobin (at least 5 g/dl). It is uncommon in the anaemic patient and is more common in the polycythaemic patient. Cyanosis may be central or peripheral. *Central cyanosis* occurs when the tongue, lips and conjunctivae are cyanosed. Its presence indicates the mixing of venous and arterial blood. It is improved by breathing oxygen. *Peripheral cyanosis* is observed in the extremities and is due to vasoconstriction and stasis of blood in these areas with a concomitant increased oxygen extraction. It will occur when there is an inadequate peripheral circulation as in shock, exposure to cold, and in severe low cardiac output, as in cardiac failure.

The arterial pulse

The rate, rhythm, character and volume of the arterial pulse should be examined.
- *Rate*. The radial pulse should be examined for not less than 30 s. *Bradycardia*, which could be physiological, due to heart block or drug-induced, e.g. digitalis overdosage, is a pulse rate of less than 60 beats/min. *Tachycardia* is a pulse rate of over 100 beats/min and may be caused by emotion, fever, thyrotoxicosis or an abnormal rhythm. In cases of atrial fibrillation, the rate counted at the wrist does not indicate the true rate of ventricular contraction. In this case the actual heart rate should be counted by auscultation at the apex, and the difference between this and the rate at the

wrist is recorded as the *pulse deficit*. This phenomenon is the result of a varying length of diastole in patients with atrial fibrillation. When diastole is short, the heart barely fills and consequently the stroke volume will be small and as such will not be felt at the wrist, although the heart will have in fact contracted.

- *Rhythm*. The examiner should next decide whether the rhythm is regular or irregular. If it is irregular the next decision is whether it is regularly irregular (usually the result of *ectopic beats*) or irregularly irregular (*atrial fibrillation*). In normal patients the pulse may be felt to quicken slightly in inspiration, and to slow slightly in expiration — so-called *sinus arrhythmia*.
- *Character*. This is best determined by palpation of the carotid pulse. The normal pulse has a moderately rapid upstroke coinciding with left ventricular ejection. As the left ventricular pressure falls, the aortic and ventricular pressure fall to their different diastolic levels.

In certain situations the character of the pulse is detectably abnormal.

(a) *Slow-rising 'plateau' pulse* is typically found in aortic stenosis. It is small in volume and slow in rising to a peak, as a result of the prolonged ejection phase of the left ventricle.

(b) *Collapsing, 'water hammer' or Corrigan's pulse* is typically found in aortic regurgitation; it is characterized by a rapid upstroke and rapid descent of the arterial pressure wave. The rapid upstroke is due to an increased stroke volume consequent upon a leaking or regurgitant valve. The rapid decline in pressure is due to the leak back into the left ventricle and also to a reduced systemic vascular resistance.

(c) *Bisferiens pulse* is a combination of the slow-rising and collapsing pulse and is found in mixed aortic valve disease (stenosis and incompetence) and hypertrophic obstructive cardiomyopathy. This is in fact a 'double pulse'. When the left ventricle is obstructed or empties slowly, the elastic recoil of peripheral vascular bed which normally occurs in diastole (and produces the dicrotic notch) occurs in late systole and is felt as a double pulse. In the case of mixed aortic valve disease it is the increased volume loading produced by a regurgitant aortic valve which causes prolonged emptying, and it is this together with an obstructed aortic valve that cause a double waveform.

(d) *Bigeminal pulse or 'pulsus bigeminus'* occurs as a result of a premature ectopic beat following a sinus beat. There is a compensatory pause following the extra systole which makes the sinus beat larger than normal.

(e) *Pulsus paradoxus* is an exaggerated normal response. Deep inspiration causes a reduction in intrathoracic pressure. This has a twofold effect — right ventricular volume increases and pooling of blood occurs within the pul-

monary circulation. The overall result is that with inspiration there is diminished return to the left ventricle, resulting in a lower stroke volume and a decreased pulse volume. Pulsus paradoxus is an exaggeration of this response.

In patients with *cardiac tamponade* the fluid within the pericardium exerts its own pressure and the normal physiological response is exaggerated by further compromising the volume of the left ventricle. It is also an important sign in patients with *severe asthma*; in this situation severe airflow limitation produces a sudden and increased negative intrathoracic pressure which exacerbates the normal physiological response. The paradox is that the heart may still be auscultated although there may be no pulse palpable at the wrist.

- *Volume*: with *pulsus alternans* the pulse volume alternates between strong and weak with successive beats; its presence is an indication that there is severe damage to the left ventricular muscle mass.

The jugular venous pulse

A measure of right atrial pressure may be attained from the jugular venous pulse (JVP). It does not measure volume but its level may give the observer an indication of the level of 'filling' of the cardiovascular system. It is an indicator of the competence of the right heart to accept and deliver blood (Fig. 18.2).

The a wave is distinguished from the v wave by palpation of the carotid artery. The a wave occurs immediately before the carotid pulsation.

Measurement of the JVP The patient should recline at an angle of 45° with the head supported and the neck muscles relaxed. In the normal subject the peaks of the JVP waves are just visible in the internal jugular vein. Without distinguishing the three separate waves, there is a mean level which is the perpendicular height of the blood column above the right atrium. The JVP is measured as the vertical distance between the manubrial sternal angle and the top of the venous column. It is usually less than $3 \, cmH_2O$.

Variations in the JVP These are as follows:
- A *low JVP* occurs in hypovolaemic states. It cannot be measured clinically, but the central venous pressure can by pressure transduction of the internal jugular vein. The JVP is defined by three waves (a, c, v) and two negative descents (x and y).
- A *raised JVP* is seen in:
  (a) heart failure;
  (b) cardiac tamponade;

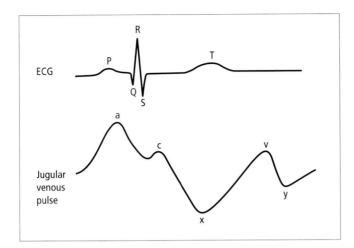

Figure 18.2 The jugular venous pulse in relation to the electrocardiogram; *a wave*, produced by atrial systole; *x descent*, occurs when atrial contraction finishes; *c wave*, interrupts the x descent and is caused by displacement of the tricuspid annulus into the right atrium as the right ventricular pressure rises — it is synchronous with ventricular systole; *v wave*, results from continued filling of right atrium during ventricular systole; *y descent*, represents the fall in right atrial pressure when the tricuspid valve opens and enters the right ventricle.

(c) fluid retention, including fluid overload;

(d) constrictive pericarditis; and

(e) superior vena caval obstruction.

Kussmaul's sign is an elevation of the JVP on inspiration, seen in patients with cardiac tamponade or constrictive pericarditis in whom ventricular filling is impeded.

• *Changes in wave pattern a waves are absent* in atrial fibrillation as there is no atrial contraction while *frequent a waves* are seen with atrial flutter. *Large a waves* occur when there is increased resistance to ventricular filling, e.g. tricuspid stenosis, pulmonary stenosis, pulmonary hypertension, all of which result in right ventricular hypertrophy. Commonly in tricuspid stenosis the patient is in atrial fibrillation and therefore the waves are not noticed. *Cannon waves* occur when the right atrium contracts against a closed tricuspid valve in complete heart block. *Large v waves* result from tricuspid regurgitation as the ventricular contraction is transmitted directly to the internal jugular veins.

Examination of the precordium

Inspection Deformities of the chest wall should be noted, for example, *pectus excavatum* (funnel chest), *pectus carinatum* (pigeon chest). Attention should also be paid to the spinal curvature e.g. *kyphoscoliosis*. Gross thoracic skeletal deformities may produce functional embarrassment of the heart as well as making surgery and anaesthesia more difficult.

Palpation The *apex beat* is the most lateral and inferior point of cardiac pulsation. It is felt in the mid calvicular line at the level of the left fifth intercostal space. The position of the apex beat is subject to great variability and it may be displaced as a result of thoracic cage deformities or lung disease. In many cases palpation of the left and right ventricle may be of greater value. It will yield information as to which ventricle is under strain, and whether the load is due to an increased stroke volume or is obstructive in nature.

• *Left ventricular impulse*: The examiner's palm locates the apex beat. As mentioned previously, it is the nature of this impulse which is of greater value than its position. In aortic stenosis the left ventricle is obstructed and hence the myocardium hypertrophies. This will be felt as a powerful heaving impulse. In aortic regurgitation, the ventricle deals with increased volumes of blood, and the resulting impulse will be turbulent and hyperdynamic. The left ventricular enlargement will produce a rather more diffuse impulse.

• *Right ventricular impulse* is palpable to the left of the sternum. If the right ventricle is hypertrophied, e.g. in atrial septal defect or pulmonary stenosis, a definite 'lift' may be felt.

Thrills These are palpable murmurs felt with the flat of the hand. They are caused by turbulent flow produced by blood flowing through stenosed valves or large volumes of blood passing through normal valves. Thrills indicate a definite abnormality. Systolic thrills in the aortic area are commonly due to aortic stenosis, and at the apex due to mitral regurgitation. A diastolic thrill at the apex is usually due to mitral stenosis. A thrill from aortic regurgitation is uncommon.

Auscultation By the time the examiner uses a stethoscope there should be well-founded clinical suspicion of the diagnosis. It should thus be regarded as a confirmatory diagnostic tool. However, once the mechanics underlying the heart sound are understood, further information may be elicited.

There are four areas where the normal heart sounds and added sounds (including murmurs) are most easily heard:

1 aortic area — second right intercostal space just to right of sternum;

2 pulmonary area — second left intercostal space just to left of sternum;

3 tricuspid area — fourth intercostal space to the left of the sternum (left sternal edge);

4 mitral area — point at which apex beat is heard.

The heart should be auscultated in all areas (aortic, pulmonary, mitral and left sternal edge) and the neck and axilla should also be listened to. The patient is turned on to the left side to listen for mitral stenosis, and sat forward on expiration to listen for aortic regurgitation. Listen first for sounds, then added sounds and finally murmurs. The bell picks up low-pitched sounds, e.g. third and fourth sounds and murmur of mitral stenosis. The diaphragm picks up high-pitched sounds, e.g. first and second heart sounds and most murmurs. The heart sound and any murmurs should always be timed with the carotid pulse.

Heart sounds There are four main heart sounds as follows:
• The *first heart sound* is caused by closure of mitral (M1) and tricuspid (T1) valves. The cessation of mitral valve flow might also contribute to the sound. Electrical and mechanical events on the left side of the heart slightly precede those on the right. Therefore mitral valve closure slightly precedes tricuspid closure. However, the observer may not hear this split. It is best heard over the mitral and tricuspid areas.
• The *second heart sound* is due to closure of aortic and pulmonary valves. The second sound is also normally split and is best heard in the corresponding aortic and pulmonary areas. The presence of two distinct components indicates that both valves are present and working. The aortic (A2) components slightly precede the pulmonary component (P2).

The gap between the first and second heart sounds represents the systolic phase of the cardiac cycle.
• The *third heart sound* is due to rapid expansion of the left ventricle in early diastole and therefore closely follows the second sound. It is a normal finding in patients with hyperdynamic states and in individuals under 30 years of age. Later in life a dilated left ventricle, mitral and aortic regurgitation will give rise to a third heart sound.
• The *fourth heart sound* is also due to ventricular filling and results from atrial contraction and hence immediately precedes the first heart sound. It occurs when the ventricle is non-compliant as in cardiac hypertrophy secondary to systemic hypertension or aortic stenosis. It has been observed as a normal finding in young athletes but is much more commonly associated with underlying pathology.

Additional sounds
• An *opening snap* of the mitral valve strongly suggests that the valve is thickened and fibrotic. It is heard just after the second sound and indicates mitral stenosis. It is heard best just medial to the apex beat. In surgical terms it signifies pliability of the valve, which may be suitable for a valve conservation procedure known as valvotomy (division of fused leaflets). This does not occur with a heavily calcified valve.
• *Friction rubs* are scratching/crunching noises produced by movement of the inflamed pericardium. As they are high-

Table 18.5 Heart murmurs.

SYSTOLIC MURMURS

Ejection systolic murmurs
Aortic stenosis
Aortic sclerosis
Pulmonary stenosis
Atrial sepal defect

Pansystolic regurgitant murmurs
Mitral regurgitation
Tricuspid regurgitation
Ventricular septal defect

DIASTOLIC MURMURS

Mid diastolic murmurs
Mitral stenosis
Tricuspid stenosis
Austin Flint murmur

Early diastolic murmur
Aortic regurgitation
Pulmonary regurgitation
Graham Steel murmur

pitched sounds they are best heard with the diaphragm in systole.

Murmurs Turbulent flow causes heart murmurs. Turbulence may be produced when there is high flow through a normal valve, or normal blood flow through an abnormal valve. The murmurs which may be heard in the heart are listed in Table 18.5.
• *Grading* of murmurs should be carried out to indicate the intensity of the murmur in question. This is arbitrary, either 1–4 or 1–6. A grade of 1 is very soft and heard only in good circumstances. The top end of the range indicates a very loud murmur associated with a palpable thrill.
• *Loudness and length* are proportional to the pressure gradient along which the blood passes. They are not good indicators of severity of the lesion. This is because, with a severely stenotic valve, the blood flow will be so little that no murmur will result.
• *Character*
(a) mitral/tricuspid — diastolic — low-pitched and rumbling;
(b) aortic/pulmonary — diastolic — high-frequency, decrescendo;
(c) mitral/tricuspid — systolic — blowing quality;
(d) aortic/pulmonary — systolic — harsher; rushing.
• *Ejection systolic murmurs.* Aortic stenotic murmurs are harsh and radiate to the neck. They are best heard over the aortic area. Pulmonary stenosis and atrial septal defect (ASD) are best heard at the left sternal edge on inspiration.
• *Pansystolic regurgitant murmurs.* Mitral regurgitation is

best heard at the apex, and radiates to axilla. Tricuspid regurgitation and ventricular septal defect (VSD) are best heard at the left sternal edge.

• *Mid diastolic murmurs*. Mitral stenosis is best heard at the apex. There is a loud mitral first sound, opening snap and low-pitched rumbling diastolic murmur. The patient should be rolled to the left side, and the murmur is accentuated on exertion. A presystolic murmur may also be heard. The latter is caused by the cusps almost closing together at the end of diastole. Tricuspid stenosis is best heard at the left sternal edge. The Austin Flint murmur is sometimes heard in aortic regurgitation (incompetence); it is produced where the flow of blood back into the left ventricle partially closes and obstructs the mitral valve.

• *Early diastolic murmur*. Aortic regurgitation is best heard at the left sternal edge and apex with the patient sitting forward and in expiration. Pulmonary regurgitation is best heard to the right of the sternum and is louder on inspiration. The Graham Steel murmur is heard in pulmonary hypertension when it is due to mitral stenosis which leads to pulmonary regurgitation.

Investigations

Cardiac enzymes

When myocardial muscle cells are damaged, a number of enzymes escape into the circulation. These can be detected in the serum and their presence used to confirm that tissue damage (e.g. myocardial infarction) has occurred. The commonly used enzymes are listed in Table 18.6.

Chest radiograph (see Chapter 19)

Attention should be paid to the bony outline, cardiac contour, areas of calcification and lungs. The size of the heart is compared with the diameter of the chest; the ratio should be no more than 50%.

Table 18.6 Cardiac enzymes.

Enzyme	Time of peak level after MI
Creatine phosphokinase (CPK) (CK-MB isoenzyme is more specific for MI)	Within 24 h
Aspartate aminotransferase (AST)	24–48 h
Alanine aminotransferase (ALT)	24–48 h
Lactic acid dehydrogenase (LDH)	3–4 days

MI, Myocardial infarction.

Electrocardiogram (ECG)

The ECG records the electrical activity generated by the myocardium. It is of value because it can identify myocardial ischaemia and infarction, ventricular hypertrophy and disturbances of rhythm. *Exercise electrocardiography* is a technique used to assess the cardiac response to exercise. The ECG is recorded whilst the patient is walking or running on a treadmill, and the work rate is gradually increased. The test is terminated when the patient complains of chest pain, dyspnoea, or if there are significant ST changes or the emergence of an arrhythmia. Myocardial ischaemia provoked by exertion results in ST segment depression of greater than 1 mm in the leads facing the affected area. During the exercise test full resuscitation equipment should be available.

Holter monitoring is a technique whereby a 24-h record of a patient's ECG is obtained. The ECG leads are placed on the patient and the ECG is recorded on a tape in a small recorder which the patient wears on a belt at the waist. The recording is analysed later, specifically looking for runs of arrhythmias.

Echocardiography and Doppler ultrasound

In this technique echoes of ultrasound waves are used to map the heart and study its function.

M-mode echocardiography

This utilizes a single ultrasound beam directed towards the heart to detect movement of structures within the heart (hence M-mode). These tracings are limited by the smallness of the area which can be visualized at any given time. M-mode images require considerable expertise to interpret correctly.

Cross-sectional or 2D echocardiography

This method visualizes a wedge, from which the relationships of various cardiac structures can be observed. Multiple ultrasound beams convey a moving image that is more easily recognized as an anatomical representation of a slice through the heart. It is well-suited to demonstrating malformation of the cardiac valves, septal defects, size of cardiac chambers and the presence of fluid or blood within the pericardium.

Doppler echocardiography

This provides knowledge about the velocity and direction of blood flow within the heart by utilizing the Doppler principle; if sound is reflected from a moving object, its frequency increases if the object is moving towards the observer and decreases if the object is moving away. With Doppler echocardiography ultrasonic beams are reflected from the red blood cells with a frequency that is proportional to the velocity of the blood flow. It is thus possible to detect a jet of blood passing across a regurgitant or leaking valve. In addition further information may be obtained by applying the Bernoulli equation to estimate the pressure difference which generated the velocity of blood. It is therefore possible to estimate the pressure differences across the heart valves.

Transoesophageal echocardiography (TOE)

In this technique, M-mode and cross-sectional imaging transducers as well as Doppler transducers are incorporated into the end of a flexible endoscope. The procedure is performed as per gastroscopy; the pharynx is sprayed with local anaesthetic and the patient is given a small amount of sedative intravenously. As the oesophagus is traversed by the scope, the heart is seen anteriorly and the descending thoracic aorta posteriorly. Although this procedure takes a long time and requires operator skill, the images obtained are of a very high quality as the heart is imaged with little intervening tissue and its important structures are near the transducer. TOE is very valuable in the diagnosis of infective endocarditis because of its ability to pick up very small vegetations. It will also enable the ascending and descending aorta to be visualized, as well as regurgitation through a mitral valve prosthesis. Hyperinflated lungs do not interfere with the images obtained by TOE and the technique may be used to image the heart during cardiac surgery.

Nuclear imaging

These techniques are primarily used in the assessment of ischaemic heart disease.

Thallium imaging

Thallium behaves like potassium, with healthy myocardium taking it up and ischaemia or infarction producing a 'cold spot'. A cold spot which appears on exercise and that is reversed by rest implies ischaemia on exertion, whereas a persistent cold spot implies infarction.

Pyrophosphate imaging

Pyrophosphate labelled with technetium will produce a 'hot spot' in an infarcted area. Disadvantages include uptake into other tissue, and complete occlusion of an artery causing the infarction will not distribute the isotope.

Radionucleotide imaging—MUGA scan

Multigated acquisition or MUGA is obtained by the injection of technetium 99. This radioisotope attaches to the erythrocytes of the patient and can therefore outline the ventricle, and estimate the volume of ventricular ejection — *left ventricular ejection fraction (LVEF)*.
- Normal: greater to or equal to 60%;
- Depressed: 40–50%;
- Severely depressed: less than 30%.

A deterioration on exercise is suggestive of coronary disease or an abnormality of the myocardium.

Computed tomography and magnetic resonance imaging

Computed tomography (CT) will show clearly the size and shape of the cardiac chambers as well as the thoracic aorta and mediastinum. The development of magnetic resonance imaging (MRI) has lagged behind its other applications due to the movement of the heart and because of the continued development of CT and echocardiography. The significant development of ECG-synchronized images has led to a wider application by producing images in systole and diastole. MRI is particularly useful in the investigation of pericardial disease, cardiac tumours, prosthetic valve pathology and thoracic aortic disease.

Cardiac catheterization and angiography

This technique is performed to measure intracardiac pressures, blood oxygen content in the various heart chambers and cardiac output.

The right heart is catheterized by introducing the catheter into a peripheral vein and advancing it through the right atrium and ventricle to the pulmonary artery. The left heart is catheterized via the brachial or femoral artery. The catheter then traverses the aortic valve to enter the left ventricle. Direct-pressure measurements may be made of the right heart chambers, aorta, left ventricle and pulmonary artery. The left atrial pressure may be measured by indirect means. This is by wedging the catheter into the distal pulmonary artery. The pressure from the right ventricle is obstructed by the catheter and only the pulmonary venous and left atrial pressures are measured. This value is the pulmonary capillary wedge pressure (PCWP). A simplified version of this manoeuvre, in which a balloon-tipped (Swan–Ganz) catheter is floated into the pulmonary circulation and the balloon is inflated to obtain a wedge pressure, has widespread application in intensive therapy unit monitoring of patients with heart failure (Fig. 18.3).

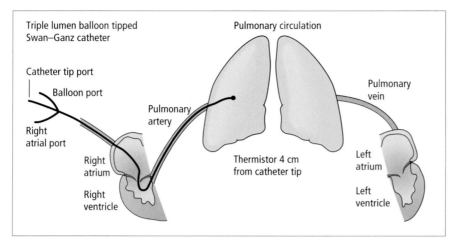

Triple lumen balloon tipped
Swan–Ganz catheter

Catheter tip port

Balloon port

Right
atrial port

Right
atrium

Right
ventricle

Pulmonary
artery

Pulmonary circulation

Thermistor 4 cm
from catheter tip

Pulmonary
vein

Left
atrium

Left
ventricle

(a)

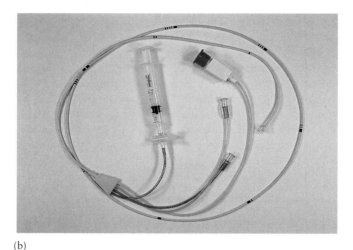

(b)

Figure 18.3 a,b (a) Schematic representation of a Swan–Ganz catheter. The catheter is passed via the superior vena cava through the right atrium and ventricle into the pulmonary artery. The right atrial pressure (= central venous pressure; CVP) is measured via the right atrial port. The pulmonary artery pressure (PAP) is measured via the catheter tip port when the balloon at the tip of the catheter is deflated. Inflating the balloon occludes the peripheral branch of the pulmonary artery and measures pulmonary capillary wedge pressure (PCWP), which reflects left atrial pressure. Cardiac output (CO) can be measured using a thermodilution technique. A 10 ml bolus of saline at 0°C is injected via the right atrial port and the temperature change is detected by the thermistor at the catheter tip. From this dilution the CO can be calculated. (b) Swan–Ganz catheter.

Cardiac catheterization allows the selective injection of radiopaque contrast material so that patterns of blood flow can be observed and recorded. The dye may be injected down the orifices of the left and right coronary arteries to identify abnormalities within these arteries. This process is called *angiography* and is an essential prerequisite for coronary bypass surgery by identifying the coronary anatomy and distribution of the disease. Different views are taken to provide a three-dimensional impression of the coronary arterial circulation. Angiography is not entirely without risk and as such it should only be performed when other non-invasive techniques of investigation are unable to provide the information required.

Perioperative care

Preoperative preparation

Following clinical assessment and informed consent, the cardiac surgical patient is ready for operation. Blood is drawn for preoperative biochemical, haematological investigations and blood is cross-matched. All preoperative medication should be given prior to surgery, with the exception of aspirin which should be discontinued at least 10 days beforehand. Because of its antiplatelet effects, bleeding may be a problem peroperatively if the patient is taking

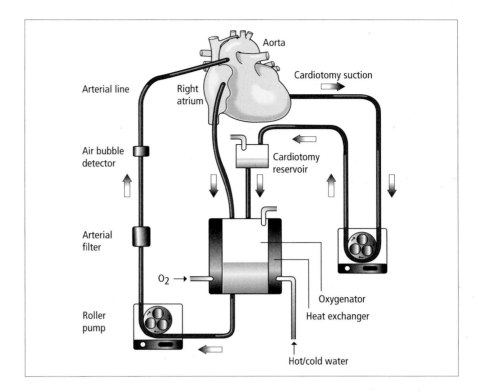

Figure 18.4 Cardiopulmonary bypass circuit.

aspirin. Prophylactic antibiotic cover is mandatory in all procedures. The antibiotics of choice differ between cardiothoracic units but should cover *Streptococcus* and *Staphylococcus* species. Antibiotics should be continued into the postoperative period for 2 days or until central lines are removed, which ever is longer.

The cardiac operation

Cardiac operations differ from other types of surgery in that the heart has to be stopped (arrested) so that the operation may be performed and the work of the heart and lungs has to be taken over by a machine (cardiopulmonary bypass; Fig. 18.4). Furthermore, as the heart itself is not being perfused during the operation it becomes ischaemic and must therefore be protected (myocardial protection).

Cardiopulmonary bypass

It is necessary to support the circulation during a variety of cardiac surgical procedures. This is because the heart needs to remain still for accurate placement of sutures, and also because in many cases, the heart has to be disturbed from its normal functional position. The elements of a cardiopulmonary bypass circuit are:

- a venous reservoir;
- a heat exchanger;
- an oxygenator;
- a roller pump; and
- an arterial filter.

The circuit is maintained and operated by a trained *perfusionist*. Blood is drained from the right atrium under the force of gravity. It passes to an oxygenator which takes over the function of the lungs and so ventilation can be discontinued. The blood is returned to the systemic circulation by roller pumps, having passed through a heat exchanger for cooling and rewarming and an arterial filter to remove any microemboli. Venous drainage is accomplished by either one or two cannula(e) placed into the right atrium or superior and inferior vena cavae, respectively. Arterial return is by a cannula placed within the ascending aorta. The bypass circuit will activate the patient's clotting cascade and in order to prevent this, the patient is heparinized (3 mg/kg).

Complications of cardiopulmonary bypass

Side-effects from cardiopulmonary bypass may occur even after short-term use.
- *Clotting factor activation and consumption* occur when blood comes into contact with foreign surfaces. Heparin

prevents this but has to be reversed with protamine at the end of the procedure to prevent excessive bleeding. If a coagulopathy persists then additional clotting factors may be necessary.

- *Destruction of blood components*: Haemolysis and platelet destruction occur as a result of the shearing forces encountered during bypass.
- *Immunological derangements*: All components of the cellular and humoral divisions of the immune system are depressed during cardiopulmonary bypass. Of particular importance is the additional activation of the complement system which results in vasoconstriction, whole-body inflammation and capillary leakage.
- *Oedema*: The combination of haemodilution and a decrease in plasma colloid osmotic pressure together with the fluid-conserving response to surgery results in postoperative oedema.
- *Cerebral dysfunction*: Stroke occurs in 1–2% of patients. However, neuropsychological tests will show minor abnormalities in a high proportion of patients. These tend to disappear within the first few months following surgery. These effects may in part be explained by microemboli of air and formed elements within the blood stream, as well as the presence of pre-existing extra- or intracranial vascular disease.

Myocardial protection

To prevent the heart from beating, a cross-clamp is applied between the aortic valve and the arterial cannula. This renders the heart ischaemic, and two methods have evolved to limit ischaemic damage:

- *Defibrillation*: Following application of the aortic cross-clamp, the heart is fibrillated using an electrical fibrillator. This arrests the pulsatile movement of the heart; however the 'safe' period of ischaemia is only about 15 min. Following the removal of the cross-clamp the heart is allowed to reperfuse in sinus rhythm, which is obtained by defibrillation. This method is used by some surgeons when performing the distal anastomosis of a coronary bypass graft.
- *Cardioplegia*: This method has superseded the former for the majority of cardiac operations. Following application of the aortic cross-clamp an infusion of a cold, hyperkalaemic solution is made via a small cannula in the aortic root (below the cross-clamp). The fluid flows into the ostia of the left and right coronary arteries. The high potassium content produces a rapid diastolic arrest and the cold temperature gives reliable protection to the myocardium for long periods of ischaemia. Cooling via the heat exchanger to 28–32°C provides additional myocardial protection by slowing the metabolic rate.

Postoperative management

Transfer from the operating theatre to the intensive care unit is a dangerous period. Mechanical ventilation and monitoring are maintained and sedation, inotropes and vasodilators are continued by infusion pumps. As a general rule most patients are ventilated overnight, although routine noncomplex cases are increasingly being extubated earlier. Too early extubation will provide additional stresses to the myocardium. In the immediate postoperative period, continuing diuresis, rewarming and blood loss will require volume expansion using either blood or plasma expanders.

This depends on the haematocrit of the patient's blood, which should ideally be kept to 0.30–0.35. There may be a large requirement for electrolytes, particularly potassium as a result of the postoperative diuresis, large infused volumes of crystalloid, and preoperative status. Postassium should be maintained in the range of 4.5–5.0 mmol/l. Following extubation the patient is transferred to a high-dependence unit where invasive monitoring continues for another 24 h in uncomplicated cases.

Cardiac physiology

An understanding of circulatory physiology is essential for the management of the cardiac surgical patient. Changes induced by disease or surgery will not be appreciated unless the principles which govern cardiovascular responses in the normal individual are understood. Table 18.7 highlights the haemodynamic parameters commonly used to assess circulatory function and provides some understanding of their derivation. Most of the parameters listed are measured routinely in cardiac patients postoperatively.

Invasive monitoring

The routine measurements that are made on the intensive care unit are urinary output, central venous pressure, arterial blood pressure and arterial blood gases. Measurement of hourly urinary output is a simple way to assess that the kidneys and, by inference, the rest of the peripheral tissues are being adequately perfused. A urinary output of 0.5 ml/kg per h (i.e. >30 ml/h for most people) indicates adequate perfusion. Frequently, more sophisticated assessment of cardiac function is required and for this a Swan–Ganz catheter has to be placed.

Pulmonary and systemic vascular resistance are calculated by computer with a knowledge of the measured cardiac output, and the patient's body surface area, venous and arterial pressures and heart rate.

Specific problems following cardiac surgery

- *Bleeding* may be due to a coagulopathy as a result of cardiopulmonary bypass or to poor surgical technique. The patient should be returned to theatre if the bleeding is not arrested by additional clotting factors.

Table 18.7 Some commonly used haemodynamic parameters.

Parameter	How derived	Normal value
Direct measurements		
Heart rate	Direct measurement, usually from ECG	72–88 beats/min
Arterial pressure	Direct measurement via radial artery cannula	120/80 mmHg
Mean arterial pressure (MAP)	Diastolic blood pressure + one-third (pulse pressure)	70–105 mmHg
Central venous pressure (CVP)	Direct measurement via central venous line	0–9 cmH$_2$O
Mean pulmonary arterial pressure (MPAP)	Direct measurement via Swan–Ganz catheter	9–16 mmHg
Pulmonary capillary wedge pressure (PCWP)	Direct measurement via Swan–Ganz catheter	8–12 mmHg
Derived measurements		
Pulse pressure	Systolic blood pressure – diastolic blood pressure	40–60 mmHg
Stroke volume	End-diastolic volume – end-systolic volume	75–80 ml/beat
Cardiac output (CO)	Stroke volume × heart rate	5.5–6.0 l/min
Cardiac index (CI)	Cardiac output/body surface area	3.0 l/min per m^2
Systemic vascular resistance (SVR)	Mean arterial pressure–right atrial pressure/cardiac output	900–1400 dyn/s per cm^5
Pulmonary vascular resistance (PVR)	PAP – PCWP/cardiac output	150–250 dyn/s per cm^5

• *Low cardiac output state* is manifested by hypotension, cool extremities, tachycardia, oliguria and obtundation. The cause may be primary cardiac failure which may be due to intraoperative myocardial infarction, poor revascularization (in the case of coronary artery bypass graft or CABG) and poor myocardial protection. In addition, compression of the heart from blood within the pericardial cavity will cause tamponade. In this case the central venous pressure (CVP) will usually be high. Other causes include hypoxia, hypovolaemia or the development of arrhythmias. In most cases pharmacological treatment is directed at the cause. Surgical reopening may be necessary in some cases to exclude the presence of a tamponade.

• *Hypertension* is common in patients with pre-existing hypertension and good left ventricles. Before treatment is commenced, pain, hypoxia and hypercarbia should be excluded.

• *Arrhythmias*: The development of an arrhythmia requires prompt treatment. The commonest arrhythmia is atrial fibrillation. Hypoxia, hypercarbia and electrolyte abnormalities should be sought and treated, although commonly no cause is found.

• *Hypoxia*: It is essential that the patient remains adequately oxygenated. As well as oxygen therapy, a cause should be sought, e.g. pneumothorax, lobar collapse, consolidation, atelectasis, position of endotracheal tube and pulmonary oedema.

• *Hypothermia*: The patient is frequently cooled in theatre. Hypothermia is deleterious as it may lead to hypertension, myocardial irritability and shivering, with increased oxygen requirements. Humidified ventilation, space blankets and warmed intravenous fluid should be used.

• *Renal failure*: A diuresis is common following cardiopulmonary bypass. It may be due to pre-existing disease, haemolysis, hypoperfusion, renal vasoconstriction, long cardiopulmonary bypass and toxins. Treatment is along conventional lines.

• *Neurological deficits*: Investigations include CT or MRI scans along with Doppler studies of the external carotid arteries. Treatment may include heparinization, but is usually expectant and supportive.

Cardiac surgery for specific diseases of the heart

Surgery for ischaemic heart disease

Coronary artery disease

Introduction

Ischaemic heart disease is the commonest cause of death in the western world, claiming more than 3000 deaths per million each year in the UK. It results from atheromatous narrowing of the coronary arteries and may present as sudden death or an acute myocardial infarction, but more commonly presents as *angina pectoris*. This is typically provoked by exertion and relieved by rest.

Physical examination is frequently normal, although the stigmata of hypercholesterolaemia of diabetes may be present. The auscultation of a heart murmur or carotid bruit will require further investigation.

Investigations

Resting and exercise ECGs will demonstrate evidence of exercise-induced ischaemia, previous infarction or arrhythmias. This test provides objective evidence, so that medical therapy may be instituted, monitored and the need for further intervention assessed.

Coronary angiography is performed when it is felt that patients need revascularization, whether this is by angioplasty or coronary bypass surgery.

Indications for surgery

Medical therapy is recommended when ischaemia is prevented by anti-ischaemic drugs that are well-tolerated. With one- or two-vessel disease not involving the left anterior descending artery, medical therapy (or angioplasty) is recommended first, with CABG being reserved for refractory ischaemia. With limited coronary artery disease refractory to medical therapy, angioplasty should be considered before recommending surgery, unless there is a compelling reason such as left main disease. If angioplasty is high-risk or the lesions are technically unsuitable, CABG is the correct way to proceed.

Coronary artery surgery may benefit the patient both in terms of providing symptomatic relief and in many cases is of prognostic benefit. Data accumulated from three large prospective randomized trials have shown that surgery is better than medical therapy for improving survival in left main or triple-vessel disease (i.e. stenosis in each of the three main arteries; right, left anterior descending and circumflex), double-vessel disease involving the left anterior descending artery, and chronic ischaemia leading to left ventricular dysfunction.

Surgical procedure

• Following the institution of *cardiopulmonary bypass* and application of the aortic cross-clamp, the heart is *arrested in diastole* and protected from ischaemic damage by the administration of cardioplegia. Usually 1 litre is infused in the first instance, followed by further infusions at further time intervals thereafter. Topical cooling in the form of ice is applied to the myocardial surface, and the patient is also systemically cooled by the heat exchanger on the bypass machine.

• The graft of choice is the internal *mammary* (*internal thoracic*) *artery*. It is anastomosed most commonly to the left anterior descending artery. In this situation it confers greater protection from subsequent cardiac events (angina, myocardial infarction and sudden death). Its patency rates are superior to long saphenous vein (95%

and 85% patency at 5 and 10 years respectively can be expected).

• Reserved long saphenous vein is also used extensively as a conduit. However, vein grafts are prone to occlusion at a rate of 10–20% in the first year, with an occlusion rate of 2–3% per year thereafter. Treatment with low-dose aspirin following the operation enhances patency.

An arteriotomy is made distal to the coronary artery stenosis. The reversed saphenous vein is then anastomosed using a fine Prolene suture. All distal anastomoses are performed in this fashion, and if the internal mammary artery is being used it is anastomosed last. When all distal anastomoses have been performed, the aortic cross-clamp is removed, allowing the heart to reperfuse and beat. As the patient rewarms, the proximal anastomoses to the aorta are performed.

• Following completion of all anastomoses and warming of the patient, ventilation is recommenced, and providing the patient is in a stable rhythm, cardiopulmonary bypass is discontinued. Following removal of venous and arterial cannulae, protamine is given to reverse the anticoagulant effects of heparin.

Outcome

The hospital mortality following CABG is 1–4% and this is likely to be a reflection of operating on older patients and those with impaired left ventricular function. Although the majority of patients get relief from angina, recurrent angina is most likely to occur within the first year following surgery. This is usually due to graft failure as a result of poor anastomotic technique, or an inadequate distal vessel. Only 50% of vein grafts are patent at 10 years. The internal mammary artery has a superior patency rate. Approximately 10% of patients will have a second operation within the ensuing 10 years. Reoperation is associated with an increased operative mortality and is reserved for patients with severe symptoms refractory to maximal medical therapy.

Complications of myocardial infarction

Most complications of acute myocardial infarction occur in the early post myocardial infarction period. The patient is frequently in cardiogenic shock. The aetiology of the circulatory collapse must be ascertained before a management plan can be formulated. As a general rule the earlier the occurrence of the complication, the higher is the overall mortality.

The surgically correctable complications of myocardial infarction are:
• VSD;
• mitral regurgitation;

- left ventricular aneurysm;
- ventricular arrhythmias; and
- ruptured ventricle.

The patient is normally profoundly unwell and is admitted directly to the intensive care unit. Full invasive monitoring, including the insertion of a Swan–Ganz catheter (which may demonstrate an interventricular shunt), will be necessary. Cardiogenic shock is treated by inotropic drugs, vasodilators and diuretics. Shock refractory to these therapies will frequently require a mechanical device to assist the failing heart. Such a device is known as an intra-aortic balloon pump. If arrhythmias are the cause of heart failure they should be treated by the use of antiarrhythmics, pacing or direct current cardioversion.

An ECG will demonstrate the presence and extent of an infarct, and associated arrhythmias. Echocardiography will demonstrate mitral regurgitation, VSD, left ventricular aneurysm, left ventricular dysfunction and a ruptured left ventricle.

If the patient is stable, then angiography can proceed so that revascularization may be performed in association with any other corrective procedure. This is often not possible as

Ischaemic heart disease at a glance

DEFINITION

Ischaemic heart disease is a common disorder caused by acute or chronic interruption of the blood supply to the myocardium, usually due to atherosclerosis of the coronary arteries, i.e. *coronary artery disease*

EPIDEMIOLOGY

M>F before age 65. Increasing risk with increasing age up to 80 years. Commonest cause of death in the western world

AETIOLOGY

- Atherosclerosis and thrombosis
- Thromboemboli
- Arteritis (e.g. periarteritis nodosa)
- Coronary artery spasm
- Extension of aortic dissecting aneurysm
- Syphilitic aortitis

RISK FACTORS

- Cigarette smoking
- Hypertension
- Hyperlipidaemia
- Type A personality
- Obesity

PATHOLOGY

- Reduction in coronary blood flow is critical when lumen is decreased by 90%
- Angina pectoris results when the supply of oxygen to the heart muscle is unable to meet the increased demands for oxygen, e.g during exercise, cold, after a meal
- Thrombotic occlusion of the narrowed lumen precipitates acute ischaemia
- The heart muscle in the territory of the occluded vessel dies — myocardial infarction. May be subendocardial or transmural

CLINICAL FEATURES

Angina pectoris
- Central chest pain on exertion, especially in cold weather, lasts 1–15 min
- Radiates to neck, jaw, arms
- Relieved by glyceryl trinitrate (GTN)

Myocardial infarction
- Severe central chest pain for >30 min duration
- Radiates to neck, jaw, arms
- Not relieved by GTN

- Usually no signs

- Signs of cardiogenic shock
- Arrhythmias

INVESTIGATIONS

Angina pectoris
- FBC for anaemia
- Thyroid function tests
- CXR heart size
- ECG ST-segment changes
- Exercise ECG
- Coronary angiography

Myocardial infarction
- ECG: Q waves, ST segment and T-wave changes
- Cardiac enzymes: LDH/CPK, CPK-MB
- CXR
- FBC, U&E

MANAGEMENT

Angina pectoris
- Lose weight
- Avoid precipitating factors (e.g. cold)
- GTN (sublingual)
- Calcium-channel blockers
- ß-Blockers, nitrates, aspirin
- Rx hypertension and hyperlipidaemias
- Coronary angioplasty or coronary artery bypass surgery (CABG)

Indications for CABG
- Left main stem disease
- Triple-vessel disease
- Two-vessel disease involving left anterior descending (LAD)
- Chronic ischaemia + LV dysfunction

Myocardial infarction
- Bedrest, oxygen, analgesia
- Thrombolysis
- Aspirin
- Rx heart failure (diuretics)
- Rx arrhythmias

COMPLICATIONS OF MYOCARDIAL INFARCTION

- Arrhythmias
- Cardiogenic shock
- Myocardial rupture
- Papillary muscle rupture causing mitral incompetence
- Ventricular aneurysm
- Pericarditis
- Mural thrombosis and peripheral embolism

the risks of catheterization may be prohibitive. In this situation surgery may proceed in the absence of CABG.

Transplantation should be considered for some patients with poor left ventricular function and heart failure, rather than correction of the defect with or without revascularization.

Surgery for valvular heart disease

Introduction

The number of operations for valvular heart disease has not risen as dramatically as those for coronary artery disease. The function of the heart valves is to maintain the forward flow of blood through the chambers of the heart. Disease may affect a valve by making the orifice smaller (*stenosis*) or by allowing backflow or leakage (*regurgitation* or *incompetence*) through the valve. Both stenosis and incompetence may coexist.

A stenotic valve produces a *pressure load* on the cardiac chamber immediately proximal to it. This chamber responds by becoming hypertrophied. Back-pressure on other chambers and vessels may follow. An incompetent valve produces a *volume load* which has effects both upstream and downstream from the valve. The proximal heart chamber will enlarge predominantly by dilatation, but also to some extent by hypertrophy.

Aetiology of heart valve disease

Rheumatic fever

In the UK rheumatic fever has largely disappeared. However, in developing countries its incidence is still high. The pathology of rheumatic fever is an immune-mediated acute inflammatory reaction which affects predominantly the heart valves (although the epicardium and myocardium may also be involved). It is due to cross-reaction between surface antigens of group A β-haemolytic streptococci and certain cardiac proteins. In the acute phase a valvulitis occurs which is followed by further haemodynamic trauma, resulting in progressive valve failure with fibrosis and calcification. The initial valvulitis may be diagnosed by detecting the presence of a murmur. Stenosis results when there is fusion of the valve leaflets and regurgitation occurs when there is retraction and shortening of the scar tissue.

Congenital valve abnormalities

Several valve abnormalities may occur as part of the spectrum of congenital heart disease, e.g. Fallot's tetralogy (Fig. 18.5) but detailed discussion of the various congenital abnormalities is beyond the scope of this book.

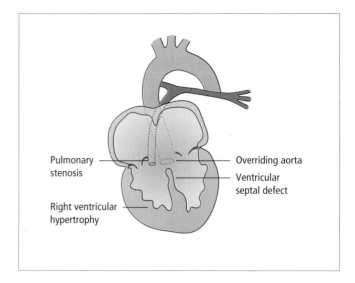

Figure 18.5 The tetralogy of Fallot is the commonest type of cyanotic congenital heart disease in older children and adults. Because of the pulmonary stenosis the shunt is from right to left and the patient is cyanotic. These patients often have marked finger clubbing.

The aortic valve is normally tricuspid, but in 1–2% of individuals it has only two cusps. A functional disturbance presents in middle adult life related to long-term turbulent flow associated with the bicuspid valve. The disturbance is related to progressive calcification of the valve which leads to stenosis and incompetence.

Degenerative valve disease

Degenerative valve disease is caused by progressive 'wear and tear' of the valvular apparatus. It is being increasingly recognized as a feature of the elderly population. A syndrome described as the mitral floppy valve syndrome is a particular form of degenerative valve disease. Not only is there cystic change within the mitral valve leaflets but the chordal apparatus becomes increasingly elongated. It leads to mitral regurgitation.

Infective endocarditis (see below)

Pathophysiology of heart valve abnormalities

Aortic valve

Aortic stenosis

A narrowed aortic office results in increased pressure in the left ventricle. Because the valve is stenosed, the pressure in the ventricle will be higher than the pressure in the root of the aorta during systole, i.e. a gradient exists across the valve. As the ventricle has to work more to overcome the obstruction, it hypertrophies. As the size of the ventricle increases there is a corresponding increase in myocardial oxygen requirements. When supply exceeds demand the patient experiences *angina*. Syncopal attacks may also occur, particularly on exertion. *Syncope* occurs because the left ventricle is unable to increase its output in response to exercise-induced systemic vasodilatation. Left ventricular hypertrophy is a compensatory mechanism. However, there is a limit to the amount of compensation that can be achieved and as the stenosis becomes tighter the compensatory mechanisms begin to fail, resulting in progressive ventricular dilatation and *heart failure*. Operation is performed to improve prognosis and to relieve symptoms, particularly if the aortic valve gradient is in excess of 60 mmHg.

Aortic regurgitation

When the aortic valve is incompetent blood floods back into the ventricle during diastole. Thus the ventricle has to deal with an increased volume load which it does by dilatation. Aortic regurgitation is usually better tolerated than aortic stenosis but will progressively lead to *left ventricular failure*.

Mitral valve

Mitral stenosis

A pressure load is placed on the left atrium. This is transmitted to the pulmonary circulation which responds by progressive *pulmonary hypertension*. The left atrium is not usually dilated. As pulmonary arterial pressure increases there is an increasing load on the right ventricle. In due course the tricuspid valve, right atrium and liver suffer the effects of back-pressure (*congestive cardiac failure*). In the early stages of mitral stenosis acute pulmonary oedema may occur, often as *paroxysmal nocturnal dyspnoea*. This will occur when the left atrial pressure exceeds the oncotic pressure in the pulmonary circulation. In some cases this may be precipitated by the development of an atrial arrhythmia, characteristically *atrial fibrillation*. In long-established cases, pulmonary oedema occurs less frequently. Surgery is performed for symptomatic deterioration, particularly New York Heart Association (NHYA) class III or IV. A valve area of less than 1.0 cm is a further indication for operation. The left atrium may contain thrombus, which makes *systemic embolization* particularly likely, especially if atrial fibrillation has developed. This constitutes a further reason for operation.

Mitral regurgitation

A volume load is produced on the left atrium and is also associated with dilatation of the left ventricle. When this occurs slowly, large increases in cardiac chamber size may occur before any increase in pulmonary artery pressure develops. In the situation where regurgitation develops suddenly due to rupture of a papillary muscle or chorda (e.g. after a myocardial infarction), the left atrial volume is small, with the result that the pulmonary vascular pressure rises abruptly, causing *pulmonary oedema* and severe *hypoxia*. In the acute situation surgery may be life-saving. The case is more complex for the patient with chronic mitral regurgitation. Valve replacement in this situation will not affect the damaged and dilated ventricle, which will still continue to require a high filling pressure. Overall, the timing of surgery should be judged on the basis of left ventricular function as well as symptoms.

Tricuspid valve

The majority of patients with tricuspid valve disease have tricuspid regurgitation secondary to right ventricular failure (e.g. caused by mitral valve disease) with long-term dilatation of the tricuspid valve annulus. The clinical signs are those of congestive cardiac failure, prominent jugular venous pulsations, liver congestion, ascites and peripheral oedema. In a small number of cases the pathological process is rheumatic fever. Operations for these conditions are uncommon in the UK and are frequently performed only in association with other valve replacements.

Pulmonary valve

Pulmonary valve disease is almost always a paediatric condition and as such is beyond the scope of this book.

Investigations of patients with heart valve disease

As has been stressed earlier in this chapter, the history and clinical examination of the patient are of great importance. Whilst the symptoms and physical signs of mitral valve disease frequently mirror the severity of the valvular defect, the symptoms of aortic valve disease may present at a later state when the point of optimal surgical intervention has been passed.
• The *ECG* will define the cardiac rhythm and will give an indication of heart hypertrophy.
• The *chest radiograph* will demonstrate cardiac size, heart chamber size (in some cases) and evidence of pulmonary oedema.

- *Echocardiography* (*transthoracic* and *transoesophageal*) is increasingly being used to provide evidence of chamber enlargement, imaging of the heart valve and calcification.
- *Doppler techniques* provide a measure of valve gradients and of regurgitation.

These assessments negate in many circumstances the need for cardiac catheterization.

In certain situations, *cardiac catheterization* may be required. It allows imaging of the coronary arteries, which is important in elderly patients, particularly with the symptoms of angina. It also allows direct measurement of transvalvular gradients and visualization and quantification of the degree of valvular regurgitation.

Surgery for heart valve disease

Virtually all operations are now performed with cardiopulmonary bypass and cardioplegia. The heart chambers are opened, allowing the surgeon to see the valves.

Valve replacement versus valve conservation

Artificial heart valves are non-physiological. Therefore, if possible, the patient's diseased valve should be remodelled. This is usually only possible with the mitral and sometimes the tricuspid valve. The criteria for valve repair are as follows:
- valve damage is minimal;
- the valve leaflets are mobile; and
- there is no calcification.

Artificial heart valves

There are three main groups of artificial heart valves:
- *Prosthetic valves*: Prosthetic valves are the most popular choice for the majority of patients. These valves are either of the ball-and-cage variety or use a tilting disc occluder or bileaflet mechanism. The initial use of metal alloys and plastics is now being superseded by pyrolytic carbon. A sewing ring made of Dacron allows suture of the valve to the native valve annulus. Patients with prosthetic valves implanted are at risk from *thromboembolism, endocarditis* (which may also produce septic emboli) and *'valve wear-out'*.

Because of the risk of thromboembolism, lifelong anticoagulation is required in patients with prosthetic heart valves. Warfarin is commenced within 48 h of operation. Anticoagulation is carried on for life. The currently recommended range of international normalized ratio (INR) in the UK has been arbitrarily set at 3–4.5. Any interventional procedures on patients with prosthetic heart valves should be performed with antibiotic cover to prevent valve endocarditis occurring (see below).

- *Bioprosthetic valves*: Animal tissue is mounted on a synthetic frame or stent. A common tissue used is *porcine aortic valve*, which is treated with glutaraldehyde to reduce antigenicity. For patients with bioprosthetic valves, anticoagulation is carried on for 3 months until the valve has become epithelialized.
- *Biological valves*: These contain only biological tissue. Cadaveric tissue is used to create a *homograft* valve. In the hands of enthusiastic proponents they give excellent haemodynamic performance and are relatively free from thromboembolic risk.

Anticoagulation is not required for biological valves.

Infective endocarditis

Introduction

Infective endocarditis affects 6–7 individuals per 100 000 annually in the UK, with a male to female ratio of 2:1. It usually results from a *bacterial infection* originating on the endocardium or vascular endothelium, although infection may be caused by *rickettsiae* and *fungi*. The use of prophylactic antibiotics in patients with known valve lesions is of extreme importance in negating the bacteraemic effect of potential sources of infection, e.g. dental procedures, urinary infections or prostatectomy. The disease may occur as a fulminating or acute infection but more commonly runs an insidious and protracted course known as subacute (bacterial) endocarditis. Infective endocarditis is typically associated with a preceding valvular or intracardiac abnormality. However, patients with normal valves (especially those with impaired immunity) may be affected by highly virulent organisms.

Before the advent of antibiotics, bacterial endocarditis was uniformly fatal; with the introduction of penicillin the mortality was reduced to 30–40%.

Aetiology

The most common organisms responsible for infective endocarditis are listed below.
- *Streptococcus viridans* forms part of the bacterial flora of the pharynx and upper respiratory tract. Any instrumentation of these areas (dental procedures, tonsillectomy, etc.) is liable to cause a transient bacteraemia which will initiate the infection.
- *Streptococcus faecalis* is found in faecal and perineal flora. As a consequence, manipulation of the genitourinary tract may predispose to infection.

Valvular heart disease at a glance

DEFINITION

Valvular heart disease is defined as a group of conditions characterized by damage to one or more of the heart valves, resulting in deranged blood flow through the heart chambers

EPIDEMIOLOGY

Rheumatic fever is still a major problem in developing countries, while *congenital heart disease* occurs in 8–10 cases per 1000 live births worldwide

AETIOLOGY

- Congenital valve abnormalities
- Infective endocarditis
- Rheumatic fever
- Degenerative valve disease

PATHOLOGY

- *Rheumatic fever*: *immune-mediated acute inflammation* affecting the heart valves due to a cross-reaction between antigens of group A β-haemolytic streptococcus and cardiac proteins
- Disease may make the valve orifice smaller (*stenosis*) or unable to close properly (*incompetence* or *regurgitation*) or both
- Stenosis causes a *pressure load*, while regurgitation causes a *volume load* on the heart chamber immediately proximal to it with upstream and downstream effects

CLINICAL FEATURES

Aortic stenosis
- Angina pectoris
- Syncope
- Left heart failure
- Slow upstroke arterial pulse
- Precordial systolic thrill (2nd Rt ICS)

Aortic regurgitation
- Congestive cardiac failure
- Increased pulse pressure
- Water-hammer pulse
- Decrescendo diastolic murmur (lower Lt sternal edge)

ICS, intercostal space.

- Harsh mid systolic ejection murmur (2nd RtICS)

Mitral stenosis
- Pulmonary hypertension
- Paroxysmal nocturnal dyspnoea
- Atrial fibrillation
- Loud first heart sound and opening snap
- Low-pitched diastolic murmur with presystolic accentuation at the apex

Tricuspid stenosis
- Fatigue
- Peripheral oedema
- Liver enlargement/ascites
- Prominent JVP with large a waves
- Lung fields are clear
- Rumbling diastolic murmur (lower Lt sternal border)

Mitral regurgitation
- Chronic fatigue
- Pulmonary oedema
- Apex laterally displaced hyperdynamic precordium
- Apical pansystolic murmur radiating to axilla

Tricuspid regurgitation
- Chronic fatigue
- Hepatomegaly/ascites
- Rt ventricular heave
- Prominent JVP with large v waves
- Pansystolic murmur (subxyphoid area)

INVESTIGATIONS

- ECG
- CXR
- Echocardiography and colour Doppler techniques
- Cardiac catheterization with measurement of transvalvular gradients

MANAGEMENT

- *Medical*: Treat cardiac failure, diuretics, restrict salt intake, reduce exercise, digitalis for rapid atrial fibrillation and anticoagulation for peripheral embolization
- *Surgical*: Repair (possible in mitral and tricuspid valve only) or replace diseased valve. *Prosthetic* (lifelong anticoagulation), *bioprosthetic* (animal tissue on prosthetic frame, 3 months' anticoagulation) and *biological* (cadaveric homografts, no anticoagulation) valves available

---

- *Staphylococcus aureus* is an organism of high virulence. Cellulitis or skin abscesses often provide the source of the infection. Patients with intravenous lines (particularly central lines), feeding lines, temporary pacemaker electrodes, catheters, etc. are at risk.

Pathophysiology

Continuous bacteraemia combined with local pathological change are the prerequisites for endocarditis. A pre-existing valve lesion produces an abnormal blood flow with turbulence and jet effects. This traumatizes the endocardium and a platelet and fibrin thrombus (vegetation) is formed which acts as a nidus for colonization. Deposition of microorganisms from the blood stream on to the thrombus initiates the infection. Injection of particulate matter by drug abusers will also cause endothelial damage, usually on the tricuspid valve, which may subsequently become colonized. The valve most commonly affected is the tricuspid valve. Infection may also occur on normal valve, particularly by organisms of high virulence.

Clinical presentation

The patient will frequently demonstrate the clinical features of sepsis: fever, rigors, malaise, anorexia, weight loss, myalgia and arthralgia. This may lead to anaemia and splenomegaly. A heart murmur is common but is not a pre-requisite for diagnosis.

Other manifestations include:
• *heart failure* secondary to regurgitation due to perforation of a valve leaflet or fistula into another cardiac chamber;
• *complete heart block* or *pericarditis* secondary to an annular or myocardial abscess;
• *disordered haemodynamics* secondary to further valve distortion due to vegetations; and
• *pulmonary* or *peripheral arterial emboli*. Well-recognized clinical manifestations of peripheral emboli include: splinter haemorrhages, Roth's spots, Janeway lesions and Osler's nodes. Emboli may also produce ischaemia of the peripheral or mesenteric circulation, mycotic abscesses and neurological syndromes. Renal infarction and infection may also occur, as may pneumonia from septic pulmonary emboli.

Investigation and evaluation

Blood cultures are of extreme importance, not only in achieving a diagnosis but also to monitor the effect of antibiotic therapy. Cultures may be negative in up to 20% of patients; this may reflect prior antibiotic therapy. False-negative cultures may result from *Chlamydia* and fungi.

A *normochromic, normocytic anaemia* is a common feature in association with a mild elevation of the white count together with a moderately raised erythrocyte sedimentation rate (ESR) and high C-reactive protein. Red blood cell casts and protein may be found in the urine. The ECG may be non-specific, or show prolonged PR interval or complete heart block. The latter is an ominous occurrence. Chest radiology may demonstrate heart failure, a pericardial effusion or evidence of septic pulmonary emboli. Echocardiography is able to demonstrate vegetations, regurgitation and the presence of an abscess.

The role of surgery

Surgery should follow a standard 4–6 weeks of antibiotic therapy with two synergistic antibiotics. Ideally, the patient should receive antibiotics for at least 1 week prior to surgery, but if there is evidence of haemodynamic deterioration or severe sepsis, urgent surgery is indicated.

Other indications for surgical intervention include:
• moderate to severe congestive heart failure;

• persistent sepsis;
• abscess, conduction disturbance, fistulae;
• systemic emboli;
• progressive renal dysfunction;
• enlarging vegetations or persistence following an embolic event; and
• prosthetic valve endocarditis.

At operation all the infected valve tissue is excised and any abscess cavities are drained and debrided. Damaged valves are repaired or replaced along with any associated pathology, e.g. septal defects. The operative mortality is high (20%), with a 4% incidence of developing infection on the newly replaced valve. This is higher if the operation is performed during active endocarditis.

Following operation the patient should be maintained on intravenous antibiotics until all investigations, both radiological and serological, show no evidence of continuing sepsis. This is commonly for a period of 6 weeks and is followed by a longer period of oral antibiotic therapy.

Aortic dissection

Pathophysiology

Aortic dissection usually occurs in the region of the aortic arch and is caused by an intimal tear; blood then enters the media which is cleaved proximally and distally into its inner two-thirds and outer third. The tear is the result of shear stress forces generated by the left ventricular ejection velocity and systemic arterial pressure. These forces cause fractional movement of aortic intima over media. Medial degeneration from hypertension, eccentric jet of blood from a bicuspid aortic valve or ageing predisposes to aortic dissection. Risk factors include hypertension, Marfan's syndrome, bicuspid aortic valve, pregnancy and surgery to the ascending aorta (as in aortic valve replacement). Traumatic aortic dissection following blunt injury to the chest is a well-recognized but rare event. It is often associated with a left first rib fracture.

A diastolic murmur may indicate aortic annulus involvement, leading to severe incompetence of the aortic valve, in which case a valve replacement or resuspension procedure will be required. The dissection may extend into or shear off aortic side branches. Rupture may occur of the false lumen through the thin outer media and adventitia. Death is due to rupture or ischaemia of viscera.

Classification

Stanford

• Type A: Ascending aorta involved, regardless of whether descending aorta is involved.

• Type B: Dissection confined to the descending thoracic aorta.

Clinical presentation and investigation

Patients usually present with sudden severe chest pain radiating into the back, neck or arms. They may also be shocked, either from external rupture or severe aortic incompetence. If the latter, a diastolic murmur will be heard. The chest radiograph will usually show widening of the mediastinum. Further investigation should aim to provide confirmatory evidence of an aortic dissection, identify whether the ascending aorta is involved, and whether the dissection has disrupted other arterial branches.

For many years *aortography* was the only accurate diagnostic procedure for the evaluation of patients with suspected aortic dissection. More recently, CT, MRI, TOE, and transthoracic echocardiography (TTE) have also been shown to be useful. For patients who are haemodynamically stable, CT or MRI should be the investigation of choice, with TOE reserved for patients who are haemodynamically unstable, as it can be performed at the bedside.

Management

• For type B dissections, conservative management should be instituted, as surgery confers no additional benefit in the absence of complications. Complications requiring operative intervention are: bleeding, visceral ischaemia, uncontrollable hypertension, neurological deficits, persistent pain, arterial compromise, expansion or rupture. The main features of conservative management are careful monitoring of the patient, provision of haemodynamic support and control of blood pressure. Of paramount importance is the lowering of the arterial pressure of a hypertensive patient and the velocity of ventricular ejection. Sodium nitroprusside is an arterial vasodilator but increases the velocity of ventricular election as a result of the reflex tachycardia. It may however be combined with a β-adrenergic blocker, which will decrease the ejection velocity, and an end-point of a heart rate of 60 beats/min may be used. Intravenous β-blockers should be used. Labetalol is an α- and β-blocker which effectively lowers the arterial blood pressure as well as reducing the velocity of left ventricular ejection due to the negative chronotropic and inotropic effects.
• Type A dissections require surgery with use of cardiopulmonary bypass. The patient should be monitored on a high-dependence or intensive care unit until transfer to a cardiothoracic unit can be made. Blood pressure should be controlled as above.

The ascending aorta (± the aortic valve) is replaced using a Dacron graft and the arch of the aorta may also have to be re-placed if flow into the carotid or subclavian vessels has been compromised or if rupture is likely. These operations have a very poor outcome with an in-hospital mortality of 70–90%.

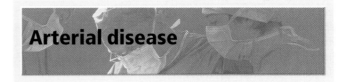

Arterial disease

Peripheral occlusive arterial disease (POAD)

Peripheral occlusive arterial disease predominantly affects the lower limb and is caused by atherosclerosis (thrombosis and embolism), vascular trauma, the complications of diabetes and Buerger's disease. The patient presents with intermittent claudication, rest pain, ulceration or gangrene. The symptoms and signs reflect the severity of ischaemia; thus clinical features may only be present when there is increased demand for blood supply, e.g. when exercising (intermittent claudication), or there may be complete loss of function and cell death at rest (gangrene).

Chronic lower limb ischaemia

Clinical features

Symptoms

Chronic lower limb ischaemia classically occurs in elderly male patients who are or have been cigarette smokers and may have other manifestations of atherosclerosis, e.g. coronary or cerebral vascular disease. Intermittent claudication is the mildest symptom of arterial insufficiency to the lower limb. It is characterized by pain or discomfort on walking, usually in the calf or buttocks, but occasionally in the thigh or foot. The pain will always appear in the segment just distal to the site of obstruction of the artery. Thus femoropopliteal obstruction will produce calf claudication while common iliac disease will produce buttock as well as calf claudication. Aortic occlusion produces buttock pain and loss of erection in the male (Leriche's syndrome). The pain steadily increases until the patient is compelled to stop. Resting rapidly relieves the pain, usually within a few minutes. Resumption of walking will reproduce the pain at exactly the same distance as before; this is called the claudication distance. Some patients will also report coldness, numbness or paraesthesia of the foot with muscle pain. This is thought to be due to shunting of blood from the skin to the ischaemic muscle.

Rest pain is characterized by a continuous aching severe pain and is indicative of critical ischaemia, i.e. arterial insufficiency severe enough to threaten the viability of the foot or leg. Elderly smoking men are the usual sufferers and often a history of intermittent claudication can be elicited. In general, patients with rest pain are older and less active than typical claudicants. Rest pain usually occurs in the most distal part of the limb, i.e. the toes and forefoot, and is often associated with tissue destruction, either ulceration or gangene. The pain is worse at night when the foot becomes warm underneath the bedclothes; thus the patient seeks relief by hanging the leg over the side of the bed or sleeping in a chair.

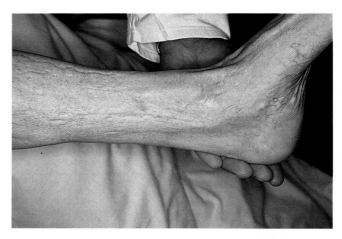

Figure 18.6 Venous guttering in a patient with arterial disease. Because of poor inflow there is not enough blood to fill the veins when the limb is elevated.

Physical examination

The clinical examination should be performed in a warm room. The entire cardiovascular system should be examined, including the heart and abdominal aorta, measuring blood pressure and auscultating the carotid arteries. The main points to be considered in physical examination of the legs are given in Table 18.8.

Inspection

In the early stages of the disease the leg will look remarkably normal. With more severe disease the leg may look pale at or on elevation from the horizontal and a dusky reddish purple when it hangs down. This observation is the

Table 18.8 Examination of the legs in a patient with peripheral vascular disease.

Inspection
Colour
Buerger's test
Posture of the limb
Venous guttering
Gangrene
Ulceration

Palpation
Temperature
Capillary refilling
Pulses
Sensation and movement

Auscultation
Bruits

basis of Buerger's test. The limb is raised for a minute or two. With a normal peripheral circulation the toes should remain pink at 90°. In an ischaemic limb, because the arterial pressure is unable to overcome gravity, the elevated leg becomes a waxy, cadaveric white colour, best seen on the sole of the foot. The venous blood in the leg drains away leaving (like the canals on Mars) the empty venous channels on the dorsum of the foot as 'gutters' (Fig. 18.6). The angle to which the leg must be raised before it becomes white is the vascular angle or Buerger's angle, usually less than 30° in an ischaemic limb. When the limb is hung down it gradually becomes a bluish/red colour due to reactive hyperaemia. If the patient has been sitting with the knee flexed in an attempt to relieve the pain of severe ischaemia, there may be a fixed flexion deformity of the hip or knee.

Gangrene means digestion of dead tissue by saprophytic bacteria, i.e. bacteria which are incapable of invading and multiplying in living tissue. In severe peripheral vascular disease tissue death is produced by ischaemia and gangrene results from subsequent saprophytic invasion. This is usually dry gangrene or mummification initially. Clinically dead tissue looks brown or black and contracts into a shrunken, crinkled mass. The junction between gangrenous and living tissue is often distinct and is known as the line of demarcation. If left alone the dry dead tissue may fall off. However, if the gangrenous area becomes infected (wet gangrene) the tissues become boggy and ulcerated, the gangrene spreads proximally and the patient becomes toxic. An urgent amputation is required in that situation. Gangrene may affect patches of skin (think of microemboli; Fig. 18.7), a digit, the foot or the distal limb (Fig. 18.8).

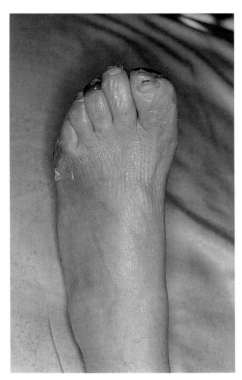

Figure 18.7 Patches of dry gangrene over pressure points in the foot.

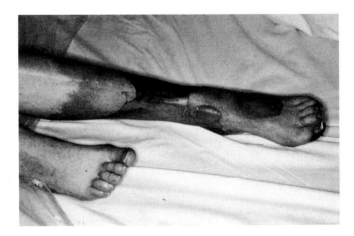

Figure 18.8 Gangrene of the lower limb following a neglected arterial embolus. This patient requires an urgent above-knee amputation.

Ischaemic ulcers are often present in severe peripheral vascular disease. They are usually very painful and are found over pressure areas (the heel, the heads of the first and fifth metatarsals) and the toes. They vary in size from a few millimetres to several centimetres in diameter; they are punched

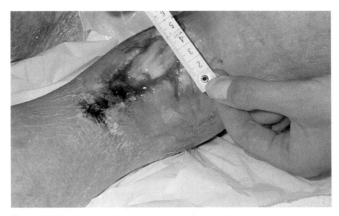

Figure 18.9 Arterial ulcer on the lower limb with gangrene and an exposed tendon in a patient with diabetes mellitus. This patient's ulcer healed following a bypass operation, debridement of the ulcer and skin grafting.

out, there is usually no evidence of healing and often tendons or bone are exposed in the base of the ulcer (Fig. 18.9).

Palpation

The ischaemic leg, regardless of its colour, feels cold. It is always surprising to find that a red dependent foot is stone cold. To assess the temperature properly, both legs should be exposed for 5 min. The capillary refilling time gives a crude estimation of capillary blood flow. Press the tip of a toenail or the pulp of a toe for 2–3 s and observe the time taken for the blanched area to return to its normal pink colour after releasing pressure. Capillary refilling should be almost instantaneous with a normal circulation but will be retarded in an ischaemic limb.

Examination of the peripheral pulses reveals the anatomical site of arterial obstruction. The pulses will be present proximal to and absent distal to the site of obstruction. The peripheral pulses to be examined are the femoral, popliteal, dorsalis pedis and posterior tibial. The femoral pulse lies midway between the symphysis pubis and the anterior superior iliac spine and is easily felt if present. The popliteal pulse is more difficult to feel (Fig. 18.10).

The dorsalis pedis pulse is found in the middle third of a line drawn from the mid-point of the malleoli to the cleft between the first and second toes and just lateral to the extensor hallucis longus tendon. This artery is congenitally absent from its usual position in 10% of patients. The posterior tibial artery lies halfway between the posterior margin of the medial malleolus and the medial border of the tendo Achilles. The peroneal artery is occasionally palpable

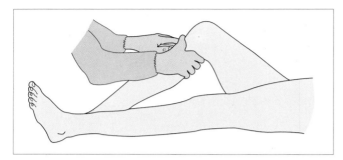

(a)

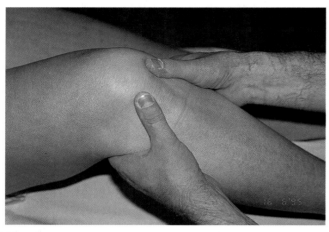

(b)

Figure 18.10 a,b Palpation of the popliteal pulse. The usual method of palpating this pulse is to flex the knee partially, to about 140°. With your thumbs on the tibial tuberosity and your fingers over the lower part of the popliteal fossa, compress the artery between your thumbs and the upper end of the tibia. Occasionally you will have to place the patient prone and feel along the course of the artery. If the popliteal pulse is very easily palpable the patient may have a popliteal aneurysm.

(and usually audible with Doppler) and should be sought 1 cm medial to the lateral malleolus.

Auscultation

Turbulent flow over a roughened artery wall produces vibration, which can be heard as a bruit on auscultation. For a bruit to occur, there must be sufficient flow through a roughened vessel. The loudness of a bruit does not grade a stenosis. It is convenient to record the pulses and bruits in diagrammatic form (Fig. 18.11).

Non-invasive tests of peripheral vascular disease

Non-invasive tests are part of the clinical evaluation and should be undertaken after history and physical examina-

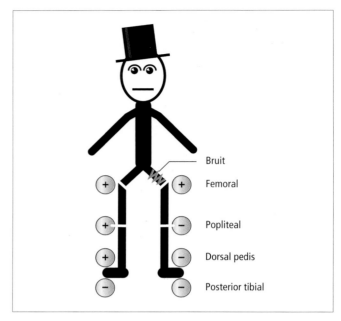

Figure 18.11 'A picture is worth a thousand words'. It is convenient to record the peripheral pulses and bruits in diagrammatic form.

Table 18.9 Non-invasive tests for assessment of peripheral vascular disease.

Indirect tests
Doppler velocimetry
    Ankle pressure measurement
    Segmental pressure measurement
    Waveform analysis
    Exercise response
Plethysmography
    Pulse volume recording
    Digital plethysmography

Direct tests
Duplex colour ultrasonography

tion. They can be classified as indirect tests which measure the haemodynamic characteristics of the disease, and direct rests which evaluate the artery and define precisely the location of the atherosclerotic lesions. These are listed in Table 18.9. However, only Doppler velicometry and digital plethysmography are currently widely used in the assessment of peripheral vascular disease. Duplex colour ultrasonography is used extensively in the assessment of carotid disease.

The simplest non-invasive test to perform is ankle pressure measurement. A pneumatic cuff, attached to a sphygmomanometer, is applied immediately above the malleoli

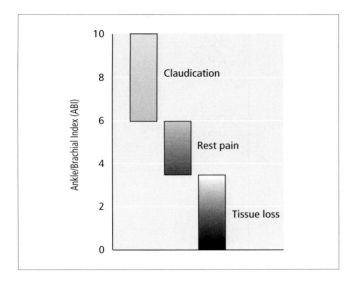

Figure 18.12 Relationship between the ankle/brachial index (ABI) and the clinical features of peripheral occlusive arterial disease.

and the posterior tibial arterial signal is located with a Doppler probe. The cuff is inflated and the pressure at which the signal disappears is noted. The cuff is then deflated and the pressure at which the signal reappears is also noted. The mean of the two readings is the ankle pressure. The dorsalis pedis pressure should also be measured and the highest ankle measurement taken as the reference. Because systemic arterial pressure varies from patient to patient, the ankle pressure is expressed as a percentage of the brachial systolic pressure — the ankle/brachial index (ABI). The relationship between the ABI and the clinical symptoms of peripheral occlusive disease is shown in Fig. 18.12.

Segmental pressures record the arterial systolic pressure along the length of the limb and give a more precise determination of the anatomy of the occlusion. The sites of measurement are high thigh, above knee, below knee and above the ankle. In the normal arterial tree pressures should decrease by about 10 mmHg from one segment to the next. A gradient of more than 20 mmHg is considered an abnormal finding. If the patient's symptoms are present only on exercise then measurements at rest may not show any abnormality. It is therefore important to repeat the ABI and segmental pressures after exercise. Such a stress test is best achieved with a treadmill. Walking at 2 miles per hour (approx. 3 km/h) with a 10% gradient usually yields an abnormal result in most claudicants.

Doppler waveform analysis and pulse volume recordings (PVR) are useful adjuncts to ABI and segmental pressure measurement and give more information in patients with rigid arteries and proximal aortoiliac disease. Digital plethysmography, which measures the increase in volume of the digit which occurs with systole, is useful in the evaluation of diabetic patients in whom abnormally high ankle pressures may be recorded due to medial calcification.

Investigation and management

The management of chronic lower limb ischaemia ranges from simple advice about smoking and exercise to detailed assessment of the vascular tree prior to reconstructive surgery. The management plan is based on the clinical assessment, having regard for the severity of the disease and the impact it has on a given patient's lifestyle. Three groups are recognized:
- patients with non-disabling claudication;
- patients whose lifestyle is seriously curtailed by claudication; and
- patients with critical ischaemia.

Non-disabling intermittent claudication

The natural history of patients with intermittent claudication is that one-third will get better, one-third will remain about the same and one-third will progress to rest pain and critical ischaemia. Thus, over 60% of claudicants improve or remain stable and only about 7% come to amputation after 5 years. Patients who have intermittent claudication which does not seriously interfere with their lifestyle should have simple non-invasive tests (ABI and segmental pressures) to quantify their disease and then be given a trial of non-operative therapy (Table 18.10).

A full blood count should be performed to exclude polycythaemia and thrombocythaemia, both of which will exacerbate the symptoms of peripheral occlusive disease. β-Adrenergic blocking agents may also worsen intermittent

Table 18.10 Management of non-disabling claudication.

Investigation
History (β-blockers)
Physical examination
ABI and segmental pressures
FBC (exclude polycythaemia and thrombocythaemia)

Treatment
Stop smoking completely
Exercise programme
Aspirin
Pentoxifylline (?)

ABI, Ankle/brachial index; FBC, full blood count.

claudication by their negative inotropic and peripheral vasoconstrictor effects.

Non-operative treatment of chronic lower limb ischaemia consists of cessation of smoking, exercise and drug therapy. Cessation of all tobacco use is the foundation of non-operative therapy of chronic lower limb ischaemia and this must be emphasized to the patient at every opportunity. Most smokers are aware of an increased risk of lung cancer and heart disease with smoking but are ignorant of the connection between smoking and peripheral vascular disease. Patients who stop smoking usually experience a doubling of their walking distance and do better than patients who continue to smoke. A walking exercise programme should also be initiated. Patients should be advised to walk for 1 h each day, repeatedly approaching the point of claudication. Attempts to walk through the claudication are misguided and may induce arrhythmias. Exercise does not, as was previously thought, enhance collateral circulation but, analogous to athletic training, probably results in more efficient oxygen extraction from the limited blood supply.

Numerous pharmacological agents have been evaluated for possible benefit in chronic lower limb ischaemia with generally mixed results. Pentoxifylline, which reduces blood viscosity, gives a modest improvement in walking distance. However, patients with POAD should receive aspirin 75 mg/day because of its general beneficial effects on survival in patients with atherosclerotic disease.

Disabling claudication and critical ischaemia

Claudication which is rapidly worsening despite good non-operative therapy or produces marked exercise restriction in young people is defined as disabling claudication. In addition to non-invasive assessment these patients should undergo arteriography prior to surgical or radiological intervention. Patients with critical ischaemia require similar investigation prior to surgical treatment.

Arteriography

This provides a two-dimensional map of the arterial system indicating the site and severity of the vessel occlusions and stenoses. It does not measure blood flow or circulatory dynamics and should only be used in patients in whom interventional radiology or surgery is being considered. Where possible, the safer per-femoral approach should be used and the arterial tree from the renal arteries to the pedal arches should be demonstrated (Fig. 18.13). Digital subtraction arteriography (DSA) is a technique which 'subtracts' the bony image and enhances the arteriographic profile. DSA also permits the use of much smaller doses of contrast than in standard arteriography (Fig. 18.14a).

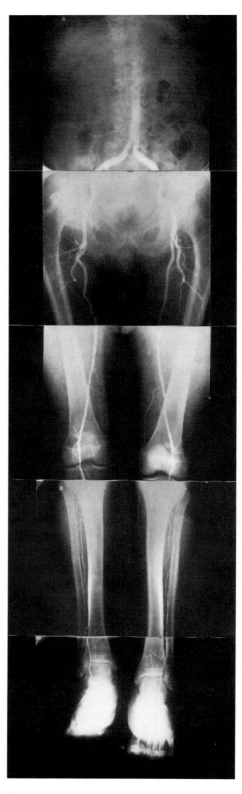

Figure 18.13 A standard arteriogram demonstrating the arterial tree from the renal to the pedal arteries.

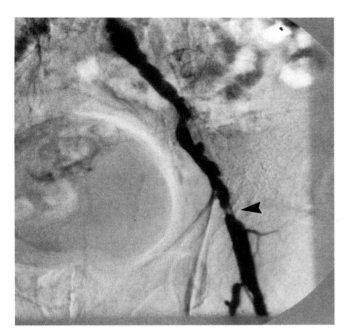

(a)

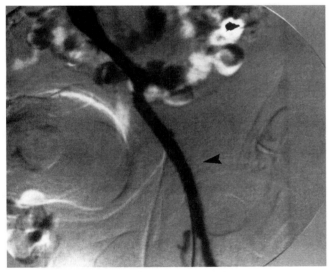

(b)

Figure 18.14 (a) A digital subtraction angiogram (DSA) demonstrating a diseased left iliac arterial tree with a tight stenosis (arrow) in the external iliac artery. Note the absence of the internal iliac artery and the 'ghost' outline of the pelvic bones and hip joint. (b) The same patient following percutaneous transluminal angioplasty. The strictured areas have been completely dilated.

The direct treatment of the critically ischaemic limb consists of percutaneous catheter procedures and surgical treatment (Table 18.11).

Table 18.11 Direct treatment of the critically ischaemic leg.

Intravenous pharmacotherapy
Pentoxifylline
Prostanoids

Percutaneous catheter procedures
Balloon angioplasty
Expandable stent placement

Surgery
Reconstructive operations
    Bypass grafting
    Endarterectomy
Amputation

Parenteral drug therapy for rest pain or tissue loss

Most limbs with ischaemic rest pain and tissue loss will be lost unless arterial inflow can be restored either radiologically or surgically. However, temporary relief of symptoms and possibly improved ulcer healing can be achieved in some patients by a small improvement in tissue perfusion and oxygenation. The agents which show most promise in achieving this goal are pentoxifylline, which decreases plasma viscosity, diminishes platelet aggregation and increases extremity blood flow, and prostanoids (PGI_2, PGE_1 and prostacyclin analogues) which cause vasodilation and inhibit platelet aggregation. However, none of the drugs investigated to date has shown a significant benefit.

Percutaneous transluminal angioplasty

This is a technique where under fluoroscopy a balloon catheter is introduced over a guidewire into the lumen of an artery. The balloon is advanced over the guidewire until it lies across the stenosis or occlusion. The balloon is then inflated to a high pressure, crushing the atheroma into the arterial wall. The technique is most effective for short, ≤5 cm proximal stenoses but total occlusion can also be recanalized. On average there is a >85% initial success rate with balloon angioplasty and a 1-year patency rate of 70% (Fig. 18.14b). Newer techniques include the placement of metal expandable stents across the stenosis/occlusion after angioplasty.

Surgical procedures

Reconstructive surgery, including bypass grafting and occasionally endarterectomy, is the usual treatment for patients with critical limb ischaemia. Endarterectomy is a procedure whereby an atheromatous plaque is removed by direct operation on the artery. Its use is now almost confined to carotid

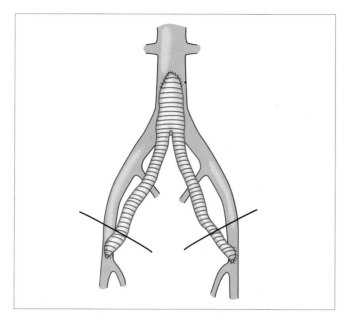

Figure 18.15 A bifurcated tube-graft has been inserted from the aorta to the femoral arteries, bypassing the diseased lower aorta and iliac arteries.

Table 18.12 Patency rates of surgical bypass procedures for lower limb ischaemia.

Bypass operation	Patency at 1 year (%)
Aortobifemoral	90
Above-knee femoropopliteal (vein)	75
Above-knee femoropopliteal (synthetic)	65
Below-knee femoropopliteal (vein)	70
Below-knee femoropopliteal (synthetic)	60

Lumbar sympathectomy

This can be performed surgically or chemically (by injecting phenol or absolute alcohol) in patients with peripheral vascular disease. The rationale behind the procedure is that sympathetic blockade may improve the blood flow to the skin, thereby relieving pain and promoting ulcer healing. A sympathectomy may be performed in patients in whom there is no possibility of reconstruction and in some patients with thromboangiitis obliterans (see below). In some patients it may lead to warming of the foot and subjective improvement but there is no evidence that sympathectomy significantly alters the outcome for the patient.

Amputation

While the majority of patients with peripheral vascular disease are amenable to limb salvage procedures, an amputation will be required in patients with critical ischaemia in whom reconstruction fails or is not possible and who do not respond to maximum medical therapy, e.g. iloprost infusions. An amputation should be performed through healthy tissue and the stump should facilitate early fitting of a prosthesis and rehabilitation. The most frequently performed amputations are: toe amputations, transmetatarsal, Syme's, below-knee and above-knee amputations (Fig. 18.16). Amputees have a very poor prognosis for survival and 40% will die within 2 years of amputation. A major amputation of the other leg is required in 30% of patients and full mobility is achieved in only 50% of below-knee and 25% of above-knee amputees.

Acute lower limb ischaemia

Pathophysiology

Embolism, thrombosis and vascular injury are the causes of acute lower limb ischaemia. The usual sources of arterial embolus are given in Table 18.13.

Emboli usually impact at branching points in the arterial tree, particularly at the bifurcation of the aorta (saddle embolus), the common femoral bifurcation and the popliteal

artery stenosis but occasionally it is performed for an isolated peripheral lesion, e.g. an iliac stenosis. However, most patients require some form of bypass procedure.

Aortoiliac occlusive disease is treated by inserting a synthetic polyester (Dacron) bifurcated graft from the aorta to the femoral arteries (Fig. 18.15), bypassing the diseased lower aorta and iliac arteries. If the patient is not fit for an aortic procedure then blood flow to the legs can be restored by placing a bifurcated graft subcutaneously from one axillary artery to the femoral arteries. This is an example of an extra-anatomical bypass procedure.

Femoropopliteal occlusion is relieved by using the patient's own saphenous vein to bypass the obstruction. Duplex ultrasonography may be helpful in evaluating the suitability of a vein before operation. The vein is removed completely, reversed so that the valves do not obstruct the flow, and then anastomosed to the femoral artery above the obstruction and the popliteal artery below the obstruction. Alternatively, the vein may be left *in situ* so that a more distal bypass, e.g. to the tibial arteries, can be performed. The diameter of the distal saphenous vein matches that of the small tibial arteries, facilitating anastomosis. However, with this technique the valves have to be destroyed with valvulotome. If the ipsilateral saphenous vein is not satisfactory, a vein may be harvested from the other leg or arm and, if all else fails, a synthetic (usually polytetrafluoroethylene (PTFE)) graft may be used. However, the best results will be obtained with the patient's own saphenous vein (Table 18.12).

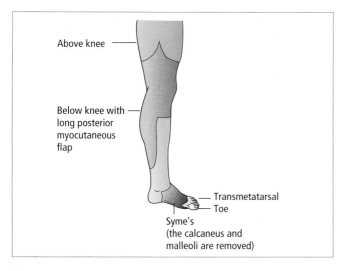

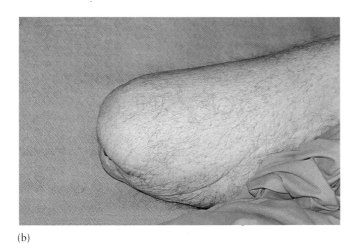

(a)

(b)

Figure 18.16 (a) The sites of commonly performed amputations of the lower limb. (b) An above-knee amputation stump.

Table 18.13 Sources of arterial emboli.

Heart (90%)
Arrhythmias (e.g. atrial fibrillation)
Valvular heart disease
Prosthetic heart valves
Mural thrombus post myocardial infarction
Ventricular aneurysm
Atrial myxoma

Great vessels (9%)
Atherosclerotic aorta
Aortic aneurysm
Popliteal artery aneurysm
Internal carotid artery plaque

Other (1%)
Paradoxical
Malignant tumour emboli

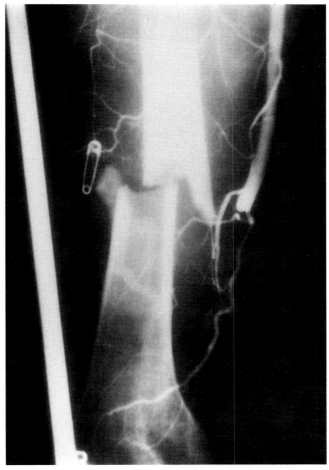

Figure 18.17 Complete disruption of the superficial femoral artery at the adductor canal in association with a comminuted fracture of the femur following a road traffic accident.

trifurcation. *Thrombosis* of a pre-existing atherosclerotic lesion may also cause acute ischaemia. Occasionally, thrombosis in a relatively normal artery can occur in patients with hypercoagulable states, e.g. patients with malignancy, polycythaemia or patients taking high doses of oestrogen. *Vascular injury* can be caused by penetrating or blunt trauma (Fig. 18.17). Trauma may cause complete disruption of an artery or only fracture the intima. The blood flow may dissect the torn intima from the media, creating a small flap which impedes flow. Even if no flap develops, a thrombus forms over the torn intima, causing an acute occlusion of the artery.

Regardless of the cause, sudden interruption of the blood supply to the lower limbs causes acute ischaemia. Two phases

Peripheral occlusive vascular disease (POAD) at a glance

DEFINITION

Peripheral occlusive vascular disease is a common disorder caused by acute or chronic interruption of the blood supply to the limbs, usually due to atherosclerosis

EPIDEMIOLOGY

M>F before age 65. Increasing risk with increasing age

AETIOLOGY

- Atherosclerosis and thrombosis
- Embolism
- Vascular trauma
- Buerger's disease

RISK FACTORS

- Cigarette smoking
- Hypertension
- Hyperlipidaemia
- Diabetes mellitus

PATHOLOGY

- Reduction in blood flow to the peripheral tissues results in ischaemia which may be acute or chronic. *Critical ischaemia* is present when the reduction of blood flow is such that tissue viability cannot be sustained

CLINICAL FEATURES

Chronic ischaemia
- Intermittent claudication in calf (femoral), thigh (iliac) or buttock (aortic occlusion)
- Cold peripheries
- Prolonged capillary refill time
- Rest pain, especially at night
- Venous guttering
- Absent pulses
- Arterial ulcers
- Gangrene over pressure points
- Knee contractures

Acute ischaemia
- Pain
- Pallor
- Pulselessness
- Paraesthesia
- Paralysis
- 'Perishing' cold
- Pistol-shot onset
- Mottling ⎫ late
- Muscle rigidity ⎭ signs

INVESTIGATIONS

Chronic ischaemia
- Ankle/brachial index (ABI) measurement (normal ABI>1.0) at rest and post-exercise on treadmill
- FBC (exclude polycythaemia)
- Doppler waveform analysis
- Digital plethysmography (in diabetes)
- Per-femoral angiography

Acute ischaemia
- ECG, cardiac enzymes
- Angiography (?), may be performed peroperatively
- Find source of embolism:
  (a) Holter monitoring
  (b) Echocardiograph
  (c) US aorta for AAA

MANAGEMENT

Non-disabling claudication
- Stop smoking
- Exercise programme
- Avoid ß-blockers
- Aspirin 75 mg/day
- Pentoxifylline (?)

Disabling claudication/ critical ischaemia
- Balloon angioplasty ± intravascular stent
- Bypass surgery
- Amputation
- Intravenous Rx: Iloprost

Acute ischaemia
- Heparin anticoagulation
- Surgical embolectomy
- Thrombolytic therapy (streptokinase, t-PA, urokinase)

PROGNOSIS

Non-disabling claudication
- >65% respond to conservative management. The rest require more aggressive treatment

Disabling claudication/ critical ischaemia
- Angioplasty and bypass surgery overall give good results. The more distal the anastomosis, the poorer the result

Acute ischaemia
- Limb salvage 85%
- Mortality 10–15%

US, Ultrasound; AAA, abdominal aortic aneurysm; Rx, prescription; t-PA, tissue plasminogen activator.

---

of cellular injury are recognized. Acute *ischaemia* alone rapidly causes cell damage but further injury occurs if and when the blood supply is restored to the ischaemic tissues. This second phase of injury is called *reperfusion* injury. It is caused by the production of toxic oxygen radicals (superoxide, O_2^-, hydrogen peroxide, H_2O_2, and the hydroxyl radical, OH^-) in the tissues when the blood flow is re-established. Some drugs, e.g. mannitol and allopurinol, help to protect the cell from reperfusion injury by inhibiting the production of oxygen radicals or scavenging them as they are produced.

Compartment syndromes are also a consequence of acute ischaemia. The muscles of the lower limb are in osseofascial compartments (i.e. compartments bounded by bone and fascia). Ischaemia (and reperfusion) cause the muscles to swell within these rigid compartments. The result is an increase in pressure in the compartment greater than the capillary perfusion pressure; thus the blood supply to the muscle is interrupted and further ischaemia and swelling occur. The muscle cells break down, releasing myoglobin which will in turn cause renal damage and myoglobinuria which can be recognized clinically by a characteristic black/brown urine. To break this cycle of injury the muscle compartment has to be opened surgically by dividing the fascia and allowing the muscle to expand; this operation is called a fasciotomy (Fig. 18.18).

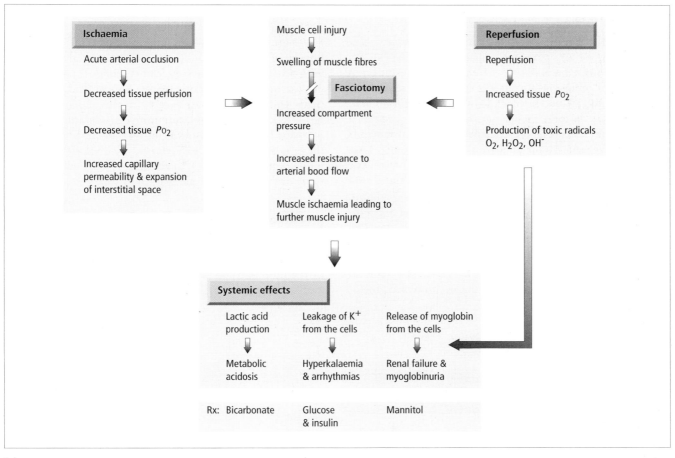

Ischaemia

Acute arterial occlusion

Decreased tissue perfusion

Decreased tissue Po_2

Increased capillary permeability & expansion of interstitial space

Muscle cell injury

Swelling of muscle fibres

Fasciotomy

Increased compartment pressure

Increased resistance to arterial bood flow

Muscle ischaemia leading to further muscle injury

Reperfusion

Reperfusion

Increased tissue Po_2

Production of toxic radicals O_2, H_2O_2, OH^-

Systemic effects

Lactic acid production

Metabolic acidosis

Rx: Bicarbonate

Leakage of K^+ from the cells

Hyperkalaemia & arrhythmias

Glucose & insulin

Release of myoglobin from the cells

Renal failure & myoglobinuria

Mannitol

(a)

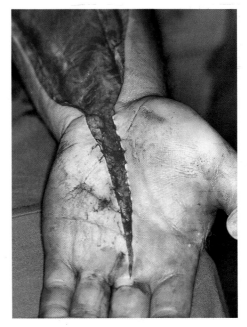

(b)

Figure 18.18 (a) The pathophysiology of compartment syndrome and the systemic consequences that may follow reperfusion of an ischaemic limb. Fasciotomy may break the cycle, preventing further muscle cell injury and thereby decreasing the systemic consequences of reperfusion, the myonephropathic metabolic syndrome, i.e. metabolic acidosis, arrhythmias, renal and respiratory failure. (b) Fasciotomy of the forearm and the hand in a patient following a gunshot injury to the axillary artery. Note that the separation of the skin edges is entirely due to the degree of swelling that occurred in the muscle compartment.

Clinical features

The classical manifestations of acute ischaemia are pain, paraesthesia, pallor, paralysis, pulselessness (the five Ps) and a cold foot. Pain is the most frequent manifestation of acute arterial occlusion. Its onset is sudden, it is severe and progressive and effects the most distal part of the limb first. As the nerves become ischaemic, pain is replaced by a feeling of numbness. The presence of paraesthesia demands immediate treatment as it indicates severe ischaemia. Loss of two-point discrimination is a significant prognostic sign. Pallor is manifested as a white waxy colour and is seen early with acute ischaemia. Stagnant capillary circulation leads to mottling, which is the herald of blistering and gangrene. Paralysis and sensory deficits are late findings in acute ischaemia and indicate severe ischaemia. Diffuse muscle rigidity usually indicates an unsalvageable limb. On examination there is often tenderness over the femoral artery and the pulses will be absent in the embolized limb.

Clinical assessment can usually establish whether acute ischaemia is due to an embolus or a thrombus and this differentiation has therapeutic implications (Fig. 18.19). If a history of previous claudication can be elicited in a patient with no obvious cardiac source of embolus, thrombosis of a pre-existing atherosclerotic plaque is most likely. These patients will require bypass surgery. If the patient, however, has atrial fibrillation or a recent myocardial infarction, has no prior history of claudication and has normal pulses in the opposite limb then a diagnosis of embolus can be made with confidence. These patients will do well with embolectomy or in some cases lytic therapy.

Investigation and management

The outcome of acute arterial occlusion depends on the medical condition of the patient, the degree of ischaemia of the limb and the promptness of revascularization. The aim of therapy is early revascularization of the limb after

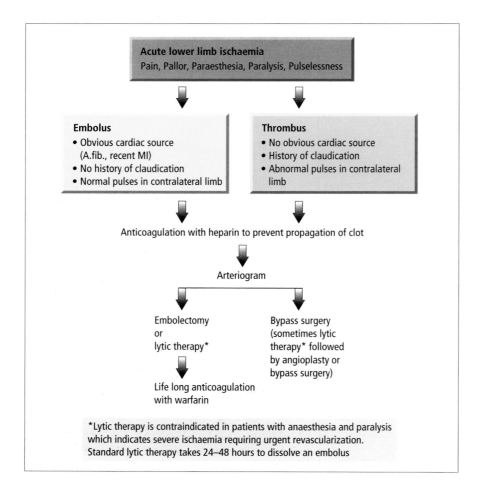

Figure 18.19 The clinical differentiation between an embolus and acute thrombosis is important as it has therapeutic implications.

stabilization and control of coexisting medical problems. In patients with a recent myocardial infarct or atrial fibrillation, assessment of haemodynamics is important and adequate urinary output should be established. Patients with acute ischaemia should be anticoagulated with heparin as soon as the diagnosis is made. This prevents propagation of thrombus and distal thrombosis and is achieved by giving a bolus of 10 000 units of heparin intravenously and an infusion of about 1000 units of heparin per hour after that.

In patients in whom thrombosis is thought to be the diagnosis, arteriography should be considered to define the extent of the problem before revascularization. To avoid delay in revascularization this can be performed per-operatively. Once the embolus has been dealt with the patient should be investigated (ECG, cardiac enzymes, Holter monitoring, echocardiography and abdominal ultrasonography for aneurysm) to establish the source of embolus.

Surgical management

Embolectomy

Since 1963 the standard approach to a peripheral embolus has been embolectomy. This operation is usually performed under local anaesthetic as the patients often have a medical problem which precludes general anaesthesia, e.g. recent myocardial infarction. A groin incision is made and the common femoral artery is opened. Often clot is found in the artery at the site of arteriotomy. A Fogarty balloon catheter is passed in turn into the proximal and distal arteries, the balloon is inflated and the catheter is withdrawn, removing the clot. An arteriogram should be done to ensure that the distal circulation is clear. If it is not, then a more distal arteriotomy and further embolectomy may be required with or without thrombolytic therapy, or an immediate bypass operation if one is dealing with an acute atherosclerotic thrombus. *Percutaneous aspiration embolectomy* is a technique of embolectomy where a percutaneous catheter is advanced into the embolus and the embolus is aspirated through the catheter. A small number of patients present having had an embolus a number of days or weeks previously. Their symptoms are obviously mild and they have a viable limb. These patients can be treated electively by *delayed embolectomy*.

Thrombolytic therapy

Percutaneous intra-arterial thrombolytic therapy may be used to manage some patients with non-limb-threatening ischaemia. Systemic thrombolytic therapy is not used because of the risks of bleeding. The agents available are streptokinase, urokinase and tissue plasminogen activator (t-PA; Table 18.15). All of these agents activate the body's own fibrinolytic system; they convert plasminogen to plasmin, which is the active lytic agent. Lytic therapy takes approximately 12–72 h to dissolve the clot and the patients require careful monitoring during therapy (Fig. 18.20).

Table 18.15 Agents currently used for thrombolytic therapy.

	Streptokinase	t-PA	Urokinase
Discovered	1933	1940s	1947
Source	Haemolytic streptococcus	Vascular endothelium	Urine
Speed of lysis	++	+++	++
Risk of haemorrhage	+	+	+
Allergic reactions	+	–	–
Cost	+	+++	+++

t-PA, Tissue plasminogen activator.

Myonephropathic metabolic syndrome

This is a systemic process characterized by metabolic acidosis, hyperkalaemia, myoglobinaemia and pulmonary dysfunction. It is caused by the outpouring of the products of anaerobic metabolism into the venous circulation following revascularization of an ischaemic limb. It is a potentially lethal condition; patients may die from severe acidosis (lactic acid), arrhythmias (hyperkalaemia), renal failure (myoglobinaemia) or respiratory failure (activated white cells). Patients with clearly non-viable extremities (such as the patient in Fig. 18.8) should have early amputation to avoid this devastating complication (Fig. 18.18a).

Results

Early aggressive treatment of acute limb ischaemia and its complications is associated with limb salvage rates of 85–90% and mortality rates of 10–15%.

The diabetic foot

Pathophysiology

Vascular disease in the patient with diabetes takes two forms. *Macroangiopathy* is atherosclerosis affecting the larger arteries, while *microangiopathy* is a thickening of the basement membrane of smaller vessels and affects the arterioles and capillaries. Microangiopathy is responsible for the renal, ophthalmic and neural complications of diabetes. There are three distinct processes involved in the aetiology of what is called the diabetic foot: ischaemia (caused by both micro- and macroangiopathy), neuropathy (sensory, motor and autonomic) and sepsis (the glucose-rich environment favours bacterial growth). Undetected repeated trauma is the usual cause of ulceration in the diabetic foot. Foot problems account for 20% of all hospitalizations of diabetics and patients with diabetic foot problems are incapacitated for an average of 16 weeks.

Clinical features

The diabetic foot usually presents with predominantly neuropathic features or a combination of neuropathic and ischaemic features. Diabetic neuropathy presents with sensory disturbances, trophic skin lesions, plantar ulceration and degenerative arthropathy (Charcot's joints; Fig. 18.21). Neuropathic ulcers are deep and painless and situated on the plantar aspect of the foot or big toe. The pedal pulses are present and one will find an obvious sensory deficit in the foot. Autonomic neuropathy is manifested by a warm foot (Table 18.16).

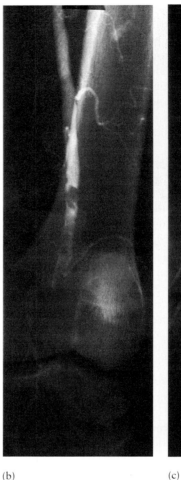
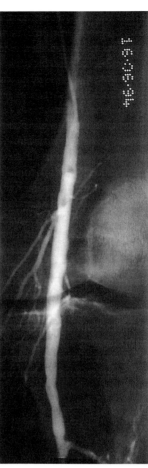

(b)   (c)

(b) After 24 h the embolus is beginning to lyse and some contrast is seen flowing around the embolus. (c) At 72 h there is complete clot lysis with recanalization of the popliteal artery.

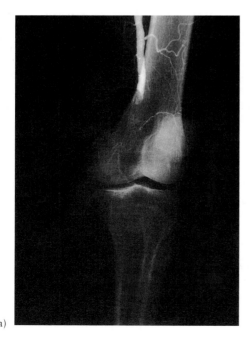

(a)

Figure 18.20 (a) Intra-arterial thrombolysis with streptokinase 500 IU/h was commenced in this patient who presented with an acutely ischaemic limb due to an arterial embolus.

Ischaemic diabetic foot problems present with rest pain and usually there is a history of intermittent claudication. Ischaemic ulcers are painful and are present over the toes or pressure areas, e.g. the medical aspect of first and fifth metatarsals. The foot may be cold and usually there is a history of intermittent claudication. Both neuropathic and ischaemic ulcers may be complicated by sepsis, characterized by cellulitis, deep tissue abscesses, osteomyelitis and, if unchecked, gangrene. Often sepsis begins as a fungal (mycotic) infection, which leads to maceration and ulceration between the toes and secondary bacterial infection. The usual organisms found are staphylococci, streptococci, colonic organisms and anaerobic bacteria. Gas gangrene may occasionally occur.

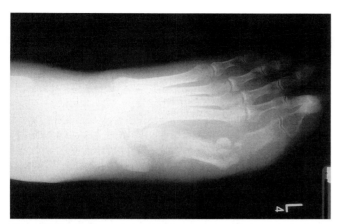

Figure 18.21 A Charcot's joint. This patient's ankle joint was completely destroyed as a consequence of diabetes. Note also the bony destruction in the first metatarsal and the metatarsophalangeal joint.

Table 18.16 Features of neuropathic and ischaemic diabetic ulcers.

Neuropathic ulcer	Ischaemic ulcer
Painless	Painful
Normal arterial pulses	Reduced or absent pulses
Loss of sensation	Variable sensory findings
Warm foot	May be cold foot
Plantar ulceration	Toe ulceration
No intermittent claudication	Intermittent claudication
Treated by local measures	Requires reconstructive surgery

Investigation and management

The presence of a palpable pedal pulse in warm pink foot is a good indicator of adequate perfusion and ulcers in this situation will probably heal with local treatment. *Non-invasive vascular tests*, including ABI, segmental pressures and digital pressure, are helpful. Because of medial calcification, the arteries in diabetes mellitus are relatively incompressible, leading to falsely elevated segmental pressures, usually 20 mmHg higher than the non-diabetic patient. Thus, most diabetic patients require an ankle pressure of least at 80–90 mmHg to heal minor amputations. Because digital blood vessels are frequently spared from medial calcification, a better estimate of foot blood flow is obtained by measuring digital blood pressure by Doppler ultrasound or plethysmography. A digital pressure of 30–40 mmHg is required to heal wounds.

When non-invasive tests indicate inadequate perfusion, an *arteriogram* should be performed to demonstrate the entire vascular tree from the aorta to the pedal vessels. Patients with diabetes have an increased risk of contrast nephrotoxicity and they should be well-hydrated pre-arteriography and a DSA technique should be performed.

Prevention

In no place is prevention better than cure than in the management of the diabetic foot. A large percentage of patients with established disease ultimately have some form of amputation. Patients with diabetes should be given detailed advice on foot care (Table 18.17) and they should have rapid access to specialist care for even minor lesions.

Neuropathic disease can usually be treated by *controlling infection* and local removal of necrotic tissue. Plain X-rays of the foot may show gas in the tissues indicative of severe anaerobic infection, or bony destruction indicative of osteomyelitis. Intravenous antibiotics are required to control infection and the choice depends on the results of culture. Several organisms are often isolated and aerobic and anaerobic antibiotic cover has to be given, e.g. metronidazole, ampicillin and an aminoglycoside or a third-generation cephalosporin if there is renal impairment. Deep infection in the foot is not uncommon and should be managed by wide incision, drainage and debridement, which will often include amputation of toes or the forefoot. These measures usually result in complete healing.

If ischaemic disease is present an arterial bypass using autogenous saphenous vein should be performed either prior to or in conjunction with local treatment. Usually a distal bypass is required, often to the pedal arch, before healing of an ischaemic ulcer can occur. It should be remembered that sepsis may precipitate ketoacidosis in diabetic patients. The patient with a diabetic foot should, therefore, be managed jointly by surgeons and specialist physicians in diabetes mellitus.

Table 18.17 Advice on foot care for diabetic patients.

Do
Carefully wash and dry feet daily
Inspect feet for injury daily
Take meticulous care of toenails
Apply antifungal powder to your feet daily

Don't
Walk barefoot
Wear ill-fitting shoes
Use a hot-water bottle
Ignore *any* foot injury

The diabetic foot at a glance

DEFINITION

The term diabetic foot refers to a spectrum of foot disorders ranging from ulceration to gangrene occurring in diabetics as a result of peripheral neuropathy or ischaemia or both

PATHOPHYSIOLOGY

Three distinct processes lead to the problem of the diabetic foot:

- *Ischaemia* caused by macro- and microangiopathy
- *Neuropathy* — sensory, motor and autonomic
- *Sepsis* — the glucose-saturated tissue promotes bacterial growth

CLINICAL FEATURES

Neuropathic features

- Sensory disturbances
- Trophic skin changes
- Plantar ulceration
- Degenerative arthropathy (Charcot's joints)
- Pulses often present
- Sepsis (bacterial/fungal)

Ischaemic features

- Rest pain
- Painful ulcers over pressure areas
- History of intermittent claudication
- Absent pulses
- Sepsis (bacterial/fungal)

INVESTIGATIONS

- Non-invasive vascular tests
  ABI, segmental pressure, digital pressure
  ABI may be falsely elevated due to medial sclerosis
- X-ray of foot may show osteomyelitis
- Arteriography

MANAGEMENT

Should be undertaken jointly by surgeon and physician as diabetic foot may precipitate diabetic ketoacidosis

Prevention

Do
- Carefully wash and dry feet daily
- Inspect feet daily
- Take meticulous care of toenails
- Use antifungal powder

Don't
- Walk barefoot
- Wear ill-fitting shoes
- Use a hot-water bottle
- Ignore any foot injury

Neuropathic disease

- Control infection with antibiotics effective against both aerobes and anaerobes
- Carry out wide local excision and drainage of necrotic tissue
- These measures usually result in healing

Ischaemic disease

- Formal assessment of the vascular tree by angiography and reconstitution of the blood supply to the foot (either by angioplasty or bypass surgery) has to be achieved before the local measures will work
- After restoration of blood supply, treat as for neuropathic disease

Thromboangiitis obliterans (Buerger's disease)

Pathophysiology

Thromboangiitis obliterans is a clinical syndrome characterized by segmental thrombotic occlusions of small and medium-sized arteries in the lower and often the upper limb, accompanied by a dense inflammatory infiltrate which affects the arterial wall and often the adjacent veins and nerves as well. Its exact aetiology is unknown but it occurs mostly in men (90%) and there is a clear association with smoking. It is particularly prevalent in Mediterranean, East European and oriental countries.

Clinical features

The symptoms and signs of thromboangiitis obliterans are those of peripheral occlusive arterial disease, but the upper limb may be involved and frequently there is superficial venous thrombosis and thrombophlebitis migrans.

However, the following specific criteria have been proposed for the diagnosis of thromboangiitis obliterans (Table 18.18).

Investigation and management

Digital plethysmography may yield some useful information but arteriography is indicated in patients with threat-

Table 18.18 Features of thromboangiitis obliterans.

Clinical
Males under 45 at onset of disease
Upper and lower limb involvement
Heavy smokers
Absence of embolic source, trauma, autoimmune disease, diabetes or hyperlipidaemia
Arteriogram
Normal proximal arteries
Distal occlusions
Corkscrew collaterals

ened limb loss. The cornerstone of treatment is *complete cessation of all tobacco use*. No further tissue loss will occur if the patient stops smoking completely. Various drugs, including aspirin, prostacyclin analogues, nifedipine and pentoxifylline have been tried but at present no drug is of proven benefit. Lumbar sympathectomy may occasionally be helpful but reconstructive surgery is rarely possible. Thromboangiitis obliterans is associated with a 30% major amputation rate over 5–10 years.

Raynaud's syndrome

Raynaud's syndrome is defined as episodic digital vasospasm occurring in response to cold or emotional stimulus. It usually affects the digits of the hand and is characterized by sequential colour changes in the fingers — white (ischaemia), blue (cyanosis), and red (hyperaemia). There may also be associated pain and paraesthesia.

Pathophysiology

There are two mechanisms of inducing Raynaud's syndrome in patients. *Vasospastic* Raynaud's syndrome is an exaggerated digital artery contraction in response to cold or an emotional stimulus. This contraction overcomes the digital perfusion pressure causing ischaemia. This is the basis of the syndrome in 40% of patients. In *vaso-obstructive* Raynaud's syndrome, digital perfusion is already compromised by obstructive disease. This form of the syndrome may be associated with a long list of disorders, a small sample of which are listed in Table 18.19. However, collagen vascular disease is eventually found in about 30% of patients. Ischaemia is produced when the normal arterial contraction response to cold overcomes the compromised digital arterial perfusion pressure.

Table 18.19 Disorders associated with Raynaud's syndrome.

Abnormal circulating globulins, e.g. cold agglutinin
Arteritis, e.g. polyarteritis nodosa
Autoimmune connective tissue diseases, e.g. rheumatoid arthritis
Malignancy
Myeloproliferative disorders, e.g. leukaemia
Peripheral embolization, e.g. proximal subclavian disease
Trauma, e.g. vibrating tools

Clinical features

Vasospastic disease typically occurs in young females with a long history of cold sensitivity. There may be a positive family history and usually it is the hands rather than the feet which are affected. All or only some of the fingers may be involved. Tissue loss rarely occurs in this group and the symptoms are more of a nuisance than disabling.

Patients with vaso-obstructive disease are older and do not have a long history of cold sensitivity. The digital involvement is asymmetrical and trophic changes or tissue loss may be present in the involved digits. The patient may have other manifestations of the underlying disease.

Investigation and management

If the history and examination give a clue to underlying pathology then the patient should be investigated appropriately, e.g. unilateral Raynaud's syndrome should make one consider subclavian embolic disease and the patient should have arteriography. However, routinely, bloods should be drawn for an ESR, a serum rheumatoid factor and antinuclear antibody titre to screen for collagen vascular disease.

Non-invasive testing, including measurement of digital systolic pressure and plethysmographic waveform analysis, is useful to detect vaso-obstructive disease. Abnormal vasospastic activity can be elicited by cold challenge (i.e. immersion of hands in ice water for 30 s) and measuring the digital temperature recovery time (normally 5 min) with a thermistor.

Treatment consists of *education* and *reassurance*, especially about tissue loss and amputation. As with all other vascular disorders, patients should *stop smoking*. Cold should be avoided and the *hands* should be *protected* when cold exposure is unavoidable. Mittens should be worn in preference to gloves. Fewer than 50% of patients will require drug therapy and then only during the cold months. Several *sympatholytic agents* which produce vasodilatation have been used with variable results. However, many are associated with unpleasant side-effects at the doses required to give relief of vasospasm. The calcium-channel blocking agent *nifedipine*, which produces vasodilatation by inhibiting calcium ingress into cells, gives good relief of symptoms at a dose of 10 mg twice or three times daily depending on the severity of symptoms. To date, nifedipine has proved the most successful drug therapy for Raynaud's syndrome. For severe prolonged attacks a course of intravenous *prostacyclin analogue (Iloprost)* is very effective. This drug inhibits platelet aggregation, increases red cell deformability, decreases blood viscosity and affects neutrophil function. Its effect can last for up to 16 weeks. Surgical sympathectomy has little or no role in the modern management of Raynaud's syndrome.

Aneurysms

An aneurysm can be defined as a permanent localized dilatation of an artery to the extent that the affected artery is 1.5 times its normal diameter. Aneurysms commonly affect the abdominal aorta, the iliac, femoral and popliteal arteries. Cerebral and thoracic aortic aneurysms are less common and occasionally patients present with false or pseudoaneurysms following penetrating trauma. The majority of abdominal aortic aneurysms (AAA) extend from just below the renal arteries to the bifurcation of the aorta. The incidence of AAA in the western world is rising and is now about 2–3% in men aged between 65 and 80 years. This increase appears to be real and not merely a reflection of increased longevity and improved methods of diagnosis. Multiple aneurysms are common in the same individual and patients with popliteal or femoral aneurysms have a 50% incidence of AAA.

Pathophysiology

AAAs are fusiform in shape and their aetiology is probably multifactorial. The traditional view is that AAA is caused by atherosclerosis and there is a higher incidence of AAA in patients with atherosclerosis and in smokers. However, biochemical studies have shown that there are decreased quantities of elastin and collagen in the wall of aneurysms, suggesting abnormal collagenase or elastase activity, and there is a marked familial tendency for aneurysmal disease. (An AAA will be found in 10–20% of first-degree relatives of patients with AAA.)

Thoracic aneurysms, which tend to be saccular (Fig. 18.22), were commonly caused by syphilis while *cerebral* aneurysms (*berry* aneurysms), which occur usually at the circle of Willis, are due to a congenital weakness of the arterial wall. *Mycotic* aneurysms are caused by a bacterial aortitis secondary to septic emboli, usually from bacterial endocarditis. A *pseudo* or *false* aneurysm develops after penetrating trauma and is an expanding pulsating haematoma in contact with an arterial lumen (Fig. 18.23).

Once an aneurysm develops, regardless of its cause, its enlargement is governed by a simple physical law: the law of Laplace ($T = RP$). This quite simply states that the tension on the wall of an artery (T) is proportional to the radius of the artery (R) and the blood pressure (P). Put another way, the higher the blood pressure and the wider the lumen, the more likely an aneurysm is to rupture. While control of blood pressure, especially with β-blockers, may be helpful, serial ultrasound examination shows that AAAs increase in size by 0.3–0.5 cm per annum; it is only a matter of time before most aneurysms rupture. Thrombus develop-

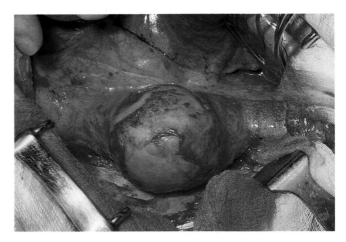

Figure 18.22 Thoracic aortic aneurysm. These aneurysms were often caused by syphilis in the past.

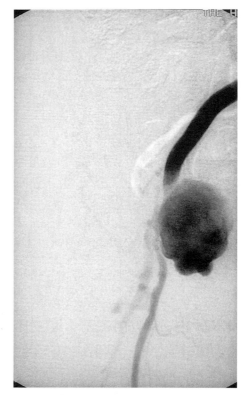

Figure 18.23 A pseudo aneurysm seen here at the right distal anastomosis of an aortobifemoral graft bypass, such as is shown in Fig. 18.15.

ing within an abdominal aortic aneurysmal sac may act as a source of peripheral embolus and frequently popliteal

Table 18.20 Risk of rupture of abdominal aortic aneurysm related to size.

Size of aneurysm (cm)	5-year rate of rupture (%)
≥7.0	>75
6.0	35
5.0–5.9	25
≤5.0	~10

aneurysms undergo complete thrombosis and the patient presents with an acutely ischaemic limb.

Autopsy studies indicate that 64% of patients with ruptured aneurysms die at home. These are probably patients who have free intraperitoneal rupture. Most patients who get to hospital have a contained leak, i.e. the aneurysm has ruptured through its left posterolateral wall into the retroperitoneum. The leak is tamponaded in the retroperitoneum for up to 6–10 h. This is the explanation for survival in patients transferred over long distances to a vascular unit with a ruptured/leaking aneurysm.

Screening for AAA

The arguments for screening for AAA are compelling. There is an increasing incidence of aneurysms in identifiable groups (e.g. males over 65, patients with other vascular disease and first-degree relatives of patients with AAA). The mortality following ruptured AAA is 85%, while elective repair carries a 5% mortality and is followed by good quality of life. A simple non-invasive screening test is available in B-mode ultrasonography (see below).

Clinical features

Asymptomatic

The vast majority of AAAs (75%) are asymptomatic when discovered. Often they are detected at routine physical examination or during an ultrasonographic or radiological procedure for other reasons. The distinctive feature of an aneurysm on physical examination is expansile epigastric pulsation, i.e. it expands outwards when digital pressure is applied gently to each side of the mass. This finding differentiates it from transmitted pulsation such as might occur with a stomach neoplasm. It is usually possible to palpate between the upper border of the aneurysm and the costal margin and this finding indicates that the AAA is infrarenal — an important surgical consideration.

Symptomatic

AAA can cause symptoms as a result of pressure on adjacent structures, expansion, rupture or embolization. Back pain is a common symptom as the aneurysm presses on and in some cases erodes the spine. However, compression on adjacent viscera may produce abdominal or flank pain and sometimes nausea.

Rapid expansion (but not rupture) of aneurysms occurs in a small number of patients, producing severe flank or back pain. Expansion is usually the herald of rupture. Free intraperitoneal rupture is characterized by sudden abdominal pain, collapse and rapid death. Patients with *ruptured/leaking* aneurysms typically present with severe back or flank pain, shock and an ill-defined left-sided mass, which may or may not be pulsating.

More rarely, an aneurysm may erode into the inferior vena cava, producing a characteristic clinical picture: congestive cardiac failure, a loud abdominal bruit, lower limb ischaemia and gross oedema. An aneurysm may also erode into the duodenum, although this is more often seen as a long-term complication of aneurysm repair but it can occur primarily. These patients have a minor herald gastrointestinal bleed initially, followed 24–48 h later by exsanguinating haemorrhage.

Investigation and management

AAAs increase in size until they rupture. Two-thirds of patients with ruptured AAAs die at home and, of those who reach hospital, 50% die. Thus, the overall mortality for ruptured AAA is in excess of 85%. By contrast, the operative mortality for elective AAA repair is less than 5%. Therefore, elective repair of AAA should be performed. There is some argument over the size an AAA should have reached before it is repaired but most vascular surgeons agree that an AAA of 5.0 cm should be repaired and many advocate repair at 4.0 cm. However, before repair the diagnosis has to be confirmed and the patient assessed for fitness for operation.

Diagnostic methods

Physical examination is not a very exact method of detecting or determining the size of an AAA. A plain abdominal and lateral spine X-ray may show the calcified rim of an aneurysm but it is only useful in 50% of patients (Fig. 18.24). The diagnostic methods currently used to confirm the diagnosis of AAA are ultrasonography, CT and MRI.

Real-time or B-mode ultrasonography is a non-invasive investigation which gives anatomical detail of the vessel wall and provides an accurate measurement of aneurysm

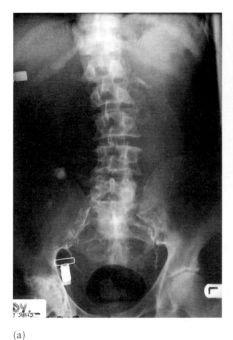

(a)

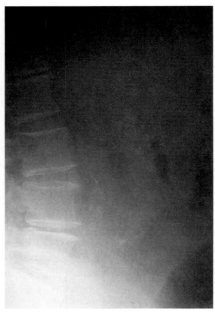

(b)

Figure 18.24 Plain abdominal (a) and lateral spine (b) radiographs may demonstrate calcification in the wall of an abdominal aortic aneurysm.

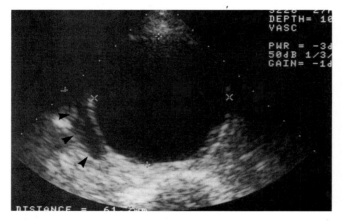

Figure 18.25 A real-time or B-mode ultrasound scan demonstrating an abdominal aortic aneurysm which measures 6.17 cm in diameter. Note the small compressed inferior vena cava to the right of the aneurysm (arrow).

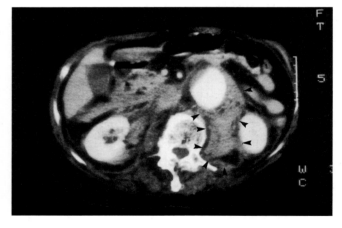

Figure 18.26 A contrast-enhanced computed tomography scan demonstrating a contained left posterior rupture of an abdominal aortic aneursym (arrows).

size (Fig. 18.25). It is the modality of choice for initial evaluation of pulsatile abdominal masses and for screening for AAA. It is less reliable for evaluation of the renal and iliac arteries.

CT with or without contrast enhancement provides more information than ultrasonography; in particular, the relationship between the renal arteries and the AAA can be established. This modality is also useful to de- tect retroperitoneal haematoma and contained rupture (Fig. 18.26). Disadvantages are expense and radiation exposure.

MRI employs radiofrequency energy and a strong magnetic field to produce images. It is probably better than CT in demonstrating involvement of branch arteries and it does not expose the patient to radiation. Recently, better signal

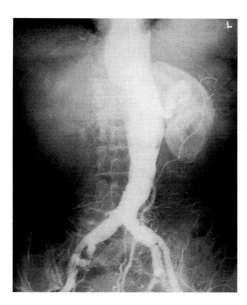

Figure 18.27 Suprarenal abdominal aortic aneurysm seen on angiography.

Table 18.21 Problems which increase mortality during elective AAA repair.

Cardiac
Unstable angina
Angina at rest
Congestive cardiac failure
Ejection fraction <30%

Pulmonary
Po_2 <8.0 kPa

Renal
Serum creatinine >260 μmol/l

acquisition and computing provide MRI images similar to conventional angiograms — MRI angiography. However, it is expensive and the presence of metal in the patient (e.g. metallic surgical clips) precludes its use.

Because AAAs are often filled with layers of mural thrombus, the lumen through which the blood flows is often much smaller than the true lumen of the aneurysm. *Aortography*, therefore, cannot be relied upon to establish the presence of or the size of an AAA. However, arteriography is useful to determine the relationship of the renal arteries to the AAA (Fig. 18.27) and it may be indicated if a correctable occlusive lesion is suspected, e.g. occlusive iliofemoral disease.

Preoperative assessment

Thorough preoperative evaluation is important prior to elective repair of AAA. High-risk patients are those with cardiac disease, pulmonary disease and renal disease and it is imperative to detect these patients and optimize the function of these systems prior to operation (Table 18.21).

Coronary artery disease, which may be completely asymptomatic, is prevalent in patients with AAA and most deaths occurring with elective AAA repair are due to ischaemic heart disease. Radionuclide angiography or echocardiography can be used to estimate the left ventricular ejection fraction at rest but stress testing (either by exercise thallium or dipyridamole-thallium 201 scanning) is probably a better means of preoperative functional cardiac assessment. If a reversible myocardial defect is detected then coronary angiography and bypass grafting should be undertaken prior to or simultaneously with AAA repair. Similarly, patients with symptomatic carotid artery disease should be treated prior to AAA repair.

Pulmonary complications are common after aortic surgery and preoperative pulmonary function tests (especially FEV_1, $FEV_{25\text{-}75}$ and vital capacity) should be obtained. Pre- and postoperative physiotherapy and epidural analgesia help to reduce pulmonary complications. A raised creatinine preoperatively is a risk factor for mortality after aortic surgery. In these patients maintainence of haemodynamic stability and meticulous care with fluid balance are essential. Mannitol may be needed in some patients.

Principles of aneurysmal surgery

Elective repair of AAA

Extensive monitoring is required during aortic surgery, as clamping and unclamping the aorta are associated with profound haemodynamic changes. Thus, large-bore intravenous cannulae, urinary catheter and rectal temperature probe as well as a Swan–Ganz catheter (to measure CVP, pulmonary artery pressure, PCWP and cardiac output) are placed. Radial arterial pressure is also monitored. Autotransfusion techniques minimize the need for blood transfusion during the operation.

The aorta can be approached through the peritoneal cavity via a midline longitudinal incision or extraperitoneally via a retroperitoneal incision (Fig. 18.28). The aim of the operation is to open the aneurysm along its length, remove any contained thrombus and inlay a synthetic graft (Dacron) into the aorta (Fig. 18.29). The native aneurysm sac is then closed back over the graft. Occasionally, as with aortoiliac occlusive disease, a bifurcated graft has to be placed.

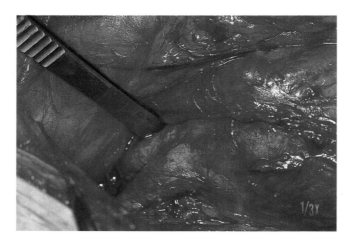

Figure 18.28 Retroperitoneal exposure of aortic and iliac artery aneurysms.

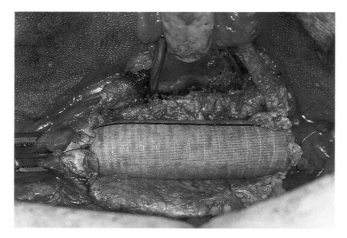

Figure 18.29 A Dacron tube graft which has been inlaid into an opened abdominal aortic aneurysm sac.

Repair of ruptured AAA

A ruptured/leaking AAA is the quintessential surgical emergency. As soon as the diagnosis is established (usually on clinical grounds but occasionally with ultrasound or CT scanning), and blood has been sent for cross-matching, the patient is taken to the operating theatre where resuscitation continues while the monitoring lines are being inserted. The patient is not anaesthetized until the surgeons are ready to make the incision as the administration of muscle relaxant will remove the tamponading effect of the anterior abdominal wall; the aneurysm/haematoma will expand rapidly and the patient may die. The operative approach is through a midline abdominal transperitoneal incision. Once a clamp

has been placed on the aorta the operation continues as for an elective repair.

Complications of aneurysm surgery

The most frequent complications following AAA repair are cardiac, pulmonary and renal, as discussed above. However, there are some other specific problems which may occur. These are presented in Table 18.22.

Table 18.22 Specific complications of abdominal aortic aneurysm (AAA) surgery.

Early complications	Comment
Bleeding	Peroperative bleeding from veins can be very troublesome but arterial bleeding is the commonest reason for re-exploration in the early postoperative period
Clotting abnormalities	May develop as a consequence of bleeding, especially after repair of a ruptured AAA
Acute limb ischaemia	Is usually caused by embolism of thrombus from the aneurysmal sac. The fragments enter the small distal vessel, producing the characteristic 'trash foot'
Colonic ischaemia	Occurs in 5% of patients but it is usually subclinical. However, one of the internal iliac arteries or the inferior mesenteric artery should be preserved
Spinal cord ischaemia	Rarely seen after infrarenal AAA repair. It is much more likely following suprarenal or thoracoabdominal aneurysmal repair
Late complications	
Graft infection	A devastating complication which occurs in 1–2% of patients. Prevention is by controlling infection preoperatively and careful antiseptic technique and prophylactic antibiotics peroperatively. Bowel surgery at the same time as aortic surgery should be avoided. Treatment of an established graft infection may require graft removal and axillobifemoral grafting. Aortic graft infection is a lethal condition
Aortoenteric fistula	The most common cause of gastrointestinal haemorrhage after an aortic graft. Infection is probably the underlying cause and this complication carries a poor prognosis
Anastomotic aneurysm	A false aneurysm which develops at the site of a graft/artery anastomosis. It is most frequently seen in the groin following aortobifemoral anastomoses. Fortunately, most can be managed successfully by a local interposition graft
Sexual dysfunction	Not uncommon with aortic surgery due to damage to the autonomic nerves or the pelvic blood supply through the internal iliac arteries

Aneurysms at a glance

DEFINITION

An *aneurysm* is a permanent localized dilatation of an artery to the extent that the affected artery is 1.5 times its normal diameter. A *pseudo* or *false* aneurysm is an expanding pulsating haematoma in continuity with a vessel lumen. It does not have an epithelial lining

SITES

Abdominal aorta, iliac, femoral and popliteal arteries
Cerebral and thoracic aneurysms are less common

AETIOLOGY

- Atherosclerosis
- Familial (abnormal collagenase or elastase activity)
- Congenital (cerebral or berry aneurysm)
- Bacterial aortitis (mycotic aneurysm)
- Syphilitic aortitis (thoracic aneurysm)

RISK FACTORS

- Cigarette smoking
- Hypertension
- Hyperlipidaemia

PATHOLOGY

- Aneurysms increase in size in line with the law of Laplace ($T = RP$, where T = tension on the arterial wall, R = radius of artery and P = blood pressure). Increasing tension leads to rupture
- Thrombus from within an aneurysm may be a source for peripheral emboli
- Popliteal aneurysms may undergo complete thrombosis
- Aneurysms may be fusiform (AAA, popliteal) or saccular (thoracic, cerebral)

CLINICAL FEATURES OF ABDOMINAL AORTIC ANEURYSM

- *Asymptomatic*: The vast majority have no symptoms and are found incidentally. This has led to the description of an AAA as 'a U-boat in the belly'
- *Symptomatic*:
  (a) Back pain from pressure on the vertebral column
  (b) Rapid expansion causes flank or back pain
  (c) Rupture causes collapse, back pain and an ill-defined mass
  (d) Erosion into IVC causes congestive cardiac failure (CCF), loud abdominal bruit, lower limb ischaemia and gross oedema

INVESTIGATIONS

Detection of AAA
- Physical examination (not accurate)
- Plain abdominal X-ray (aortic calcification)
- Ultrasonography (best way of detecting and measuring aneurysm size)
- CT scan (provides good information regarding relationship between AAA and renal arteries)
- Angiography — not routine for AAA

Determination of fitness for surgery
- History and examination
- ECG ± stress testing
- Radionuclide cardiac scanning (MUGA or stress thallium scan)
- Pulmonary function tests
- U&E and creatinine for renal assessment

MANAGEMENT

- Surgical repair is the treatment of choice for AAA
- AAAs ≥5 cm should be repaired *electively* as they have a high rate of rupture (perioperative mortality for elective AAA repair = 5%)
- Surgical repair with *inlay of a synthetic graft* is the standard method of repair
- Endovascular repair with graft/stent devices is indicated in selected patients
- *Ruptured AAAs* require immediate surgical repair (perioperative mortality 50%, but 70% of patients die before they get to hospital so that overall mortality = 85%)

PROGNOSIS

- Most patients do well after AAA repair and have an excellent quality of life

---

While a long list of complications may occur, most patients do well following elective aneurysm repair and have a good quality of life.

Extracranial arterial disease

Stroke continues to be a major worldwide health problem. In the USA approximately 500 000 people suffer from stroke annually and at any given time there are about 1 000 000 disabled stroke victims in the USA needing care at a cost of billions of dollars. The causes of stroke are cerebral haemorrhage, lacunar infarcts, emboli from cardiac sources and extracranial arterial disease.

Pathophysiology

The carotid arterial system is the most frequent site of extracranial arterial pathology followed by the vertebral arteries and the great vessels. Pathological lesions produce symptoms either by emboli or, much more rarely, flow restriction. By far the commonest extracranial lesion is an atherosclerotic plaque at the bifurcation of the carotid artery. Turbulence over an irregular plaque stimulates platelet aggregation and cerebral or ocular symptoms develop with embolization of the platelet aggregates into the brain or eye, respectively. Bleeding into the plaque may lead to intraluminal rupture and discharge of the plaque contents (e.g. cholesterol, fibrin and atheromatous debris) as emboli into the blood stream. Sometimes cholesterol emboli will be detected in the retinal vessel on fundoscopy. If the emboli break up quickly then symptoms will be transient but failure of the embolic material to disperse leads to a focal infarct. TIAs often precede a major stroke.

Flow-related symptoms are rare because of the excellent collateral circulation to the brain via the circle of Willis. This explains how complete occlusion of both internal carotid arteries can occur without any symptoms in some patients. However, postural related basilar artery insufficiency may be present in patients with diseased vertebral arteries, e.g. neck extension produces cerebellar symptoms. In the subclavian steal syndrome, the origin of the subclavian artery is occluded and the arm is perfused by reversed blood flow from the vertebral artery into the distal subclavian artery, thus 'stealing' from the posterior cerebral circulation. Symptoms may be present only when the arm is exercised.

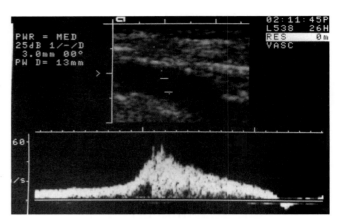

Figure 18.30 A duplex scan of the internal carotid artery (ICA). Real-time or B-mode ultrasonography is used to produce an anatomical picture of the vessel (top). In this patient there is a plaque at the origin of the ICA, causing 50–79% stenosis. Doppler ultrasonic velocimetry assesses the flow through the stenosis, which is represented by a tracing (lower picture).

Clinical features

Patients with carotid disease may be asymptomatic or present with TIAs or stroke. *TIAs* are temporary focal neurological or ocular deficits lasting not more than 24 h with complete recovery. An embolus from a carotid source will produce ischaemia of the ipsilateral cerebral hemisphere resulting in neurological deficits on the contralateral side of the body. Symptoms may be motor (weakness, clumsiness, paralysis), sensory (numbness, paraesthesia) or speech-related (receptive or expressive dysphasia). Transient visual loss is usually described by the patient as a curtain coming down over the visual field. This symptom is called *amaurosis fugax*.

Careful physical examination of the patient is very important as demonstration of a neurological deficit indicates the presence of a cerebral infarct and early cerebral reperfusion (by carotid endarterectomy) could precipitate a haemorrhage into the infarct. A bruit may be heard on auscultation over the carotid arteries but this finding is not helpful. Significant lesions can occur in the absence of a bruit and a bruit can occur in the absence of significant lesions.

Investigation

Patients with TIAs, stroke and some asymptomatic patients (e.g. those undergoing aneurysm repair) should have non-invasive assessment of their carotid arteries. This is best achieved by Duplex ultrasonography or colour ultrasonography. Patients being considered for surgery should have CT brain scanning or MRI of the brain as well as carotid angiography.

Duplex scanning incorporates real-time B-mode scanning, which provides anatomical detail of the structures being scanned, and Doppler ultrasonic velocimetry, which assesses blood flow through the vessel being examined (Fig. 18.30). Recently, colour has been added to this system so that blood flowing in one direction is assigned a red colour while blood flowing in the opposite direction appears blue. Duplex scanning is an excellent test for detecting and grading stenoses at the carotid bifurcation. The result is usually expressed as percentage stenosis: <50%, 50–79%, 80–99%. Detection of a complete occlusion, i.e. 100% stenosis, can sometimes be difficult.

Carotid angiography is an invasive technique to demonstrate pathology in the carotid arterial tree (Fig. 18.31). It carries a small risk of stroke and should therefore be reserved for patients in whom surgery is contemplated; some vascular surgeons have dispensed with angiography prior to carotid endarterectomy. DSA is now the preferred angiographic technique for imaging the carotid arteries.

CT or MRI brain scanning will differentiate between a haemorrhagic and an ischaemic cerebral infarct (Fig. 18.32). These scans are necessary to detect asignomatic infarcts and they help in the timing of operation in stroke patients who have made a good recovery.

Management

The management of extracranial carotid disease includes medical (antiplatelet therapy) and surgical (carotid endarterectomy) therapy. The indications for carotid endarterectomy have been clarified recently and depend on

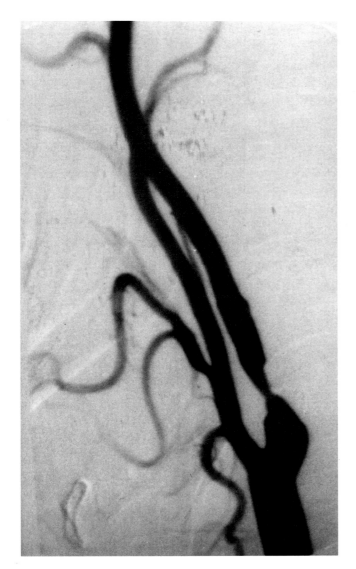

Figure 18.31 A digital subtraction angiography carotid angiogram showing a tight stenosis at the origin of the internal carotid artery.

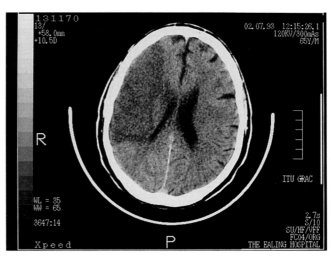

Figure 18.32 Computed tomography scan showing large infarct in right hemisphere.

Table 18.23 Indications for carotid endarterectomy.

Carotid distribution TIAs
>70% ipsilateral stenosis
>50% ipsilateral stenosis with ulceration

Stroke with good recovery after 1-month delay
>70% ipsilateral stenosis
>50% ipsilateral stenosis with ulceration

Controversial indications
Asymptomatic carotid stenosis
Vertebrobasilar symptoms with combined vertebral and carotid disease
Acute stroke within first few hours of occurrence

TIAs, Transient ischaemic attacks.

symptoms and the degree of narrowing in the artery (Table 18.23).

Medical therapy

Medical therapy has centred on drugs that inhibit platelet aggregation for carotid disease and full anticoagulation for cardiac sources of embolus.

Aspirin has its therapeutic action by the irreversible inactivation of platelet cyclo-oxygenase, preventing the production of thromboxane A_2 (TXA_2) and thus inhibiting platelet aggregation for the duration of the life of the platelets, i.e.

7–10 days. Aspirin results in a 20–30% decrease in stroke after TIA. Doses ranging from 1300 to 70 mg/day have been given but it seems prudent to prescribe smaller doses. *Dipyridamole* is ineffective in preventing TIAs or strokes and its use in combination with aspirin is no better than aspirin alone. *Ticlopidine* is a new drug which inhibits platelet activity without interfering with the synthesis of prostaglandins or cyclo-oxygenase. Initial studies are promising and this drug may have a major role in the management of cerebrovascular disease in future. *Anticoagulation* with heparin and warfarin is indicated in patients who have cerebral symptoms as a result of cardiac embolic disease. The presence of a haemorrhagic infarct has to be excluded by CT scan before initiating therapy.

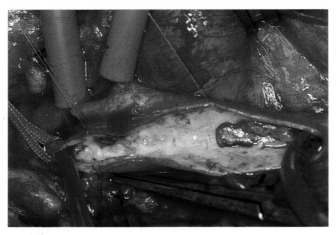

Figure 18.33 A large loose plaque in the common carotid artery seen during carotid endarterectomy.

Surgical therapy

Surgical therapy consists of carotid endarterectomy (Fig. 18.33) and this has been shown to be superior to medical therapy in the management of patients with symptomatic high-grade (>70%) carotid stenoses. The operation consists of opening the carotid bifurcation longitudinally and 'scooping' out the atheromatous plaque from the arterial wall. The blood supply to the brain is obviously interrupted during this procedure and, if there is not adequate collateral blood flow, a shunt (a simple plastic tube) has to be placed to maintain cerebral perfusion. Cerebral function is usually monitored during the operation by electroencephalographic (EEG) or transcranial Doppler monitoring. Carotid endarterectomy is a very successful operation but it does have a small mortality (1%) and morbidity (5%).

Extracranial arterial disease at a glance

DEFINITION

Extracranial arterial disease is a common disorder characterized by atherosclerosis of the carotid or vertebral arteries resulting in cerebral-ocular (stroke, TIA, amaurosis fugax) or cerebellar (vertigo, ataxia, drop attacks) ischaemic symptoms

EPIDEMIOLOGY

M>F before age 65. Increasing risk with increasing age

AETIOLOGY

- Atherosclerosis and thrombosis
- Thromboemboli
- Fibromuscular dysplasia

RISK FACTORS

- Cigarette smoking
- Hypertension
- Hyperlipidaemia

PATHOPHYSIOLOGY

- The commonest extracranial lesion is an atherosclerotic plaque at the carotid bifurcation. Platelet aggregation and subsequent *platelet embolization* cause ocular or cerebral symptoms
- Symptoms due to *flow reduction* are rare in the carotid territory but vertebrobasilar symptoms are usually flow-related. Reserved flow in the vertebral artery in the presence of ipsilateral subclavian occlusion leads to cerebral symptoms as the arm 'steals' blood from the cerebellum — subclavian steal syndrome

CLINICAL FEATURES

- Cerebral symptoms (contralateral):
  (a) Motor (weakness, clumsiness or paralysis of a limb)
  (b) Sensory (numbness, paraesthesia)
  (c) Speech-related (receptive or expressive dysphasia)
- Ocular symptoms (ipsilateral): Amaurosis fugax (transient loss of vision described as a veil coming down over the visual field)
- Cerebral (or ocular) symptoms may be transitory (a *TIA* is a focal neurological or ocular deficit lasting not more than 24 h) or permanent (a *stroke*)
- Vertebrobasilar symptoms: Vertigo, ataxia, dizziness, syncope, bilateral paraesthesias, visual hallucinations
- A *bruit* may be heard over a carotid artery but it is an unreliable indicator of pathology

INVESTIGATIONS

- Duplex scanning: B-mode scan and Doppler ultrasonic velocimetry; method of choice for assessing degree of carotid stenosis
- Carotid angiography: Not essential any more prior to surgery
- CT or MR brain scan: Demonstrates the presence of a cerebral infarct

MANAGEMENT

Medical therapy
- Aspirin (75 mg/day) inhibits platelet aggregation for the life of the platelet
- Ticlopidine has similar action to aspirin
- Anticoagulation is indicated in patients with cardiac embolic disease

Surgical therapy
- Carotid endarterectomy (+ aspirin)
Indications for carotid endarterectomy
- Carotid distribution TIA or stroke with good recovery after 1-month delay
  >70% ipsilateral stenosis
  >50% ipsilateral stenosis with ulceration
- Asymptomatic carotid stenosis >80%
- Carotid endarterectomy has about 5% morbidity and mortality

Arterial miscellany

Renovascular hypertension

Renovascular hypertension (RVH) is the cause of hypertension in approximately 5–10% of all hypertensive patients and is commoner in patients with severe hypertension. The essential lesion in RVH is a stenosis of one or both renal arteries. RVH affecting children and young women is often caused by fibromuscular dysplasia while RVH in the elderly is usually due to atherosclerosis. Hypertension results from activation of the renin–angiotensin system in unilateral disease and, in addition, expansion of the plasma volume in bilateral disease. A renal artery bruit may be heard but the diagnosis is made by isotope renography, angiography and renal vein renin assays.

Treatment consists of dilating, removing or bypassing the stenosed segment of renal artery. Percutaneous transluminal angioplasty is successful for some lesions, particularly fibromuscular dysplasia. The surgical approaches to RVH are thromboendarterectomy or aortorenal bypass. Improved renal function and beneficial blood pressure response can be expected in most patients and some, especially those with fibromuscular dysplasia, will be cured following surgical therapy.

Mesenteric ischaemia

Acute mesenteric ischaemia (AMI) is caused by a sudden occlusion of the superior mesenteric artery due to thrombosis or embolism, or an acute thrombosis of the mesenteric veins. Non-occlusive mesenteric ischaemia occurs when there is splanchnic vasoconstriction in response to hypotension. Clinically the patient presents with abdominal pain, which is often severe. Initially there is a paucity of abdominal findings but later the signs of an acute abdomen will develop and there may be gastrointestinal bleeding. Most patients have a leukocytosis and severe metabolic acidosis. These are very ill patients. Therapy is directed at resuscitating the patient, treating the underlying cause, e.g. cardiac failure, and revascularizing or resecting the ischaemic bowel. In spite of aggressive management, the mortality from AMI is still over 70%.

Chronic mesenteric ischaemia is 'intermittent claudication' or 'angina' of the bowel. Symptoms develop after meals, when the increased energy demands of the bowel for digestion cannot be met by an impoverished blood supply. The result is postprandial abdominal pain. Atherosclerotic involvement of the mesenteric vessels is almost always the cause. The anatomical diagnosis is made by angiography. Symptoms can be relieved by an aortosuperior mesenteric artery bypass in properly selected patients.

Thoracic outlet compression syndrome

The subclavian artery passes out of the chest through a crowded narrow space over the first rib and under the clavicle. The artery is surrounded by the brachial plexus and passes over the first rib between the attachments of the anterior scalene muscle (in front) and the middle scalene muscle (behind). Narrowing of this space results in compression of the artery and the brachial plexus. This may be caused by a cervical rib, which is an extra rib cephalad to the first rib, or more commonly, by congenital fibrocartilaginous bands. Long-standing compression on the artery may lead to post-stenotic dilatation and aneurysm formation.

Symptoms are often neurological and are made worse when the arms are abducted and externally rotated (the 'hands-up' position). The first presentation may be a digital embolus from a subclavian aneurysm. An Adson manoeuvre (assessment of the radial pulse during hyperabduction and external rotation of the arm) and an elevated arm stress-test (rapid opening and closing of the fists while the arms are held overhead) are the two most useful clinical tests. Objective tests include cervical spine X-rays for detection of arthritic/degenerative vertical spine changes, thoracic inlet X-rays for the presence of a cervical rib, chest X-ray to detect apical lung pathology, nerve conduction studies and arteriography of the abducted externally rotated arm. Relief of symptoms can be obtained by scalenotomy or scalenectomy and resection of a cervical rib if present. If a subclavian aneurysm is present resection is mandatory.

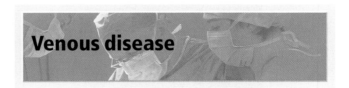

Venous disease

Introduction

While congenital abnormalities of veins exist (Klippel–Trenaunay syndrome; Fig. 18.34) and occasionally veins are involved by inflammation (thrombophlebitis), by far the greatest venous problem is thrombosis (phlebothrombosis) and its sequelae. Acute thrombosis manifests clinically as deep vein thrombosis (DVT) or, more seriously, iliofemoral thrombosis (Fig. 18.35). Migration of the thrombus to the lungs (pulmonary embolism) may be fatal, while local destruction of the valves in the deep venous system of the leg results in venous hypertension and ulceration (postphlebitic

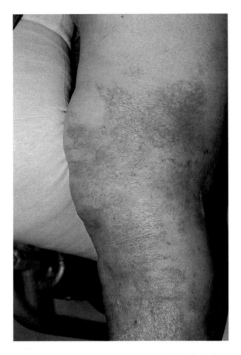

Figure 18.34 Skin changes seen in a patient with Klippel–Trenaunay syndrome.

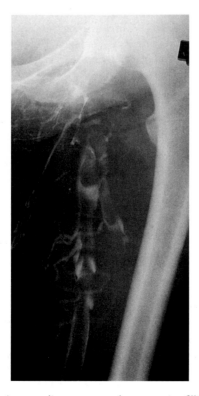

Figure 18.35 An ascending venogram demonstrating filling defects in the femoral vein due to thrombus.

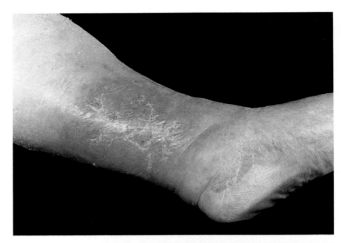

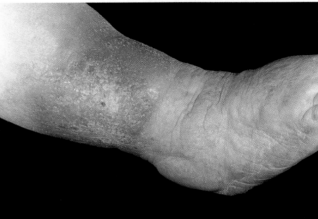

Figure 18.36 Typical changes seen in a postphlebitic limb.

limb; Fig. 18.36). Chronic venous insufficiency is a source of considerable morbidity and is a major health care problem. Finally, varicose veins continue to plague humanity as they have done for centuries.

Venous thrombosis

Pathophysiology

Blood is maintained in its normal state by the interaction of several processes which prevent bleeding (haemostasis) and, simultaneously, prevent the accumulation of clot within the circulation (anticoagulation/fibrinolysis). Haemostasis is achieved by blood vessel wall contraction, platelet adhesion and aggregation and coagulation, which may be activated by the intrinsic and extrinsic pathways. The major naturally occurring anticoagulant is antithrom-

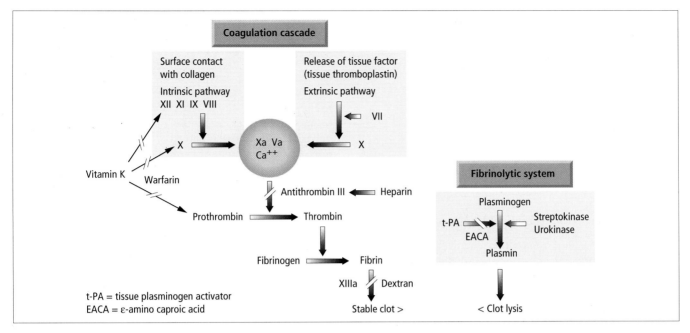

Figure 18.37 A schematic representation of the clotting and lytic systems and the sites of action of the commonly used anticoagulants and thrombolytic agents.

bin III (ATIII). Others of less importance are proteins C and S. Fibrinolysis is achieved by the action of plasmin which is activated by plasminogen activators, the most important of which is t-PA (Fig. 18.37).

Virchow suggested that venous thrombosis resulted from a triad of factors — stasis, endothelial injury and hypercoagulability of the blood. Venous thrombosis usually begins with aggregation of platelets in vein valve pockets, where maximum stasis occurs, or on a damaged vein wall. Activation of the clotting cascade, e.g. by surgical trauma, produces fibrin at a rate which cannot be controlled by the anticoagulant/fibrinolytic system and a venous thrombus develops.

Risk factors for venous thrombosis include increasing age, trauma, immobilization, sepsis (particularly with endotoxin), obesity, heart disease, malignancy, pregnancy and oestrogen therapy, and previous history of venous thromboembolic disease. Recently a number of congenital deficiencies of anticoagulant proteins have been recognized. AT III deficiency is the commonest of these, with an incidence of 1 : 2000–5000 in the general population. Heparin resistance may be the first manifestation of this disorder. Fibrinolytic deficiencies also occur.

DVT, which is very common in both medical and surgical patients, can have devastating consequences. An analysis by the National Hospital Discharge Survey suggests that DVT accounts for 10 000 deaths per annum in the USA. The natural history of DVT includes:
- complete resolution (the vein recanalizes and the valves remain competent);
- pulmonary embolism (clot migrates and causes a pulmonary infarct);
- development of chronic venous insufficiency (either the vein does not recanalize at all or the valves are destroyed when recanalization occurs).

The importance of DVT as a cause of mortality and morbidity cannot be overstated.

Clinical features

DVT in the lower limbs is often silent and is clinically apparent in only 40% of cases. Moreover, only 50% of patients with clinical evidence of DVT actually have a venous thrombosis. However, when symptoms and signs are present two groups can be defined:

1 Patients with DVT in the calf veins may have calf tenderness, ankle oedema, low-grade pyrexia and increase in leg temperature. Calf pain on passive dorsiflexion (Homan's sign) is a well-known dangerous physical sign. Attempting to elicit it may cause a pulmonary embolus.

2 Iliofemoral thrombosis, which occurs predominantly on the left side, produces pain, extensive pitting oedema and

blanching of the limb. This is *phlegmasia alba dolens* and, as it was often seen in puerperal women, it was also called 'the milk leg of pregnancy'. Progression of thrombosis impedes most of the venous return, producing a painful blue leg, *phlegmasia caerulea dolens*. Without aggressive treatment this will lead to venous gangrene.

Investigation

Because the clinical diagnosis of DVT is so inexact and its complications so serious, considerable effort has gone into the development of diagnostic tests for DVT.

Bilateral ascending venography (phlebography)

This is the gold standard for the diagnosis of DVT. The patient is tilted to a 45–60° angle with the feet down. A dorsal vein in the foot is cannulated and 200 ml of dilute contrast is injected. Venous tourniquets are placed at the knee and ankle to direct the contrast preferentially into the deep venous system. The result will give information about the site, size and extent of thrombosis and its propensity for embolization. Disadvantages are that venography is expensive and invasive (Fig. 18.35).

Doppler ultrasound

Venous obstruction distorts blood flow and this can be detected using a Doppler velocimeter probe. A normal vein gives a phasic signal with respiration. Compression of the vein distal to the probe causes flow augmentation while compression proximally stops flow and abolishes the signal. With a DVT the respiratory variation is lost and there is no flow augmentation on distal compression. While this test can be very accurate, it is very operator-dependent.

Duplex imaging

The combination of Doppler ultrasound velocimetry and B-mode ultrasound images (i.e. duplex imaging) is a very accurate non-invasive method for diagnosing DVT, especially in the proximal veins. The anatomy of each segment of the deep venous system is defined by B-mode imaging and thrombus can be detected by altered echogenicity. Doppler evaluation is performed as before. Both Doppler ultrasound and duplex imaging are very useful in pregnancy where venography is contraindicated. While the equipment is expensive and operator-dependent, duplex scanning may eventually displace venography as the gold standard for the diagnosis of DVT.

125I-Fibrinogen scanning

The incorporation of radioactive fibrinogen into a forming thrombus is the basis of this test. An injection of ^{125}I-fibrinogen is given and counts are obtained from marked locations on the legs and expressed as a percentage of the radioactivity measured over the heart. An increase of 20% or more indicates an underlying thrombus. Thrombi in pelvis veins cannot be detected. It is useful as a screening test and in assessment of methods of DVT prophylaxis, but is of little value in the clinical setting.

Impedance plethysmography

This test assesses the change in volume in a limb by measuring changes in electrical resistance. Two pairs of electrodes are placed on the calf and a pneumatic veno-occlusive tourniquet is placed around the thigh. The normal leg will rapidly swell when the tourniquet is inflated and rapidly return to normal when the occlusive tourniquet is released. Both responses are abolished or considerably slowed if a DVT is present. Disadvantages are that it is cumbersome to use and it cannot detect small, non-occlusive thrombi. More recently, photoplethysmography and air plethysmography have been used to assess deep vein function.

Management

Prophylaxis

Adequate methods of prophylaxis against DVT are available and their use saves lives. All patients over 40 and those with the risk factors listed in Table 18.24 should have prophylaxis for DVT.

General prophylactic measures include adequate hydration, mobilization pre- and postoperatively and avoidance of oestrogen therapy for 6 weeks prior to elective surgery. Specific measures are aimed at reducing venous stasis by mechanical techniques and pharmacologically countering hypercoagulability.

Mechanical prophylaxis

Mechanical measures aim at diminishing venous stasis in the legs. Such measures include elevation of the foot of the bed 10–15° and compression stockings, which are properly called antithrombotic rather than antiembolic. Pneumatic-graded sequential compression devices have been shown to inhibit venous stasis and enhance fibrinolytic activity. Electrical stimulation of calf muscles has also been used peroperatively. One of the most important prophylactic

Table 18.24 Risk factors for deep vein thrombosis.

Age (>40 years)
Prior history of deep venous thrombosis
Surgery
Trauma
Sepsis (particularly with endotoxin)
Recumbency/immobilization
Obesity
Malignancy
Heart disease
Pregnancy
Oestrogen administration
Inflammatory bowel disease
Blood disorders
  Thrombocytosis
  Polycythaemia
  Antithrombin III deficiency
  Fibrinolytic deficiencies

measures is early ambulation postoperatively, which does not mean sitting in a chair!

Pharmacological prophylaxis

Three agents have been used for prophylaxis against DVT: warfarin, dextran and heparin. Aspirin, which inhibits platelet aggregation, does not prevent postoperative venous thrombosis.

• *Warfarin sodium* is an effective prophylactic oral antithrombotic agent and its use reduces the incidence of DVT and pulmonary embolus. It acts by inhibiting the synthesis of vitamin K-dependent coagulation factors (II, VII, IX, X; Fig. 18.37). However, because of its slow delay in action and reversal in the event of bleeding, warfarin has not found much favour with surgeons as a prophylactic anticoagulant. Recently, minidose warfarin (1 mg/day without laboratory control) has been used successfully for prophylaxis in gynaecology.

• *Dextran 70* in 500 ml of 5% dextrose, given as an intravenous infusion at the time of operation and for 2 days postoperatively, reduces proximal vein thrombosis and pulmonary embolus. Low-molecular-weight dextran interferes with platelet function and fibrin polymerization (Fig. 18.37) and is associated with less bleeding than heparin. It is used extensively in elective orthopaedic surgery, especially hip arthroplasty.

• *Subcutaneous heparin*: Low-does or minidose heparin is the most widely used agent for DVT prophylaxis. In 1975, Kakkar showed that subcutaneous minidose heparin reduced the incidence of DVT from 24.6 to 7.7%. Heparin acts by accelerating AT III inhibition of activated factor X

(Fig. 18.37). The prophylactic regimen consists of 5000 units administered 2 h preoperatively followed by 5000 units every 8–12 h postoperatively. Heparin (5000 units) in combination with dihydroergotamine (0.5 mg), which increases venous flow by constricting capacitance vessels, has also been used for venous thrombosis prophylaxis and this combination reduces the incidence of wound haematoma. Recently, low-molecular-weight heparin has been used for prophylaxis. Its advantage is that only one injection is required per day and it may have fewer haemorrhagic side-effects.

Treatment of an established DVT

The aims of management of an established DVT are to minimize the risk of pulmonary embolism, to limit further thrombosis, to facilitate complete resolution of the DVT and to avoid a postphlebitic limb. General measures include adequate hydration, bedrest for the initial 4–5 days and then ambulation with support stockings. Standing still and sitting should be avoided as they promote venous stasis. Specific measures are anticoagulation, thrombolysis and thrombectomy.

Anticoagulation

The mainstay of therapy for DVT is adequate anticoagulation. This is achieved initially with *intravenous heparin*, which prevents clot propagation and subsequently warfarin, which protects against recurrent thrombosis. A bolus intravenous dose of heparin, 100–150 units/kg (usually 10 000 units) should be given initially. Thereafter, heparin may be administered by continuous infusion or intermittent intravenous bolus doses regulated by the activated partial thromboplastin time (APTT), which should be maintained at about twice normal. Complications of heparin therapy include bleeding, hypersensitivity and thrombocytopenia. Bleeding should be managed by cessation of heparin and administration of fresh frozen plasma. Rarely is the specific antagonist protamine sulphate required. Heparin-induced thrombocytopenia (HIT) is due to an immune reaction and is rapidly reversed by stopping the drug. Patients on heparin should have regular platelet counts performed.

Oral anticoagulation with warfarin is begun early in the treatment as it usually takes several days to achieve the optimal antithrombotic effect, i.e. a prothrombin time (PT) of 1.5–2 times the control value. Complications of warfarin therapy include bleeding, dermatitis and skin necrosis and several drugs (e.g. barbiturates, alcohol) interact with warfarin. Most problems resolve with discontinuation of the drug and, if necessary, vitamin K can be administered to restore the PT. After an episode of uncomplicated DVT, anticoagulant therapy should be continued for 6–8 weeks.

Thrombolysis

While the use of thrombolytic agents (streptokinase, urokinase and t-PA) to dissolve intravenous thrombus is theoretically attractive, in practice these agents have very little role in the management of venous thrombosis. Their use does not give better results than adequate anticoagulation with heparin and haemorrhage is a major complication. Only in patients with phlegmasia alba or caerulea dolens should their use be considered at all, and then only in consultation with a haematologist. Streptokinase is associated with allergic reactions in 10% of patients.

Thrombectomy

This is achieved by a direct operation on the common femoral vein and the removal of thrombus with a Fogarty catheter. There is a high incidence of rethrombosis and, as with thrombolysis, removal of the thrombus does not improve the outlook for valve function. The procedure is seldom performed today and is reserved for patients with impending gangrene.

Pulmonary embolism

Pulmonary embolism is the most serious complication of venous thrombosis. Approximately one in five patients with a DVT will develop a pulmonary embolism and 50% of those will be fatal. If no prophylaxis is given, 0.5–3.4% of patients will have a fatal pulmonary embolism following major surgery of any kind. Pharmacological prophylaxis (see above) with heparin or dextran reduces the incidence of fatal pulmonary embolism by 50%.

Pathophysiology

The lower limb is the source of embolus in 85% of patients. Five per cent arise in the pelvic veins and vena cava and the remaining 10% come from the right atrium. Thrombi which become detached from their site of origin migrate through the great veins, through the chambers of the right heart and lodge in the pulmonary arteries. The result depends on the amount of the pulmonary circulation obstructed. Thus, a large embolus which blocks the major pulmonary arteries interrupts the circulation and causes death. A massive pulmonary embolus has been defined as embolic obstruction of 40–50% of the pulmonary vasculature. Smaller emboli interrupt the circulation to isolated areas of lung tissue and produce infarction of those areas. As the infarcted lung tissue rubs against the parietal pleura, *pleuritic* pain is produced and clinically pleural rub can be detected on auscultation. An exudate from the infarct may collect in the pleural cavity and be detected as a pleural effusion. Bleeding into and destruction of the infarct lead to haemoptysis and superimposed infection may result in a lung abscess. Multiple small emboli may cause enough destruction to produce pulmonary hypertension and, as a consequence, right heart failure (cor pulmonale).

Clinical features

Symptoms

The classical presentation of massive pulmonary embolism is crushing substernal chest pain, dyspnoea, circulatory arrest and death. Pulmonary embolism was said to occur at a week to 10 days postoperatively but in reality it may occur at any time in the postoperative period. Non-fatal emboli also present with sudden chest pain (occasionally epigastric pain) and dyspnoea. The chest pain is classically pleuritic (i.e. made worse by coughing, sneezing and deep breathing) and is followed by haemoptysis in only about 15% of patients. Less obvious presentations include unexplained pyrexia, tachycardia or tachypnoea in the postoperative or postpartum period.

Physical examination

Signs of DVT may be present but usually examination of the legs is unrewarding. Tachycardia and tachypnoea are frequently observed and the patient may be cyanosed if there is a large embolus. A pleural friction rub (which has been likened to the sound of a finger being slid hard over a pane of glass), may be present with peripheral emboli. Rales may be heard over the infarcted area and a pleural effusion may be detected in some patients.

Investigations

The ECG and chest radiograph may provide useful pointers to the diagnosis of pulmonary embolism. The classical ECG (S-wave in lead I and Q-waves and inverted T-waves in lead III; S1QT3) findings are found in only 10–20% of patients. Decreased vascularity, dilated pulmonary veins or a pleural effusion may be seen on the chest film. If infarction is present, wedge-shaped infiltrates may be detected.

However, chest X-rays rarely show specific changes. Most laboratory tests are unhelpful but a low Pa_{O_2} (<10.4 kPa; 80 mmHg) with hypocarbia (Pa_{CO_2} <4.6 kPa; 36 mmHg) and alkalosis (pH >7.44) may indicate embolism. A firm diagnosis of pulmonary embolism requires more specific investigation.

Ventilation–perfusion (V/Q) lung scan

Ventilation–perfusion scanning is an isotope study designed to identify ventilation–perfusion mismatch in lung tissue. In the normal lung the perfusion pattern should match the ventilation pattern exactly. Two isotopes are used. Technetium-labelled microspheres or macroaggregates are injected intravenously into the patient and its distribution throughout the lung detected by a camera. As there is no circulation through the area of lung tissue blocked by a pulmonary embolus, no radioactivity will be emitted from that area and it will appear as a filling defect on the perfusion scan (Fig. 18.38). The patient then inhales a radioactive gas (krypton, xenon) or aerosol (technetium-labelled diethylene triaminepenta acetic acid or DTPA) and its distribution throughout the airways is again detected by a γ-camera. The ventilation scan in acute pulmonary embolism is usually normal. In areas of atelectasis or pneumonia the perfusion scan is normal, while the ventilation scan will demonstrate filling defects.

Pulmonary angiography

Pulmonary angiography provides the most effective means of diagnosing pulmonary embolism and it is most helpful in diagnosing the presence and extent of massive pulmonary embolus. It is indicated if the diagnosis cannot be established by any other means and is essential prior to embolectomy or thrombolytic therapy. Pulmonary arteriography is achieved by inserting a catheter through the

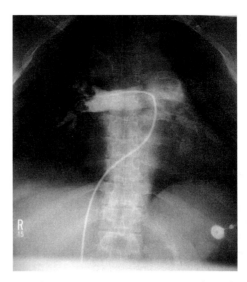

Figure 18.39 Pulmonary angiogram in a patient with a pulmonary embolus. Note the filling defect at the bifurcation of the right pulmonary artery.

right heart into the pulmonary artery and injecting contrast directly into the pulmonary circulation (Fig. 18.39). Pressure measurements in the pulmonary circulation can be obtained simultaneously and haemodynamic monitoring established.

Management

The therapeutic approaches to pulmonary embolism include anticoagulation, thrombolysis and physical removal of the embolus by open operation or embolectomy.

Anticoagulation

The majority of patients with pulmonary embolism are treated with anticoagulation therapy alone. The lung has the highest concentration of t-PA in the body and thus the capacity for spontaneous thrombolysis of pulmonary emboli is high. A large bolus dose of heparin (10 000–15 000 units) should be administered initially and thereafter heparin is administered as a continuous infusion at a dose to maintain the APTT between 50 and 80 s. Continuous infusion is associated with fewer bleeding complications than intermittent bolus injections but infusion requirements of up to 1500 units/h may have to be given. Warfarin therapy can be instituted early and there is no advantage in continuing heparin therapy for a week or 10 days. Warfarin therapy is continued for 3–6 months but in patients who have idiopathic pulmonary embolism or those

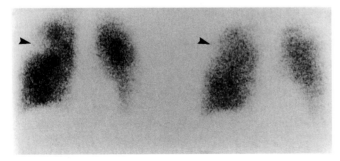

Figure 18.38 Ventilation–perfusion scan showing a perfusion defect (left) in the absence of a ventilation defect (right) in the right upper lobe, indicating a pulmonary embolism.

who suffer recurrent pulmonary embolism lifelong anticoagulation may be indicated.

Thrombolytic therapy

Thrombolytic therapy results in greater improvement and normalization of the haemodynamic responses to pulmonary emboli than heparin alone. Thrombolytic therapy should be considered in all patients with an established diagnosis of pulmonary embolism with haemodynamic compromise. However, there are many contraindications to its use (Table 18.25).

Streptokinase, urokinase and t-PA are the three agents used for thrombolysis. Allergic reactions may occur with streptokinase and it should be avoided if the patient has had a recent streptococcal infection or has received streptokinase within 6 months.

Pulmonary embolectomy

Attempts to remove pulmonary emboli by thoracotomy and direct operation on the pulmonary arteries (Trendelenburg procedure), with or without bypass, are associated with a high mortality from uncontrollable pulmonary parenchymal haemorrhage. More recently, pulmonary emboli have been aspirated from the pulmonary arteries by a special steerable cup catheter which is introduced via the femoral vein and steered through the right heart into the pulmonary artery. The embolus is suctioned into the cup and the whole apparatus is withdrawn through the femoral venotomy Several passages may be required to clear an embolus and filter (see below) should be left in the vena cava at the end of the procedure to prevent recurrent embolism. This technique should be considered in haemodynamically unstable patients in whom thrombolytic therapy is contraindicated.

Recurrent pulmonary embolism

Adequate anticoagulation is usually effective in managing pulmonary embolism and it usually prevents further em-

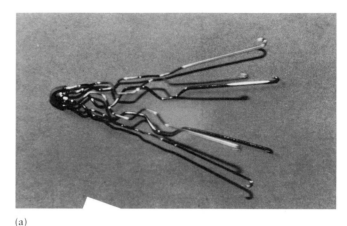

(a)

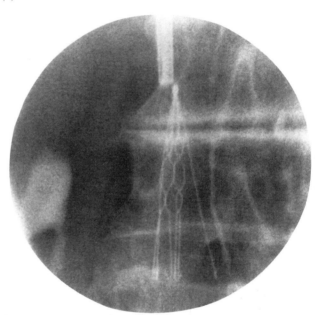

(b)

Figure 18.40 (a) A Greenfield filter. (b) This Greenfield filter has just been placed into the inferior vena cava to prevent migration of thrombus from the leg veins to the pulmonary circulation.

Table 18.25 Contraindications to thrombolytic therapy.

Intracranial or spinal cord pathology
Recent brain, eye or spinal cord injury
Malignant hypertension
Recent major surgery or trauma
Active internal bleeding
Active peptic ulcer
Recent childbirth
Pregnancy

bolization from a DVT. However, if recurrent embolization occurs during *adequate* anticoagulation or there is a contraindication to anticoagulation then surgical prophylaxis is indicated. The operative placement of clips (e.g. De Weese clip) on the inferior vena cava (IVC) has been superseded by transvenous placement of filters (e.g. Greenfield filter; Fig. 18.40) which are positioned in the IVC below the level of the renal veins. The filter traps migrating thrombus and protects the pulmonary circulation from embolism.

Postthrombotic (postphlebitic) limb

The postthrombotic limb is a common sequel to deep venous thrombosis and is a major source of morbidity and expense worldwide. A knowledge of venous anatomy and physiology is essential to understand this condition.

Venous anatomy of the lower limb

Venous blood is drained from the lower limb by deep and superficial vein systems. The deep system consists of the soleal plexus of veins in the soleal muscle, and the popliteal and femoral veins. The long and short saphenous veins make up the superficial system and they drain into the femoral and popliteal veins, respectively. The superficial system also communicates with the deep system through a series of perforating veins along the medial side of the leg at the mid-thigh and at 5, 10 and 15 cm above the medial malleolus. Normal venous flow is unidirectional from the foot to the groin and from the superficial to the deep venous systems. Contraction of the soleal and gastrocnemius muscles during walking compresses the blood and pumps it towards the heart. Reverse flow is prevented by the action of numerous valves throughout both systems. One of the most important is at the junction of the saphenous and femoral veins. Trouble begins when the valves are destroyed or become incompetent.

Pathophysiology of postthrombotic limb

The venous pressure at the ankle while standing is approximately 125 cmH_2O, i.e. the distance from the diaphragm to the ankle. On walking, this pressure falls to 30% of the resting pressure. This response is dependent on calf muscle contraction and competent valves to prevent blood regurgitating back into the deep system. If the deep valves are incompetent or, worse still, if the deep system is occluded as a sequela to DVT, venous ankle pressure will remain elevated and will actually rise with calf compression, producing venous hypertension. Continued back-pressure on the valves in the perforator veins renders them incompetent, resulting in inefficient drainage of blood from the superficial system. This may manifest as secondary varicose veins.

It has been suggested that venous hypertension results in loss of plasma protein (especially fibrin) from the capillaries in the tissues around the ankle; *pericapillary fibrin cuffs* develop which interfere with the transfer of oxygen to the tissues, leading to hypoxic injury. A second theory suggests that *trapping of white cells* and release of cytokines may be the underlying cause of tissue injury. A reduction in fibrinolytic activity in the tissues and blood has also been observed in patients with venous hypertension. Whatever the exact mechanism of injury, the result is the same: varicose eczema, lipodermatosclerosis and, eventually, venous ulceration.

Clinical features

The typical postthrombotic sequelae appear at 2–30 years after the thrombotic episode. Consequently, many patients do not remember that they had a thrombus and many patients may have had a silent DVT in any case. The patient may complain of an aching sensation in the limb. The postthrombotic leg is typically chronically swollen and may have secondary varicose veins with incompetent perforators. Usually there is varicose eczema above the medial malleolus (Fig. 18.36). This is due to haemosiderin deposition and indicates chronic venous stasis and red cell destruction in the tissues. The subcutaneous tissues may be thickened and contracted around the ankle (lipodermatosclerosis), giving the characteristic inverted champagne-bottle appearance to the leg. The most serious problem associated with the postthrombotic leg is venous ulceration (Fig. 18.41). The term varicose ulcer is a misnomer as many patients do not have varicose veins.

Venous ulceration is usually seen in elderly female patients. The ulcer is usually on the medial side of the leg just above the ankle. They can be of any shape and size, but are commonly shallow with a sloping edge. A raised or thickened edge in a chronic venous ulcer should raise the suspicion of malignant change (Marjolin's ulcer). The base of the ulcer is usually covered with pink granulation tissue and often the surrounding tissues are indurated and pigmented. Occasionally, cellulitis may be present.

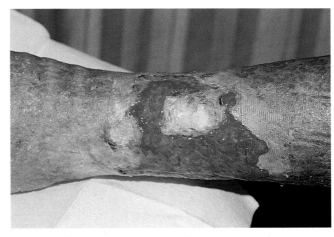

Figure 18.41 A typical venous ulcer (the term varicose ulcer is incorrect).

Investigation

Proper investigation of a patient with a suspected post-thrombotic limb is important as treatment will depend on the findings. *Ascending venography* is again the gold standard against which other non-invasive techniques have to be measured. It will demonstrate the anatomy of the deep venous system, determine the site of any obstruction that may be present and, if the veins are patent, determine the competence of the deep and perforating valves. If surgery is being considered, *descending venography* is also indicated.

The *Doppler ultrasound* probe can be used to assess the deep venous system. If an obstruction is present, the same findings are elicited as in an acute DVT (see above). If, however, the deep system is patent but incompetent, then compression distal to the probe produces minimal flow augmentation and compression proximally produces flow augmentation as the blood regurgitates down the leg.

Perforator vein competence can easily be assessed by placing the probe over the perforator, occluding the superficial vein above and below the probe and compressing the leg. Flow augmentation indicates an incompetent perforator. *Duplex scanning* provides additional anatomical information while *photoplethysmography*, in which changes in the volume of the microcirculation are detected by the transmission of light through the superficial layers of the skin, indicates the overall effect of venous insufficiency. *Ambulatory venous pressure* at the ankle can also be measured using direct cannulation. High venous pressure during calf exercise is typical of a postthrombotic limb.

Management

Patient education is important and time is well spent in explaining the disease process to the patient. The patients will then understand why there is no 'quick-fix' operation

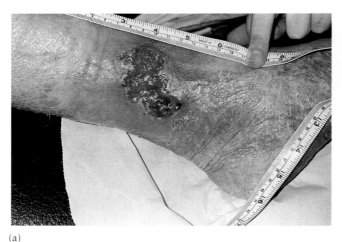

(a)

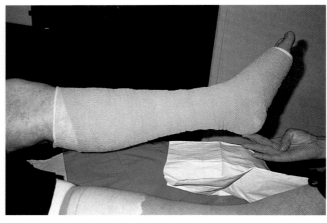

(b)

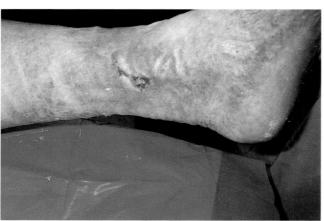

(c)

Figure 18.42 The Charing Cross four-layer compression bandaging has revolutionized the management of venous ulcers. (a) A typical venous ulcer prior to treatment; (b) four-layer bandage in place; (c) the ulcer after 12 weeks of bandaging.

for their disease, why they should elevate their legs above the level of the heart when sitting or reclining and why they must put on elastic compression stockings before they get out of bed in the morning. Compression is the mainstay of non-operative treatment and elastic graduated compression stockings and compression bandaging are the principal methods of applying compression (Fig. 18.42). A graduated stocking is one that applies the greatest pressure at the ankle and progressively less pressure up along the limb. Elevation reduces venous pressure, promotes reabsorption of oedema fluid and prevents the calf muscle pump acting and producing ambulatory venous hypertension.

Leg ulcers

When managing a patient with a presumed venous ulcer, it is important first to exclude other causes of leg ulcer, including arterial disease, vasculitis and diabetes mellitus. In some patients there may be a combination of pathology, e.g. both venous hypertension and arterial insufficiency, and all elements will require treatment. However, an established venous ulcer can be healed with careful treatment. Surrounding cellulitis should be treated with a course of systemic antibiotics and after gentle debridement the ulcer should be treated with a mild antiseptic solution until clean, when saline dressings should be used. Elevation and com-

---

Deep venous thrombosis at a glance

DEFINITION

A *deep venous thrombosis* (DVT) is a condition in which the blood in the deep veins of the legs or pelvis clots. Embolization of the thrombus results in a *pulmonary embolus* (PE), while local venous damage may lead to chronic venous hypertension and the *postphlebitic limb* (PPL)

EPIDEMIOLOGY

DVT is extremely common among medical and surgical patients, affecting 10–30% of all general surgical patients over 40 years who undergo a major operation. PE is a common cause of sudden death in hospital patients (0.5–3.0% of patients die from PE)

AETIOLOGY

Risk factors
- Increasing age >40 years
- Immobilization
- Obesity
- Malignancy
- Inflammatory bowel disease
- Anticoagulant protein (e.g. antithrombin III, protein C, protein S) deficiency
- Trauma
- Sepsis
- Heart disease
- Pregnancy/oestrogens

Virchow's triad
- Stasis
- Endothelial injury
- Hypercoagulability

PATHOLOGY

- Aggregation of platelets in valve pockets (areas of maximum stasis or injury)
- Activation of clotting cascade producing fibrin
- Fibrin production overwhelms the natural anticoagulation fibrinolytic system
- Natural history:
  - Complete resolution
  - PE
  - PPL

CLINICAL FEATURES

DVT
- Asymptomatic

PE
- Substernal chest pain

PPL
- History of DVT

- Calf tenderness
- Ankle oedema
- Mild pyrexia
- Phlegmasia alba/Caerulea dolens
- Dyspnoea
- Circulatory arrest
- Pleuritic chest pain
- Haemoptysis
- Aching limb
- Leg swelling
- Venous eczema
- Venous ulceration
- Inverted-bottle-shaped leg

INVESTIGATIONS

- Duplex imaging
- Ascending venography
- ECG — S1QT3
- CXR
- Blood gases
- Ventilation–perfusion lung scan
- Pulmonary angiography
- Ascending ± descending venography
- Duplex scanning
- Plethysmography
- Ambulatory venous pressure

MANAGEMENT

Prophylaxis against DVT

Indications
- Presence of risk factors (see above)

Methods
- Mechanical — compression (TED) stockings
- Pharmacological — subcutaneous heparin 5000 IU sc bd (warfarin 1 mg/day, dextran 70 i.v., 500 ml/day)

Definitive Rx

DVT	PE	PPL
• Anticoagulation for 6–8 weeks	• Anticoagulation for 3–6 months	• Limb elevation
		• Compression
i.v. heparin (check efficacy with APTT) Warfarin (check efficacy with PT)		• Four-layer bandaging to achieve ulcer healing
(• Thrombolysis)	• Thrombolysis	• Graduated compression stockings to maintain limb compression
(• Thrombectomy)	• Pulmonary embolectomy	
	• IVC filters for recurrent PE	(• Venous valve reconstruction)

pression bandaging are essential in the management of venous ulcers. An effective bandaging regime known as four-layer bandaging has revolutionized the management of this difficult problem (Fig. 18.42b). In the USA a gauze boot (Unna's boot) impregnated with zinc oxide, gelatin and glycerin, wrapped around the lower leg, is frequently used to treat venous ulceration. The boot has to be changed twice weekly.

Several drugs have been used in the treatment of venous ulceration. Stanozolol, an anabolic steroid which enhances fibrinolysis, helps to reduce lipodermatosclerosis but does not improve ulcer healing. Defibrotide, a new antithrombotic and profibrinolytic agent, improves ulcer healing in combination with compression therapy. Prostaglandin E_1, which has to be given parenterally, and pentoxifylline (400 mg t.d.s.) have both improved ulcer healing in combination with compression therapy.

Surgical intervention is indicated if a large varicose vein is seen draining from the ulcer. Before ligating it, however, it has to be established that the deep system is patent. If it is not, then ligating the varicose vein may disrupt the only venous drainage of the limb. Occasionally, perforating veins under the ulcer are ligated and, even more rarely, attempts at deep vein valve reconstruction or valve transplantation from the axillary vein are undertaken.

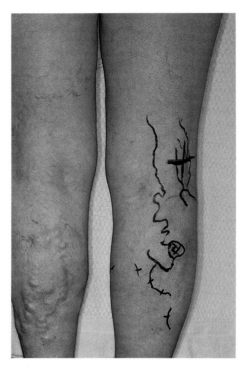

Figure 18.43 Varicose veins.

Varicose veins

Varicose veins are tortuous, dilated, prominent superficial veins in the lower limb, often in the anatomical distribution of the long and short saphenous veins. Descriptions of varicose veins exist from the earliest medical writings. They are exceedingly common and in the western world they are found in half of the adult male and two-thirds of the adult female population. However, only 10–15% of those affected have symptoms or complications (Fig. 18.43).

Pathophysiology

While the exact aetiology of varicose veins remains elusive, various types have been recognized. These are primary or familial, secondary or postthrombotic (see above), congenital malformations of veins alone (Klippel–Trenaunay syndrome): varicose veins, limb hypertrophy and port-wine staining (see Fig. 18.33)) or in combination with arteriovenous malformations (Parkes–Weber syndrome). Finally, varicosities are deliberately created by arteriovenous fistulae in patients with renal failure to facilitate repeated cannulation for haemodialysis.

Primary or familial varicose veins usually appear early in life and more than one family member is affected. Pregnancy is often the precipitating event. Progesterone, the principal hormone of pregnancy, causes passive dilatation of veins, facilitating the development of varicose veins. Secondary varicose veins occur with the postphlebitic limb and are usually caused by perforator valve failure.

Venous valve failure is the essential factor in developing varicose veins. In most patients with primary disease the process begins with failure of the valve at the saphenofemoral junction. The pressure in the femoral vein is then transmitted into the proximal long saphenous vein, causing dilatation and progressive distal valvular incompetence. As with the postthrombotic limb, an incompetent long saphenous vein disrupts the capillary circulation around the ankle, which may lead to varicose eczema, lipodermatosclerosis and sometimes ulceration. However, unlike the postthrombotic limb, surgical removal of the varicose vein reverses the microcirculatory changes and allows the ulcer to heal.

Clinical features

Varicose veins may be totally asymptomatic but common symptoms are dull, aching leg pain and a sensation of heaviness in the leg. The symptoms are absent in the early morning and are most severe in the evening. They are exacerbated by long periods of standing and relieved by lying down, leg elevation and elastic support stockings. Cutaneous itching and night cramps may also occur. Patients frequently seek treatment because of poor cosmetic appearance and occasionally they may give a history of repeated superficial thrombophlebitis. The complications of varicose eczema, venous ulceration or haemorrhage may also be presenting features.

The patient should be examined standing up. On inspection, obvious varicose veins are seen usually, but not exclusively, associated with the tributaries of the long and short saphenous systems. Pigmentation or ulceration may be present around the ankle. Many patients have unsightly spidery vascular markings composed of small clumps of dilated superficial venules. These are not really varicose veins and camouflage is the best policy in their management, as no therapy is satisfactory.

Varicose veins feel tense on palpation and a cough impulse may be elicited at the saphenofemoral junction. A *saphena varix* is a soft compressible dilatation of the saphenous vein just adjacent to the saphenofemoral junction. A thrill may be elicted over a saphena varix on coughing (Cruveilhier's sign) and an impulse will be felt if the saphenous vein distally is percussed. Palpation along the medial side of the leg may reveal defects in the deep fascia at the site of perforating veins.

The *tourniquet tests* identify clinically the sites of reflux from the deep to the superficial vein systems. A tourniquet is applied to the elevated limb just below the groin. The patient stands up. If there is no filling of the veins below the tourniquet then the incompetence is above the tourniquet (i.e. at the saphenofemoral junction; Fig. 18.44), while rapid filling of the veins below the tourniquet indicates an incompetent perforator distally. To identify such an incompetent perforator a tourniquet is placed on the elevated limb just above the suspected incompetent perforating vein. Digital pressure directly over the perforator with the tourniquet in place prevents reflux. However, the vein fills immediately on removal of the digit (Fig. 18.45). Direct digital pressure over the saphenofemoral junction preventing retrograde filling of the saphenous vein is called the Trendelenburg test. Assessment of varicose veins has become much more precise with the advent of hand-held Dopplers and in complex cases plethysmography and duplex scanning. Regurgitation following calf compression can easily be detected over the saphenofemoral junction using a hand-held Doppler probe.

Investigation

While most patients with simple varicose veins do not need elaborate investigation, any suggestion that they have a postthrombotic limb warrants full investigation, as described previously. However, as autogenous vein should be preserved for peripheral or coronary artery bypass grafting, it is important to evaluate patients who have equivocal clinical findings. The most useful methods to determine

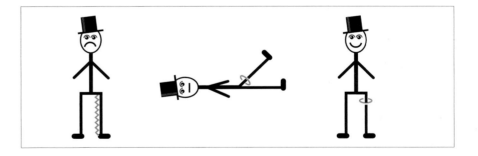

Figure 18.44 Trendelenburg test. A tourniquet is applied to the elevated limb just below the groin. The patient stands up. If there is no filling of the veins below the tourniquet then the incompetence is above the tourniquet, i.e. at the saphenofemoral junction.

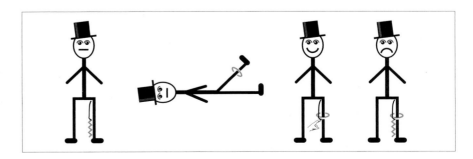

Figure 18.45 To identify an incompetent perforator in the lower leg, a tourniquet is placed on the elevated limb just above the suspected incompetent perforator. Digital pressure directly over the perforator with the tourniquet in place prevents reflux. However, the vein fills immediately on removal of the digit.

whether or not there is saphenofemoral or perforator incompetence are Duplex scanning and photophlethysmography. Detection of reflux with a Valsalva manoeuvre is a very specific test for venous valvular insufficiency. Rarely, varicography is used to detect incompetent perforators. With more precise diagnosis, more precise treatment can be planned and valuable venous segments can be preserved.

Management

Many patients simply need to be advised to elevate their legs when sitting and to wear elastic stockings. The indications for more specific treatment, i.e. sclerotherapy or surgery, are: appearance, pain and heaviness, superficial thrombophlebitis and external bleeding. Impending or established ulceration in association with varicose veins is an indication for ablative treatment provided the patient does not have a postphlebitic limb. Anaphylaxis and local ulceration are complications of sclerotherapy.

Sclerotherapy

Injection sclerotherapy is useful for treating small varicose veins below the knee but it not suitable for large varicosities, particularly above the knee. The principle of the technique is that sclerosant (sodium tetradecyl) injected into a vein produces a superficial thrombophlebitis and obliteration of the vein. Compression with a foam pad has to be applied over the injection site and compression bandaging has to be maintained for 3–6 weeks. Patients are also advised to walk several miles per day.

Surgical ablation

This is quite a successful treatment for varicose veins. Prior to surgery, with the patient standing up, the varicose veins to be removed should be marked with an indelible marker by the surgeon who is going to perform the operation. The veins are removed by making a small stab incision of only 2–3 mm over the vein. A hook or fine artery forceps is used to hook the vein out through the wound, where it is avulsed. Steristrips or fine sutures are used to close the skin. If long or short saphenous incompetence is present, a formal exploration of the saphenofemoral or saphenopopliteal junction has to be made and the superficial vein disconnected from the deep system. It is useful to identify and mark the skin over the saphenopopliteal junction by duplex scanning preoperatively. If a long segment of vein is varicose, it may be stripped out (from above downwards to avoid lymphatic and cutaneous nerve damage) and the best results are probably achieved by stripping the above-knee segment of the long saphenous vein. Postoperatively, the leg is bandaged firmly from the toes to the groin and an elastic support stocking is applied at 24 h. The bandages may be removed at a week, when stitches are removed, but the stocking should be worn for several weeks. Patients are encouraged to walk 1–2 miles (2–3 km) per day and should keep their legs elevated when sitting.

Venous miscellany

Superficial thrombophlebitis

Superficial thrombophlebitis is characterized by local inflammation of a segment of superficial vein. The usual cause is prolonged cannulation (< 72 h) of the vein for intravenous administration of fluids or drugs. Administration of acidic fluids (e.g. dextrose and some antibiotics) predisposes to thrombophlebitis. It is often associated with varicose veins and may follow injection of contrast material into a vein. Thrombophlebitis migrans is a condition of recurrent episodes of superficial thrombophlebitis and is associated with malignancy and collagen vascular disease. With thrombophlebitis the vein feels like a cord, and the surrounding skin is red and tender. Aseptic thrombophlebitis, which is common, usually responds to removal of the cannula, warm compresses and simple analgesia. However, septic thrombophlebitis, either bacterial or fungal, can be a serious condition requiring antibiotics and excision of the infected peripheral vein.

Subclavian or axillary vein thrombosis

Subclavian vein thrombosis is most likely to be due to cannulation of the vein for diagnostic or therapeutic purposes (e.g. cardiac catheterization or indwelling cannula). Subclavian or axillary vein thrombosis can occur as a primary event in a fit athletic person following prolonged arm exercise (effort thrombosis). Repetitive intermittent venous compression is thought to be the precipitating cause. The patient presents with aching arm pain, swelling and bluish discoloration of the arm. Prominent superficial collateral veins are seen over the shoulder, arm and chest wall. Treatment consists of arm elevation and anticoagulation and an underlying cause, e.g. a cervical rib, should be sought. There is a 10% incidence of pulmonary emboli with subclavian vein thrombosis.

Superior vena cava thrombosis

Superior vena cava (SVC) obstruction is usually secondary to a neoplastic process – usually bronchogenic carcinoma — in

Varicose veins at a glance

DEFINITION

Varicose veins are tortuous, dilated prominent superficial veins in the lower limbs, often in the anatomical distribution of the long and short saphenous veins

EPIDEMIOLOGY

Very common in the western world, affecting about 50% of the adult population

PATHOPHYSIOLOGY

Venous valve failure, usually at the saphenofemoral junction (and sometimes in perforating veins), results in increased venous pressure in the long saphenous vein with progressive vein dilatation and further valve disruption

AETIOLOGY

- Primary or familial varicose veins
- Pregnancy (progesterone causes passive dilatation of veins)
- Secondary to postphlebitic limb (perforator failure)
- Congenital: Klippel–Trenaunay syndrome
  Parkes–Weber syndrome
- Iatrogenic: following creation of an arteriovenous fistula

CLINICAL FEATURES

- Asymptomatic
- Cosmetic appearance
- Dull aching leg pain   ⎫ symptoms worse in the evening or
- Heaviness in the leg   ⎭ on standing for long periods
- Itching and eczema
- Superficial thrombophlebitis

- Bleeding
- Saphena varix
- Ulceration

INVESTIGATIONS

- Clinical assessment by Trendelenburg tourniquet tests
- Doppler velocimetry
- Duplex scanning

MANAGEMENT

- Symptomatic veins should be treated

General
- Avoid long periods of standing
- Elevate limbs
- Wear support hosiery

Specific
Injection sclerotherapy with sodium tetradecyl
- Suitable for small veins and usually only below the knee
- Patients are encouraged to walk several miles per day
- Anaphylaxis and local ulceration may occur
Surgical ablation
- With the patient standing, the dilated veins are carefully marked with an indelible marker
- The saphenous vein is surgically disconnected from the femoral vein and the perforators are also ablated
- The elongated veins are removed via multiple stab incisions and long segments above the knee are removed using a 'vein stripper'
- Postoperatively, compression stockings are worn for several weeks and exercise is encouraged
- Surgery is the most effective treatment for large varicose veins but recurrence rates are high

the mediastinum. In the past mediastinal saccular syphilitic aneurysms were a common cause of SVC obstruction and occasionally fibrosing mediastinitis is a cause. Symptoms include headache, swelling of the face and eyelids and chemosis. Lying down exacerbates the symptoms. Prominent neck veins, cyanosis and oedema are frequent findings. The diagnosis is usually obvious from the clinical findings but venography is sometimes required. The finding of a venous pressure of 200–500 cmH$_2$O confirms the diagnosis. Patients with SVC obstruction from malignancy usually have a very poor prognosis but palliation can sometimes be achieved with radiotherapy and, more recently, self-expanding stents have been inserted transvenously into the obstructed SVC.

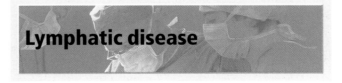

Lymphatic disease

Introduction

The lymphatic system consists of a network of capillary-like vessels which coalesce to form collecting lymphatics which,

like veins, have valves and drain via the lymph node groups, the cysterna chyli and thoracic duct into the venous circulation. The function of the lymphatic system is:
• to drain some of the macromolecular protein (mostly albumin) lost from the capillary circulation;
• to remove bacterial and foreign material from tissues;
• to transport specific materials (e.g. vitamin K and long-chain fatty acids) from the gut.

The spectrum of lymphatic disease consists of inflammatory conditions (e.g. lymphangitis), failure of lymph drainage (lymphoedema) and tumours of the lymphatic system. Lymphangitis is usually caused by streptococcal infection and often follows cellulitis.

Lymphoedema

Lymphoedema results from the accumulation of protein-rich fluid in the tissues and is caused by failure of lymph transport. Lymphangitis is a frequent complication and produces fibrosis, which makes the oedema worse. Lymphoedema may be primary, for which no obvious cause can be discerned (Fig. 18.46), or secondary, when lymphoedema follows a well-defined event (Table 18.26).

Primary lymphoedema

This type of oedema is congenital in origin but three distinct times of onset are recognized. *Congenital lymphoedema* presents at birth. Milroy's disease is a specific subgroup of congenital oedema characterized by hypoplasia of the lymphatic trunks and a familial sex-linked incidence. *Lymphoedema praecox* presents in adolescence and accounts for 80% of all patients with primary lymphoedema. *Lym-*

Table 18.26 Classification of lymphoedema.

Lymphoedema	Lymphatic defect
Primary	
Congenital (Milroy's disease)	Aplasia
Praecox	Hypoplastic
Tarda	Hyperplastic/varicose
Secondary	
Infection*	
Surgery	Hyperplastic/varicose
Radiation therapy	
Trauma	

*Filariasis, tuberculosis, lymphogranuloma, actinomycosis, chronic lymphangitis.

phoedema tarda presents in middle age. Patients with primary lymphoedema have three different congenital lymphatic abnormalities: *aplasia* (15%), in which there are no lymphatic trunks; *hypoplasia* (70%), in which there are only a few rudimentary trunks; and *hyperplastic* (15%) or varicose, in which there are several dilated lymphatic trunks secondary to lymphatic valve incompetence.

Secondary lymphoedema

The removal or destruction of inguinal or axillary nodes by surgery, radiation therapy, infection or tumour infiltration results in secondary lymphoedema. The commonest worldwide cause of secondary lymphoedema is infestation of the lymph nodes by filarial worms, *Wuchereria bancrofti*. Anatomically, secondary lymphoedema has a hyperplastic (varicose) pattern.

Clinical features

Lymphoedema usually starts at the ankle and ascends up the leg over a period of months, giving a characteristic 'tree-trunk' appearance. Lymphoedema can be differentiated from venous oedema by the absence of pigmentatory changes. Pitting can occur with lymphoedema but is related to the degree of fibrosis present. The diagnosis can be established clinically and detailed investigations such as lymphangiography should be reserved for those patients for whom surgery is being considered.

Management

There is no cure for lymphoedema and the chronic nature of this condition should be explained to the patient. The aims

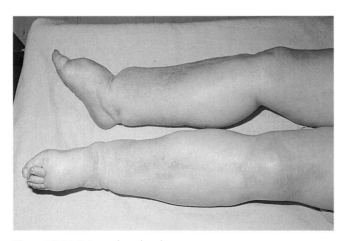

Figure 18.46 Primary lymphoedema.

of therapy are to preserve skin quality, soften subcutaneous tissue, prevent lymphangitis and reduce limb size. The key elements of treatment are limb elevation, graduated compression hosiery (which needs to be renewed every 3 months) and external pneumatic compression (e.g. Flowtron pump).

Surgical therapy is only considered in a small number of patients for recurrent lymphangitis, functional impairment and cosmesis. Attempts to anastomose lymphatic channels to veins have not been very successful and most surgery now involves excision of subcutaneous tissue and redundant skin.

Tumours of lymphatics

Lymphangiomas

Lymphangiomas are benign tumours of the lymphatics which are usually present at birth. These are sequestered portions of the lymphatic system which can produce lymph. The commonest is the *cystic hygroma* (see Fig. 1.8), which is found typically around the head and neck and presents as a soft, non-tender cystic mass which transilluminates. Treatment is by surgical excision.

Lymphangiosarcoma

Lymphangiosarcoma is an aggressive malignant tumour of the lymphatics which is associated with lymphoedema. It generally appears 10 years after the onset of lymphoedema and has an average survival rate of 19 months. Lymphangiosarcoma presents as a reddish-purple discoloration or nodule and early radical amputation remains the mainstay of therapy.

19 Pulmonary Disorders

The ancient inhabitants of this island were less troubled with coughs when they went naked and slept in caves and woods than men now in chambers and feather beds. (Sir Thomas Brown 1605–82)

Introduction

Diseases of the respiratory system are a major cause of illness and are frequently encountered in surgical practice. Many patients require detailed assessment of their pulmonary function prior to surgery and postoperative respiratory complications are not uncommon. Bronchial carcinoma is the commonest cancer to cause death and the lung is often the site of secondary deposits from tumours elsewhere in the body, e.g. renal carcinoma. The complications of 'benign' pulmonary disease sometimes require surgical treatment (e.g. drainage or decortication of the lung for empyema or resection of emphysematous bullae for persistent pneumothorax) and chest injury (see Chapter 9) is also a serious problem which requires skilful management.

Evaluation of the patient

Patients with acute or chronic disorders of the chest have specific symptoms and signs. The elucidation of the underlying problem is achieved by good history-taking, followed by complete physical examination and the performance of certain specific investigations. Some of the latter are needed in all patients with chest problems. Others are dictated by the details of the individual case.

Clinical assessment

Symptoms

The history often provides the most important piece of information leading to the diagnosis of a pulmonary disorder. General points to be considered in the history are listed below.
- *Smoking*: an attempt should be made to calculate the quantity of cigarettes smoked by calculating the 'pack-year' history. Smoking 20 cigarettes per day for 1 year represents 1 pack-year. Smoking 40 cigarettes per day for 1 year would be 2 pack-years.
- *Foreign travel*: tuberculosis (TB) is still common in certain parts of the world.
- *Exposure to asbestos*: bronchial carcinoma or pleural mesothelioma may develop years after exposure to asbestos.
- *Risk factors for human immunodeficiency virus (HIV) infection*: pneumonia is often the first indication of HIV infection.

The important symptoms of chest disease are outlined in Table 19.1.
- *Cough*: This may be dry or productive of sputum. It may occur in the morning only, as in chronic smokers, or be nocturnal (asthma, heart disease). In some disorders, the patient develops attacks of coughing when lying supine. This is encountered in patients with oesophageal disease and in those suffering from lung abscess. A 'bovine' cough suggests left recurrent laryngeal nerve palsy, often secondary to bronchial carcinoma.

Table 19.1 Symptoms of chest disorders.

Cough
Sputum production
Chest pain
Dyspnoea
Wheezing
Fever/rigors
Weight loss
Hoarseness
Dysphagia
Joint and bone pain

• *Sputum*: In patients suffering from chronic bronchitis the sputum is white and tenacious. A purulent nature is indicative of acute infections. In patients with bronchial carcinoma the sputum is often both purulent and blood-stained while bronchiectasis results in copious amounts of yellow or green sputum.

• *Chest pain*: This may originate from disorders of the chest, oesophagus (reflux disease and motility disorders) or ischaemic heart disease. The exact location, distribution, radiation and precipitating factors must be determined in the individual patient. Pulmonary pain is usually deep-seated and dull, whereas pleuritic pain encountered in pulmonary embolism and infection of the pleural space is sharp, synchronous with respiration and often accompanied by a pleural rub.

• *Dyspnoea*: Breathlessness may be acute (e.g. pneumonia, pulmonary embolism, pneumothorax, pulmonary oedema, asthma) or chronic (e.g. obstructive airways disease, emphysema, fibrosing alveolitis). Breathlessness on lying flat is called orthopnoea and occurs with pulmonary oedema and asthma. Paroxysmal nocturnal dyspnoea is characteristic of left ventricular failure and is relieved by sitting up. Dyspnoea may be accompanied by wheezing in patients with asthma and it is painful in patients suffering from lobar pneumonia.

• *Wheeze and stridor*: A wheeze is a high-pitched noise produced when the patient exhales. It denotes intrathoracic airway obstruction. It may be unilateral (bronchial foreign body, bronchial adenoma) or bilateral, as in patients suffering from an asthmatic attack and those who develop pulmonary embolism. Stridor is a low-pitched noise produced on inspiration and usually indicates obstruction to the trachea or a major bronchus.

• *Fever/rigors*: These are indicative of pulmonary sepsis such as pneumonia, bronchiectasis, TB (characteristically, patients with TB have night sweats) and lung abscess which may be caused by aspiration, postpulmonary infarction or bronchial occlusion from carcinoma of the lung.

• *Weight loss*: This is encountered in chronic pulmonary sepsis and in bronchial carcinoma.

• *Hoarseness and dysphagia*: This may be encountered in patients with intrathoracic malignancy (bronchial carcinoma or secondary mediastinal node involvement) and these symptoms always signify advanced disease. The hoarseness is due to involvement of the recurrent laryngeal nerve. The dysphagia is caused by compression or invasion of the oesophagus and may progress to malignant tracheo-oesophageal fistula. The patient then develops significant respiratory problems due to flooding of the bronchial tree by saliva and ingested liquids. Involvement of the phrenic nerve leading to unilateral diaphragmatic paralysis is also a sign of advanced inoperable intrathoracic tumour.

• *Joint and bone pain*: Patients with bronchial carcinoma most commonly experience bone pain as a result of osseous metastases. Less frequently, some patients develop a syndrome of hypertrophic pulmonary osteoarthropathy which causes persistent bone and joint (wrists and ankles) pain and marked finger clubbing. In this condition (which is quite unrelated to metastatic disease) there is thickening of the bones near the affected joints due to subperiosteal deposition of osteoid tissue.

• *Haemoptysis*: This is always significant and may be due to neoplasms (bronchial carcinoma), infections (pneumonia, lung abscess, TB, bronchiectasis, fungal, parasitic) or cardiovascular disorders. Pulmonary embolic disease and pulmonary infarction also cause haemoptysis.

Physical examination

The important physical signs of pulmonary disease are cyanosis, finger clubbing (Fig. 19.1), pyrexia, altered respiratory pattern and rate, supraclavicular lymph node enlargement and the specific chest signs elicited by inspection, palpation, auscultation and percussion (Table 19.2). Cyanosis is present when about 5 g/100 ml of haemoglobin is in the reduced state within the skin blood vessels. Peripheral cyanosis is usually due to a local circulatory slowing and the part (e.g. hand) is generally cold. Central cyanosis is associated with hypoxaemia (arterial Pao_2 will be <6 kPa or 45 mmHg in the presence of central cyanosis). However, cyanosis may not be detectable clinically if the patient is anaemic with a haemoglobin level of <5 g/100 ml. By contrast, the patient may appear to be cyanotic if he or she is polycythaemic. The latter may be secondary to chronic hypoxia or develop as a primary disease (polycythaemia rubra vera). Cyanosis may also be due to the presence of significant amounts of circulating altered haemoglobin, e.g. methaemoglobinaemia and sulphhaemoglobinaemia. Inspection of the sputum should be part of the clinical examination. The amount of sputum produced, the colour (white,

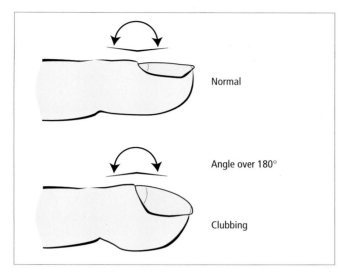

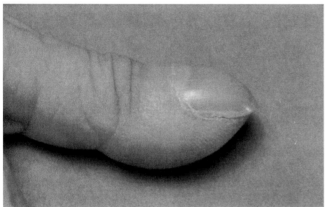

Figure 19.1 Finger clubbing. There is an increase in the nail bed angle, increased curvature of the nail and swelling of the tip of the finger.

yellow or green) and the presence or absence of blood should all be noted.

Investigations

The investigations commonly used for assessing patients with pulmonary disease are given in Table 19.3. The initial essential investigations for patients with pulmonary disease include a chest radiograph (posteroanterior and lateral films), full blood count (FBC) and erythrocyte sedimentation rate (ESR). Specific things to look at on the radiographs are listed in Table 19.4. The FBC may show secondary polycythaemia in response to chronic hypoxia and a raised ESR may indicate infection. If the patient has a productive cough, sputum culture and cytology are also performed routinely. An electrocardiogram (ECG) is indicated to detect underlying heart disease.

Imaging

Other imaging tests such as computed tomographic (CT) scanning are carried out to obtain better definition of pulmonary and mediastinal lesions encountered on the chest X-ray. Ventilation–perfusion scanning (V/Q scan) is used in the diagnosis of pulmonary embolism. The scan uses a γ-camera to compare the distribution of radioactivity in the lung when a patient breathes radiolabelled xenon gas (the ventilation scan) and after injection of radiolabelled albumin (the perfusion scan). Normally the two scans should match perfectly and this test is most reliable when normal in excluding pulmonary embolism. It may be highly suggestive of pulmonary embolism if the ventilation scan (V) is normal and the perfusion scan (Q) abnormal (no

Table 19.2 Examination of a patient with a suspected pulmonary disorder.

Inspection	Palpation	Percussion	Auscultation
Hands			
Nicotine staining	Pulse		
Clubbing			
Peripheral cyanosis			
Tremor or flap			
Face and neck			
Conjunctiva (anaemia)	Lymph nodes	Supraclavicular fossae	Supraclavicular fossae
Lips and tongue (central cyanosis)			
Accessory muscles of respiration			
Jugular venous pressure			
Chest			
Deformities	Ribs	Compare two sides of	Nature of sounds
Breathing rate and pattern	Trachea	chest wall	Added sounds
Accessory muscles of respiration	Apex beat	Note hepatic and cardiac dullness	Vocal resonance

Table 19.3 Investigations available for assessment of patients with pulmonary disease.

Investigation	Comment
Haematology	
Full blood count	Secondary polycythaemia
Microbiology	
Sputum culture and direct staining	ZN staining for tuberculosis
Imaging	
Chest radiography	Both PA and lateral films
Computed tomography of the thorax	Identifies small lesions
Bronchography	Used now only for bronchiectasis
Ventilation–perfusion scan	Diagnosis of pulmonary embolus
Endoscopy	
Indirect laryngoscopy	Assess vocal cords
Bronchoscopy	Visualize and biopsy bronchial tree
Mediastinoscopy	Assess lymph node status in bronchial carcinoma
Thoracoscopy	Examine pleural cavity
Pulmonary function tests	Detect and define abnormal lung function
Biochemistry	
Arterial blood gas analysis	Respiratory failure
Biopsy for histopathology	
Bronchoscopy	Biopsy of bronchial tree to fourth or fifth divisions
Bronchoalveolar lavage	Collects fluid for cytology and culture
Percutaneous fine-needle biopsy	For discrete lung lesions beyond bronchoscopic range and pleural biopsy
Thoracocentesis	Drains pleural effusion and provides cells for cytology
Open or thoracoscopic lung biopsy	Lung tissue is removed via a thoracotomy or thoracoscopy

ZN, Ziehl–Neelsen; PA, posteroanterior.

filling) in several segments (see Chapter 18.3). Otherwise the test is indeterminate as perfusion defects may be caused by a variety of chest disorders.

Endoscopy

Endoscopic visualization of the bronchial tree includes indirect laryngoscopy, which assesses vocal cord function, bronchoscopy and mediastinoscopy. Bronchoscopy allows visualization of the endobronchial tree down to the fourth or fifth divisions. It is performed using a fine flexible endoscope (Fig. 19.2) which has now replaced the rigid bronchoscope. Bronchoscopy may be diagnostic when the entire tracheobronchial tree is inspected and any lesions encountered are biopsied; or therapeutic for the removal of thick retained secretions and extraction of foreign bodies. Medi-

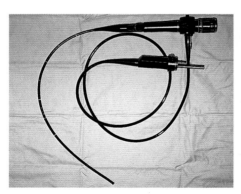

(a)

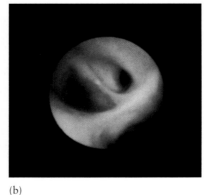

(b)

Figure 19.2 (a) Flexible bronchoscope. (b) A view of the right upper lobe obtained at bronchoscopy.

Table 19.4 Specific things to look at on a chest radiograph.

Penetration and rotation
Overpenetrated films are very dark
Underpenetrated films are white
The vertebral spines should be midway between the costoclavicular joints

Bony skeleton
Collapse or secondary deposits in the vertebrae
Fractures or metastases in ribs

The heart
Size, shape and cardiothoracic ratio (<0.5 normally)

Trachea and major bronchi
Position of trachea and bronchi

Hilar regions
Abnormal configuration may indicate lymphadenopathy

Lung fields
Pneumothorax
Collapse
Consolidation
Shadows
Effusion

Diaphragm and pleura
Position of diaphragms
Costophrenic angles for fluid
Air under diaphragm
Pleural thickening

astinoscopy is performed under general anaesthetic and is used to sample mediastinal lymph nodes in patients prior to surgery for bronchial carcinoma. Thoracoscopy is a technique whereby a rigid scope is passed into the pleural cavity. A number of operative procedures may be performed using this technique, e.g. transthoracic sympathectomy for hyperhidrosis, pulmonary biopsy and even pulmonary lobectomy.

Pulmonary function tests

In the elective situation, a good indication of global pulmonary function is obtained by assessing the exercise tolerance of the patient, i.e. distance walked before development of breathlessness and ability to climb a flight of stairs. Dyspnoea at rest always indicates severe compromise of pulmonary function.

The peak expiratory flow rate (PEFR) can easily be measured with a peak expiratory flow meter. PEFR is the flow over the first 10 ms on maximal expiration after a maximum inspiration. It correlates well with the forced expiratory volume in 1 s (FEV_1) and is reduced by airway narrowing (asthma, bronchitis) or muscle weakness (Fig. 19.3). Lung volume measurements (Fig. 19.4) are used to estimate functional lung volumes. The best parameters for detection and quantitation of airflow obstruction in chronic obstructive disease (e.g. chronic bronchitis) are FEV_1 and forced vital capacity (FVC). The ratio between these (FEV_1/FVC $\times$

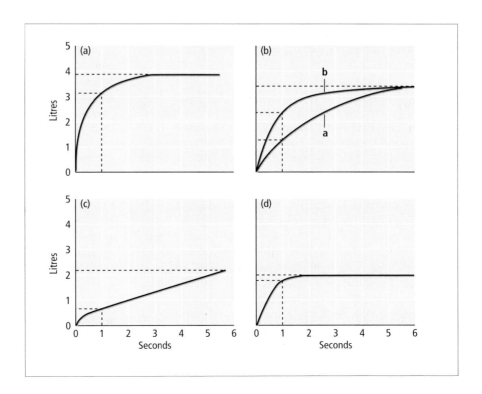

Figure 19.3 Spirogram tracings obtained from a vitalograph.
(a) Normal: FEV_1 3.1l, FVC 3.8l, FEV_1/FVC 82%. (b) Obstructive reversible defect (asthma): **a** before bronchodilator: FEV_1 1.4l, FVC 3.5l, FEV_1/FVC 40%; **b** after bronchodilator: FEV_1 2.5l, FVC 3.5l FEV_1/FVC 71%. (c) Obstructive irreversible defect (chronic bronchitis and emphysema): unchanged with bronchodilator FEV_1 0.5l, FVC 2.2l, FEV_1/FVC 23%. (d) Restrictive defect (fibrosing alveolitis): unchanged with bronchodilator FEV_1 1.8l, FVC 2.0l, FEV_1/FVC 90%.

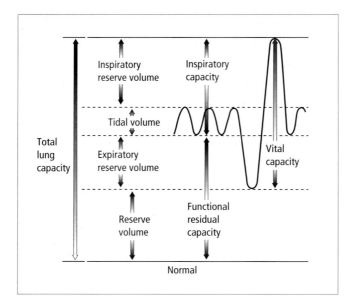

Figure 19.4 Subdivisions of total lung capacity.

100 = 70–80% normally) can be used to distinguish between obstructive (decreased ratio <60%) and restrictive (increased ratio >80%) lung disease (Fig. 19.3). However, the best indicators for restrictive lung disease (e.g. interstitial pulmonary fibrosis) are the vital capacity (VC) and total lung capacity (TLC). Transfer factor (T_{LCO}), also called diffusing capacity (D_{LCO}), is a measurement which uses small amounts of inert gases or carbon monoxide to test the diffusion capacity of the alveolar–capillary membrane.

Blood gas analysis

This is performed on a sample of arterial blood (usually obtained by a femoral stab). The analysis gives valuable information on the state of oxygenation, presence of pulmonary injury or disease, the acid–base balance and the cause of acidosis or alkalosis. The arterial oxygen tension (Pa_{O_2}) reflects the amount of oxygen dissolved in the blood at sea level. Hypoxaemia is said to be present when this falls below 10.4 kPa (80 mmHg). However, the oxygen in solution only represents 1–2% of the blood's total oxygen content, 98% of which is carried by haemoglobin. What is more important is the realization that adequate oxygenation of the blood does not ensure adequate tissue oxygenation to the vital organs. This necessitates efficient transport to (by nutrient flow) and extraction by the tissues. The difference between the oxygen tension in the alveolar space (PA_{O_2}) and in the arterial tree (Pa_{O_2}) is used to distinguish the pulmonary origin of the hypoxaemia from extrapul-

monary causes (e.g. hypoventilation and low inspired oxygen tension). This difference, $P(A-a)_{O_2}$, is increased in pulmonary disease from any cause and is normal in patients with extrapulmonary impairment. The PA_{O_2} can be calculated by the alveolar air equation: $PA_{O_2} = P$ inspired $O_2 - (Pa_{CO_2} \div 0.8)$. A Pa_{CO_2} greater than 7.1 kPa (55 mmHg) is always indicative of severe respiratory impairment. The relationship between pH, bicarbonate and the arterial carbon dioxide tension (Pa_{CO_2}), is outline in Chapter 6.

Biopsies for histopathology or cytology

These may be obtained by thoracoscopy, thoracocentesis, percutaneous techniques or, in the last restort, thoracotomy.

Thoracocentesis is a technique that entails aspiration of pleural fluid to relieve dyspnoea and to obtain samples of pleural fluid for bacteriology and cytology. Percutaneous lung or pleural biopsies are obtained using conventional or CT imaging to guide the needle to the correct site for the diagnosis of primary pleural disorders (e.g. mesothelioma) or solitary accessible lung lesions (on the periphery of the pulmonary parenchyma). Nowadays, most wedge lung biopsies are performed via the thoracoscopic approach which has replaced open thoracotomy for this purpose.

Pulmonary embolism, collapse and infections

Pulmonary embolism (see Chapter 18)

The types of emboli which may lodge in the main pulmonary trunk or pulmonary arteries or their branches are: thromboemboli, tumour emboli, foreign-body emboli (venous cannulae), air emboli (exogenous air inadvertently introduced into the venous system) and fat emboli (after multiple fractures). Of these, by far and away the commonest is thromboembolism and this is the condition that is commonly referred to as pulmonary embolism. It can be immediately fatal and is often accompanied by significant morbidity. The complications of pulmonary embolism consist of pulmonary infarction and pneumonia. Both are serious and may contribute to death of the patient. Pulmonary infarction tends to occur if the obstruction occurs in a peripheral branch and is associated with hypotension or heart failure. Pulmonary embolism has been fully discussed in Chapter 18.

Pulmonary collapse

Pulmonary collapse results from alveolar hypoventilation such that the alveolar walls collapse and become deaerated.

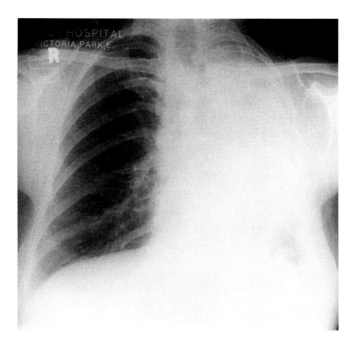

Figure 19.5 Complete collapse of the left lung due to a mucus plug in the main bronchus.

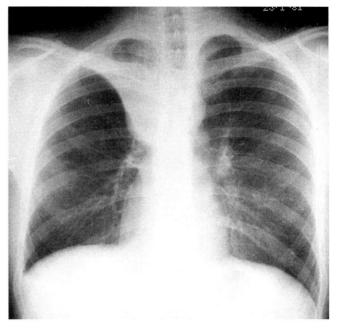

Figure 19.6 Right upper lobe collapse. Note the elevation of the right hilum and spreading of the right lower zone blood vessels.

The term is often used synonymously with atelectasis which, strictly speaking, is incorrect; pathologically atelectasis refers to alveoli which have never been filled with inspired air. Pulmonary collapse is due to proximal bronchial occlusion which may be organic or secretional in origin. Examples of the former include obstruction by bronchogenic carcinoma. Secretional airway obstruction leading to collapse is the commonest cause in the postoperative period and is encountered predominantly in chronic smokers and patients with chronic bronchitis (Fig. 19.5). Aside from the increased airway resistance, these patients develop a bronchorrhoea after surgery and general anaesthesia. This consists of thick viscid mucus which plugs various segments of the bronchopulmonary tree leading to patchy segmental or lobar collapse. In addition, ciliary activity is impaired in these patients so that movement of the secretion into the upper reaches of the bronchial tree where it can be expectorated is impaired. Following bronchial obstruction the residual air trapped in the alveoli is absorbed and the resulting deaerated area becomes prone to infection — bronchopneumonia. This is the commonest type of postoperative chest infection.

Diagnosis of pulmonary collapse

The collapse of a pulmonary segment is associated with pyrexia and clinical manifestations of a chest infection: tachypnoea, productive sputum, diminished air entry and bronchial breathing. A more severe ventilatory disturbance is exhibited by patients who develop lobar or pulmonary collapse when respiratory difficulty and significant hypoxaemia are present. The diagnosis of pulmonary collapse is confirmed by a chest X-ray (Fig. 19.6).

Treatment of pulmonary collapse

As in pulmonary embolism, prophylaxis is important. This consists of deep breathing exercises started preoperatively, adequate pain relief and early ambulation. The treatment of established pulmonary collapse is by intensive physiotherapy. Antibiotics are administered in the presence of infection. If the secretional airway obstruction is major (as in the patient in Fig. 19.5), bronchoscopic suction is necessary. Patients with severe disease with persistence of excessive bronchial secretion are nowadays managed by minitracheostomy.

Pulmonary infections

Pneumonia

Pneumonia is an infection with consolidation of the pulmonary parenchyma and may be caused by bacterial (Table

Table 19.5 Microorganisms causing bacterial pneumonia.

Streptococcus pneumoniae (commonest)
Staphylococcus aureus (children and elderly)
Haemophilus influenza (children, chronic lung disease, alcoholism)
Gram-negative organisms (severely ill and immunocompromised patients)
Legionella species
Myobacteria (malnutrition, poor social conditions)

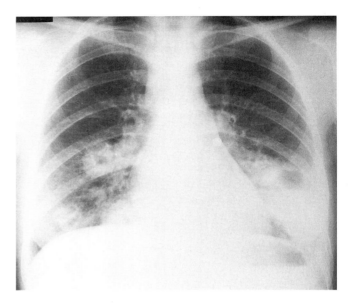

Figure 19.8 Bilateral cavitating pneumonia due to staphylococcal pneumonia. Note the air fluid levels in the cavities.

19.5), viral (influenza, cytomegalovirus, varicella), fungal (*Candida*, *Aspergillus*, *Cryptococcus*) and protozoal infections (*Pneumocystis*, *Toxoplasma*).

The commonest variety of pneumonia is bacterial, due to *Streptococcus pneumoniae* (Fig. 19.7). When serious, it carries a high mortality from acute pulmonary failure. Certain groups of people are especially prone to develop life-threatening pneumonia (Table 19.6).

Pneumonia causes obvious respiratory distress with dyspnoea, which is painful, and tachypnoea. In addition, breathing is laboured with recruitment of the accessory muscles of respiration. If the resulting hypoxia is profound, the patient becomes confused or stuporous. Coughing is usually productive and purulent and haemoptysis may occur. Physical signs include pyrexia, cyanosis, tachycardia and hypotension (in severe pneumonia). The chest signs are those of diminished air entry, and consolidation over a lobe or whole lung. The chest X-ray is usually diagnostic. Aside from the consolidation, pleural effusion, interstitial infiltrates and air–fluid cysts may be present (Fig. 19.8). Sputum culture is essential for effective antibiotic therapy.

Treatment

The management of the usual streptococcal pneumonia entails respiratory support and specific medication. Respiratory support consists of oxygen therapy, ensuring adequate tissue perfusion by administration of crystalloid solutions and physiotherapy. If hypoxaemia is severe with obvious acute pulmonary failure, endotracheal intubation with mechanical ventilation becomes essential.

In the absence of the results of sputum culture, microscopical examination of the sputum with Gram staining can yield valuable information on the nature of the infecting organism and hence guide the selection of the appropriate antibiotic regimen. Penicillin remains the antibiotic of choice for streptococcal pneumonia, vancomycin for staphylococcal disease and ampicillin for *Haemophilus influenzae* infection. Most of the hospital-acquired pneumonias are due to

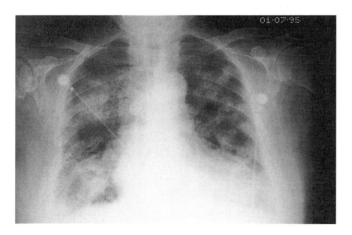

Figure 19.7 Bronchopneumonia which developed postoperatively in a patient after laparotomy.

Table 19.6 Patient groups prone to severe pneumonia.

Elderly
Patients with chronic lung and heart disease
Chronic alcoholics
Debilitated individuals
Diabetics
Immunodeficiency from any cause
Asplenic state
Cerebrovascular accident victims

Gram-negative organisms and for these the best-guess antibiotic regimen is a combination of an aminoglycoside and a cephalosporin. β-Adrenergic bronchodilators as aerosols or intravenous aminophylline are administered in patients with chronic obstructive airways disease and to those who have associated acute bronchospasm.

Lung abscess

The causes of lung abscess are outlined in Table 19.7.

Table 19.7   Types of lung abscess.

Aspiration
Secondary to specific pneumonias: *Staphylococcus, Klebisella*
Metastatic
Malignant
Postpulmonary infarction
Specific: amoebic, tuberculous

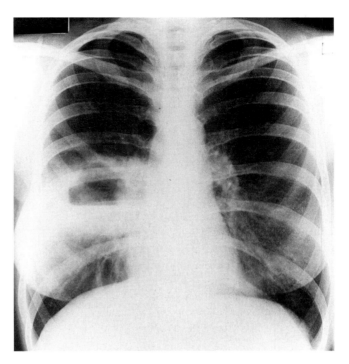

Figure 19.9   Lung abscess in the right lower lobe. Note the air fluid level in the cavity.

Aspiration lung abscess is most commonly located in the apical segment of the left lower lobe as the left bronchus is more in line with the trachea and this segment is in the dependent position when the patient is supine. It is due to aspiration and infection by organisms from the oropharynx during episodes of loss of consciousness, e.g. epileptic fit, alcoholic stupor, etc. Lung abscess may develop as a complication of specific pneumonias, e.g. staphylococcal pneumonia, or be metastatic when the infection is carried to the lung from a focus of sepsis elsewhere in the body. Malignant lung abscess may arise in two ways: from bronchial obstruction by the tumour or as a result of central necrosis with superadded infection. An abscess may burst into the bronchial tree and discharge its contents (e.g. coughing-up of 'anchovy sauce' in amoebic lung abscess) or into a branch of the pulmonary artery (e.g. tuberculous abscess), when it may cause fatal exsanguination and drowning. Fungal infection of an abscess cavity (*Aspergillus*) may occur and can be very difficult to eradicate.

The symptoms of a lung abscess include malaise, intermittent fever and sweating, weight loss and cough. The diagnosis is usually established by a chest X-ray (Fig. 19.9). An associated pleural effusion is common. An abscess may resolve with antibiotic therapy but when it becomes chronic, drainage is essential.

Pulmonary tuberculosis

Most tuberculous infections involve the lungs only or in association with extrapulmonary lesions such as TB of the skin (once known as scrofula), lymph nodes, bones and joints, genitourinary system, abdomen, intestines and the central nervous system. In the western hemisphere the disease is rare as a result of improved nutrition and housing, pasteurization of milk, tuberculin testing in cattle and eradication of positive reactors, and human bacillus Calmette–Guérin (BCG) vaccination. Most of the infections in these countries are caused by *Mycobacterium tuberculosis*. They are acquired by inhalation of organisms present in fresh droplets or dust that has been contaminated with dried sputum from a patient with open pulmonary tuberculosis, i.e. a patient with myobacteria in the sputum. In economically deprived countries, infections caused by *M. bovis* are common. These are acquired by both ingestion and inhalation.

Pulmonary TB in childhood is characterized by marked involvement of the regional lymph nodes which, together with the solid pulmonary focus usually in the lung midzone (Ghon focus), is referred to as the primary complex. Particularly in malnourished individuals the disease may spread to both lungs in miliary fashion.

In adults pulmonary TB extends locally by caseation (coagulative necrosis) with cavitation and healing is by fibrosis (Fig. 19.10). Apart from the chest symptoms and signs, pulmonary TB is accompanied by malaise, asthenia, weight

Pulmonary collapse and pneumonia at a glance

DEFINITION

Pulmonary collapse or *atelectasis* results from alveolar hypoventilation such that the alveolar walls collapse and become deaerated. *Pneumonia* is an infection with consolidation of the pulmonary parenchyma

AETIOLOGY/PATHOPHYSIOLOGY

Postoperatively, patients frequently develop atelectasis which may develop into a pneumonia

Pulmonary collapse
- Proximal bronchial obstruction
- Trapped alveolar air absorbed
- Common in smokers
- Common with chronic bronchitis

Pneumonia
- Infection with microorganisms
  - (a) *Bacteria* — *Streptococcus pneumoniae staphylococcus, Haemophilus influenzae*
  - (b) *Viral* — influenza, cytomegalovirus
  - (c) *Fungal* — *Candida, Aspergillus*
  - (d) *Protozoal* — *Pneumocystis, Toxoplasma*

Predisposing factors
- *Secretional airway obstruction*
  - (a) Bronchorrhoea postsurgery
  - (b) Mucus plugs block bronchi
  - (c) Impaired ciliary action
  - (d) Postoperative pain prevents effective coughing
- *Organic airway obstruction*
  - (a) bronchial neoplasm

Patients prone to severe pneumonia
- The elderly
- Alcoholics
- Chronic lung and heart disease
- Debilitated patients
- Diabetes
- Post CVA
- Immunodeficiency states
- Postsplenectomy
- Atelectasis postsurgery

CLINICAL FEATURES

Pulmonary collapse
- Pyrexia
- Tachypnoea
- Diminished air entry
- Bronchial breathing

Pneumonia
- Respiratory distress
- Painful dyspnoea
- Tachypnoea
- Productive cough ± haemoptysis
- Hypoxia — confusion
- Diminished air entry
- Consolidation
- Pleural rub
- Cyanosis

INVESTIGATIONS

- CXR — consolidation, pleural effusion, interstitial infiltrates, air–fluid cysts
- Sputum culture — essential for correct antibiotic treatment
- Blood gas analysis — diagnosis of respiratory failure

MANAGEMENT

Prophylaxis
- Preoperative deep breathing exercises
- Incentive spirometry
- Adequate analgesia postoperatively
- Early ambulation

Treatment
- Intensive chest physiotherapy
- Respiratory support:
  - (a) Humidified oxygen therapy
  - (b) Adequate hydration
  - (c) Bronchodilators if bronchospasm is present
- Specific antimicrobial therapy based on sputum culture

COMPLICATIONS

- Respiratory failure
- Lung abscess

---

loss, fever and night sweats. Diagnosis is made by identifying the tubercule bacillus; the presence of alcohol and acid-fast bacilli on Ziehl–Neelsen staining of a sputum smear indicates TB. Frequently surgeons are asked to biopsy lymph nodes to confirm the diagnosis. TB is curable by modern chemotherapy which has eliminated the need for sanatorium management. The drugs available include streptomycin, para-aminosalicylic acid, isoniazid, rifampicin, pyrazinamide and ethambutol.

Disorders of the pleura

The pleural space is outlined by the pleural membrane which covers the inner chest wall (parietal pleura), the mediastinum and the lung surface (visceral pleura). In the normal state the intrapleural pressure is negative such that only a thin film of fluid separates the two opposing pleural surfaces. Various pathological states result in abnormalities of the pleural lining and these are accompanied by accumulation of fluid, blood or air within the pleural cavity itself.

Traumatic disorders of the pleura

The traumatic disorders are pneumothorax (air in the pleural cavity), haemothorax (blood in the pleural cavity) and haemopneumothorax. The cause is most commonly fracture of the ribs. The fragments may lacerate the intercostal vessels as well as the subjacent lung. Rarely, open chest wounds can result in air entering the pleural cavity

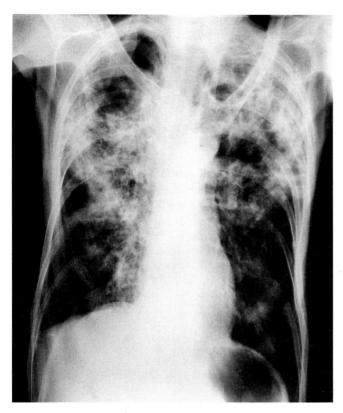

Figure 19.10 Extensive bilateral cavitating tuberculosis. This patient died in spite of aggressive and appropriate antituberculous chemotherapy.

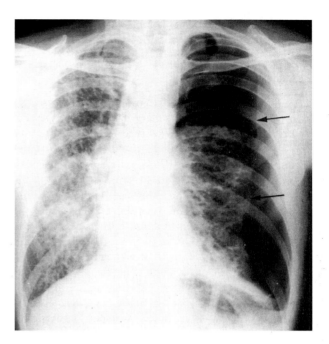

Figure 19.11 Left-sided pneumothorax in a patient with extensive bilateral pulmonary fibrosis following a percutaneous drill biopsy.

through the wound itself. This is referred to as sucking pneumothorax. Pneumothorax is also encountered in patients with rupture of the bronchi (Chapter 9).

Pathophysiology of pneumothorax

When the pressure inside a pneumothorax is static, the condition is called a *simple pneumothorax* and, although this condition requires treatment, it is not usually serious (Fig. 19.11). By contrast, *a tension pneumothorax* is always life-threatening. In these patients, the pulmonary laceration acts as a one-way valve, admitting inspired air into the pleural cavity with each inspiration, but closing during expiration. The consequence is a progressive build-up of air with rising pleural pressure on the affected side. The result is total lung collapse, and a shift of the mediastinum including the heart and great vessels to the contralateral side. Thus, in addition to the respiratory distress and hypoxaemia, the patient may develop cardiovascular collapse (Fig. 19.12).

The symptoms of pneumothorax are anxiety, breathlessness and cyanosis. The trachea may be deviated. Percussion of the chest wall reveals hyperresonance and on ausculta-

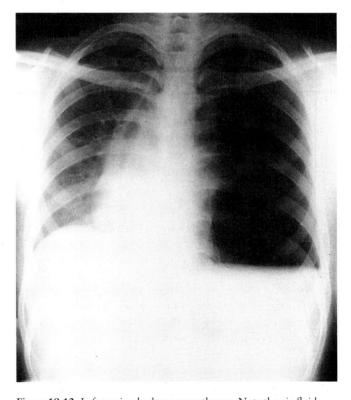

Figure 19.12 Left tension hydropneumothorax. Note the air-fluid level and the absence of lung markings on that side. The heart and trachea are shifted to the right. This patient requires urgent treatment to release the pneumothorax.

tion, air entry is diminished or absent. The diagnosis is confirmed by a portable chest radiograph.

Treatment

The treatment of a patient with tension pneumothorax must be immediate. If the patient is very distressed, a large-bore hypodermic needle is inserted into the second or third interspace anteriorly to decompress the pleural cavity until the equipment for underwater seal drainage becomes available.

The principle of underwater seal drainage is that a liquid trap is interposed between the tubing exiting from the pleural cavity and the atmosphere. If the pressure in the pleural cavity is greater than atmospheric pressure, air, fluid or blood will drain out through the water-immersed tube (A in Fig. 19.13). On the other hand, when the pleural pressure becomes negative, atmospheric air is prevented from being sucked into the pleural space by the water level (B in Fig. 19.13). The underwater seal bottle or disposable equivalent

(such as the Pleurivac) must always be kept at a lower level than the chest and during changes or emptying of the bottle, the exit tubing from the chest cavity must be clamped.

For treatment of a pneumothorax, the chest drain is inserted into the apex of the pleural cavity, either anteriorly through the second intercostal space in the mid clavicular line or, preferably, through the fourth interspace in the mid axillary line. A basal drain is necessary for drainage of blood or fluid. This is inserted posterolaterally through the fifth interspace. Patients with haemopneumothorax require both apical and basal chest drains.

The chest drain is maintained until there is full lung expansion and any blood or fluid has drained away. A persistent air leak is easily recognized by bubbling through the water of the underwater seal drain. Lung expansion is signified by cessation of movement of the fluid column but this must be confirmed by a chest radiograph. The tube is then clamped for several hours and if a repeat radiograph shows that the lung remains expanded, the drain is removed and the chest wound sutured and dressed.

Spontaneous pneumothorax

The causes of pneumothorax are listed in Table 19.8.

Table 19.8 Causes of pneumothorax.

Spontaneous rupture of a congenital pleural bleb
Rupture of an emphysematous bulla
Trauma
    Penetrating injury
    Fractured ribs
    Iatrogenic (e.g. following central line insertion or after lung biopsy)
Rupture of intrapulmonary cavity (e.g. staphylococcal pneumonia)
Positive-pressure ventilation
Resuscitation and ventilation of the newborn
Asthma
Cystic fibrosis
Rare connective tissue disorders (Marfan's syndrome, Ehlers–Danlos syndrome)

Spontaneous pneumothorax arises in the absence of trauma. There are two groups of patients who are most at risk. The first consists of fit young adults (often tall, thin young men) in whom apical blebs, often bilateral, rupture and cause pneumothorax. In this group pneumothorax is often recurrent unless specific surgical treatment is undertaken. These blebs were thought to result from childhood TB in the past but they are now considered to be due to congenital defects in the alveolar wall. The other group of patients who commonly develop spontaneous pneumothorax

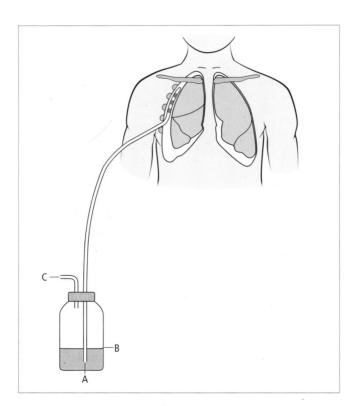

Figure 19.13 Principle of underwater seal drainage. A is the drainage point situated under water, B is the water level which separates the pleural pressure from the atmosphere, C is the exit tube which is exposed to atmospheric pressure and to which low pressure suction may be applied.

are those suffering from emphysema with air trapping and bullae formation. Due to impaired pulmonary reserve, pneumothorax induces severe respiratory distress in these patients.

Other causes of pneumothorax include hyperinflation of the lung during intermittent positive-pressure ventilation, α_1-antitrypsin deficiency-related pulmonary disease and staphylococcal pneumonia in children. This pneumonia leads to the formation of tense cystic spaces within the area of consolidation. These cystic lesions may rupture and cause a pyopneumothorax.

Initially the management of spontaneous pneumothorax is with intercostal drainage as described above. Lung expansion may be expedited by low negative suction to the outlet of the underwater seal (C, Fig. 19.13). If the lung does not expand or the pneumothorax is recurrent, surgical treatment designed to obliterate the bullae and excise or abrade the parietal pleura is required. Pleurectomy or pleural abrasion is undertaken to encourage the formation of adhesions between the lung surface and the chest wall. This is now performed via the thoracoscopic approach.

Pleural effusions

A pleural effusion signifies the presence of fluid within the pleural cavity. The effusion may consist of:
* transudate — congestive cardiac failure;
* exudate — infections and tumours;
* blood-stained fluid — trauma, tumour, tuberculosis, pulmonary infarction, pancreatitis, trauma;
* turbid fluid — empyema;
* chyle — chylothorax due to rupture of thoracic or right lymphatic duct.

Clinically a pleural effusion is detected by stony dullness on percussion and diminished breath sounds on auscultation. Radiologically, effusions appear as basal areas of uniform shadowing without distinct (Fig. 19.14) margins unless the effusion is loculated. An air–fluid level signifies either a leak from the lung or exogenous air introduced during chest aspiration (Fig. 19.15).

The management of pleural effusion consists of treating the underlying cause and relieving symptoms caused by the effusion. A sample of the fluid, obtained by aspiration, is submitted for culture, biochemical analysis and cytological examination. If the pleural effusion is massive and symptomatic, evacuation by aspiration (thoracocentesis) is performed. Malignant pleural effusions are caused by secondary involvement of the pleural lining or by primary pleural tumours. They often require aspiration. Reaccumulation may be prevented by the intrapleural instillation of a pleural sclerosing agent such as tetracycline, bleomycin or *Corynebacterium parvum*.

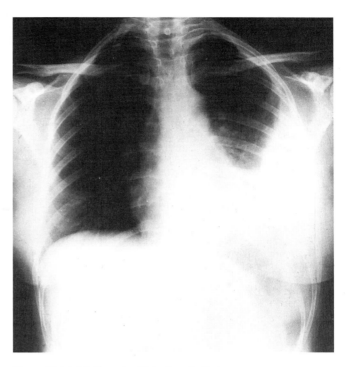

Figure 19.14 Medium sized left pleural effusion.

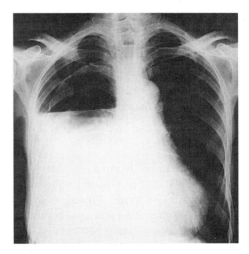

Figure 19.15 Air–fluid level in a patient with haematopneumothorax.

Empyema

Empyema is defined as an infection within the pleural cavity with formation of purulent exudate or frank pus. It is always secondary to spreading infection from the underlying lung or elsewhere. The causes of empyema are shown in Table 19.9. A neglected empyema may burst through the chest wall and discharge externally (empyema necessitatis).

Table 19.9 Causes of empyema.

Pulmonary infections
Pneumonia
Lung abscess
Bronchiectasis
Tuberculosis

Trauma and postoperative
Chest injuries
Oesophgeal perforations
Leaking intrathoracic anastomosis

Subdiaphragmatic infections
Subphrenic abscess
Hepatic abscess

Osteomyelitis
Ribs and vertebrae

Metastatic infection
Septicaemia

Irrespective of cause, pleural inflammation results in the formation of fluid rich in fibrin and polymorphonuclear leukocytes. The fibrin is continually deposited on the pleural surfaces which become progressively thickened. The deeper layers of this pyogenic membrane become fibrotic and contract down, trapping the lung parenchyma and preventing expansion of the alveoli. Untreated, the process continues until the empyema becomes chronic and the underlying lung totally collapsed. The transition from acute to chronic empyema takes 6–12 weeks from the onset of the disease. A chronic empyema may become calcified.

Clinical features

The usual clinical picture is that of a patient who develops a chest infection which fails to respond to treatment or relapses soon after. The situation following oesophageal perforation or leaking intrathoracic anastomosis is more dramatic and the patient rapidly becomes acutely ill. The symptoms of empyema include toxicity with fever, malaise and dyspnoea. The physical findings are similar to those of a pleural effusion except in patients with perforated/leaking oesophagus who exhibit a pyopneumothorax. This may also be encountered in victims of staphylococcal pneumonia. Radiologically, an empyema resembles a pleural effusion and, if large, the entire hemithorax may become opaque. A marked leukocytosis is invariably present.

Treatment

An acute empyema is treated by the appropriate antibiotics, repeated chest aspirations and vigorous physiotherapy. If the fluid is or becomes too thick for aspiration, an intercostal underwater seal drain is inserted. Failure of such treatment or the presence of chronic empyema are indications for surgical treatment, i.e. decortication. Decortication is an operation whereby the chest cavity is opened via a thoracotomy and the thickened inflamed pleura is stripped off the surface of the lung, thus allowing the lung to expand. Antibiotics are continued until the infection has been eradicated. During surgery, any underlying lung pathology is also dealt with. This often involves resection of the affected lung parenchyma.

Chylothorax

Chylothorax signifies the presence of lymph fluid in the pleural space. The condition is readily diagnosed by chest aspiration when the nature of the opalescent milky fluid becomes apparent. Chylothorax most commonly arises from trauma to the thoracic duct or right lymphatic duct during thoracic operations such as oesophagectomy. Other causes include malignant obstruction of the thoracic duct by metastatic lymph nodes.

Although conservative measures such as repeated chest aspiration with the instillation of intrapleural sclerosants may be employed, these are often ineffective and open or thoracoscopic surgical ligation of the affected duct is usually necessary.

Tumours of the pleura

The primary tumour which affects the pleural membrane arises from mesothelial tissue and is therefore known as a mesothelioma. Histologically the tumour consists of a mixture of epithelial and connective tissue components in varying proportions. The important aetiological factor is exposure to asbestos, usually 20–40 years prior to the development of the tumour. There are two macroscopic types of mesothelioma: localized and diffuse lesions. Malignant diffuse mesothelioma is a prescribed industrial disease and should be reported to the appropriate authorities for compensation.

Localized lesions

These are well-encapsulated tumours and may affect the visceral or parietal pleura. They usually form thickened plaques but occasionally may be nodular or even pedunculated. They are often of low-grade malignancy and some are benign.

Diffuse malignant mesothelioma

This tumour carries a poor prognosis. It forms a thick spreading sheet of tumour tissue which infiltrates the underlying lung, chest wall, mediastinum, opposite pleura and even the peritoneum by direct extension. A blood-stained pleural effusion may be present initially but in time, the entire pleural space becomes completely obliterated by tumour. Spread to the regional mediastinal lymph nodes is present in the majority of patients at the time of diagnosis.

Treatment

Localized disease is readily amenable to surgical excision with good results in terms of long-term survival. The diffuse mesothelioma may be operable when a radical pleuropneumonectomy is performed. Often, however, the disease is inoperable. There is little that can be done aside from analgesia and terminal care in these patients as the tumour does not respond to radiotherapy or chemotherapy.

Bronchial neoplasms

The commonest pulmonary tumours are secondary deposits but primary bronchial neoplasms are frequent with an incidence of 40–110 per 100 000 of the population above the age of 45 years. Primary pulmonary lymphomas are rare, although secondary involvement from Hodgkin's and non-Hodgkin's disease is common. Benign lung tumours (e.g. hamartoma, chondroma, angioma) are uncommon and produce symptoms by local effects. Bronchial adenomas are also uncommon and cause bronchial obstruction and distal collapse. They present with cough and haemoptysis. Histologically the majority are bronchial carcinoids but carcinoid syndrome is rare and suggests the presence of metastases. These tumours are slow-growing and locally invasive, but 10% show malignant features. Treatment is by surgical excision.

Secondary pulmonary deposits

The extensive capillary bed of the pulmonary parenchyma is the main reason for the common occurrence of pulmonary metastases from a variety of malignant neoplasms. Although virtually any malignant tumour may metastasize to the lungs, some tumours have a special predilection for this spread. These include cancer of breast, hypernephroma, melanoma, neuroblastoma and osteogenic sarcoma. The pulmonary deposits are usually multiple and bilateral (Fig. 19.16). Less frequently, a solitary metastasis is encountered and this may be amenable to surgical resec-

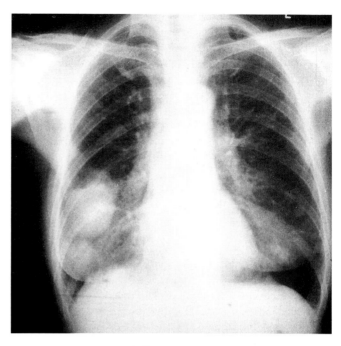

Figure 19.16 Two cannonball metastases in the right lower lobe.

Table 19.10 Histological types of bronchial carcinomas.

Squamous cell carcinoma
Small cell carcinoma
Adenocarcinoma
Large cell carcinoma
Adenosquamous carcinoma
Carcinoid tumour
Bronchial gland carcinoma

tion. When the secondary nodules involve the pleura, malignant pleural effusion occurs. Pulmonary deposits indicate advanced incurable disease, although modern chemotherapy may result in significant regression in some patients.

Primary bronchial neoplasm

Bronchial carcinoma remains one of the major killer diseases and 80% of victims die within 1 year of diagnosis. The mean age at presentation is in the seventh decade and men are affected 4 to 5 times more commonly than women. The important aetiological factor is cigarette smoking which increases the risk of death from bronchial carcinoma by a factor of 10. Other aetiological factors include atmospheric pollution and industrial exposure to uranium, chromium, arsenic, hematite and asbestos. The various histological types of bronchial tumours are shown in Table 19.10.

Squamous cell lesions are the commonest and account for 60% of all bronchial carcinomas. They occur centrally in the main bronchi and have a tendency to undergo central necrosis. Small cell carcinomas include the oat cell tumours and other cell types. These lesions are responsive to chemotherapy. Adenocarcinomas tend to be peripheral tumours and may arise in relation to scars. They carry the best prognosis after resection. The commonest sites for metastases from bronchial carcinomas are the brain, bone, liver and contralateral lung.

Clinical features

The early symptoms are non-specific and include tiredness, cough, anorexia and weight loss. The cough may be productive and the sputum is often purulent due to secondary infection. Haemoptysis is usually minor but persistent. Often the presentation is with an acute chest illness — bronchopneumonia due to infection within the collapsed lung parenchyma following bronchial occlusion by the tumour. Pleuritic pain may be secondary to the infection or result from invasion of the chest wall. Other manifestations include neuropathy and myopathy, hypertrophic osteoarthropathy and endocrine syndromes. The latter are usually caused by

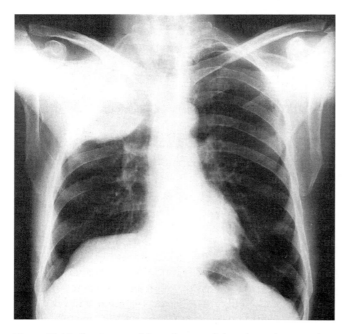

Figure 19.17 Carcinoma of the right upper lobe. This is the type of lesion that produces the Pancoast syndrome (lower brachial plexus lesion, Horner's syndrome, rib erosion and an apical lung shadow).

oat cell tumours which may secrete adrenocorticotrophic hormone (ACTH) causing adrenal cortical hyperplasia, parathormone (hypercalcaemia) and ADH.

Other symptoms and signs are produced by direct invasion and these signify inoperability. Invasion of the cervical sympathetic chain causes Horner's syndrome. Hoarseness is due to involvement of the left recurrent laryngeal nerve and breathlessness may be caused by paralysis of the diaphragm following invasion of the phrenic nerve. The Pancoast syndrome is particularly distressing. It results from an apical tumour which invades the sympathetic trunk and brachial plexus causing a Horner's syndrome, severe brachial neuralgia and paralysis of the upper limb (Fig. 19.17). Dysphagia signifies invasion of the oesophagus and this may progress to a malignant broncho-oesophageal fistula. Finally, mediastinal involvement, particularly of the lymph nodes, results in superior vena caval obstruction. In the physical examination of patients with bronchial carcinoma, the neck must be examined for supraclavicular lymph node enlargement and the abdomen for hepatomegaly.

Investigations

The essential investigations for establishing the diagnosis of bronchial carcinoma are chest radiograph, sputum cytology and bronchoscopy with biopsy. Other tests, such as CT scanning of the thorax and abdomen, liver ultrasound examination, etc., are used to stage the disease and detect inoperability (Fig. 19.18). Lung function tests are performed to establish whether the patient has enough pulmonary reserve to tolerate the lung resection.

Treatment

The best results follow excision via a thoracotomy. The extent of the resection depends on the size and location of the tumour. It may involve a lobe (lobectomy) or a whole lung (pneumonectomy). Adjuvant (additional) treatment with chemotherapy (especially for small (oat) cell tumours) and radiotherapy is used in some centres.

Surgery is contraindicated for advanced inoperable disease and in patients with poor respiratory function. These patients are treated by supervoltage radiotherapy and combination chemotherapy. Small cell carcinomas are the most radiosensitive, whereas adenocarcinomas respond poorly to this treatment. The best results with combination chemotherapy (vincristine, methotrexate and cyclophosphamide) are obtained in patients with small cell carcinomas.

Palliation of symptoms such as breathlessness can be achieved by destroying tumour which is narrowing a major bronchus with laser therapy applied via a bronchoscope. Superior vena caval obstruction may be helped by steroids

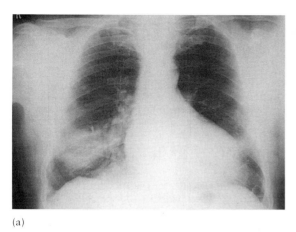
(a)

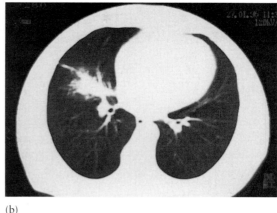
(b)

Figure 19.18 (a) Chest radiograph showing a large bronchial neoplasm in the right lower lobe. (b) A CT scan of the same lesion. This was a squamous carcinoma and as there was no evidence of metastatic disease the patient underwent a right lower lobe lobectomy.

and more recently it has been relieved by endovascular stenting. Pain control and relief of distressing symptoms such as cough and shortness of breath are important and hospice care either in a hospice or at home should be provided for all terminally ill patients with cancer.

Prognosis

The prognosis for lung cancer is grim. Most patients will be dead within 12 months of diagnosis. Following 'curative' resection, 5-year survival rates are approximately 20–30% but overall 5-year survival is only about 6%. Chemotherapy may produce a response in 60–80% of patients with small cell carcinoma but survival is not greatly improved, although 10% remain disease-free at 2 years.

Lymphomas

Secondary involvement of the lung from primary extrapulmonary lymphomas (Hodgkin's and non-Hodgkin's) is commoner than primary disease. Primary pulmonary Hodgkin's disease arises in peribronchial lymph nodes, usually in young patients. The symptoms include pyrexia, cough, asthenia, haemoptysis and itching. The lesion appears as a well-circumscribed shadow. If the diagnosis is established, treatment is by radiotherapy and chemotherapy. When the diagnosis remains in doubt, thoracotomy and excision of the lobe containing the lesion are performed (Fig. 19.19).

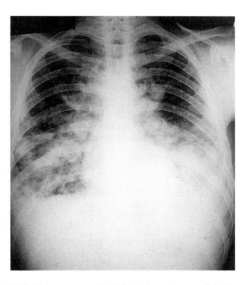

Figure 19.19 Primary non-Hodgkin's lymphoma of the lung.

Mediastinal lesions

The mediastinum, the intrathoracic space between the two lungs, is anatomically divided into four regions (Fig. 19.20). The mediastinum contains the heart and great vessels, the oesophagus, trachea and main bronchi, the thymus, the azygous system of veins, the thoracic and right lymphatic ducts, lymph nodes and nerves — recurrent laryngeal, vagal, phrenic and autonomic.

The disorders of the mediastinum are classified as:
- infection — mediastinitis;
- syndromes arising from ectopic endocrine tissue;

Bronchial carcinoma at a glance

DEFINITION

Malignant lesion of the lung

EPIDEMIOLOGY

M/F = 5 : 1 Uncommon before age 50. Most patients are in their 60s. Accounts for 40 000 deaths per annum in the UK

AETIOLOGY

Predisposing factors are:
- Cigarette smoking
- Air pollution
- Exposure to uranium, chromium, arsenic, hematite and asbestos

PATHOLOGY

- Histology:
  - (a) Squamous carcinoma   50%
  - (b) Small cell (oat cell) carcinoma   35%
  - (c) Adenocarcinoma   15%
- Spread:
  - (a) Direct to pleura, recurrent laryngeal nerve, pericardium, oesophagus, brachial plexus
  - (b) Lymphatic to mediastinal and cervical nodes
  - (c) Haematogenous to liver, bone, brain, adrenals
  - (d) Transcoelomic pleural seedlings and effusion

CLINICAL FEATURES

- History of tiredness, cough, anorexia, weight loss
- Productive cough with purulent sputum
- Haemoptysis
- Finger clubbing
- Bronchopneumonia (secondary infection of collapsed lung segment distal to malignant bronchial obstruction)
- Pleuritic pain
- Neuropathy, myopathy, hypertrophic osteoarthropathy
- Endocrine syndromes (ACTH is secreted by oat cell tumours, parathormone secreted by squamous carcinoma — hypercalcaemia)
- Pancoast tumour   { Horner's syndrome
  (apical tumour invading   { Brachial neuralgia
  sympathetic trunk and   { Paralysis of upper limb
  brachial plexus)
- Dysphagia and broncho-oesophageal fistula
- Superior vena caval obstruction

INVESTIGATIONS

Diagnostic
- CXR — PA and lateral (lung opacity, hilar lymphadenopathy)
- Sputum cytology
- Bronchoscopy and cytology

Assess operability
- CT thorax/abdomen
- Bone scan
- Liver ultrasound
- Lung function test
- Mediastinoscopy

MANAGEMENT

Surgery
- Indicated only when tumour is confined to one lobe or lung; there is no evidence of secondary deposits; carina is tumour-free on bronchoscopy
- Operation: lobectomy or pneumonectomy

Palliation
- Radiotherapy (small cell carcinoma most radiosensitive)
  - (a) Stop haemoptysis
  - (b) Relieve bone pain from secondaries
  - (c) Relieve superior vena caval obstruction

PROGNOSIS

- Following 'curative' resection, 5-year survival rates are approximately 20–30% but overall 5-year survival is only about 6%

- tumours; and
- idiopathic mediastinal fibrosis.

Mediastinitis

This is a suppurative inflammation of the mediastinal space and is usually encountered as a complication of oesophageal perforation (Chapter 13). Much less commonly, it is secondary to infection of the mediastinal lymph nodes (from a focus in the lungs) or vertebral osteomyelitis. The condition is always serious. The clinical features include chest pain, rigors, pyrexia and dyspnoea. When secondary to oesophageal perforation, it is accompanied by surgical emphysema in the neck and mediastinal air on the chest X-ray. Treatment is surgical with measures to deal with the underlying perforation, drainage and broad-spectrum antibiotic therapy.

Syndromes from ectopic endocrine tissue

Truly ectopic thyroid tissue deriving its blood supply from the mediastinum is exceedingly rare and is usually a chance radiological finding. Symptomatic mediastinal thyroid tissue is the result of a retrosternal extension of a large multinodular goitre which derives its blood supply from the neck. The rounded mediastinal extension is best visualized by the lateral film.

In some 5% of patients with hyperparathyroidism (Chapter 15), the adenoma causing the disease arises from a genuinely ectopic gland. These patients usually come to

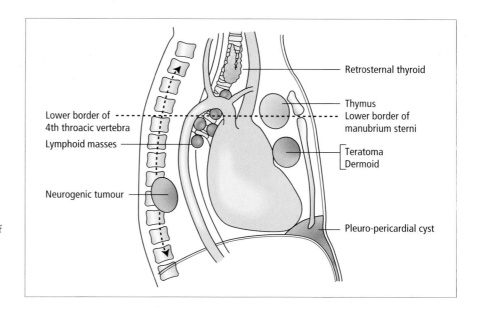

Figure 19.20 Diagrammatic representation of the mediastinum. The mediastinum is divided into four regions for diagnostic purposes: (i) superior; (ii) anterior; (iii) middle; and (iv) posterior. The sites of the commoner mediastinal tumours are also shown.

Table 19.11 Tumours of the mediastinum.

Secondary deposits in mediastinal lymph nodes

Primary lymphomas

Primary tumours of
Oesophagus
Trachea and main bronchi
Heart and great vessels

Specific mediastinal tumours
Thymic cysts and tumours
Teratomas and extragonadal germcell tumours
Neurogenic tumours
Thoracic meningocoele
Pleuropericardial cysts (coelomic, spring-water cysts)
Cystic duplications of the foregut
   Bronchogenic cysts
   Enterogenous cysts

light after neck exploration performed by an expert fails to reveal the tumour.

Tumours of the mediastinum

These are shown in Table 19.11.

It is important to stress that the important common tumours are secondary deposits in the mediastinal lymph nodes (usually from lung, oesophagus, stomach and breast) and primary lymphomas. Thus, mediastinal involvement occurs in 50% of patients with Hodgkin's disease and in 10–20% of patients with non-Hodgkin's lymphoma. Both secondary nodal deposits and mediastinal lymphomas may present with compression of the superior vena cava, oesophagus and trachea, requiring urgent treatment.

Thymomas

These are the most common anteriorly situated specific mediastinal tumours. Their histology is often very difficult to interpret, especially in terms of whether the tumour is benign or malignant. They are composed of a mixture of epithelial and lymphocytic components, often with one of these elements predominating. These tumours have a propensity to recur after excision irrespective of their histological appearance.

Thymomas may be clinically silent (detected on a chest film) or cause non-specific symptoms if large (chest pain, cough, breathlessness) or be accompanied by myasthenia gravis. In myasthenia gravis an antibody is present which blocks the effect of acetylcholine at the motor end-plate. Although the thymus is often abnormal in these patients, thymic tumours are only found in 10–20% of patients. Thymic tumours should be removed whether symptomatic or not. About 75% of patients with myasthenia gravis derive some benefit from thymectomy (irrespective of the presence or absence of thymic tumour) and half obtain a satisfactory remission. Radiotherapy is administered after resection of thymic tumours to reduce the risk of recurrence and in patients with irresectable lesions.

Teratomas

Teratomas are developmental tumours composed of tissue elements from all the germinal layers. They are always situated in the anterior mediastinum and may be cystic or solid.

Although benign, teratomas may undergo malignant change, particularly those that are solid. About one-third of these lesions are calcified at the time of diagnosis, which is usually made by chest X-ray. Some may exhibit recognizable teeth and the cystic variety may communicate with the tracheobronchial tree when a fluid level is visible on the chest film. Symptoms, when they arise, are largely due to compression. The treatment of teratomas is excision through a median sternotomy or posterolateral thoracotomy.

Extragonadal germ-cell tumours

These are similar in nature to the germ cell tumours that affect the testis and, like their testicular counterparts, they secrete tumour surface antigens which are used as tumour markers (Chapter 20). They are always malignant and may be seminomas or teratomas. Treatment is by excision, radiotherapy and chemotherapy.

Neurogenic tumours

Neurogenic tumours occur in the posterior mediastinum and are often associated with rib and vertebral abnormalities.

They are classified in accordance with the neural tissue of origin (Table 19.12). The benign nerve sheath tumours are the neurilemmoma and the neurofibroma with malignant schwannoma and neurogenic sarcoma being respectively their malignant counterparts. Ganglioneuromas are benign tumours arising from the autonomic ganglia and have the propensity to extend to the spinal canal via the intervertebral foramina (dumb-bell tumours). Neuroblastoma is a malignant tumour of ganglionic tissue which occurs in children, usually in the upper posterior mediastinum and is not encapsulated and infiltrative. It secretes catecholamines and a specific tumour antigen (neuron-specific enolase) which are used for establishing the diagnosis preoperatively. The equivalent malignant tumour in adults is the ganglioneuroblastoma. This has a better prognosis and is encapsulated. For this reason it is also known as differentiated neuroblastoma. Phaeochromocytoma occurs very rarely in the mediastinum (Chapter 15).

Table 19.12 Neurogenic mediastinal tumours.

Benign	Malignant
Neurilemmoma	Malignant schwannoma
Neurofibroma	Neurogenic sarcoma
Ganglioneuroma (dumb-bell)	Neuroblastoma
Phaeochromocytoma	Ganglioneuroblastoma
	Phaeochromocytoma

All neural tumours should be removed surgically. Children suffering from neuroblastomas receive preoperative radiotherapy. In addition, following excision pulsed chemotherapy using cis-platinum-based regimens is administered.

Idiopathic mediastinal fibrosis

This is a condition of unknown aetiology (currently thought to be immunological) and is related to retroperitoneal fibrosis and Riedel's thyroiditis. It is characterized by dense fibrous infiltration of the mediastinum (especially the superior), eventually leading to obstruction of the trachea, vena cava, oesophagus and pulmonary vessels.

Ventilatory failure

Ventilatory failure is defined as the inability of the respiratory system to oxygenate the blood and remove carbon dioxide. This section should be read in conjunction with Chapters 3, 6 and 7. Clinically, ventilatory failure may assume several forms (Table 19.13).

Table 19.13 Types of ventilatory failure.

Acute pulmonary: hypoxaemia with elevated $P(A-a)o_2$*
Acute extrapulmonary: hypoxaemia with normal $P(A-a)o_2$
Chronic: compensated hypoxaemia and hypercarbia
Acute decompensation of chronic ventilatory failure

* Difference between alveolar (PAo_2) and arterial (Pao_2) oxygen tension.

Thus ventilatory failure may be acute, where the dominant feature is severe life-threatening hypoxaemia (<6.5 kPa; 50 mmHg; see Chapter 3) or chronic, where the hypoxaemia is accompanied by carbon dioxide retention but survival in a state of chronic respiratory insufficiency is possible because of certain body compensatory mechanisms. However, these patients may decompensate suddenly into acute insufficiency. Acute ventilatory failure is further classified into pulmonary and extrapulmonary.

Chronic respiratory failure

This occurs in chronic heavy smokers and in patients with chronic airway obstruction (emphysema and chronic bronchitis). These patients have chronic pulmonary insufficiency (chronic hypoxia and hypercarbia) but often can compensate for this, although their exercise tolerance is limited to varying degrees and their life expectancy is reduced. They require long-term specific medication, including supportive oxygen therapy, although the latter has to be administered with care because these patients' respiration is predominantly stimulated by the hypoxic drive rather than the $Pa\text{CO}_2$. They may decompensate rapidly and develop life-threatening ventilatory failure with $Pa\text{O}_2$ below 7.2 kPa (55 mmHg) and $Pa\text{CO}_2$ greater than 7.2 kPa (55 mmHg) as a result of superadded acute chest disorders or surgical intervention. The common conditions which precipitate this acute decompensation are shown in Table 19.14. Thus, acute-on-chronic ventilatory failure requires support with endotracheal intubation and mechanical ventilation, although recovery may not occur and the mortality is high.

Table 19.14 Conditions which precipitate decompensation in patients with chronic pulmonary insufficiency.

Acute bronchitis (viral or bacterial)
Acute lobar pneumonia (viral or bacterial)
Left ventricular failure
Spontaneous pneumothorax
Pleural effusion
General anaesthesia and surgery
Pulmonary embolism

Acute pulmonary failure

Acute pulmonary failure is caused either by the adult respiratory distress syndrome (ARDS) or severe lobar pneumonia. ARDS is essentially a rapidly progressing pulmonary oedema due to increased permeability of the alveolar capillary membrane (high-permeability pulmonary oedema or alveolar capillary leak syndrome) as distinct from the pulmonary oedema associated with heart disease which is caused by alterations in the hydrostatic or osmotic pressure gradients across the membrane (normal-permeability pulmonary oedema or cardiogenic). ARDS is a serious and increasingly common emergency in both surgical and medical practice. The syndrome is of multiple aetiology (Table 19.15).

The pathogenesis of ARDS is being unravelled. It is thought that activation of the complement system (e.g. by endotoxin or followng ischaemia/reperfusion) produces activation of neutrophils which are sequestered in the lungs. These then release reactive oxygen species (superoxide (O_2^-), the hydroxyl radical (OH^-) and hydrogen peroxide H_2O_2), proteolytic enzymes (elastase) and eicosanoids (thromboxane, leukotrienes and prostaglandins). These cause extensive damage to the endothelium of the lung cap-

Table 19.15 Causes of adult respiratory distress syndrome (ARDS).

Common causes
Shock (of any type)
Pulmonary infections
Severe sepsis
Severe pancreatitis
Severe trauma
Drug overdose
Aspiration (gastric juice, drowning; Fig. 19.21)

Other causes
Massive blood transfusions
Cardiopulmonary bypass
Fat and air embolism
Smoke inhalation
Poisoning: paraquat and inhaled toxins
Oxygen toxicity
Neurogenic

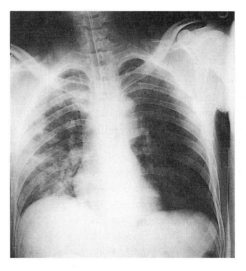

Figure 19.21 Areas of consolidation in the right lung are due to inhaled vomitus. The regurgitation of gastric contents and aspiration during general anaesthesia resulting in bronchospasm, atelectasis, oedema and hypoxia is called Mendelson's syndrome.

illaries, resulting in increased permeability of the capillary–alveolar membrane and gross pulmonary oedema (see Chapter 7).

In contrast to cardiogenic oedema, ARDS is usually sudden in onset. The physical signs in the chest are minimal, despite obvious respiratory distress (tachypnoea and laboured breathing) and refractory hypoxaemia. Initially the chest radiograph may be normal or show an interstitial infiltrate but as the condition progresses, diffuse alveolar

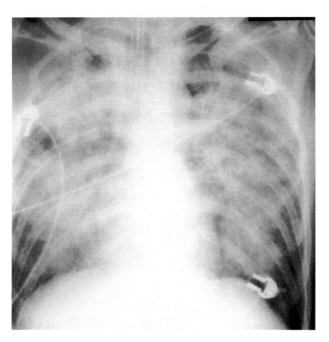

Figure 19.22 Non-cardiogenic pulmonary oedema in a patient with ARDS.

infiltrates ('white-out', Fig. 19.22) become evident. The cardiac shadow is normal in shape and size, and pleural effusion is absent. The cardiac output in ARDS is normal at the onset but often falls during the course of the disease. The blood gas analysis shows a severe hypoxaemia (PaO_2 <6.5 kPa; 50 mmHg) with a low $PaCO_2$ and low pH (mixed respiratory alkalosis and metabolic acidosis).

Patients with ARDS require treatment in the intensive care unit with detailed continuous haemodynamic (blood pressure, central venous pressure, pulmonary arterial pressure, wedge pressure and measurement of cardiac output via a Swan–Ganz catheter), ECG and blood gas monitoring. Adequate oxygenation can only be maintained by mechanical ventilation after the insertion of an endotracheal tube. Careful intravenous fluid management with crystalloid solutions is essential to maintain adequate circulation without overload. Often diuretics are needed to prevent the latter complication. When the cardiac output is reduced, inotropic agents (e.g. dopamine) are administered. Antacids or H_2-blockers are given by some as a prophylaxis against stress-induced erosive gastritis. The lung recovery is to a large extent dependent on correction of the underlying condition. This applies especially to the treatment of intra-abdominal sepsis. Antibiotics are used for suspected or established infection.

Extrapulmonary ventilatory failure (EPVF)

In this type of ventilatory failure, the lungs are normal, the acute respiratory insufficiency being the result of extrapulmonary disorders. The distinguishing feature of this type of ventilatory failure is hypoxaemia in the presence of a normal gradient between alveolar and arterial oxygen tension (normal $P(A - a)O_2$). The causes of EPVF fall into three main categories:
• decreased ventilatory drive (depression of the respiratory centre by drugs, head injury or central nervous system disease);
• neural or muscular dysfunction (poliomyelitis, myasthenia gravis, muscular dystrophies, flail chest, tetanus, etc.);
• increased impedance: stiffening or compression of the lungs within the thoracic cavity.

The increased impedance group is important in surgical practice because of its common occurrence. The conditions associated with EPVF due to increased impedance are shown in Table 19.16.

Table 19.16 Causes of extrapulmonary ventilatory failure due to increased impedance.

Morbid obesity
Chest trauma with massive haemo-/pneumothorax, or tension
    pneumothorax
Ruptured diaphragm with extensive herniation of abdominal contents
Massive pleural effusion from any cause
Massive ascites
Pregnancy with hydramnios
Ankylosing spondylitis
Kyphoscoliosis

Patients with EPVF may present with agitation, confusion, stupor or coma. The essential emergency investigations in all these patients are a full blood gas analysis and portable chest X-ray. If the patient is comatose, naloxone is administered intravenously. When this is followed by recovery of consciousness and improvement of the respiratory pattern and rate, supportive management including oxygen therapy is maintained. Lack of response to naloxone or a respiratory rate of less than 10 breaths/min or a blood pH lower than 7.2 (severe acidosis) are indications for assisted mechanical ventilation via an endotracheal tube.

'When I makes tea I makes tea, as old mother Grogan said. And when I makes water I makes water so I do, Mrs Cahill', says she. 'Begob, ma'am', says Mrs Cahill, 'God send you don't make them in the one pot'.   (James Joyce, *Ulysses*)

Introduction

Disorders of the genitourinary system are very common and encompass a huge spectrum of pathology, including con-genital anomalies, infections, stone disease, benign and ma-lignant tumours and disorders of sexual function. The consequences of disorders of the kidney and urinary tract range from local discomfort (e.g. a quiescent renal cal-culus) to life-threatening situations (e.g. septicaemia). The management of patients with genitourinary problems also ranges from very simple treatments to extremely complicated and sophisticated management strategies and these treatments are undertaken by a wide range of physicians including general practitioners, paediatricians and paediatric surgeons, radiologists, general surgeons, gynaecologists, nephrologists and urologists.

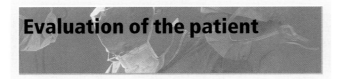

Evaluation of the patient

Clinical assessment

Symptoms

A number of general points need to be considered in a patient presenting with a genitourinary problem:
- In women the obstetric history, with special reference to difficult deliveries, is crucial, previous gynaecological procedures are also relevant.
- The occupational history of the patient is especially relevant in patients suspected of having urothelial cancer. Employment in the dye, rubber, cable or sewage industries exposes the patient to industrial carcinogens. There is a long latent period (15–20 years) between exposure and development of cancer.
- Similarly, a smoking history is germane as certain byproducts of cigarette smoke have been implicated in the pathogenesis of urothelial tumours.
- Allergies and drug history are also relevant as a large number of drugs affect the urinary tract.

The important symptoms of genitourinary disease are outlined in Table 20.1.
- *Micturition* It is important to assess how often the patient passes urine by day and by night (frequency and nocturia). Daytime frequency should be quantified by the period of time, in minutes or hours, between each episode of micturition. Nocturia is quantified by the number of times during a night's sleep that the patient wakes to pass urine. In addition, the nature of the voiding pattern should be ascertained by asking the following questions. Does the patient experience a delay in starting to pass urine (hesitancy)? Is the force or calibre of the stream diminished? Does urine dribble out when micturition is finished (postmicturition dribble)? Is there a burning discomfort (dysuria) on voiding? Is there gas (pneumaturia) or faecal material (faecaluria) in the urine?

Table 20.1 Symptoms of genitourinary disease.

Disordered micturition
Frequency
Nocturia
Hesitancy
Force and calibre of the stream
Postmicturition dribble
Dysuria
Pneumaturia
Faecaluria

Incontinence
Continuous or intermittent
Stress or urge or both
Enuresis

Haematuria
Painful or painless
Gross or microscopic
Timing of haematuria with micturition
Haemospermia

Pain
Site, radiation and periodicity
Acute or chronic
Relieving, aggravating or precipitating factors

Non-specific symptoms
Headache and visual disturbance
Sweating and rigors
Oedema, dyspnoea, orthopnoea
Malaise, nausea, vomiting
Weight loss

- *Incontinence* If the patient complains of involuntary loss of urine, is this continuous or intermittent? Is it associated with coughing, sneezing, laughing or lifting (stress incontinence) or does it occur because of urgency with involuntary voiding before the patient reaches the toilet (urge incontinence)? Is there associated nocturnal incontinence (enuresis)? The degree of wetting can be quantified as a few drops, damp or soaked.
- *Haematuria* Blood in the urine is an ominous symptom. Is the haematuria associated with pain or is it painless? Is the haematuria obvious to the patient (gross haematuria) or has it been detected by urinanalysis? Is the blood mixed throughout the stream or does it occur at the beginning or the end? Is the blood in the urine or is it in the semen (haemospermia)?
- *Pain* It is important to establish the site, radiation and periodicity of the pain. Is it acute or chronic? Is it constant or intermittent? Are there associated symptoms? Are there relieving, aggravating or precipitating factors?
- *Non-specific symptoms* A number of general symptoms may be associated with urological disease and a careful

Table 20.2 Physical examination of the genitourinary system.

General
Anaemia, jaundice, cachexia
Pulse, blood pressure

Abdomen
Renal mass
Loin
Palpable bimanually
Ballottable
Distended bladder
Mass arising from pelvis
Dull to percussion

External genitalia
Prepuce
Urethral meatus
Scrotum (see Fig. 20.1)

Rectal
Anal tone
Prostate
    Size
    Contour
    Consistency

Perineum
Sensation

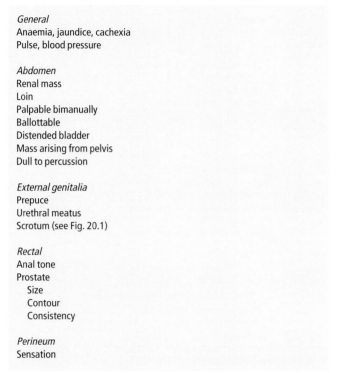

Figure 20.1 Algorithm for the assessment of a scrotal mass.

systems review is an important part of a urological history. Non-specific symptoms include: headaches and visual disturbances (hypertension), sweating and rigors (infection), peripheral oedema and dyspnoea or orthopnoea (renal disease), general malaise (infection or renal disease), nausea, vomiting and weight loss (malignancy).

Physical examination

The major signs of genitourinary disease to be sought for by physical examination are given in Table 20.2.

Examination commences with a general inspection of the patient for anaemia, jaundice and cachexia. Estimation of pulse rate and blood pressure and a brief assessment of the cardiovascular and respiratory system are then undertaken. The abdomen should be inspected for previous surgical incisions and masses. The abdomen is gently palpated for tenderness and intra-abdominal masses. A renal mass arises from the loin and is palpable bimanually and ballottable. An enlarged bladder may be palpable as a mass arising from the pelvis and can be confirmed by percussion which will reveal suprapubic dullness. The inguinal and femoral areas should be inspected for hernia.

Examination of the external genitalia in the male commences with retraction of the prepuce and inspection of

the external urinary meatus. The scrotum is inspected for masses. It is important to determine if the mass arises in the scrotum or is coming from above. If it is scrotal in origin, one can get above it. Next it is important to decide if the mass arises from the testis (solid swelling) or if it is a hydrocele or epididymal cyst (cystic swelling). Transillumination in a darkened room will help differentiate between the two. Finally, the scrotum should be examined with the patient in the standing position for a varicocele. In the female patient, a vaginal examination for prolapse is essential.

Rectal examination is a crucial part of the urological examination. The anal tone is assessed. The prostate is assessed for size, contour and consistency. Assessment of prostate size comes with experience. Does the finger feel a bi-lobed gland with a median sulcus? Does the prostate feel firm or hard in consistency? A hard gland with loss of the median sulcus is likely to be malignant. Equally, malignancy may be felt as a discrete area of hardness (a nodule) in an otherwise firm benign gland. Finally, perineal sensation should be tested and also the leg reflexes as an assessment of bladder innervation.

Table 20.3 Investigations for assessment of the urinary tract.

Type of investigation		Comment
Urinalysis		
Dipstix	pH, glucose, protein, blood, bilirubin, ketones, nitrates	Useful screening test for diabetes and renal and hepatic disease
Microscopy and Gram stain	RBCs, WBCs, casts, crystals, bacteria	May indicate infection or renal disease
Urine culture	Number and type of bacteria	Diagnosis of urinary tract infection
Blood analysis		
	Hb, WBCs, platelets	May detect anaemia or polycythaemia
	Urea, creatinine, electrolytes	Raised in patients with renal failure
	Ca²+, phosphates, uric acid, albumin	Used for screening for metabolic disorders in patients with renal caluli
	Serum acid phosphatase, prostate-specific antigen (PSA)	Tumour markers for prostatic cancer
	α-Fetoprotein (AFP)	Tumour markers for testicular cancer
	Human chorionic gonadotrophin (HCG)	
Imaging		
Structure	Abdominal radiograph (KUB) (Fig. 20.2)	Detect bony metastases, Paget's disease, soft-tissue masses, abnormal calcification
	Intravenous urogram	Delineates the entire urinary tract
	Ultrasonography	Assessment of renal and scrotal masses and bladder emptying
	Transrectal ultrasound (TRUS)	Useful in assessing prostatic disease
	Contrast-enhanced CT scan	Preoperative staging of renal carcinoma
Function	Radioisotope renography DPTA, DMSA	Assess function of each kidney independently
Urodynamics		
	Urine flow rates	Useful in assessing degree of obstruction to micturition, e.g. benign prostatic hyperplasia
	Cystometry (static and ambulant)	Differentiates between urge and stress incontinence
Endoscopy		
	Cystoscopy	Assessment of urinary tract for neoplastic or stone
	Ureteroscopy	disease
	Ureterorenoscopy	

RBCs, Red blood cells; WBCs, white blood cells; Hb, haemoglobin; KUB, kidney, ureter, bladder; CT, computed tomography; DTPA, diethylenetriaminepentaacetic acid; DMSA, dimercaptosuccinic acid.

Investigations

The investigations commonly used in the assessment of a patient with genitourinary problems are given in Table 20.3.

Urinalysis

The most appropriate urine specimen for laboratory analysis is a freshly voided midstream specimen of urine. This urine sample can be tested using dipstix, which are strips coated with chemicals that indicate urine pH, the presence of glucose, protein, blood, bilirubin, ketones and nitrates (see Chapter 2). If the dipstix test is positive, full urinalysis is necessary. However, for patients presenting with urinary symptoms, it is better to proceed to a formal analysis of the urine specimen in the hospital laboratory by microscopy, culture and sensitivity testing.

Microscopy is performed on the urinary sediment after centrifugation. Specifically, the urine is examined for red blood cells, white cells, casts, crystals and bacteria. The

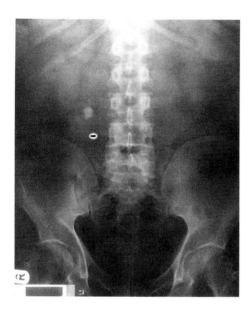

Figure 20.2 KUB (kidney, ureter, bladder) film showing stone in right ureter.

presence of more than three red blood cells per high-powered field examined is a significant finding that warrants further investigation. The presence of more than five white blood cells per high-powered field (pyuria) is also a significant finding. Bacteria may also be noted on examination and should be examined by Gram stain to aid identification. In addition, the urine should be cultured. If pyuria exists without bacteria (sterile pyuria), tuberculosis should be considered and the urine should be stained by the Ziehl–Neelsen technique. If sterile pyuria is noted urine should be obtained for culture of *M. Tuberculosis*. Three early-morning urine samples are examined. The presence of casts in the urine, which are formed in the distal tubules and collecting ducts, may indicate renal disease.

The presence of bacteria in the urine may indicate urinary tract infection (UTI) but may result from an improperly collected urine sample. To confirm a diagnosis of infection, urine culture is necessary. A significant infection exists if the culture reveals more than 100 000 organisms per millilitre.

Blood investigation

A full blood count may show anaemia, polycythaemia, a raised white cell count, abnormal erythrocyte sedimentation rate (ESR) and platelet abnormalities. Renal function is assessed by measurement of serum urea, creatinine and electrolytes. In patients with stone disease, serum calcium, phosphates, uric acid and albumin should also be estimated. In patients with suspected prostate cancer, serum acid phosphatase and prostate-specific antigen are measured as tumour markers. In patients suspected of having testicular neoplasia, α-fetoprotein and β human chorionic gonadotrophin are measured as tumour markers.

Imaging

The basic urological radiological investigation is the plain film of abdomen, frequently referred to as a KUB — kidneys, ureter and bladder. Examination of this radiograph consists of evaluation of the bony skeleton for areas of increased density (osteoblastic prostatic metastases; Paget's disease); soft-tissue masses and abnormal calcification (stones, phleboliths, calcified mesenteric nodes, gallstones).

An intravenous urogram (IVU) is performed by injecting intravenously an iodine-containing contrast medium that is excreted by the kidneys. Serial radiographs are taken to show passage of the contrast through the glomeruli and tubules (nephrogram); passage through the collecting system which outlines the calyces, renal pelvis and ureters. Films are taken before and after bladder emptying. In patients with iodine allergies a renal ultrasound may be performed instead. In patients with a suspected kidney lesion renal ultrasound is particularly helpful and will distinguish between solid and cystic lesions (Fig. 20.3). Ultrasound examination is also helpful in the evaluation of scrotal masses. Computed tomography (CT) combined with contrast injection gives great detail and is an essential part of staging tumours prior to surgery. These investigations give information about structure.

For detailed assessment of function, radioisotope renography is required. Renal scanning is simple to perform and can give detailed information on the function of each

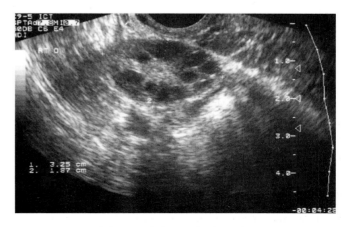

Figure 20.3 Renal ultrasound showing hydronephrosis.

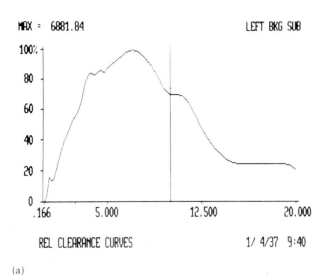
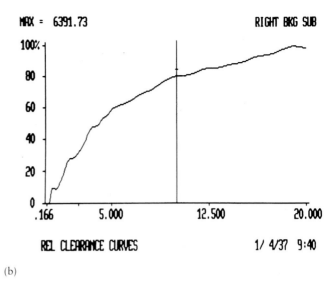

Figure 20.4 (a) Renogram showing a normal tracing. The line in the middle indicates the timing of an injection of frusemide which is followed by rapid excretion of isotope. (b) Abnormal renogram. There is a continually rising trace which is not affected by frusemide. This indicates the presence of obstruction.

kidney. Technetium-labelled diethylenetriaminepentaacetic acid (DTPA) is excreted in the urine-like contrast material. DTPA scans provide information on renal perfusion, function and the presence of obstruction (Fig. 20.4). Renal scanning with technetium-labelled dimercaptosuccinic acid (DMSA), which is taken up by the renal tubules and accumulates in cortical tissue, allows assessment of renal size and function. Radioisotope scanning is also used to detect bony secondaries. Technetium-labelled methylene diphosphonate is taken up into areas of increased osteoblastic activity.

Urodynamics

Urodynamics is a dynamic assessment of the storage and voiding functions of the urinary tract. The simplest test is the urine flow rate which assesses the rate and pattern of voiding. Ranges of normal values for age and sex aid in the interpretation of results. Cystometry involves the measurement of intravesical pressure during filling and voiding and is useful in differentiating between stress and urge incontinence. By filling the bladder with contrast medium during cystometry it is possible to watch bladder activity on a fluoroscope during the filling and voiding phases (videocystometry). Ambulatory measurements of bladder function are now possible.

Endoscopy

Almost the entire urinary tract can be visualized using various endoscopes. The urethra and bladder can be exam-

ined with a cystoscope, which may be either rigid or flexible. Traditionally, rigid scopes were used but flexible scopes have the advantage that the examination can be performed with minimal anaesthesia. The ureters can be examined by ureteroscopy and a flexible ureterorenoscope can be used to examine the ureter and renal pelvis.

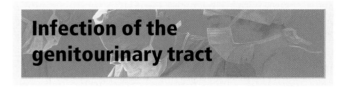

Infection of the genitourinary tract

Introduction

By employing a systematic approach, the diagnosis and treatment of infections of the genitourinary tract can be simplified using basic principles of infectious disease and genitourinary physiology. Many factors play a role in this approach; in particular, age, sex, location of infection, the agent causing infection, the state of the patient's immunocompetence and the presence or absence of obstruction. Bacteriuria is defined as the presence of bacteria in the urine. Although colony counts greater than 100 000/ml are considered significant, counts less than that do not rule out infection.

Laboratory diagnosis

The laboratory diagnosis of a UTI relies on the proper collection of the urine specimen, avoidance of contamination and prompt culturing of the urine. Refrigeration of the specimen will enable accurate results to be obtained when immediate culturing is not possible. The method of collection of urine samples is also important to ensure reliable results. In adult males, urine should be collected prior to prostatic examination and the clean-catch midstream method should be used. Uncircumcised men must retract the foreskin and clean the meatus with an antiseptic solution to avoid contamination. After the first 25–50 ml has passed, a sterile container is used to collect the specimen. A similar technique is used for women with attention to separating the labia and cleansing the meatus. If difficulty arises in obtaining an uncontaminated specimen, sterile catherization of the bladder must be used. In young children, urine is usually collected by applying a sterile bag over the cleansed penis or vulva. If this method appears unreliable, suprapubic needle aspiration of the bladder is often employed.

It is often difficult to distinguish urinary infection isolated to the lower tract from that of the upper tract. Several non-invasive tests have been developed to make this distinction, including the presence of antibody-coated bacteria, urinary β_2-microglobulin and lactic acid dehydrogenase (LDH) levels. However, these tests are non-specific and of limited clinical value. More reliable methods include cystoscopy with catheterization of each ureter to collect urine and percutaneous needle aspiration of urine in the renal pelvis.

Urinalysis and Gram stain techniques can provide immediate information regarding the presence of UTI. This is particularly helpful in acute symptomatic infections when early antibiotic treatment is necessary while awaiting urine culture results. Interpreting urine culture results depends on several factors: method of collection, type of organisms isolated, patient's symptoms and the number of colony-forming units per millilitre of urine. The organism *Escherichia coli* has been cultured in over 80% of urine samples received from patients with uncomplicated cystitis or pyelonephritis. *Enterobacter* and *Klebsiella* are more likely to be found with nosocomial (hospital-acquired) infections. *Pseudomonas* and *Candida* UTIs often appear in patients with lowered host resistance or those who have been receiving antibiotics. *Staphylococcus aureus* can be a urine pathogen, usually in the presence of obstruction, while *Proteus* infection (a urea-splitting organism) suggests the existence of urinary calculi (struvite stones). Multiple organisms are cultured from urine in only about 5% of true infections, usually indicating contamination of the specimen in asymptomatic patients.

Classification

A classification system for UTIs has been suggested to define and simplify many frequently used terms.
• A patient's first *UTI* is the first documented episode of significant bacteriuria.
• *Unresolved bacteriuria* refers to an infection that is never totally eliminated from the urine during and after treatment. Among the causes are stones or foreign bodies in the urinary tract, obstruction, bacterial resistance or insufficient concentration of drug used at the site of infection. Inadequate drug concentrations may result from renal insufficiency, poor drug absorption or non-compliance on the part of the patient in taking the drug.
• The third category in the Stamey classification is *bacterial persistence*, a term used to signify that the urine is sterilized by the treatment implemented but a persistent source of infection remains in the urinary tract. Included in this category are foreign bodies, infected stones, bladder or urethral diverticula, renal abscess and chronic bacterial prostatitis.
• The final term used is *reinfection*, which means that the urine is sterilized by initial treatment but a new infection with a new organism has developed. This accounts for approximately 80% of all recurrent UTIs.

Bacteraemia and sepsis

The mortality rate from Gram-negative bacteraemia approaches 15%. Septic shock develops in 25% of bacteraemic patients and carries a mortality of 50% (Chapter 7). Gram-negative sepsis commonly occurs in hospitalized patients after instrumentation of the genitourinary tract or from a primary focus in the genitourinary tract. Aerobic Gram-negative bacteria (*E. coli*, *Klebsiella*, *Enterobacter*, *Serratia*, *Pseudomonas* and *Proteus*) are the usual causes of sepsis originating from the genitourinary tract. Anaerobic bacteria can also produce sepsis as a result of transrectal biopsy of the prostate, while Gram-positive sepsis can result from enterococcus infection. Any patient with bacteriuria is at risk for sepsis if obstruction of the genitourinary tract exists or if the patient undergoes instrumentation.

The diagnosis of bacteraemia can be made on symptoms, signs and laboratory data. The development of pyrexia, especially with rigors, is evidence of bacteraemia in any patient after recent instrumentation. However, bacteraemia must be ruled out in a patient who is found to be ill after instrumentation, as 10% of patients will be hypothermic initially, while another 5% will be unable to mount a febrile response. Along with pyrexia, early signs of bacteraemia include tachycardia, tachypnoea, oliguria and hypotension. Confusion, agitation or other changes in mental status often ensue and later the patient will become lethargic or comatose while the skin becomes cold, moist and clammy. Laboratory findings commonly include leukocytosis, while thrombocytopenia will develop in more than 50% of patients. Later stages of sepsis can be associated with disseminated intravascular coagulation (DIC), hypoxia, azotaemia and jaundice.

Septic shock generally develops within the first 8–12 h after the development of bacteraemia. What is termed warm shock occurs early in the process and refers to a state of vasodilatation, increased cardiac output and mild hypotension. As the process continues, cold shock develops; this is distinguished by pronounced hypotension, peripheral vasoconstriction, diminished cardiac output and oliguria.

Treatment measures should be implemented immediately upon suspicion of bacteraemia or septic shock. Both urine and blood cultures should be obtained with Gram staining of the urine to determine whether Gram-negative or Gram-positive bacteria exist. Serum determinations of white blood cell count, platelets, creatinine, electrolytes and coagulation status should be made as well as arterial blood gas analysis. If sensitivities of specific bacteria to antibiotics are known, the appropriate drugs should be delivered intravenously immediately. However, as is usually the situation, if the offending organism is not immediately known, empirical antibiotic therapy should commence until specific sensitivities are known. Coverage should include antibiotics effective against Gram-negative, Gram-positive and anaerobic bacteria and must be administered intravenously. Once the organism is isolated and treated, intravenous therapy should continue for at least 5 days after the patient is apyrexial. If sepsis develops, cardiovascular support should be instituted rapidly with placement of a central venous pressure line or Swan–Ganz catheter. This allows close monitoring of the patient's haemodynamic status and also enables resuscitation with the administration of crystalloids and colloids for volume expansion. If patients fail to respond to these measures, pressor agents such as dopamine may be needed to maintain blood pressure. Oxygen should be delivered by facemask during the resuscitative measures. However, if respiration becomes inadequate as sepsis continues, intubation and mechanical ventilation may be needed.

Renal infection

Acute pyelonephritis

Acute pyelonephritis is a bacterial infection causing acute inflammation of one or sometimes both kidneys. The process involves the renal parenchyma but may also involve the calyces, renal pelvis and ureter. The most common causative agents are aerobic Gram-negative bacteria, with infection of the kidney occurring generally by ascending infection from the lower urinary tract. *E. coli* is the most common organism cultured in acute pyelonephritis. *Proteus mirabilis* and *Klebsiella* are urease-splitting organisms which create an alkaline urine secondary to release of ammonia, a condition that allows the precipitation of struvite stones in the renal pelvis and calyces. Gram-positive bacteria are a rare cause of acute pyelonephritis.

Several underlying conditions can predispose a patient to acute pyelonephritis (Table 20.4). Vesicoureteral reflux is associated with an increased risk of pyelonephritis. Obstruction anywhere in the urinary tract will lead to stasis of urine with subsequent pyelonephritis. Obstruction can be of multiple aetiologies, including congenital causes such as pelviureteric junction obstruction or acquired causes, as in ureteral stricture or calculous disease. Anatomical factors can predispose patients to pyelonephritis, as this condition is more common in females, owing to the shorter length of the urethra and increased incidence of bacterial colonization of the lower urinary tract. Patients with neurogenic bladder dysfunction may develop chronically increased intravesical pressures that are transmitted to the upper tracts, leading to a functional obstruction and pyelonephritis. Although a less common cause, haematogenous spread of infection to the kidney can occur from bacteria of the gastrointestinal tract or skin, especially in the face of obstruction of the kidney. Another common condition that may increase the risk of pyelonephritis is diabetes mellitus. Contributing factors in this disease include decreased host resistance, obstruction from sloughed papillae and bladder

Table 20.4 Factors which predispose to pyelonephritis.

Vesicoureteric reflux
Obstruction
   Congenital, e.g. pelviureteric obstruction
   Acquired, e.g. urethral stricture, stone disease
Anatomical, e.g. short urethra in females
Neurogenic bladder
Haematogenous spread from skin or gastrointestinal tract
Diabetes mellitus

dysfunction. An uncommon but potentially fatal form of this disease seen in diabetes patients is termed emphysematous pyelonephritis and is caused by gas-forming organisms.

Pyrexia, rigors, flank pain and dysuria are the clinical features of acute pyelonephritis. Patients may also complain of generalized malaise and anorexia. Physical examination will often elicit significant costovertebral angle tenderness as well as abdominal pain. Laboratory findings include a marked leukocytosis, urinanalysis showing pyuria, bacteriuria and microscopic haematuria. Urine culture almost always reveals greater than 100 000 colonies per millilitre of the bacteria causing infection. Acute pyelonephritis can mimic other disease processes. Included in the differential diagnosis are acute appendicitis, acute pancreatitis, acute cholecystitis and pelvic inflammatory disease in women.

Critical to the investigation of a patient with suspected pyelonephritis is the radiological work-up, which is often diagnostic. An excretory urogram will usually show renal enlargement and a somewhat decreased nephrogram, both of which return to normal with resolution of the infection. An ultrasound study of the kidney may reveal a dilated collecting system from obstruction, the presence of urinary stones or renal abscess. Lobar nephronia, a form of pyelonephritis limited to a focal area within the kidney, can also be seen with ultrasound.

In the absence of complicating factors such as obstruction or infected stones, acute pyelonephritis is treated by intravenous antibiotic therapy (determined by urine culture and sensitivity) until the patient is apyrexial and clinically improved. This is followed by a 2-week course of oral antibiotics. If no significant improvement is seen after 2–3 days of therapy, the diagnosis of abscess or obstruction with pyelonephrosis must be considered and if necessary treated.

Chronic pyelonephritis

Chronic pyelonephritis is a condition in which active infection is not usually demonstrated; however, parenchymal scarring of the kidney is featured along with generalized chronic inflammation and glomerular fibrosis. The condition is often the result of childhood infection of the kidney, especially in the face of vesicoureteral reflux. The presentation of adults with bilateral chronic pyelonephritis is frequently that of azotaemia or hypertension rather than evidence of infection. Findings on both excretory urography and ultrasonography include polar renal scarring, typically with underlying dilated calyces. If a single kidney is involved, the contralateral normal kidney will usually show evidence of compensatory hypertrophy, while in bilateral disease both kidneys are small.

Xanthogranulomatous pyelonephritis

A form of chronic pyelonephritis known as xanthogranulomatous pyelonephritis is usually unilateral and characterized by multiple renal parenchymal abscesses, pyelonephrosis and poor renal function. Characteristic of this disease is an inflammatory response characterized by the presence of xanthogranulomas containing lipid-laden macrophages, which can be difficult to distinguish from the clear cell appearance of renal adenocarcinoma. Pyuria and bacteriuria with *E. coli* or *Proteus mirabilis* are usually present and IVU often reveals renal calculi and a non-visualizing kidney. Given that the affected kidney's function is poor or absent and given the difficulty of distinguishing this condition from renal adenocarcinoma, the treatment of xanthogranulomatous pyelonephritis is usually nephrectomy.

Renal abscess

A renal abscess may develop by several mechanisms: it may arise as a direct result of pyelonephritis or occur by haematogenous spread from a distant site. The term perinephric abscess refers to the condition caused by rupture of a renal abscess into the perirenal space. The clinical findings of renal abscess vary depending on the cause. Patients with a haematogenous abscess will often present with pyrexia, rigors and flank pain, although no history of UTI is noted. Patients with an abscess secondary to pyelonephritis will usually have a history of previous urinary infection, obstruction or stones and are generally found to have bacteriuria.

Abscess caused by haematogenous infection usually arises from skin lesions or intravenous drug use, with *Staphylococcus aureus* being the predominant causative organism. This type of abscess is also known as a renal carbuncle and affects the cortex of the kidney. The intrarenal abscess resulting from pyelonephritis, sometimes referred to as medullary abscess, will involve both medulla and cortex and be multifocal in nature. Underlying obstruction often exists, with Gram-negative bacteria as the offending organism. Several radiological modalities are useful in diagnosing renal abscesses. Ultrasound will often reveal a well-circumscribed fluid collection differing in density from that of the surrounding parenchyma or of a simple renal cyst. IVU may show a poorly functioning kidney if an abscess is large or multifocal. Renal carbuncles can be seen as space-occupying defects in the cortex. A large perinephric abscess may obscure the renal outline and psoas shadow, making diagnosis difficult. When diagnosis is unclear or when it is necessary to distinguish renal abscess from solid masses, CT scan and magnetic resonance imaging may be required.

Treatment of renal abscess usually centres on draining the fluid collection. Localized abscesses can be drained by percutaneous or surgical means and should be accompanied by appropriate intravenous antibiotic therapy. Small abscesses, renal carbuncles and those seen in the paediatric population can often be adequately treated with antibiotic therapy alone. Prompt therapy is necessary to ensure preservation of the kidney.

Infections of the bladder

Acute cystitis

Acute bacterial cystitis refers to infection of the urinary bladder and is usually caused by coliform bacteria that ascend from the urethra to the bladder. Females are especially susceptible to ascending infections because of the short female urethra and the tendency of the rectal flora to colonize the perineum and vaginal vestibule. Sexual intercourse is also a major precipitating factor for urinary infection in women. Gram-positive bacteria and viruses are a less common cause of cystitis, although adenovirus infection can cause haemorrhagic cystitis in children.

Patients generally present with irritative voiding symptoms (dysuria, frequency and urgency). Suprapubic pain and low back pain occur commonly, as do haematuria and urge incontinence. Pyrexia occurs infrequently. Urinalysis usually shows pyuria and bacteriuria with microhaematuria. Urine cultures will reveal the infecting organism. A full blood count is often normal but occasionally leukocytosis may be present. Radiological investigation is limited to cases where renal infection is suspected. Patients found to have *Proteus* infections unresponsive to antibiotic therapy should have X-rays performed to exclude infection (struvite) stones. Cystoscopic evaluation is generally reserved for situations where haematuria is prominent but should be performed after the infection has been treated.

Complications of acute cystitis include ascending infections of the kidneys, to which pregnant women and children with vesicoureteral reflux are most susceptible. The differential diagnosis of acute bacterial cystitis varies widely but can usually be distinguished from other processes by proper examination and laboratory findings. In women, the urethral syndrome will cause frequency and dysuria but cultures generally show no growth. Vulvovaginitis can be distinguished by pelvic examination, looking for vaginal discharge. In males, acute cystitis can be differentiated from infections of the prostate, urethra and kidney by careful physical examination and specific laboratory testing. Non-infectious causes include cystitis sec-

ondary to radiation therapy, chemotherapy, bladder cancer and carcinoma-*in-situ*, eosinophilic cystitis and interstitial cystitis.

Acute uncomplicated bacterial cystitis generally responds rapidly to antimicrobial therapy. In women, short-term treatment with appropriate oral antibiotics is effective, ranging from a single dose to 1–2 days. *E. coli* causes 80% of uncomplicated, non-hospital-acquired infections and is usually sensitive to a wide array of antibiotics. Infections that do not respond appropriately to this treatment should be further investigated by urological and radiological means.

Urethral syndrome

Acute urethral syndrome is characterized by frequency, urgency and dysuria in women with urine cultures showing no growth or low bacterial counts. The urethral syndrome can vary in cause.
• Women with low bacterial counts but acute symptoms should be treated appropriately with the antibiotic to which the organism is sensitive.
• Some women will have cultures that reveal sexually transmitted organisms. Among women with acute dysuria, 7% will be found to have *Chlamydia trachomatis* and 2% will have *Neisseria gonorrhoeae*. These patients and their partners should be treated with appropriate antimicrobial agents including a tetracycline or erythromycin for *C. trachomatis* and a penicillin or tetracycline for *N. gonorrhoeae*.
• A third group of women will have no identifiable organism but many will respond paradoxically to antimicrobial therapy.

Vaginitis is a condition characterized by dysuria, pruritus and vaginal discharge that can be easily differentiated by physical examination, urine culture and vaginal culture. Urine cultures are usually sterile while vaginal infections are commonly caused by *Trichomonas vaginalis* and *Candida albicans*, although non-specific vaginitis is often associated with *Haemophilus vaginalis* infection.

Infections of the prostate

Acute bacterial prostatitis

This form of prostatitis is a bacterial infection characterized by pyrexia, rigors, low back pain, perineal discomfort, dysuria, urinary frequency and urgency. The major cause is aerobic Gram-negative bacilli, of which *E. coli* is seen in 80% of patients. *Pseudomonas* and enterococcus are also commonly found. Anaerobic bacteria are not generally seen in acute prostatitis unless infection occurs after transrectal biopsy and faecal contamination with *Bacteroides fragilis* occurs.

Possible routes of infection of the prostate include ascending organisms from the urethra, reflux of infected urine into prostatic ducts, lymphatic spread from the rectum or haematogenous spread. Acute bacterial prostatitis will often result in acute urinary retention but this usually resolves after the infection has been treated.

Rectal examination reveals an extremely tender prostate that is swollen, warm and firm. Acute cystitis will often accompany the disease, causing pyuria, bacteriuria and microhaematuria. Urine culture will usually reveal the causative bacteria and in addition prostatic massage will express pus and bacteria; however, this is generally avoided in the acute setting, owing to pain and risk of bacteraemia. Microabscesses may occur early in the disease process and develop into large abscesses if treatment is not implemented rapidly. Patients with acute bacterial prostatitis generally respond well to antimicrobial agents directed at the specific organism. Initial therapy usually includes intravenous antibiotics for acute pyrexic episodes, changing to oral agents after about 1 week. Subsequent oral therapy should continue for 1 month to prevent progression to chronic bacterial prostatitis or prostatic abscess formation.

Chronic bacterial prostatitis

Chronic bacterial prostatitis is an indolent non-acute infection of the prostatic ducts and glands. It is the most common cause of relapsing urinary tract infection in men. The causative agents are similar to those of acute bacterial prostatitis, i.e. Gram-negative aerobes. Enterococcus has been found on occasion to cause this condition; however, other Gram-positive bacteria are unusual causes. The mechanism and routes of infection are the same for acute and chronic bacterial prostatitis and in some situations chronic infection can be seen to evolve from previous acute episodes. However, it is often the case that no preceding history of acute prostatitis is found.

Symptoms vary widely; some patients are completely asymptomatic and are diagnosed only on the basis of bacteriuria found incidentally on urinalysis. However, most patients have differing degrees or irritative voiding symptoms, including dysuria, frequency and urgency, along with complaints of perineal discomfort and low back pain. Examination of the prostate may also be quite variable with its consistency ranging from normal to boggy or at times indurated. Prostatic secretions will show numerous inflammatory cells and will often have pyuria and bacteria. If urine is sterile, sequential collections of specimens from the urethra, midstream urine and prostatic secretions should be performed. The first 10 ml of voided urine represents a urethral specimen, a midstream urine sample represents a bladder specimen, and the first 10 ml of urine voided after prostatic massage represents a prostatic specimen.

The differential diagnosis of chronic prostatitis includes cystitis, which often results from prostatic infection. Also, diseases of the anus and rectum such as haemorrhoids or fissures can cause perineal pain, mimicking prostatitis. Careful physical examination and appropriate laboratory studies will usually identify the source of the problem.

Treatment of chronic bacterial prostatitis is directed at eradicating the prostatic focus of infection. Most antibiotics have been shown to diffuse poorly into prostatic tissue when it is not acutely inflamed. Trimethoprim, however, can achieve therapeutic intraprostatic levels and is recommended for patients with normal renal function. Long-term oral antibiotic therapy for 12 weeks has been shown to be more successful than short-term therapy and trimethoprim together with sulphamethoxazole in combination has the best documented success. Other treatment regimens include erythromycin, the tetracyclines and carbenicillin indanyl sodium. If elimination of the prostatic focus cannot be achieved, suppressive therapy with long-term antimicrobials can generally control recurrent infections.

Prostatic abscess

Most cases of prostatic abscesses are progressions or complications of acute bacterial prostatitis and signs and symptoms will often mimic this. Physical examination of the prostate usually reveals a swollen tender gland and fluctuation may be present. When cases of acute bacterial prostatitis do not respond appropriately to antibiotic therapy, the possibility of abscess must be entertained and investigated.

Coliform bacteria, typically *E. coli*, are the most common infecting organisms in prostatic abscesses, occurring in about 70% of cases. Laboratory data are similar to those in acute and chronic bacterial prostatitis. If the diagnosis is uncertain, transrectal ultrasound (TRUS) is a useful modality to confirm or exclude the diagnosis. Treatment consists of surgical drainage together with appropriate therapy. Drainage options include transperineal needle aspiration, transurethral resection or open perineal incision.

Non-bacterial prostatitis

Non-bacterial prostatitis is considered one of the most common syndromes affecting the prostate and often poses a diagnostic dilemma as its cause is unknown. Patients present with dysuria, perineal discomfort or low back pain, as with the other prostatitis syndromes. However, after bacteriological investigation, no urinary or prostatic infection is found. Prostatic secretions do, however, show excessive numbers of inflammatory cells, although repeated cultures fail to reveal an infectious agent. Attempts to isolate unusual organisms such as *Chlamydia*, *Ureaplasma*, *Mycoplasma*, anaerobic bacteria or viruses have been unsuccessful.

Treatment is initially directed at a possible infective cause and trials of antibiotic therapy are recommended with either a tetracycline or erythromycin. As this therapy is usually unsuccessful, treatment is then directed at symptomatic control. Anti-inflammatory and anticholinergic agents have met with limited success, as has prostatic massage or frequent ejaculation.

Infection of the testes and epididymis

Acute orchitis

In the absence of concomitant epididymitis, most cases of acute orchitis are felt to be secondary to haematogenous spread of a systemic bacterial or viral infection.

Mumps orchitis is a serious complication of mumps parotitis that typically affects adolescent boys or young men. Some 20–35% of adolescent mumps patients will develop orchitis and, of these, 10% will be bilateral. Presentation generally occurs 3–4 days after onset of parotitis with acute testicular pain and swelling noted. The scrotum becomes erythematous and oedematous. Significant pyrexia is common but urinary symptoms generally do not occur. Hydrocele can develop as a result of the inflammation.

The differential diagnosis includes acute epididymitis, torsion of the spermatic cord, trauma, tumour and granulomatous diseases, including tuberculosis. The serious complication of irreversible loss of spermatogenesis occurs in about 30% of the affected testes. Treatment of mumps orchitis centres on relief of symptoms as no specific therapy is available. Infiltration of the spermatic cord with 1% lignocaine will give rapid pain relief and may protect the testis from further damage by improving blood supply.

Acute epididymitis

Most cases of acute epididymitis develop from retrograde contamination of the epididymitis by urethral contents via the vas deferens. The increased pressure associated with voiding or straining may force infected urine from the urethra or prostate into the ejaculatory ducts, vas deferens and ultimately the epididymis. Infection starts at the distal portion or tail of the epididymis but may progress to involve the entire structure and the testis (epididymo-orchitis). Generalized inflammation often makes it difficult to distinguish the epididymis from the testis.

The aetiology of epididymitis is generally divided into two categories. The first is a sexually transmitted form due to *Chlamydia trachomatis* or *Neisseria gonorrhoeae* or both. This form of epididymitis is most commonly seen in men under the age of 35. The second form of the disease is due to a bacterial genitourinary infection and is the commonest cause of acute epididymitis seen in men over 40 years of age. Associated with UTIs and prostatitis, this form is caused by Gram-negative organisms, particularly Enterobacteriaceae and *Pseudomonas*.

Clinical findings include sudden pain in the scrotum radiating along the spermatic cord while the epididymis is exquisitely tender. Scrotal swelling occurs rapidly with erythema, oedema and occasional reactive hydrocele. Differentiation between the epididymis and testis is often difficult. High pyrexia is usually noted, while symptoms of cystitis or prostatitis may be present. Laboratory findings include a leukocytosis. Pyuria is often seen as well as bacteraemia in cases of epididymitis due to bacterial infection.

All causes of scrotal swelling are included in the differential diagnosis. Torsion of the spermatic cord can be seen in the age group susceptible to chlamydial infection. In situations where urinalysis is unrevealing, elevating the scrotum may relieve pain due to epididymitis, while increasing the pain due to torsion (Prehn's sign). Doppler flow studies and radionuclide scans may aid in diagnosis but none of these methods should cause delay in surgical exploration of potential torsion. Torsion of testicular or epididymal appendages can mimic epididymitis and torsion of the spermatic cord. Testicular tumours are generally non-tender and testicular trauma is usually diagnosed by history and lack of findings on urinalysis. Mumps orchitis and tuberculous epididymitis are less common but may have a similar presentation.

Treatment centres on the suspected or isolated organism. Sexually transmitted cases caused by *Chlamydia* are treated with a tetracycline or erythromycin. As *Chlamydia* may be difficult to isolate, therapy is often empirical once gonorrhoea has been excluded by negative culture of the urethra. Treatment for gonorrhoeal causes includes parenteral administration of a third-generation cephalosporin for penicillinase-producing strains. Non-penicillin-resistant strains can be treated with oral penicillin, tetracycline or quinolone or by intramuscular administration of penicillin. Bacterial causes of acute epididymitis generally respond to prompt treatment with oral antibiotics chosen on the basis of culture and sensitivities. Severe cases with significant pyrexia may require hospitalization and intravenous antibiotics.

Urinary tract infection at a glance

DEFINITION

A *urinary tract infection* (UTI) is a documented episode of significant bacteriuria (i.e. an infection with a colony count of >100 000 organisms per millilitre) which may affect the upper (*pyelonephritis, renal abscess*) or the lower urinary tract (*cystitis*), or both

EPIDEMIOLOGY

UTI is a very common condition in general practice (usually *Escherichia coli*) and accounts for 40% of hospital-acquired (*nosocomial*) infections (often *Enterobacter* or *Klebsiella*)

RISK FACTORS

- Urinary tract obstruction
- Instrumentation of urinary tract (e.g. indwelling catheter)
- Neurogenic bladder
- Diabetes mellitus
- Immunosuppression
- Vesicoureteric reflux
- Pregnancy

PATHOLOGY

- *Ascending infection*: Most UTIs caused in this way (bacteria from GI tract colonize lower urinary tract)
- *Haematogenous spread*: Infrequent cause of UTI (seen in i.v. drug users, bacterial endocarditis and TB)

CLINICAL FEATURES

Upper urinary tract infection
- Fever
- Rigors/chill
- Flank pain
- Malaise
- Anorexia
- Costovertebral angle and abdominal tenderness

Lower urinary tract infection
- Dysuria
- Frequency
- Urgency
- Suprapubic pain
- Haematuria
- Scrotal pain (epididymo-orchitis) or perineal pain (prostatitis)

INVESTIGATIONS

- Gram stain and culture of a 'clean-catch' urine specimen before antibiotics have been given. Usual organisms are *E. coli, Enterobacter, Klebsiella, Proteus* (suggests presence of urinary calculi)

Upper urinary tract infection
- FBC and U&E
- Serum creatinine
- Renal ultrasound
- Intravenous urogram
- CT scan
- Isotope scan (DTPA, DMSA)

Lower urinary tract infection
- FBC
- Cystoscopy only if haematuria
- If obstruction is present ultrasound scan, IVU and cystoscopy may be needed

MANAGEMENT

- The principles of management are to treat the infection with an appropriate antibiotic based on urine culture results and deal with any underlying cause (e.g. relieve obstruction). High fluid intake should be encouraged and potassium citrate may relieve dysuria
- Upper-tract UTIs, epididymo-orchitis and prostatitis require intravenous antibiotic therapy. Agents commonly used: gentamicin, cephalosporin or co-trimoxazole
- Cystitis and uncomplicated lower UTIs can be managed with oral antibiotics. Agents commonly used: trimethroprim, ampicillin, nitrofurantoin, cephalosporin
- An abscess will require drainage either radiologically or surgically
- If there is a poor response to treatment, consider unusual urinary infections: tuberculosis (sterile pyuria), candiduria, schistosomiasis, *Chlamydia trachomatis, Neisseria gonorrhoeae*

COMPLICATIONS

- Bacteraemia and septic shock
- Chronic and xanthogranulomatous pyelonephritis
- Renal and perinephric abscesses

Sexually transmitted diseases in males

Sexually transmitted diseases (STDs) form a constantly changing group of diseases influenced by mode of transmission, contraceptive practices and antibiotic treatment. Before World War II, syphilis was the most common STD but has now become somewhat rare. Gonorrhoeal infection was also quite common but its incidence is declining, while that of non-gonococcal urethritis (NGU) is increasing. Genital herpes is a disease of great concern as its prevalence has increased in both men and women. In general, male patients with STDs present with variable complaints of urethral discharge, dysuria or an ulcerative lesion of the genital skin.

Gonococcal urethritis

Gonococcal urethritis is caused by the bacteria *Neisseria gonorrhoeae*, a Gram-negative intracellular diplococcus. In men, the urethra is the most common site of infection but other sites may be involved. The oropharynx is infected in 7% of heterosexual men and 40% of homosexual men, while the rectum is infected in 25% of homosexual men.

In males, the most common presentation is acute purulent urethritis and dysuria. Symptoms generally begin

3–10 days following sexual contact but the incubation period can vary from 1 day to 3 months. The urethral discharge is diffuse and usually yellow or brown with meatal erythema and oedema.

Laboratory diagnosis is based on Gram stain and culture of the urethra. A calcium alginate swab is inserted into the urethra and rotated. The swab is then used to inoculate a Thayer-Martin agar culture plate and rolled on to a glass slide for Gram stain. The presence of intracellular Gram-negative diplococci on Gram stain is diagnostic; however, if only extracellular Gram-negative diplococci are seen, diagnosis relies on culture results.

Treatment of gonococcal urethritis has been influenced by the existence of β-lactamase-producing and other resistant strains of *N. gonorrhoeae*. Present recommendations include the third-generation cephalosporin, e.g. ceftriaxone, 250 mg intramuscularly and in addition a 7-day course of an oral tetracycline to cover the 10–35% of patients with concurrent chlamydial infections. Patients should refrain from sexual intercourse until cure is established. Complications of gonococcal infection include periurethritis, which can lead to the formation of periurethral abscess, urethral fibrosis and stricture. Prostatitis and epididymitis also develop if not treated expeditiously. Systemic infection is uncommon.

Non-gonococcal urethritis (NGU)

NGU is a syndrome with multiple microbial aetiology and is diagnosed when *N. gonorrhoeae* cannot be isolated. The most common organisms are *Chlamydia trachomatis* and *Ureaplasma urealyticum*. The typical presentation of NGU includes a thin mucoid urethral discharge, dysuria and pruritus at the meatus. Asymptomatic infections can occur. The incubation period is 7–21 days. Diagnosis of NGU is based on the presence of urethritis and exclusion of gonococcal infection. When suspected, patients should be examined several hours after last voiding to demonstrate discharge reliably. Gram stain of a urethral swab will reveal numerous polymorphonuclear leukocytes, as with that of a spun urine specimen. *C. trachomatis* is a small bacterium and intracellular parasite of columnar epithelium. To culture this organism effectively, an endourethral swab is taken and a technique using a fluorescein-conjugated monoclonal antibody is carried out. As this technique is not always available to the physician, therapy is often started impirically when NGU is suspected. Other causes of NGU include *Trichomonas vaginalis* and herpes infection.

Results of treatment for NGU are inconsistent as the syndrome can be caused by various organisms that respond to differing therapy. Patients with *C. trachomatis* infections respond best as tetracycline resistance has not been documented. *Ureaplasma* will also respond to tetracyclines but are much less sensitive than chlamydiae. Therefore, recommended therapy for NGU begins with a 7-day course of tetracycline with sexual partners treated with the same regimen. Most non-responders are due to *Ureaplasma* but those due to *T. vaginalis* should be treated with metronidazole while patients with persistent or recurrent urethritis should be given a trial of erythromycin. Complications of NGU include epididymitis, prostatitis, proctitis and Reiter's syndrome, a disorder characterized by urethritis, conjunctivitis, arthritis and mucocutaneous lesions and associated with *C. trachomatis* infection.

Genital ulcers

Genital ulcers include several disease entities that most commonly affect younger, sexually active men. It is difficult to make the diagnosis based solely on the appearance of the lesion, which can present as a papule, vesicle or pustule before developing into a true ulcer. Laboratory tests are necessary to make the diagnosis, while other factors including the presence of inguinal adenopathy and incubation time, must be taken into account.

Primary syphilis

The organism that causes syphilis is the spirochaete *Treponema pallidum*. The primary genital ulcer generally develops as a painless lesion, termed a chancre, 2–4 weeks after sexual exposure. The ulcer commonly appears on the glans penis but may form on the foreskin, shaft, suprapubic or scrotal areas. The chancre is typically a deep non-tender ulcer with indurated edges and a clean base. Inguinal lymph nodes are often enlarged but also non-tender. The diagnosis is made by the presence of spirochaetes on dark-field examination of scrapings from the base of the ulcer. Other techniques include a reagin test which has replaced the Venereal Disease Research Laboratory (VDRL) test, although both serological examinations may be negative for 1–3 weeks after appearance of the ulcer. The fluorescent *Treponema* antibody absorption test (FTA-ABS) is specific for antitreponemal antibodies and becomes positive early in the disease. Treatment for primary syphilis consists of benzathine penicillin G 2.4 million units as a single intramuscular dose. Tetracycline or erythromycin may be used for patients with penicillin allergies.

Chancroid

Chancroid is a genital lesion caused by *Haemophilus ducreyi*. The ulcer is generally soft with erythematous borders and often has purulent secretions and may be painful. Many patients may develop constitutional symptoms of pyrexia, malaise and headache. Painful inguinal adenopathy is often seen. The ulcer usually appears within a few days of sexual exposure. Diagnosis can be made with Gram stain revealing Gram-negative coccobacilli; however, culture for *H. ducreyi* is more sensitive and specific. Biopsy of the ulcerative lesion is always diagnostic. Treatment measures include erythromycin or tetracycline orally for 7–10 days or a single dose of ceftriaxone 250 mg intramuscularly. Washing the genitalia carefully is also important.

Granuloma inguinale

This is a chronic infection of the skin and subcutaneous tissue of the genitalia, perineum and inguinal areas. *Calymmatobacterium granulomatis* is the infective agent and incubation time is 2–3 months. The genital ulcer is firm, indurated and non-tender with an erythematous border. Subcutaneous inguinal granulomas cause inguinal swelling rather than true adenopathy. Chronic inguinal inflammation may produce lymphatic obstruction. The diagnosis of granuloma inguinale is made by identifying Donovan bodies within monocytes in tissue obtained from the ulcer base. A crush preparation of the tissue between two glass slides is stained with Giemsa's or Wright's stain. If diagnosis is questionable, a biopsy may be performed. However, no reliable culture for *C. granulomatis* is available.

Lymphogranuloma venereum

This is caused by immunotypes L1, L2 and L3 of *Chlamydia trachomatis*. The genital lesion is generally small, superficial and transient and may go unnoticed. The incubation period is 5–21 days. Painful lymphadenitis usually ensues and lymph nodes may become matted and suppurative. Rectal strictures may develop as a late complication. The most specific diagnostic test for lymphogranuloma venereum is culture of *C. trachomatis* from an inguinal node aspirate. Microimmunofluorescent serological tests are also very sensitive and specific. Treatment consists of tetracycline or trimethoprim–sulphamethoxazole orally until the lesion is healed.

Genital herpes

Herpes simplex virus is a double-stranded DNA virus. Most cases of genital herpes infections are caused by type 2 virus, although a small percentage may develop from type 1 virus, which more commonly produces oral infections. The incubation period is generally 2–10 days but may vary from 1 to 30 days. The herpesvirus may also cause persistent or latent infections in both men and women.

Although symptoms vary depending on prior exposure to the herpesvirus, the first clinical episode is usually most severe. Grouped vesicles on an erythematous base are pathognomonic for genital herpes. The lesions are painful and do not follow a neural distribution. Lymphadenopathy is present and painful in 80% of patients and most patients develop pyrexia and malaise. Dysuria is seen in 45% of men. The laboratory diagnosis is made on cytological techniques and viral culture. Tzanck smears of genital lesions will reveal intranuclear inclusions or multinucleated giant cells. Isolation of the virus by culture, however, is more sensitive for diagnosing herpes infections.

The treatment of genital herpes consists of the drug acyclovir, a guanine analogue that acts on viral thymidine kinase to inhibit DNA replication. Acyclovir is available in topical, oral and intravenous forms. The topical form, a 5% ointment, is less effective than the other two but when started within 6 days of developing the lesions it will decrease the time course of the disease and diminish the pain and itching. Topical treatment will not, however, decrease dysuria, vaginal discharge or systemic symptoms. The oral and intravenous forms are effective in reducing recurrences and decreasing systemic symptoms, dysuria and vaginal discharge.

Genital warts

This is an STD due to the DNA-containing papillomavirus. Also termed condyloma acuminata, the incubation period is approximately 45 days but can vary. Several subtypes exist, with visible genital warts caused by types 6 and 11. Other subtypes seen in the anogenital areas, such as 16, 18 and 31, are associated with cervical dysplasia and possible carcinoma in women. Lesions in males are typically found on the glans penis, foreskin or shaft but intraurethral lesions can develop. Involvement at the urethral meatus or persistent dysuria are indications for endoscopic evaluation. Although no treatment has been shown to eliminate the virus completely, several therapies are available. Topical podophyllin can be applied at weekly intervals. Cryosurgery or laser therapy is also effective to remove visible lesions. However, recurrences are common with all forms of treatment.

Urinary tract obstruction and urolithiasis

Obstruction of the urinary tract may occur at any level from the external urinary meatus to the ureteropelvic junction. Obstruction may be classified according to site as lower urinary tract obstruction (i.e. distal to the bladder) and obstruction of the upper urinary tract (i.e. bladder and upwards). Within each type of obstruction further subclassification according to aetiology (congenital or acquired), duration (acute or chronic) and degree of obstruction (partial or complete) is possible.

Lower urinary tract obstruction

Introduction

Outflow obstruction of the lower urinary tract remains one of the most prevalant and clinically significant diseases in urology. While there are numerous aetiologies, each specific obstructive lesion can be widely manifested ranging from minimal symptoms to urinary sepsis and renal failure. Symptoms referable to the lower urinary tract are categorized into obstructive and irritative (Table 20.5).

Obstructive symptoms include weak stream, hesitancy, intermittency, dribbling and straining to void while irritative symptoms typically include urinary frequency, urgency, nocturia, dysuria and urge incontinence. The term prostatism refers to a combination of these symptoms, including frequency, urgency, hesitancy and weak stream. While the name implies that prostatic obstruction is the cause, this is not always the case as bladder instability in patients with no evidence of obstruction can present in an identical fashion.

Table 20.5 Symptoms of lower urinary tract obstruction.

Obstructive	Irritative
Weak stream	Frequency
Hesitancy	Urgency
Intermittency	Nocturia
Dribbling	Dysuria
Straining to void	Urge incontinence

Table 20.6 Differential diagnosis of lower urinary tract infection.

Obstructive
Meatal stenosis
Phimosis
Urethral stricture
Posterior urethral valves
Benign prostatic hyperplasia
Carcinoma of the prostate
Bladder neck contracture

Functional
Neurogenic bladder dysfunction
Psychogenic voiding dysfunction

Neoplastic
Carcinoma of the bladder
Carcinoma-*in-situ* of the bladder

Infectious
Prostatitis (acute or chronic)
Prostatic abscess
Cystitis
Balanitis

Differential diagnosis

The differential diagnosis of lower urinary tract obstruction varies widely and can be classified on the basis of anatomical, functional, neoplastic and infectious causes (Table 20.6).

Obstruction of the distal urethra can result from meatal stenosis, typically seen in newborn or infant males. There is usually a congenital web of epithelial tissue permitting only a pinpoint opening at the meatus. In adults this may be the result of inflammatory processes of the glans penis (balanitis). In uncircumcised males, chronic inflammation and scarring of the prepuce or foreskin can lead to an inability to retract the prepuce (phimosis) and occasionally cause obstruction of urine. The condition of urethral stenosis in females is rare and may be related to trauma or inflammation. Urethral stricture is a frequent problem seen in adult males. Although a common sequel to gonococcal urethritis in the past, the majority of strictures now seen are the result of trauma to the urethra from instrumentation or catheterization.

Posterior urethral valves, i.e. congenital mucosal folds in the area of the membranous urethra, are the most common cause of proximal urethral obstruction in male infants. In adults, obstruction in this region can be both functional and anatomical. Failure of the external urethral sphincter to relax secondary to spasm during micturition will impede flow. Several neurological diseases, including spinal cord injury and multiple sclerosis, as well as psychogenic causes will result in this type of obstruction. The most common anatomical obstructive lesion in adult males is benign prostatic hyperplasia (see below). Carcinoma of the prostate is a less common cause of obstruction as most cancers occur in the peripheral regions of the prostate while benign prostatic hyperplasia tends to occur in the periurethral transition zone. Infectious processes of the prostate can also lead to obstructive symptoms owing to surrounding inflammation and oedema and include acute prostatitis and prostatic abscesses.

Obstruction at the level of the bladder neck can occur under several circumstances. Contracture of the bladder neck is a common cause and typically seen secondary to surgery or trauma. Neurological and idiopathic dysfunction are less common causes and are characterized by failure of the vesical neck to open completely during micturition without anatomical cause. This may mimic benign prostatic hyperplasia but usually occurs in a younger age group. In female patients who have had vaginal deliveries or pelvic surgery, cystocele may develop, causing a range of symptoms from obstruction and retention to urinary incontinence.

Several neuromuscular aetiologies of vesical dysfunction exist and can present with obstructive urinary symptoms or complete retention. Peripheral neuropathies may adversely affect detrusor muscle contraction by involving the autonomic nerve supply. Causes include diabetes mellitus, chronic alcoholism, uraemia, Guillain–Barré syndrome and trauma. Many pharmocological agents have been shown to exacerbate obstructive symptoms and precipitate retention. Drugs with anticholinergic activity such as phenothiazines and certain antianxiety medications act by inhibiting detrusor contractility. The commonly used α-adrenergic agonists pseudoephedrine, ephedrine and phenylpropanolamine increase sympathetic tone of the bladder neck and prostatic urethra. Both temporary and permanent detrusor dysfunction can be seen from prolonged overdistension or ischaemia of the bladder muscle — so-called myogenic failure.

Benign prostatic hypertrophy (BPH)

Pathophysiology

The initial change in BPH is the development of microscopic stromal nodules around the periurethral glands. Around these nodules, glandular hyperplasia originates. A review of ageing in otherwise normal males revealed the incidence of BPH to be slightly over 50% in men between 60 and 90 years of age. Early changes probably occur between the ages of 30 and 40 years. The aetiology of BPH is uncertain.

Clinical findings

BPH induces gradual changes in the urinary tract, which result from the interactions between prostatic urethral resistance and intravesical pressure. The symptoms of BPH are a combination of the obstructive and irritative symptoms discussed earlier (Table 20.5). Urethral compression from the enlarging prostate will result in a decreased force of stream, while hesitancy is due to the prolonged time required for the detrusor muscle to overcome the increased urethral resistance. Intermittency, terminal dribbling and incomplete emptying arise when the detrusor muscle can no longer maintain the increased pressure required to empty the bladder. Irritative symptoms, including frequency and nocturia, result from incomplete bladder emptying. Thus there are shortened intervals between voids, as well as increased excitability of the hypertrophied detrusor muscle leading to bladder instability. When patients are asleep, cortical inhibition is decreased, as is urethral tone, leading to nocturia. Incontinence is generally a late finding with BPH, when large volumes of residual urine accumulate in the bladder and overcome urethral resistance, often called overflow incontinence. Acute urinary retention may develop as a result of a precipitating factor aggravating existing BPH. Such factors include pharmacological agents (α-adrenergic drugs, anticholinergics and psychotropic agents), alcohol, cold temperatures and infection.

Physical signs attributable to BPH tend to occur late in the disease. Examination of the abdomen may reveal a distended bladder or occasionally a palpable kidney and flank tenderness from hydronephrosis or pyelonephritis. Rectal examination of patients with BPH usually reveals an enlarged prostate with a smooth surface. Right and left lobes are often not discernible, although asymmetry is common while the consistency of the gland may be either soft or firm, depending on whether there are more glandular or fibromuscular elements. Seminal vesicles are usually not palpable with enlarged glands. If irregularities of the prostate are felt on digital rectal examination, including firm nodules, induration or a generally hard prostate, carcinoma is more likely and further investigation including biopsy should ensue. In advanced cases signs of uraemia secondary to renal failure may be present — hypertension, tachycardia and tachypnoea from metabolic acidosis and anaemia as well as neurological changes and uraemic foetor.

Investigations

The investigation of a patient with BPH should start with urinalysis to look for evidence of infection and haematuria. If haematuria exists, other causes referable to the urinary tract should be excluded. Serum levels of electrolytes, creatinine and blood urea nitrogen should be tested. Objective signs of BPH can be evaluated using uroflowmetry and determining post-void residual volume. Diminished flow rates indicate prostatic outlet obstruction, while residual urine volumes greater than 100 ml would indicate significant failure to empty the bladder completely.

Radiological and imaging studies have an important role in the evaluation of BPH as they can assess the volume of BPH and of residual urine and exclude other urinary tract pathology. Studies typically used include ultrasonography to evaluate the kidneys and bladder while transrectal ultrasound will more accurately assess the prostate for size and evidence of cancer. IVU is a more invasive technique that will study the entire urinary tract.

Cystoscopy is an important modality to evaluate BPH and is often done prior to transurethral resection of the prostate (TURP). Bladder capacity can be evaluated as well as determining the presence of trabeculations and diverticula. This inspection also includes evaluation of the ureteric orifices, the possible presence of bladder tumours or stones, size and length of the prostate, and condition of the urethra.

Surgical treatment

BPH is most effectively treated by surgical removal of the adenomatous portion of the prostate. Surgical indications for prostatectomy vary among urologists but a number of conditions which develop as a result of BPH are widely accepted as indications for surgery. Included in this group are uraemia, hydronephrosis, acute or chronic urinary retention, bladder calculi, urinary sepsis and symptoms extremely bothersome to the patient.

TURP is the most common surgical treatment of BPH. Methods for open prostatectomy are limited to patients with extremely large glands (greater than 70 g) that are not suitable for TURP because of gland size and time required for resection. Open prostatectomy is associated with greater blood loss and higher morbidity and mortality. During TURP, the adenomatous portion of the prostate is removed via a resectoscope using electrocautery from within the prostatic urethra.

Complications of TURP

The overall complication rate of TURP is about 18%, while mortality is approximately 0.2%. During TURP, irrigation fluid composed of 3% sorbitol or 1.5% glycine is used to maintain a clear visual field. Even with constant-flow resectoscopes which allow the irrigation fluid to be removed continuously, an average of 900 ml of fluid is absorbed into the extra- and intravascular space through open venous sinuses in the prostatic capsule. This fluid is electrolyte-free and absorption of these volumes is generally well-tolerated by patients. Occasionally a hyponatraemic, hypochloraemic metabolic acidosis develops with serious complications, including hypertension, tachycardia, confusion and obtundation. This condition is termed TURP syndrome and has an incidence of approximately 2%. Other immediate complications include failure to void, postoperative haemorrhage, clot retention and UTI. Late complications include impotence, incontinence and bladder neck contractures.

Non-surgical treatment

Alternative treatment options to prostatectomy are gaining acceptance. Medical therapies include α-adrenergic blockers that act on the abundant α-adrenergic receptors present in prostatic smooth muscle and capsule. While these agents do not cause any change in the size of the prostate, nor do they alter the natural history of BPH. Flow rates have been shown to improve by approximately 50% with this therapy and 30–70% of patients report improvement in symptoms. Side-effects include hypotension and tachycardia. Other agents inhibit the conversion of testosterone to dihydrotestosterone by blocking the enzyme 5α-reductase; finasteride acts by reducing the size of the prostate by about 30% causing a mean improvement in peak flow of 1.5–2.0 ml/s. Early results of this drug, finasteride, are promising for treating BPH. Other non-surgical modalities to treat BPH include intermittent self-catheterization as a temporizing measure, transurethral balloon dilatation of the prostate, microwave hyperthermia, prostatic urethral stents, transurethral needle ablation and high intensity focused ultrasound; these are all currently under evaluation.

Upper urinary tract obstruction

Upper urinary tract obstruction may result in renal impairment, especially if the obstruction is prolonged. The kidney responds to distal obstruction, partial or complete, by a decrease in ipsilateral renal blood flow with a concomitant increase in contralateral renal blood flow. Other protective mechanisms include ureteric dilatation, which dissipates the increased pressure to some extent, urine reabsorption through the renal lymphatics and collecting ducts (pyelointerstitial back flow) and papillary shutdown. However, continued unrelieved obstruction produces renal impairment due to a combination of pressure and ischaemic atrophy. Acute obstruction is symptomatic with low pain but chronic obstruction may be asymptomatic or produce

Benign prostatic hypertrophy at a glance

DEFINITION

Benign prostatic hypertrophy (BPH) is a condition of unknown aetiology characterized by an increase in size of the inner zone of the prostate gland

EPIDEMIOLOGY

BPH is present in 50% of 60–90-year-old men

PATHOPHYSIOLOGY

- Microscopic stromal nodules develop around the periurethral glands
- Glandular hyperplasia originates around these nodules
- As the gland increases in size, it compresses the urethra, leading to urinary tract obstruction

CLINICAL FEATURES

- Weak stream
- Hesitancy
- Intermittency
- Dribbling
- Straining to void
- Acute urinary retention
- Palpable (or percussable) bladder
- Enlarged smooth prostate on digital rectal examination
- Frequency
- Urgency
- Nocturia
- Dysuria
- Urge incontinence
- Overflow incontinence

INVESTIGATIONS

- Urinalysis for evidence of infection or haematuria
- Urine culture
- FBC, U&E, serum creatinine
- Uroflowmetry
- Pressure-flow studies
- Residual volume measurement (normal <100 ml)
- Ultrasonography of kidneys and bladder
- Transrectal ultrasound to determine prostate size
- IVU
- Cystoscopy

MANAGEMENT

Medical
- α-Adrenergic blockers (e.g. phenoxybenzamine, prazosin)
- Antiandrogens acting selectively at prostatic cellular level (e.g. finasteride)
- Intermittent self-catheterization
- Balloon dilatation and stenting of prostate

Surgical
- Majority of patients are treated surgically
- Surgical removal of the adenomatous portion of the prostate
- Transurethral resection of the prostate (TURP) with electrocautery or laser
- Open prostatectomy, which may be transvesical or retropubic

Complications of surgical treatment
- TURP syndrome — in 2% of patients absorption of irrigation fluid via venous sinuses in the prostate causes hyponatraemia and metabolic acidosis
- Postoperative haemorrhage and clot retention
- Urinary tract infection
- Retrograde ejaculation
- Incontinence
- Urethral stricture

PROGNOSIS

The majority of patients have very good quality of life after prostatectomy

---

vague symptoms. Diagnosis of obstruction depends mainly on the IVU with judicious application of specialized radiographic techniques such as isotopic renography, ascending ureterography and perfusion studies (Whitaker test). On the basis of clinical and radiological findings, obstruction may be found to be unilateral or bilateral, complete or partial, acute or chronic.

Unilateral upper tract obstruction

The causes of unilateral upper tract obstruction are summarized in Table 20.7. Such obstruction may be due to lesions within the ureteric lumen, lesions within the ureteric wall or lesions outside the wall of the ureter compressing it.

Intraluminal obstruction

- The commonest intraluminal obstructing ureteric lesion is a calculus. Ureteric calculi usually present with acute ureteric colic with associated haematuria. A plain abdominal film will demonstrate the calculus in 90% of patients and the IVU will confirm the diagnosis and indicate the degree of obstruction. Treatment of ureteric calculi is dealt with elsewhere in this chapter.
- Clots from bleeding in the renal pelvis or kidney (transitional cell carcinoma, renal cell carcinoma) may mimic ureteric colic but the findings on X-ray of a filling defect in the renal pelvis or distorted calyces gives a clue to the correct diagnosis.
- Renal papillary necrosis is uncommon but the sloughed papilla may obstruct the ureter, mimicking the clinical picture

Table 20.7 Causes of unilateral ureteric obstruction.

Intraluminal
Stone
Clot
Sloughed renal papilla

Intramural
Congenital obstruction
    Pelviureteric junction
    Ureterovesical junction
Tumour
Stricture

Extraluminal
Vascular
Pregnancy
Complete procidentia
Pelvic tumours
Retroperitoneal tumours

of ureteric stone. Patients with sickle-cell disease, diabetes mellitus or those who ingest large doses of analgesics over prolonged periods are most at risk of necrosis of the renal papillae. Ureteric obstruction with superimposed infection may also cause the papillae to slough. The symptoms are pain associated with haematuria and sterile pyuria with a typical IVU which shows defects in the medulla where the papillae were and a non-calcified obstructing ureteric lesion. Sloughed papillae are managed in the same manner as ureteric calculi.

Intramural obstruction

• Congenital obstruction of the pelviureteric junction (PUJ obstruction; Fig. 20.5) is a common ureteric abnormality that occurs more frequently in males and affects the left side more often than the right side. Bilateral PUJ obstruction occurs in 15% of cases. In the majority of cases the condition is idiopathic. Associated abnormal renal vessels are not uncommon but rarely cause PUJ obstruction. The basic abnormality is a failure of transmission of peristalsis from the pelvis to the ureter. Histological examination of the PUJ shows an increased concentration of both collagen and elastin. As a result of this block to transmission of peristalsis, the intrapelvic pressure rises and the renal pelvis and calyces dilate. Gradual deterioration of renal function on the affected side is the rule.

This condition may be asymptomatic and detected serendipitously during medical investigations for unassociated complaints or it may produce loin pain, especially after an increased fluid load (Dietl's crisis). An IVU will show dilated calyces and pelvis with obstruction at the level of the PUJ. The ureter is not visible and, if it can be seen on the IVU, then the diagnosis of PUJ obstruction is incorrect. A renogram with diuretic will confirm the obstructive nature of the lesion and give a rough estimate of renal function on the obstructed side.

Treatment is surgical. If renal function is poor, nephrectomy is the most appropriate treatment provided the condition is not bilateral. If renal function is good then pyeloplasty is undertaken (Anderson–Hynes operation). In this procedure the abnormal PUJ is excised, the dilated renal pelvis is tailored and the ureter is reanastomosed to the newly fashioned pelvis. A follow-up renogram is advised at 6 months. Improvement of function occurs in only one-third of patients but 90% will have improved drainage. Reoperation may be needed in up to 5% of patients.

• Obstruction may also occur at the ureterovesical junction (obstructed megaureter; Fig. 20.6). This congenital ureteric

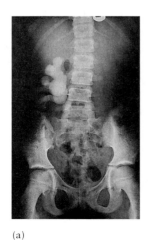

(a)

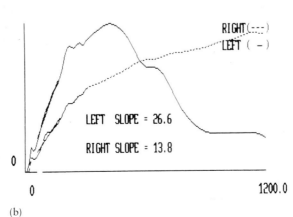

(b)

Figure 20.5 (a) Intravenous urogram film showing right pelviureteric junction (PUJ) obstruction. (b) Renogram demonstrating the presence of PUJ obstruction on the right side. There is a normal trace on the left and a rising trace on the right, confirming the presence of obstruction on that side.

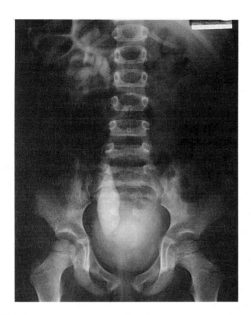

Figure 20.6 Intravenous urogram film showing congenital megaureter. Note the hydronephrosis and megaureter on the right side due to ureterovesical obstruction.

obstruction also affects boys more often than girls. It is often bilateral but one ureter is usually more severely affected than the other. Whilst the aetiology is uncertain, failure of transmission of peristalsis at the ureterovesical junction is believed to be the mechanism. Ultrastructural studies show an excess of collagen and elastin, as is the case with PUJ obstruction. Pain, haematuria and infection are the usual presenting symptoms. An IVU will show a dilated ureter with less dilatation proximally and blunting of the calyces. A diuretic renogram to confirm obstruction is indicated. Treatment consists of reimplantation of the ureter after excising the diseased distal portion.

• Ureteric strictures may occur after ureteroscopy and stone manipulation, pelvic surgery or irradiation for carcinoma of the prostate, cervix or bladder. Congenital idiopathic ureteric strictures are uncommon. Ureteric strictures may also occur with chronic inflammatory conditions such as genitourinary tuberculosis or schistosomiasis. The stricture usually affects the lower ureter. In tuberculosis stricture formation can occur during treatment if the affected area heals by fibrosis rather than resolution. The treatment of ureteric stricture depends on the site and cause. Lower ureteric strictures are best treated by reimplanting the ureter. Tuberculous strictures may be avoided by the use of ureteric stents during treatment. Short mid-ureter strictures may be treated by excision and anastomosis where possible or by swinging the proximal ureter over to the normal other side (transureteroureterostomy). Strictures in the proximal

third may require ileal loop interpositions or even renal autotransplantation if they cannot simply be treated by a pyeloplasty procedure.

• Ureteric tumours account for approximately 1% of all urothelial tumours and may present as ureteric pain with haematuria mimicking a stone. Diagnosis depends on urine for cytology and an IVU. Treatment consists of nephroureterectomy and regular follow-up cystoscopy, as recurrences in the bladder commonly occur. Ureteric obstruction may also result from ureterocele, which is a bulging dilatation of the submucosal portion of the ureter. If the ureteric orifice is stenosed, obstruction will occur with associated pain. Ureteroceles are usually unilateral but may be bilateral and they occur more frequently in girls. Ureteroceles more frequently affect ectopic ureters than normal ureters. Simple treatment involves transurethral resection (deroofing) of the bulging submucosa but if there is significant reflux then reimplantation may be required.

Extramural obstruction

• Vascular abnormalities such as aneurysms of the aorta or common iliac arteries may cause ureteric obstruction. Less common vascular causes include ovarian vein compression or retrocaval ureter.

• Pregnancy, third-degree uterine prolapse (complete procidentia) and endometriosis are also uncommon causes of extrinsic obstruction.

• Inflammatory or neoplastic disorders of the pelvic organs or retroperitoneum may also cause unilateral ureteric obstruction but more frequently involve both ureters.

Bilateral upper tract obstruction

The common causes of bilateral upper tract obstruction are listed in Table 20.8.

• Marked outflow obstruction due to BPH with bladder hypertrophy may obstruct both ureterovesical junctions, causing bilateral hydroureteronephrosis. Carcinoma of the prostate involving the trigone and bladder tumours involving the ureteric orifices may also cause bilateral ureteric obstruction.

Table 20.8 Causes of bilateral ureteric obstruction.

Bladder outflow obstruction
Pelvic tumours
Retroperitoneal tumours
Retroperitoneal fibrosis

• Tumours of the pelvis and retroperitoneum may also obstruct both ureters. Most tumours of the retroperitoneum are malignant and 70% of these tumours arise in the cervix, prostate, bladder, breast, colon, ovary or uterus. The remainder are primary retroperitoneal tumours such as lymphoma or sarcoma. Treatment is dictated by the underlying disease and prognosis. When treatment of the underlying tumour is feasible, the ureters may be reimplanted or urinary diversion may be considered. If the underlying tumour is untreatable, relief of the ureteric obstruction is not indicated.

• Retroperitoneal ureteric obstruction may also be due to retroperitoneal fibrosis. Retroperitoneal fibrosis is idiopathic in 70% of cases. Evidence suggests that in many cases of idiopathic retroperitoneal fibrosis the aetiology may be a fibrotic reaction to insoluble lipids which leak into the retroperitoneum from atheromatous plaques in the aorta. In approximately 30% of cases the retroperitoneal fibrosis is secondary to malignant disease of the retroperitoneum, irradiation-induced fibrosis or drugs such as methysergide or β-blockers. As the fibrotic plaque develops the ureters are pulled towards the midline and progressively obstructed. This may present as backache and gradual renal impairment. Hypertension and signs of distal venous occlusion are frequently associated features. The main causes of mortality in patients with idiopathic retroperitoneal fibrosis are hypertension and thromboembolic disease. Renal failure occurs in a small proportion of cases.

Men are affected more often than women and the disease usually presents in middle age. Laboratory investigation may reveal impaired renal function, anaemia and a raised ESR. An IVU will show deviation of the ureters towards the midline and hydronephrosis. A CT scan-guided biopsy of the plaque is necessary to rule out underlying malignancy. Initial treatment consists of relieving the obstruction by passing double-J stents or percutaneous nephrostomy. Once the patient is stable and underlying malignancy has been excluded, definitive surgical therapy may be undertaken. This involves a laparotomy to free the ureters from the fibrous plaque (ureterolysis), and wrapping of the ureters in omental tubes to prevent recurrence. Further biopsies of the plaque should be taken at surgery to exclude undiagnosed malignancy.

Urolithiasis

Introduction

The prevalence of urinary tract stones among Europeans is 3%, with an estimated incidence of new stone formation of between 45 and 80 per 100 000 of the population. Calculi are especially common in Europe, North America and Japan. A diet that is rich in refined carbohydrate and animal protein with a low intake of crude fibre is thought to predispose to stone formation. Urinary calculi are more common in people with sedentary occupations such as doctors. Urinary calculi usually present in early adult life and are more common in males. The exception to this statement is infective stones, which are more common in women, who are frequently middle-aged at the time of presentation.

The exact mechanism of stone formation is unclear and probably involves several mechanisms acting in concert.

• The nucleation theory proposes the presence of a crystal or foreign body which acts as the nucleus for deposition of further crystals in a urine which is supersaturated with crystallizing salts. These crystals may form on the basement membrane of the collecting tubules or the surface of the renal papillae or within the renal lymphatics.

• The stone matrix theory suggests that crystals forming in a supersaturated urine become embedded in a protein matrix secreted by the renal tubular cells. Such a matrix (matrix substance A) can be found in the urine of 85% of stone-forming patients.

• A third theory suggests that stone-forming patients have reduced urinary levels of naturally occurring inhibitors of crystallization such as glycoaminoglycans.

Some patients will have inherited renal diseases such as renal tubular acidosis, medullary sponge kidney and cystinuria which predispose them to stone formation. Other patients may suffer from inflammatory bowel disease, gout, prolonged immobilization or recurrent UTI. Certain medications such as acetazolamide, vitamin D and hydrochlorthiazide may predispose patients to stone formation. Excessive dietary calcium intake (dairy produce) may be responsible in some cases. However, in the majority of patients with urinary stones there are no associated predisposing causes but urine metabolic abnormalities can be identified in most patients. Of these, idiopathic hypercalciuria is the most common abnormality (65%), with urine infection (20%) an important second most frequent abnormality. Less common urine findings include hyperoxaluria, cystinuria and hyperuricosuria. Patients with hyperparathyroidism frequently develop urinary calculi.

Assessment of a patient presenting with urinary calculi should include a detailed history seeking evidence of familial renal disease, associated diseases and medications. Laboratory investigation should include a serum analysis of creatinine, urea, electrolytes, calcium and phosphates, urates, serum proteins (especially albumin) and alkaline phosphatase. Blood for serum calcium estimation should be taken after an overnight fast, with the patient resting and without a tourniquet. If hypercalcaemia is found, it should be confirmed on a second sample prior to sending blood for parathormone estimation. Urine microscopy for haematuria and crystals, as well as urine for culture, is a basic part of the initial assessment. Special kits are available to test for cystinuria. At least one 24-h urine collection should be performed, preferably when the patient is in his or her normal environment at home. Any stone passed by the patient, or removed surgically, should be tested for its constituents.

Radiological investigation is essential to confirm the diagnosis and aid management decisions. A plain abdominal film, which is the preliminary radiograph of an IVU, will reveal 90% of urinary calculi as they contain either calcium or cystine which are radiopaque. Approximately 70% of stones contain calcium oxalate or phosphate, whilst infective stones (20%) contain calcium, magnesium and ammonium phosphate, so-called triple-phosphate stones. The films taken after injection of contrast will confirm that the opacity seen on the plain film lies within the genitourinary tract and show what level the stone is at and whether or not it is causing obstruction. A radiolucent stone will appear as a filling defect but so will a tumour so that a CT scan may be needed to help in the differential diagnosis.

Diagnosis and management of urinary calculi

The management of urinary calculi depends on their site, size and the degree of trouble they are causing.

Renal and ureteric stones

Diagnosis

Renal stones may be situated in the calyces, renal pelvis or at the PUJ. Caliceal stones are usually asymptomatic and are found incidentally, but they may cause haematuria. Occasionally these stones may obstruct the infundibulum leading from the calyx to the pelvis, causing pain. A small stone in the renal pelvis may be asymptomatic or it may pass down the ureter causing ureteric colic. If the stone is too large to pass through the PUJ, it may cause obstruction with colic. Staghorn calculi are dealt with below.

Pain due to a stone at the PUJ, or in the ureter, is severe, colicky in nature and radiates from the groin towards the loin. The pain may radiate to the testis in males or the labium majus in females. Haematuria, gross or microscopic, is present in almost all patients with colic. If obstruction occurs and is complicated by infection, pyrexias and rigors will also be experienced. As the stone moves down the ureter, the site of pain follows the route of the stone. When the stone reaches the intramural ureter, trigonal irritation with frequency may be noted. Physical examination is usually non-contributory unless there is

gross hydronephrosis (palpable kidney) or pyelonephritis (tender kidney). Routine blood and urine testing, as described above, should be commenced. The IVU will confirm the diagnosis and reveal the size and site of the stone as well as the degree of obstruction.

Management

The first priority of management for a patient with renal or ureteric colic is pain relief. Traditionally pethidine was used but nausea, bradycardia and hypotension are unpleasant complications frequently associated with narcotic analgesics. Recent studies have shown that Voltarol is at least as effective with regard to pain relief and is not associated with unpleasant side-effects. Traditionally a high fluid intake has been advised but the value of this measure is questionable. Patients with stones in the ureter can be managed expectantly in the first instance for as many as 80% of these stones will pass, usually within the first 48 h. The indications for intervention include failure of conservative management, obstruction and infection. The size and site of the stone help in predicting the outcome of conservative management. The higher and the larger the stone, the less the likelihood of passage. Stones less than 4 mm diameter almost always pass. Stones 4–6 mm are more likely to pass if situated in the lower ureter, whilst stones greater than 6 mm are unlikely to pass. Renal stones causing pain or obstruction of the PUJ also require intervention (Table 20.9).

Interventional techniques

Renal stones
- *Extracorporeal shock-wave lithotripsy* (ESWL) is a technique whereby shock waves generated outside the body are focused on stones within the body; repeated application of

Table 20.9 Indications for intervention in a patient with a urinary calculus.

Site of stone	Indication for intervention
Kidney	Symptomatic (pain, haematuria) Obstruction (PUJ) Staghorn
Ureter	Failure to pass Large stones Obstruction Infection
Bladder	All stones

PUJ, Pelviureteric junction.

shock energy to a stone causes internal stress in the stone, leading to stone fragmentation. The fragments are then passed in the urine. Shock waves generated by a spark gap, piezoelectric crystals or an electromagnetic field are focused on the stone, which is localized in the kidney by fluoroscopy or ultrasound (Fig. 20.7). For renal stones greater than 2 cm

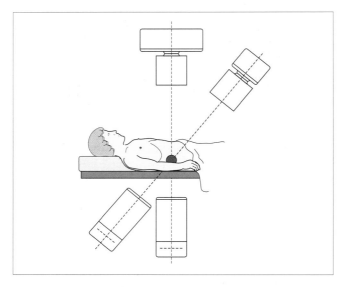

Figure 20.7 Diagram of a lithotriptor. A shock wave, generated outside the body (extracorporeal), is focused on the stone in the kidney. Repeated shocks cause the stone to disintegrate (lithotripsy), hence extracorporeal shock-wave lithotripsy (ESWL).

in size it is advisable to insert a double-pigtail ureteric stent to prevent larger fragments obstructing the ureter (Fig. 20.8). Almost all patients have haematuria after ESWL. Some patients experience colic, which may be due to fragments obstructing the ureter (steinstrasse; Fig. 20.9), and patients should be warned to return to hospital immediately if colic develops. Stone clearance rates of 95% have been reported for stones up to 2 cm in diameter. Larger stones may require multiple treatments.

• For stones that fail to break or are considered too large, a *percutaneous nephrolithotomy* may be considered. In this technique a guidewire is placed percutaneously into the renal pelvis and the tract is dilated to accommodate a nephroscope. The stone can be grasped with a forceps and extracted or, if too large, it may be fragmented using an ultrasonic lithotrite and the fragments extracted. The kidney is drained with a nephrostomy tube postoperatively for 48 h. If the patient is stone-free and a nephrostogram shows normal drainage down the ureter, the tube may be removed. Admission and general anaesthesia are required and blood should be available, as marked bleeding occasionally occurs.

• If these modalities fail, then one must resort to conventional surgery. The kidney is exposed through a loin incision and the stone is removed through an incision in the renal pelvis (pyelolithotomy).

Ureteric stones
• *ESWL*: Lithotriptors that localize stones by fluoroscopy may be used to treat ureteric calculi. For those machines

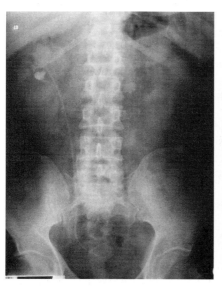

(a)

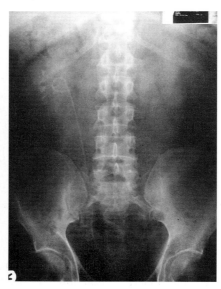

(b)

Figure 20.8 (a) A double-J stent has been placed into the right ureter prior to extracorporeal shock-wave lithotripsy (ESWL). (b) The stone has completely fragmented following one treatment with ESWL (approximately 1500 shocks in this case).

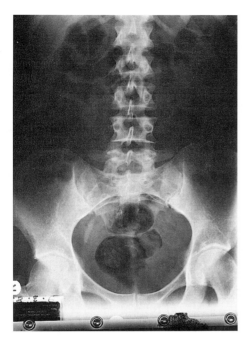

Figure 20.9 Following extracorporeal shock-wave lithotripsy (ESWL), stone fragments occasionally accumulate in the lower ureter, producing a steinstrasse. In this patient the steinstrasse is in the right lower ureter.

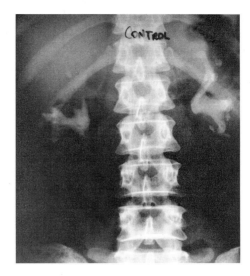

Figure 20.10 Plain film showing staghorn calculi.

depending on ultrasound for localization it is necessary to push the stone back to the kidney ureteroscopically before starting lithotripsy. Stones that lie over the bony pelvis or vertebral transverse processes on the radiograph are not suitable as they cannot be localized on fluoroscopy. Stones in the upper ureter can be cleared in 80% of cases with ESWL whilst stones in the lower ureter can be cleared in 70% of cases. Once again, colic may occur and may require endoscopic intervention.

• *Endoscopy*: If ESWL is unavailable or the stone is not suitable because of its position, endoscopy is required. For stones in the ureter above the pelvic brim two options are available. The stone may be pushed back to the renal pelvis, a double-J stent inserted and the patient referred for lithotripsy. Alternatively, the stone may be disintegrated *in situ* using an ultrasonic or electrohydraulic lithotrite passed up the ureteroscope.

For stones in the lower ureter the ureteroscope may be passed and the stone snared in a basket and gently removed down the ureter under direct vision. Alternatively, *in situ* disintegration using ultrasonic or electrohydraulic lithotripsy may be used. For smaller stones within a short distance of the ureteric orifice, a basket (dormia basket) may be passed, via a cystoscope, blindly up the ureter, attempting to ensnare and remove the stone. If these

options fail, then open surgery (ureterolithotomy) is required. This is necessary in less than 5% of cases.

Staghorn calculi

These are so called because the outline on the abdominal radiograph resembles a stag's horn (Fig. 20.10). They may be complete or incomplete. A complete staghorn fills the renal pelvis and collecting system whilst an incomplete staghorn calculus fills the pelvis and one or two of the calyces. These stones are triple-phosphate (calcium, ammonium, magnesium phosphate) stones of infective origin. Women are infected more often than men. These stones are formed by the action of bacteria (*Proteus*, *Klebsiella*) which produce an enzyme (urease) which splits urea to form ammonium ions, thereby rendering the urine alkaline. The bacteria are found within the interstices of the stone crystals and therefore the infection is very difficult to eradicate. Because of persistent infection the recurrence rate is very high. Pain is unusual but loin ache may be present. Recurrent infection (pyelonephritis) is the usual presentation. Diagnosis is obvious from a plain abdominal radiograph. However, as renal damage can frequently occur from recurrent infections and obstruction by the stone mass, an IVU and renogram should be performed.

Management

If the stone is unilateral and the renogram shows very poor function, a nephrectomy is the best option. However, if the disease is bilateral, then nephrectomy should be avoided. In this instance the poorer of the two kidneys is treated first and its function reassessed before treating the other kidney. If the kidney function is reasonable in a patient with a staghorn calculus, every effort should be made to make the patient stone-free whilst conserving the remaining functioning renal tissue.

- *ESWL*: Because of the stone size, there is a risk of ureteric obstruction from large fragments so that a double-J stent should be passed prior to commencing lithotripsy. The results with lithotripsy are disappointing, with an overall clearance rate of 45–50%. Better results can be anticipated with incomplete staghorn calculi. Multiple treatment sessions are the rule. For these reasons ESWL is not the optimum treatment for staghorn calculi.
- *Percutaneous nephrolithotomy*: The stone may be fragmented using an ultrasonic lithotrite passed through the nephroscope. Because the nephroscope is a rigid instrument it is often difficult to fragment and remove all the caliceal fragments. Fragments remaining after percutaneous nephrostomy may be dealt with by ESWL. Thus percutaneous nephrostomy is used to debulk the stone and ESWL to deal with residual fragments. Using this combined approach an 80% clearance rate has been reported.
- *Nephrolithotomy*: For complete staghorn calculi open surgical removal remains the best option. Two operative techniques are vigorously recommended by their proponents. Pyelolithotomy with radial nephrostomies is a technique where the pelvic portion of the stone is removed through an incision in the renal pelvis (pyelolithotomy) and the caliceal fragments are removed through numerous small incisions over the individual calyces (nephrotomies). The alternative approach is the anatrophic nephrolithotomy, where the kidney is bisected along its convex border in the avascular plane between the intersegmental arteries. After each technique, on-table radiographs are required to ensure stone clearance prior to closure of the incisions in the pelvis and parenchyma. Both of these procedures required a bloodless field: therefore, the renal artery must be isolated and clamped before stone removal.

The kidney is very sensitive to ischaemia, so measures must be taken to protect it during the ischaemic period. Hypothermia decreases the cellular metabolic rate greatly, increasing the period of ischaemia before functional or structural injury occurs. However, adequate constant hypothermia is difficult to achieve and the cooling device may impede access to the kidney. As an alternative, pharmacological agents have been used to minimize the ischaemic insult. Of these, inosine, a purine nucleotide administered prior to clamping, is the most successful, allowing renal artery clamping for up to 1 h without significant renal injury. Regular follow-up is required because of the high rate of recurrence. Ascorbic acid 200 mg three times daily may be given to acidify the urine. Low-dose suppressive antibiotics may also be used.

Bladder calculi

Whilst the incidence of renal calculi is increasing worldwide, the incidence of bladder calculi is diminishing, except in those areas where schistosomiasis is endemic. Some bladder calculi were originally renal calculi which have lodged and enlarged in the bladder. Most bladder calculi originate in the bladder. Bladder calculi usually result from bladder outflow obstruction but can occur due to the presence of foreign bodies in the bladder, such as urethral catheters. Bladder calculi may also form in diverticula. Patients with neuropathic atonic bladders may also develop bladder calculi.

Coexistent UTI is common and may give rise to dysuria, frequency and haematuria. In patients with bladder outflow obstruction, nocturia, hesitancy and poor flow will also be present. The classical symptom ascribed to a bladder calculus is a sudden cessation of flow with pain in the perineum and tip of the penis. This is due to the stone obstructing the bladder neck on voiding. Diagnosis may be clinched on the plain film when an opacity is noted in the bladder. However, if the opacity is poorly calcified it may not be seen on the preliminary picture. An IVU will show a filling defect in the bladder with the stigmata of outflow obstruction — detrusor hypertrophy, diverticula (possibly), a raised bladder base and residual urine. Treatment consists of removal of the stone and relief of the underlying cause. Most bladder calculi may be dealt with endoscopically but very large stones will require open surgery (cysto-lithotomy). Endoscopic removal involves passage of a lithotrite via the urethra to crush the stone and evacuate the fragments.

Management of recurrent stone disease

Patients with recurrent stone disease require a more in-depth evaluation in conjunction with a metabolic physician to determine predisposing abnormalities. Based on the findings of these investigations, dietary manipulation and medications may be used to lessen the chance of further recurrence (Table 20.10).

Table 20.10 Management of patients with recurrent urinary stone disease.

Diagnosis and possible treatments

Idiopathic hypercalciuria
Low-calcium diet
Vegetable bran to bind calcium in the intestine
Orthophosphates to decrease urinary crystallization
Thiazide diuretics
High fluid intake to dilute supersaturated urine

Uric acid stones
Allopurinol
Urinary alkalinization using oral sodium bicarbonate
High fluid intake

Cystine stones
Penicillamine to decrease urinary cystine excretion
Alkalinization of urine with oral sodium bicarbonate
High fluid intake
Dietary restriction of methionine intake

Infective stones
Urinary acidification with ascorbic acid
Low-dose suppressive antibiotics

Oxalate stones
High fluid intake
Pyridoxine
Dietary restriction (chocolate, tea, cola, spinach)

Renal tubular acidosis
Urinary alkalinization

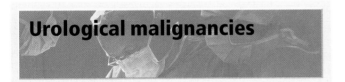

Urological malignancies

Malignancy may develop in almost any part of the urinogenital tract and a variety of tumours, including adenocarcinoma (e.g. renal carcinoma), transitional cell carcinomas (e.g. bladder carcinoma) and germ cell tumours (e.g. testicular seminomas and teratomas) may develop. Nephroblastomas (Wilms' tumour) are developmental tumours that are found in infancy or early childhood. The commonest tumours of the urinary tract are transitional cell carcinomas of the bladder and the management of these malignancies accounts for a considerable amount of urological practice.

Renal carcinoma

Incidence

Renal carcinoma (also previously called hypernephroma and Grawitz tumour) is commoner in males over the age of 40 years. It accounts for 2–3% of all tumours in adults and 85% of all renal tumours. It is the ninth commonest tumour in white adult males. The other renal tumours which can occur in adults are:
- urothelial tumours;
- adult Wilms' tumours; and
- sarcomas.

Aetiology

The cause of renal carcinoma is unknown. A large amount of work has been carried out and a number of factors which are associated with an increased incidence of the disease have been isolated.
- *Diet*: A high consumption of fat, oils and milk has been associated with an increased incidence of renal carcinoma.
- *Toxic agents*: Exposure to lead, cadmium, asbestos and petroleum byproducts have been implicated. There is a marked increase in renal carcinoma in smokers, but the reason for this association is uncertain.
- *Genetic factors*: Oncogene localization to the short arm of chromosome 3 and human leukocyte antigen (HLA) antigen types BW-44 and DR-8 has also been thought to be related to the cause of renal carcinoma.
- *Associated diseases*: There is an association between renal carcinoma and
    (a) von Hippel–Lindau syndrome;
    (b) adult polycystic renal disease (Fig. 20.11); and
    (c) acquired renal cystic disease from chronic renal failure.

Pathology

The preferred name for the condition is renal cell carcinoma. Many other less satisfactory names have been used, such as hypernephroma and Grawitz tumour, but these are no longer recommended. The tumour is an adenocarcinoma, with the cell of origin being the proximal convoluted tubular cell. Previously, well-differentiated tumours measuring less than 3 cm in diameter were given the name of renal adenomas, but subclassifying renal tumours on the basis of size is no longer considered acceptable. It is impossible to differentiate histologically the smaller tumours from the larger ones, and so the term renal

Renal calculi at a glance

DEFINITION

Renal stones are concretions formed by precipitation of various urinary solutes in the urinary tract. They contain *calcium oxalate* (60%), a mixture of *calcium, ammonium* and *magnesium phosphate* (triple-phosphate stones are infective in origin; 30%), *uric acid* (5%) and *cystine* (1%)

EPIDEMIOLOGY

M>F   Age: early adult life. Among Europeans, prevalence is 3%

PATHOGENESIS

- *Hypercalciuria*: 65% of patients have idiopathic hypercalciuria
- *Nucleation theory*: a crystal of foreign body acts as a nucleus for crystallization of supersaturated urine
- *Stone matrix theory*: a protein matrix secreted by renal tubular cells acts as a scaffold for crystallization of supersaturated urine
- *Reduced inhibition theory*: reduced urinary levels of naturally occurring inhibitors of crystallization e.g. glycoaminoglycons
- *Infection*: staghorn triple-phosphate calculi are formed by the action of urease-producing organisms (*Proteus, Klebsiella*) which produce ammonia and render the urine alkaline. *Schistosomiasis* predisposes to bladder calculi (and cancer)

PATHOLOGY

- Staghorn calculi are large, fill the renal pelvis and calyces and lead to recurring pyelonephritis and renal parenchymal damage
- Other stones are smaller, ranging in size from a few millimetres to 1–2 cm. They cause problems by obstructing the urinary tract, usually the ureter. Caliceal stones may cause haematuria and bladder stones may cause infection. Chronic bladder stones predispose to the unusual squamous carcinoma of the bladder

CLINICAL FEATURES

- Caliceal stones may be asymptomatic
- Staghorn calculi present with loin pain and upper tract UTI
- Ureteric colic: severe colicky pain radiating from the loin to the groin and into the testes or labia associated with gross or microscopic haematuria
- Bladder calculi present with sudden interruption of urinary stream, perineal pain and pain at the tip of the penis

INVESTIGATIONS

- FBC, U&E, serum creatine, calcium, phosphate, urate, proteins and alkaline phosphatase
- Urine microscopy for haematuria and crystals
- Urine culture
- Plain abdominal X-ray; 90% of renal calculi are radiopaque
- IVU confirms the presence and identifies the position of the stone in the genitourinary tract
- A renogram may be indicated with staghorn calculi to assess renal function
- 24-h urine collection when patient is home in normal environment
- Stone analysis

MANAGEMENT

- Pain relief for ureteric colic — pethidine, Voltarol. High fluid intake
- 80% of ureteric stones pass spontaneously. Stones of <4 mm in diameter almost always pass, >6 mm almost never
- Indications for intervention:
  (a) Kidney stones: symptomatic, obstruction, staghorn
  (b) Ureteric stones: failure to pass, large stone, obstruction, infection
  (c) Bladder: all stones

INTERVENTIONAL PROCEDURES

- Extracorporeal shock-wave lithotripsy (ESWL) for small/medium kidney stones
- Percutaneous nephrolithotomy for large kidney stones and staghorn calculi
- ESWL or contact lithotripsy for upper ureteric stones (above pelvic brim)
- Contact lithotripsy or extraction with a dormia basket for lower ureteric stones
- Open surgery: ureterolithotomy or nephrolithotomy
- Mechanical lithotripsy or open surgery for bladder stones

---

adenoma should no longer be used. The tumours are grossly orange or yellow, because of the high lipid content. Histologically, there are four subtypes:
- clear cell;
- granular cell;
- sarcomatoid cells; and
- oncocytoma.

Renal carcinoma may spread locally into the renal vein, extending as high as the right atrium in some cases. It may also spread through the pseudocapsule which surrounds the tumour. The tumour may metastasize to lymph nodes, most commonly the hilar nodes and the interaortocaval nodes. Distant visceral metastases may occur, most commonly to the lung (50–60%) and bone (30–40%), with the contralateral kidney being involved in 2% of cases. Bones which are involved most commonly are the vertebrae and ribs.

Staging

A number of staging methods exist and the most commonly used in Europe is the TMN classification. This is wide-based, but to describe fully the tumour it must be divided

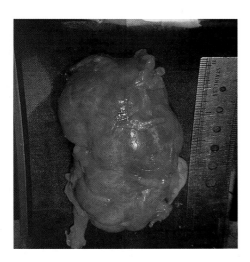

Figure 20.11 A polycystic kidney.

into five sublevels, in addition to a pre- and postsurgical classification. The basic T classification is as follows:

- T1: Small tumour with renal enlargement;
- T2: Large tumour with renal deformity;
- T3: Spread into perinephric fat or hilum;
- T4: Invasion of adjacent organs or abdominal wall.

The original staging system of Flocks and Kadesky, which was introduced in the USA in 1958, is still satisfactory, and in some ways preferable:

- Stage 1: Tumour confined to the kidney;
- Stage II: Tumour extends through capsule;
- Stage III: Tumour extends into renal vein or spreads to lymph nodes, or through Gerota's fascia;
- Stage IV: Distant metastases or invasion of adjacent organs.

Clinical features

Renal carcinoma is well-known for its association with many different symptoms and signs. There is a classic triad of haematuria, flank pain and a palpable mass, but these three features are only seen together in a small percentage of cases. Individually they constitute the commonest methods of presentation of renal carcinoma:

- haematuria in 50–60%;
- flank pain in 35–40%; and
- abdominal mass in 25–45%.

Renal carcinoma may also present in a number of different ways which indirectly point to the diagnosis. The effects of malignancy, e.g. anaemia, weight loss, pyrexia of unknown origin or ESR, or a combination of these, may indicate an underlying renal tumour. Renal carcinoma may also present with endocrine effects such as hypertension or erythrocytosis. Hypercalcaemia, or elevation of adrenocorticotrophic hormone (ACTH), antidiuretic hormone (ADH), prolactin, gonadotrophins, insulin or glucagon are much less common.

In 10% of patients, hepatic dysfunction (e.g. raised alkaline phosphatase, γ-glutamyl transferase, bilirubin and prolonged prothrombin time) may be present even in the absence of metastatic disease. Sometimes this tumour may present with evidence of widespread disease or a left-sided varicocele may be present due to left renal vein spread which blocks the insertion of the gonadal vein. Haemoptysis, with or without a pleural effusion, may indicate pulmonary metastases, and pain in the posterior region of the chest or the lumbar area of the back should suggest that bony deposits may be present.

Investigations

Routine blood and urine investigations should be performed. It is essential that these be used not only to help in diagnosis, but also as a preoperative baseline so that all postoperative events may be viewed with this in mind. They are also important as these patients are often sick and anaemic before surgery and will therefore need careful preoperative management. The liver function tests may on occasion be abnormal, even in the absence of metastatic disease, but this can be suggestive of a poor prognosis. Imaging of the kidneys must be performed. On some occasions the lesion is discovered routinely on upper abdominal ultrasound. In this instance, not only must the lesion be imaged carefully, but also the opposite normal kidney must be shown to be present and functioning. It is sufficient to proceed to a CT scan in which intravenous contrast has been administered (Fig. 20.12). This will enhance

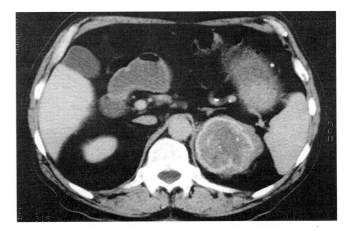

Figure 20.12 Computed tomography scan showing left renal tumour.

both kidneys in the form of a step-section IVU. The CT scan will show the size of the mass, its fixity to adjacent organs, the presence of enlarged lymph nodes, and may give an indication as to whether there is renal vein and/or vena caval involvement. An IVU may be required by some clinicians, who prefer to see the kidneys imaged antero-posteriorly rather than longitudinally.

The inferior vena cava may also be imaged by ultrasound or by a vena cavogram which is performed transfemorally if there is a suspicion of vena caval extension of the tumour. In cases where vena caval extension of the tumour throm-bus has gone as far as the right atrium, echocardiography may be required.

Management

Radical surgery offers the best chance for patients with renal carcinoma. This entails removal of the affected kidney and upper ureter with the renal vessels in addition to the adrenal gland and Gerota's fascia. Control of the vessels should be gained as early as possible in the operation, prior to excessive handling of the tumour. The kidney may be ap-proached from the front, the loin, or through the chest. If wide exposure is required for large masses, the trans-thoracic approach is the most satisfactory.

Management of metastases

A number of strategies are available for the management of metastatic renal carcinoma:

• *Surgery*: In patients with a single pulmonary metastasis, radical nephrectomy may be performed at the same time as re-section of the metastasis (for example, a pulmonary metasta-sis). If several metastases are present at the time of diagnosis it is probably unjustified to perform a radical nephrectomy. It could only be justified if the patient is in danger of bleeding to death (a very unusual situation) or if some form of adjuvant chemotherapy or immunotherapy is proposed.

The question of spontaneous regression of metastases after surgery has been raised on a number of occasions. The reported incidence of spontaneous regression is only 0.5%, but some clinicians believe that it is potentially higher. This is a very debatable point, and current clinical judgement would suggest that spontaneous regression after surgery is not a justification for radical surgery.

• *Renal artery embolization*: This does not have a role in the routine management of renal carcinoma but it would seem to be a valuable alternative to surgery for the primary lesion in patients who have multiple metastases, and who may also be bleeding from their tumour. It is performed under X-ray control through a transfemoral arterial catheter which is passed into the renal artery, and

through which gel-foam, gelatine sponge, steel springs or autologous blood clot are injected.

• *Chemotherapy*: Chemotherapy has been unsuccessful in the management of renal carcinoma. Many single-agent regimens and combinations have been used, but none has shown more than a 10–16% response rate.

• *Hormone therapy*: The stimulus for the use of hormones in metastatic renal cell carcinoma was generated by the introduction of Provera, which was reported as having a 5–10% response rate. Other hormonal agents have been introduced but none has been of significant success.

• *Immunotherapy*: It is in this area that the most exciting possibilities exist. The following methods of immunother-apy are available:

   (a) interferon;
   (b) lymphokine-activated killer (LAK) cells;
   (c) tumour-infiltrating lymphocytes (TILS).

These methods of treatment are currently under evalu-ation and are encouraging in their early response rates. They are associated with a high morbidity, and this of ne-cessity means that their use is confined to specialized units.

Nephroblastoma (Wilms' tumour)

Nephroblastoma is a malignant mixed renal tumour that occurs predominantly in children and usually appears at about 3 years of age. Approximately one-third are heredit-ary. The tumours are usually solitary, soft, lobulated and tan or gray in colour. Histologically they are made up of a mixture of epithelial, stromal and immature mesenchymal elements. Direct spread via capsular invasion occurs and the tumour also metastasizes via lymphatics and the renal vein. The lung is the commonest site for metastases.

The tumour may present with pain but many are detected serendipitiously during a well-baby examination. An abdominal mass is the usual physical finding. Ultra-sonography and enhanced CT scanning support the diag-nosis and treatment is a combination of surgery, radiotherapy and chemotherapy. The outlook for patients with Wilms' tumour has improved remarkably in recent years and an 80% cure rate can now be achieved with combination therapy.

Tumours of the renal pelvis and ureter

Incidence

These tumours are uncommon. Transitional cell tumours of the renal pelvis account for only 7% of all renal tumours,

Renal cell carcinoma at a glance

DEFINITION

Malignant lesion (*adenocarcinoma*) of the kidney (also known as *hypernephroma* and *Grawitz tumour*)

EPIDEMIOLOGY

M/F = 2 : 1 Uncommon before age 40 Accounts for 2–3% of all tumours in adults and 85% of all renal tumours. (The other renal tumours are urothelial tumours, Wilms' tumour and sarcomas)

AETIOLOGY

Predisposing factors
- *Diet*: high intake of fat, oil and milk
- *Toxic agents*: lead, cadmium, asbestos, petroleum byproducts
- *Smoking*
- *Genetic factors*: oncogene on short arm of chromosome 3; human leukocyte antigen BW-44 and DR-8
- *Other diseases*: von Hippel–Lindau syndrome, adult polycystic disease

PATHOLOGY

Histology
Adenocarcinoma (cell of origin is the proximal convoluted tubular cell)

Staging
- TNM staging
- Flocks and Kadesky stages I–IV
  - (a) Stage I: Tumour confined to kidney
  - (b) Stage II: Tumour extends through capsule
  - (c) Stage III: Tumour to renal vein, nodes or through Gerota's fascia
  - (d) Stage IV: Distant metastases or invasion of adjacent organs

Spread
Direct into renal vein and perirenal tissue
Lymphatic to periaortic and hilar nodes
Haematogenous to lung, bone and contralateral kidney

CLINICAL FEATURES

- Triad of haematuria (50–60%), flank pain (35–40%), palpable abdominal mass (25–45%). All three are present in <10% of patients
- Anaemia, weight loss, pyrexia of unknown origin (PUO)
- Hypertension, erythrocytosis
- Hypercalcaemia, ectopic hormone production (ACTH, ADH)
- Liver dysfunction (raised enzymes and prolonged PT) in the absence of metastatic disease
- Renal carcinoma is one of the 'great mimics' of medicine

INVESTIGATIONS

- FBC, ESR, U&E, liver function test (LFT)
- Urine culture
- Abdominal ultrasound: assess renal mass and IVC
- Contrast-enhanced CT scan: assess renal mass, fixity, nodes
- Intravenous urogram: image renal outline
- Cavogram and echocardiogram: assess IVC and right atrium

MANAGEMENT

Surgery
- Offers best chance for patients with renal carcinoma
- Remove kidney, renal vessels, upper ureter, adrenal and Gerota's fascia
- Isolated lung metastases should also be removed surgically

Palliation
- Renal artery embolization (may stop haematuria)
- Chemotherapy (only 10% response rate)
- Hormone therapy (only 5% response rate)
- Immunotherapy (currently under review)

PROGNOSIS

Overall survival is 40% at 5 years

---

and tumours of the ureter and renal pelvis account for only 2–4% of all transitional cell tumours of the urothelium. Patients who develop a transitional cell carcinoma of the pelvis or ureter have a 30–50% chance of developing a transitional cell tumour of the bladder in the future. The presence of a transitional cell carcinoma of the bladder is associated with only a 2–3% chance of future development of a tumour in the upper urinary tract.

Aetiology

The exact cause of transitional cell tumours of the renal pelvis and ureter is uncertain, but a number of aetiological factors have been isolated:

- Balkan nephropathy;
- analgesic nephropathy;
- inflammation and infection; and
- cigarette smoking.

Clinical features

The most common presenting symptom is painless intermittent haematuria. Other patients may present with clot colic, loin pain, anorexia and weight loss. These tumours may be found incidentally in up to 10% of patients. Physical examination may be unhelpful, with an abdominal mass palpable in only 5% of patients.

Investigations

The following investigations may be helpful in establishing the diagnosis:
- urine cytology;
- IVU;
- ultrasonography;
- retrograde ureterography;
- antegrade pyelography;
- CT scan;
- chest X-ray;
- cystoscopy; and
- ureteroscopy.

Management

Patients with tumours of the renal pelvis or ureter should be managed by nephroureterectomy and partial cystectomy. In the presence of lymph node metastases, the same chemotherapy as is given for bladder cancer is helpful.

Carcinoma of the bladder

Incidence

Carcinoma of the bladder is usually not seen before the age of 50 years. The incidence begins to rise in the fifth decade and continues thereafter. Over the last number of years in the UK there has been an increase every year in the incidence of bladder cancer and the death rate from bladder cancer is 7.6 per 100 000.

Aetiology

Transitional cell carcinoma is the commonest type of bladder cancer in the western world, and is known to be associated with certain types of occupation. Urothelial carcinogens have been related to the chemical rubber and cable industries, in addition to sewage and gas works and rodent extermination. The agents which are believed to be responsible are:
- 1 and 2-naphthylamine;
- benzidine;
- amino biphenyl.

Other aetiological agents in the genesis of bladder cancer are smoking, tryptophan metabolites and phenacetin. In areas where schistosomiasis is endemic, squamous cell carcinoma of the bladder occurs frequently. In other parts of the world, squamous cell carcinoma is uncommon and may result from prolonged irritation by infection or stones. Adenocarcinoma of the bladder may occur but is very

Table 20.11 Staging of bladder tumours.

	TIS	Carcinoma-*in-situ*
Superficial tumours	Ta	Tumour confined to the urothelium
	T1	Involvement of the lamina propria
Invasive tumours	T2	Superficial muscle invasion
	T3a	Deep muscle invasion
	T3b	Serosal involvement
Fixed tumours	T4a	Invasion of prostate, uterus or vagina
	T4b	Fixation to pelvic wall

uncommon. It virtually always develops in a urachal remnant at the dome of the bladder.

Pathology

In the UK, by far the commonest type of bladder tumour is the transitional cell carcinoma, with sqamous cell carcinoma and adenocarcinoma being very uncommon. Transitional cell carcinoma may be divided into three types, which aids in staging (Table 20.11):

Carcinoma-*in-situ*

Malignant changes take place in transitional cells with no involvement of the deeper layers. These malignant changes are subtle, comprising loss of polarity and increased pleomorphism, and are sometimes difficult to distinguish from severe dysplasia of the bladder. It is a very important condition as up to 60% of patients with flat carcinoma-*in-situ* may subsequently develop invasive bladder cancer.

Superficial bladder cancer

This term is applied to papillary tumours which have remained confined to the urothelial layer (Ta) and to tumours that have penetrated the basement membrane into the lamina propria (T1). Although the latter are classified as being superficial, they have an increased tendency to recur and to become truly invasive.

Invasive bladder cancer

These are most often solid, although on some occasions they have papillary areas. The tumour invades muscle either superficially (T2) or deeply (T3a) or through the wall to invade the serosa (T3b). It may also invade prostate, uterus or vaginal wall (T4A), or be fixed to the wall of the pelvis (T4b). Metastases occur in the internal iliac lymph nodes and then spread to the para-aortic lymph nodes. More

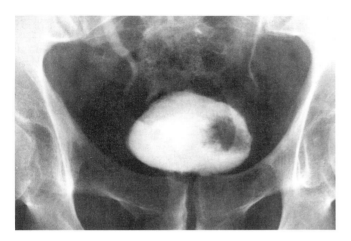

Figure 20.13 Intravenous urogram film showing bladder-filling defect secondary to bladder tumour in the left side of the bladder.

distant spread may occur to the liver, lungs and, less commonly, the brain. Local spread may occlude one or both of the ureters, leading to uraemia. Not only is the stage of the tumour important but also the grade. Tumours are graded from 1 to 3. Higher-grade tumours (grade 3 or poorly differentiated) have a worse prognosis than well-differentiated tumours (grade 1).

Clinical features

The commonest symptom of bladder carcinoma is painless intermittent haematuria; it is present in up to 95% of patients. In addition, 20% of patients with bladder cancer may have dysuria or frequency without haematuria. Microscopic haematuria is of significance if there is in excess of 8 red cells per high-power field; 10% of patients with asymptomatic microscopic haematuria have been found to have bladder carcinoma.

Investigations

The essential investigations are:
- IVU (Fig. 20.13);
- cystourethroscopy; and
- urine cytology.

If a superficial papillary tumour is found, the resected specimen and multiple random bladder biopsies should be sent for histology. If an invasive tumour is found and surgery is contemplated, a chest X-ray and CT scan of the abdomen and pelvis will be required. Transvesical ultrasound may be helpful in assessing depth of invasion, but deep resection of the tumours will be required to confirm this histologically.

Management

The treatment of bladder cancer is dictated by the stage of the tumour.

Superficial tumours (Ta, T1)

Initial treatment is by transurethral resection of the tumour and follow-up cystoscopy. Regular cystoscopic examination should be performed when following up these patients and it is recommended at every 3 months for the first year, every 6 months for the second year, and every year thereafter. If a recurrence develops, the follow-up schedule should begin again. The overall incidence of recurrences is in the region of 50–60% and the development of invasion is low. In some patients, risk factors exist for both recurrence and invasion. These are smoking, the presence of large tumours, multiple tumours, severe dysplasia or carcinoma-*in-situ* in random biopsies and high-grade superficial tumours. In any patient who is in the high-risk category, or who has had a number of recurrences, treatment with intravesical chemotherapy should be considered. Several agents, including Thiotepa, Epodyl, Adriamycin, Mitomycin C and BCG, have been used. These agents are given as once-weekly intravesical installations for 6 weeks. All have been shown to decrease the incidence of recurrence in different groups of patients.

Invasive tumours (T2, T3)

When muscle has been invaded, local treatment by transurethral resection must be supplemented by a more radical form of treatment. In carefully selected patients, particularly those with small tumours on the dome, partial cystectomy may be indicated, but most urologists would consider either radical radiotherapy or radical surgery.
- Radical radiotherapy gives a 35–40% 5-year survival rate and leaves the patient with the bladder and without an appliance. The disadvantage is that troublesome symptoms of radiation cystitis and proctitis may occur. If the patient fails to respond to radiotherapy, savage cystectomy may be difficult and associated with significant morbidity.
- Radical cystectomy is also associated with a 35–40% 5-year survival rate in patients with T3 tumours. Up until recently, a urinary diversion such as an ileal conduit has been required in these patients. At the present time some form of continent urinary diversion with the patient self-catheterizing the stoma and not requiring an appliance, or a bladder substitution procedure has become popular. Preoperative radiotherapy, either 20 Gy over 2 weeks immediately prior to surgery or 40 Gy over a 1-month period prior to surgery has been popular, but long-term

follow-up has not been as encouraging as original reports. Preoperative neoadjuvant chemotherapy, using one of the regimens listed below, is now thought to provide a higher 5-year survival rate, but is still under evaluation.

Fixed and metastatic tumours

Patients in whom the bladder tumour is fixed to either organs or the pelvic side wall, or in whom metastases to lymph nodes or distant viscera have developed, have a short life expectancy. In recent times three chemotherapeutic regimens have been introduced, and early results have encouraged clinicians to evaluate their use in advanced disease:
- MVAC: This consists of methotrexate followed by three courses of vinblastine, Adriamycin and cis-platin.
- CMV: Three to four cycles of cis-platin, methotrexate and vinblastine.
- Cisca: Cycles of cis-platin, cyclophosphamide and Adriamycin.

Carcinoma of the bladder at a glance

DEFINITION

Malignant lesion bladder

EPIDEMIOLOGY

M>F   Uncommon before age 50. Increasing incidence of bladder cancer in recent years. Death rate is 7.6/100 000

AETIOLOGY

Predisposing factors
- Exposure to carcinogens in rubber industry (1 and 2 naphthylamine, benzidine, amino biphenyl)
- Smoking, tryptophan metabolites, phenacetin
- Schistosomiasis and bladder stones

PATHOLOGY

Histology
Transitional cell carcinoma (TCC)
Squamous cell carcinoma ⎫
Adenocarcinoma   ⎬ rare

Staging for TCC

	TIS	Carcinoma-*in-situ*
• Superficial tumours	Ta	Tumour confined to urothelium
	T1	Lamina propria involved
• Invasive tumours	T2	Superficial muscle invasion
	T3a	Deep muscle invasion
	T3b	Serosal involvement
• Fixed tumours	T4a	Invasion of prostate, uterus or vagina
	T4b	Fixation to pelvic wall

Spread
Direct into pelvic viscera (prostate, uterus, vagina, colon, rectum)
Lymphatic to periaortic nodes
Haematogenous to liver and lung

CLINICAL FEATURES

- Painless intermittent haematuria (95%)
- Dysuria or frequency (10%)

INVESTIGATIONS

- Urine cytology
- Intravenous urography
- Cystourethroscopy
- FBC, U&E, creatinine
- Ultrasound
- CT scan

MANAGEMENT

Superficial tumours (Ta, T1)
- Depends on stage of tumour
- Transurethral resection of tumour (TURT) and follow-up cystoscopy
- If recurrences or increased risk of invasion (large tumours, multiple tumours, severe dysplasia or carcinoma-*in-situ*), intravesical chemotherapy (Thiotepa, Epodyl, Adriamycin, Mitomycin C, BCG)

Invasive tumours (T2, T3)
- TURT + radical radiotherapy or
- Radical cystectomy (and urinary diversion, e.g. by ileal conduit)

Fixed tumours (T4)
- Chemotherapy: *MVAC* (methotrexate, vinblastine, Adriamycin, cis-platin), *CMV* (cis-platin, methotrexate, vinblastine), *Cisca* (cis-platin, cyclophosphamide, Adriamycin)
- Radiotherapy for palliation

Carcinoma-*in-situ* (CIS)
- Intravesical chemotherapy for isolated CIS and associated with papillary tumours
- Cystourethrectomy for malignant cystitis

PROGNOSIS

- Superficial tumours: 75% 5-year survival
- Invasive tumours: 10% 5-year survival
- Fixed tumours and metastases: median survival 1 year

Carcinoma-*in-situ*

This condition can present clinically with frequency, urgency and severe dysuria. The bladder capacity is markedly reduced and haematuria is generally not a presenting symptom. There are three types of this condition:

- isolated patches of carcinoma-*in-situ*;
- areas of carcinoma-*in-situ* associated with papillary tumours;
- malignant cystitis.

The first two of these types will almost certainly respond to intravesical chemotherapy, particularly with intravesical BCG. Some patients with malignant cystitis will also respond to intravesical agents, but these and other resistant cases are likely to require radical cystourethrectomy.

Prostatic cancer

Prostate cancer is the commonest malignancy of the genitourinary tract in the male. In the USA it is the most common malignancy of all types in the male and the second commonest cause of cancer deaths. In the recent past, many new developments have taken place in the diagnosing and staging of this disease, as well as the introduction of new therapeutic modalities.

Aetiology

The presence of latent prostatic carcinoma in the aged male is a well-known autopsy finding. The disease is commonest in patients over 60 years of age but it can present in patients much younger than this, particularly in the black population. The following have been suggested as possible aetiological factors in the development of prostatic carcinoma:

- age;
- race;
- environmental factors;
- diet;
- nationality;
- endocrine environment; and
- viral infection.

Pathology

The commonest type of prostatic tumour is the adenocarcinoma, which arises from the glandular epithelium, and this comprises 95% of tumours. They arise in the outer part of the prostate gland or peripheral zone. As the tumour enlarges, it spreads medially into the remainder of the gland, and outwardly to the surrounding tissues, particularly the seminal vesicles. Invasion of the rectum is uncommon, as it is protected by the fascia of Denonvilliers. The tethering of the rectal mucosa which may occur does not indicate invasion of the rectum, but rather of the fascia beneath it.

Previous difficulties associated with the variety of tumour grades appearing within the prostate tumour have been resolved by the development of the Gleason grading system. This describes five grades of cellular arrangement. The two most common patterns seen by the histopathologist are given scores ranging from 1 to 5 (i.e. well to poorly differentiated) and the scores are added together to give a single grade on a scale of 2–10. Thus, a sum score of 8–10 indicates poor differentiation and a score of 2–4 shows a well-differentiated tumour.

Clinical features

Most patients will present with symptoms of bladder outflow obstruction, such as poor stream, hesitancy, nocturia and incomplete bladder emptying. Sometimes the tumour may present as acute urinary retention. About 40% of patients may present with symptoms of advanced prostatic carcinoma, either caused by ureteric obstruction or bony metastasis. The pain associated with bony metastasis occurs classically at night, waking the patient from sleep. The pain may be relieved by getting out of bed and walking for a while.

On physical examination the prostate may feel normal (T0). In the case of localized prostatic carcinoma, there may be a hard nodule in one of the lobes (T1) or a hard area which has spread into the opposite lobe, but with no evidence of spread outside the gland (T2). If digital rectal examination of the prostate reveals the presence of locally invasive prostate cancer, there may be a hard mass spreading outside the boundaries of the prostate and involving the seminal vesicles (T3), or the side wall of the pelvis (T4). In this instance, the examining finger may feel a hard flat prostate which may be irregular, and associated with a fixed loin and sometimes tethering of the rectal mucosa.

Investigations

In addition to full blood count and renal profile, specific markers of prostatic carcinoma must be looked for on suspicion of the disease being present. The traditional markers, such as acid and alkaline phosphatase, are still helpful, but prostate-specific antigen has been shown to be superior as a marker, stage for stage, and as a measure of disease activity.

Imaging of the prostate has now become possible with transrectal ultrasound. This is most helpful as a guide for needle biopsy of the prostate. These procedures can be done

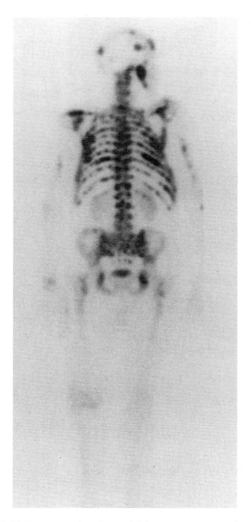

Figure 20.14 Bone scan showing multiple metastases secondary to prostatic cancer.

without anaesthesia and in an outpatient setting. A bone scan may demonstrate the presence of bony metastases (Fig. 20.14). This should be done prior to any hormonal manipulation of the patient, or before any definitive potentially curative treatment. Distant metastases to the lungs and liver may be discovered by a chest X-ray and serum liver function tests. There is no reliable method for imaging the presence of lymphatic metastasis, as this occurs first to the regional lymph nodes which are inside the pelvic brim.

Management

If a carcinoma of the prostate is suspected, tissue must be removed for histological examination and confirmation of the diagnosis. If the patient has severe outflow obstruction

in association with the tumour, a transurethral resection of the prostate (TURP) may be performed, but this is best withheld unless absolutely necessary. A needle biopsy with transrectal ultrasound guidance is the optimum method of diagnosis, after which further treatment may be carried out. As with bladder cancer, the method of treatment is dictated by the stage of the tumour.

Unsuspected carcinoma of the prostate (stage T0)

If the examining finger has found the prostate to be normal, but the specimen from TURP has revealed well-differentiated tumour in some of the removed tissue, the recommended method of treating the patient is by observation, with regular digital rectal examination of the prostate and assessment of serum prostate-specific antigen.

Localized prostatic carcinoma (stage T1 and T2)

There are three treatment options in this type of prostatic tumour:
- radical prostatectomy;
- radical radiotherapy;
- interstitial irradiation with ^{125}I or ^{198}Au.

Each of these treatments has its advocates. Radical prostatectomy is now associated with a very low incidence of urinary incontinence – in the region of 2–3%. This is acceptable, particularly since it can, if necessary, be treated by the insertion of an artificial urinary sphincter. Impotence following radical surgery is also now quite uncommon with the advent of the nerve-sparing technique. Radical radiotherapy has the advantage of leaving the patient with his prostate, but may be associated with cystitis and proctitis. The long-term survival of patients treated by irradiation or radical surgery is comparable.

Local spread (stage T3 and T4)

The treatment of choice in this stage of prostate tumour is almost certainly external-beam radiotherapy. In some cases, particularly those with incipient ureteric obstruction, endocrine therapy may be required as described below, in addition to irradiation.

Metastatic disease (stage T1–T4, M1)

The treatment options for the management of patients with metastatic disease centre on androgen deprivation as the prostate gland is very androgen-sensitive. Methods of therapy include:
- bilateral orchiectomy;
- stilboestrol;

- Luteinizing hormone-releasing hormone (LH-RH) agonists;
- antiandrogens;
- progestational agents.

It was initially felt that the best method of treating patients with bony metastases was with stilboestrol 1 mg t.d.s. Subsequent studies showed that there was a significant morbidity associated with the use of stilboestrol, in particular deep venous thrombosis, peripheral oedema and gynaecomastia. Its use is also contraindicated in patients with congestive cardiac failure and hypertension. Bilateral orchiectomy was therefore seen as preferable, and remains in many departments the treatment of choice. The introduction of LH-RH agonists has been seen by some clinicians as a preferable method of treating the disease,

particularly in association with antiandrogens such as cyproterone or flutamide. These agents create a pharmacological orchiectomy, thereby avoiding surgical castration.

Testicular cancer

Introduction

The vast majority of tumours found in the testis are primary testicular tumours (Table 20.12). Germ cell tumours are by far the most common tumours of the testis and constitute the most common solid tumour in males aged between 20 and 40. Cryptorchidism is an important predisposing

Carcinoma of the prostate at a glance

DEFINITION

Malignant lesion of the prostate gland

EPIDEMIOLOGY

Uncommon before age 60. 80% of prostate cancers are clinically undetected (latent carcinoma) and are only discovered on autopsy. The true incidence of this disease is considerably higher than the clinical experience would indicate

AETIOLOGY

- Increasing age
- Commoner in black men
- Hormonal factors: prostate cancer growth is enhanced by testosterone and inhibited by oestrogens or antiandrogens

PATHOLOGY

- Prostatic tumours are multicentric and located in the periphery of the gland

Histology
Adenocarcinoma arising from glandular epithelium; Gleason grading (2–10) is used to grade differentiation

Staging
- T0   Unsuspected
- Localized: T1   Localized to one lobe of prostate
                  T2   Spread within prostate
- Local spread: T3   Spread to seminal vesicles
                  T4   Spread to pelvic wall
- T1–4, M1   Metastatic disease

Spread
Direct into remainder of gland and seminal vesicles
Lymphatic to iliac and periaortic nodes
Haematogenous to bone (usually osteosclerotic lesions), liver, lung

CLINICAL FEATURES

- Bladder outflow obstruction (poor stream, hesitancy, nocturia)
- Symptoms of advanced disease (ureteric obstruction and hydronephrosis or bone pain from metastases, classically worse at night)
- Nodule or mass detected on rectal examination

INVESTIGATIONS

- FBC, U&E, creatinine
- Specific markers: prostate-specific antigen (PSA), alkaline and acid phosphatase
- Transrectal ultrasound
- Needle biopsy of the prostate
- Bone scan

MANAGEMENT

- Depends on stage of tumour
- T0: Observation, repeated digital (or ultrasound) examination and PSA
- T1 + 2: Radical prostatectomy or radical radiotherapy or interstitial radiation with ^{125}I or [198]Au
- T3 + 4: External-beam radiation ± hormonal therapy
- Metastatic: Hormonal manipulation
  - (a) Bilateral orchiectomy; stilboestrol
  - (b) LH-RH agonists; antiandrogens (cyproterone acetate)

PROGNOSIS

- Localized tumours: 80% 5-year survival
- Local spread: 40% 5-year survival
- Metastases: 20% 5-year survival

Table 20.12 Classification of tumours of the testis.

Germ cell tumours
Seminoma
Non-seminomatous germ cell tumour
  Embryonal carcinoma
  Teratocarcinoma
  Choriocarcinoma

Stromal tumours
Leydig cell
Sertoli cell
Granulosa cell

Metastatic tumours

factor, whether orchidopexy has been performed or not; it constitutes a 50-fold increase in that patient's chance of developing testicular cancer. Carcinoma-*in-situ* has been noticed in the contralateral testis in patients with testis cancer; the exact significance of this needs to be further elucidated, but it is certain that it is also a predisposing factor to testis cancer.

Stromal tumours occur uncommonly and arise in the cells of the testis other than the germ cells; for example, the Leydig cell tumours occur in the interstitium, and the Sertoli cells may also develop tumours. Granulosa cell tumours are the least common of the three. These stromal tumours probably rarely metastasize, and on occasion may produce hormones. Metastatic tumours may occur, particularly in the older age group, when lymphoma must be included in the differential diagnosis; this may occur bilaterally. Leukaemic infiltration of the testicle may also occur and is important when treatment schedules for this condition are being considered.

Germ cell tumours of the testis

Germ cell tumours of the testicle can be divided into two types: seminoma and non-seminomatous germ cell tumours. The latter group is subdivided into embryonal carcinoma, teratocarcinoma and choriocarcinoma (Table 20.12). These are important tumours occurring mainly between the ages of 20 and 40 years. Because of the vastly improved cure rates which can be achieved in this form of tumour, early diagnosis, aggressive treatment, and close and careful follow-up are essential. Germ cell tumours of the testicle metastasize directly to the para-aortic lymph nodes. Subsequent spread takes place to the supra-diaphragmatic lymph nodes, and to viscera such as the lungs or brain.

Clinical features

Most commonly a germ cell tumour of the testis presents as a painless swelling in the testis, which has been discovered incidentally by the patient or his partner. Sometimes there may be a vague discomfort in the region of the testicle, and on occasion the swelling may first come to the patient's notice following some mild trauma in this area. Only rarely do these tumours present with symptoms of metastatic disease or gynaecomastia. On physical examination there is generally a hard, irregular, non-tender mass occupying a part of the testis or the testis in its entirety. Trans-illumination of the scrotum will not show any evidence of fluid, thus excluding lesions such as hydrocele or epididymal cyst.

Tumour markers

If a germ cell tumour of the testis is suspected serum should be withdrawn for the following tumour marker estimations:
- α-Fetoprotein; and
- β Human chorionic gonadotrophin.

These markers are essential in the staging and follow-up of patients with germ cell tumours of the testis. Elevation of one or both of these markers will occur in 75–80% of non-seminomatous germ cell tumours (Table 20.13). Serum should be drawn prior to and after surgery. It is important to remember that the half-life of α-fetoprotein is 5–7 days, so elevation of this marker for up to 1 week after surgery may not be significant; persistent elevation at 2 weeks raises the suspicion of metastatic disease.

Imaging

- Scrotal ultrasonography is helpful in excluding cystic lesions of the intrascrotal contents, and may also be helpful

Table 20.13 Tumour markers in testicular cancer.

AFP is elevated in:
  75% of embryonal carcinomas
  65% of teratocarcinomas
It is *not* elevated in pure seminoma or choriocarcinoma

β-hCG is elevated in:
  100% of choriocarcinomas
  60% of embryonal carcinomas
  60% of teratocarcinomas
  10% of pure seminomas

AFP, α-Fetoprotein; β-hCG, β-human chorionic gonadotrophin.

in ruling out infective lesions of the testicle, particularly in association with serum tumour markers.

• Chest X-ray must be performed in order to assess the lungs and mediastinum. If a suspicion of metastatic lesions in these areas exists, CT scanning of the chest should be performed.

• Abdominal CT scan will identify the presence of enlarged lymph nodes within the abdomen. It will also show any evidence of obstruction of the ureters by a mass of lymph nodes.

Pathology

Histological examination of the tumour gives the diagnosis. Once the clinical suspicion of a testicular tumour is confirmed by elevated tumour markers and scrotal imaging, surgical removal of the testicle is undertaken. An inguinal incision is performed and the inguinal canal opened. Cross-clamping of the spermatic cord should be performed prior to handling of the testis, in order to prevent vascular spread of the tumour. Transscrotal approaches to the testis, either by needle aspiration or incision, must be avoided, because of the danger of involving the scrotal lymphatics, which drain to the inguinal lymph nodes. The spermatic cord is ligated and divided at the deep inguinal ring and the wound closed.

Staging

Staging is possible only through a combination of testicular histology, serum tumour markers (Table 20.13), and imaging of the abdominal lymph nodes, and a chest X-ray. As mentioned above, a CT scan of the chest and brain may be done if necessary. Staging of testis tumours is related to whether disease is localized to the testicle, whether there is spread to the abdominal lymph nodes, or whether there is spread to the supradiaphragmatic lymph nodes or distant viscera (Table 20.14).

Management

The primary treatment of testis tumours is, of course, removal of the affected testicle. Following histological identification of the tumour and adequate staging, further treatment is instituted as follows:

Seminoma

This tumour is highly radiosensitive and treatment strategies have been based on this fact for a number of years. It has become obvious that large tumour bulk is less radiosensitive than was previously thought and so chemo-

Table 20.14 Staging of testis tumours (Royal Marsden staging).

Stage I	Disease confined to the testis
Stage II	Retroperitoneal lymph node involvement
	IIa Nodes less than 2 cm in size
	IIb Nodes 2–5 cm in size
	IIc Nodes greater than 5 cm in size (bulky disease)
Stage III	Nodal disease above the diaphragm
Stage IV	Visceral metastases

Table 20.15 Treatment of seminoma.

Stage I	DXT to abdominal nodes	(30 Gy)
Stage II	IIa DXT to abdominal nodes	(60 Gy)
	IIb DXT to abdominal nodes	(60 Gy)
	IIc Chemotherapy	
Stage III	DXT to abdominal nodes and thoracic nodes	(60 Gy)
	or chemotherapy	
Stage IV	Chemotherapy	

DXT, Deep X-ray therapy.

therapy has a significant role to play in treating large tumours. The current treatment of seminoma is summarized in Table 20.15.

The application of deep X-ray therapy (DXT) to the abdominal nodes in stage IIc and III and to the thoracic nodes in stage III is still held by some to be the correct form of treatment. On the other hand, the incidence of recurrence of nodal disease is higher in patients treated exclusively with DXT. The role of chemotherapy, therefore, should be considered strongly in bulky or widespread disease in seminoma.

Non-seminomatous germ cell tumour

This tumour is not radiosensitive but has been found to be highly chemosensitive. The current treatment of non-seminomatous germ cell tumours is summarized in Table 20.16.

There has been controversy as to whether the correct form of management for stage I disease is careful observation or retroperitoneal lymph node dissection (RPLND). The main contraindication to RPLND has been the possibility of retrograde ejaculation, but further modified dissection on the contralateral side has lessened this as a complication. If observation is chosen, 20–30% of patients will subsequently develop obvious abdominal nodal metastases. It is essential, therefore, that careful and regular follow-up by chest X-ray, serum markers and CT scans is

Table 20.16 Treatment of non-seminomatous germ cell tumours.

Stage I	Observation or RPLND
Stage II	IIa Chemotherapy and RPLND for residual disease
	IIb Chemotherapy and RPLND for residual disease
	IIc Chemotherapy and RPLND for residual disease
Stage III	Chemotherapy
Stage IV	Chemotherapy

RPLND, Retroperitoneal lymph node dissection.

carried out. In stage II disease chemotherapy is the treatment of choice. Any residual nodal enlargement following a full course of chemotherapy should be managed by RPLND.

Chemotherapy

The exact form of chemotherapy used varies from department to department, but one of the most effective regimens is BEP: bleomycin, etoposide and cis-platin. Courses of these drugs are given every 3 weeks for three to four cycles.

Testicular cancer at a glance

DEFINITION

Malignant lesion of the testis

EPIDEMIOLOGY

Age 20–40 years. Commonest solid tumours in young males

AETIOLOGY

- Cryptorchidism — 50-fold increase in risk of developing testicular cancer. Risk is unaffected by orchidopexy
- Higher incidence in whites

PATHOLOGY

Classification of testicular tumours
Germ cell tumours (90%) (secrete (AFP) and (hCG)
Seminoma
Non-seminoma
   Embryonal carcinoma
   Teratocarcinoma
   Choriocarcinoma
Stromal tumours
Leydig cell
Sertoli cell
Granulosa cell
Metastatic tumours

Staging
- Stage I: confined to scrotum
- Stage II: spread to retroperitoneal lymph nodes below the diaphragm
- Stage III: distant metastases

Spread
- Germ cell tumours metastasize to the para-aortic nodes, lung and brain
- Stromal tumours rarely metastasize

CLINICAL FEATURES

- Painless swelling of the testis, often discovered incidentally or after trauma
- Vague testicular discomfort

- Rarely, evidence of metastatic disease or gynaecomastia
- Examination reveals a hard, irregular, non-tender testicular mass

INVESTIGATIONS

- Blood for tumour markers, i.e. AFP and hCG
- AFP is elevated in 75% of embryonal carcinomas and 65% of teratocarcinomas
- AFP is *not* elevated in pure seminoma or choriocarcinoma
- hCG is elevated in 100% of chorio-, 60% of embryonal, 60% of teratocarcinomas and 10% of pure seminomas
- Scrotal ultrasound
- Chest X-ray to assess lungs and mediastinum
- CT chest and abdomen to detect lymph nodes
- Laparoscopy (retroperitonoscopy) to assess abdominal nodes

MANAGEMENT

Orchidectomy (via groin incision) and histological diagnosis, further treatment depends on histology and staging

Seminoma
- Stage I: Radiotherapy to abdominal nodes
- Stage II: Radiotherapy to abdominal nodes
- Stage III: Chemotherapy (bleomycin, etoposide, cis-platin)

Non-seminoma germ cell
- Stage I: Retroperitoneal lymph node dissection (RPLND)
- Stage II: Chemotherapy + RPLND
- Stage III: Chemotherapy

PROGNOSIS

Overall cure rates are over 90% and node-negative disease has almost 100% 5-year survival

Cancer of the penis

Incidence

Carcinoma of the penis is uncommon in the UK, occurring in only 1 per 100 000 males. It rarely occurs in patients who have been circumcised, or in patients under the age of 45 years. It most commonly occurs in the sixth and seventh decades and in patients over 75 years of age the incidence is 8.9 per 100 000 males.

Aetiology

The aetiology of cancer of the penis is uncertain, but a number of factors associated with its development have been described (Table 20.17).

Pathology

Tumours of the penis are in nearly every case squamous cell carcinomas with keratinization, epithelial pearl formation and mitotic activity. The tumours are usually low-grade and on microscopic examination are usually papillary or ulcerating lesions. Spread occurs most commonly to the inguinal lymph nodes, with distant visceral metastatic spread being uncommon.

Clinical features

An ulcerating or papillary lesion of the penis may be found; this may be painful (Fig. 20.15). It may present as a painful swelling underneath a tight foreskin, with a foul-smelling

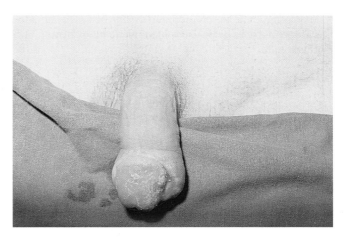

Figure 20.15 Penile cancer.

purulent and haemorrhagic discharge. Palpable lymph nodes in the inguinal region may be found, but these may be associated with infection of the tumour. If this is the case, they will disappear shortly after treatment of the primary tumour.

Management

Treatment of the primary lesion

- If the lesion is localized to the prepuce, circumcision is likely to be all that is required.
- If the glans alone is affected, and especially if the tumour is 1 cm or less in size, local radiotherapy gives excellent results.
- Where the shaft of the penis is involved, partial amputation is the preferred treatment.
- Where extensive involvement of the shaft has taken place, total amputation of the penis would probably be required, although partial amputation is possible if a 2 cm margin of normal tissue can be removed proximal to the tumour.

Management of the inguinal lymph nodes

- Impalpable nodes. Careful follow-up is required. If inguinal lymph node enlargement subsequently occurs, a radical lymph node dissection on the side of the enlargement may be carried out.
- Palpable mobile nodes at diagnosis. In many cases, the cause of the enlarged lymph nodes is inflammatory in nature and they will disappear after management of the primary tumour. If, 3 months after initial treatment, the nodes remain enlarged, radical dissection of the lymph nodes should be performed.

Table 20.17 Aetiological factors for the development of penile carcinoma.

Factor	Comment
Age	Incidence increases with age
Circumcision	Effectively prevented by circumcision
Geographic factors	Higher incidence in the Orient
Phimosis	Long known to be an aetiological factor
Venereal disease	High incidence of STD in patients with penile cancer
Socioeconomic factors	Higher incidence in poorer communities
Premalignant lesions	The following lesions predispose to penile cancer:
	Erythroplasia of Queyrat
	Bowen's disease
	Buschke-Loewenstein tumour
	Balanitis xerotica obliterans
	Leukoplakia

STD, Sexually transmitted disease.

- Fixed inguinal lymph nodes. In this instance, chemotherapy may be of help, using bleomycin, cis-platinum and methotrexate.

Incontinence and neuropathic bladder disorders

Incontinence

Incontinence is the involuntary loss of urine. Urine loss may occur through the urethra or, less commonly, from an abnormal extraurethral route such as a vesicovaginal fistula or etopic ureter. The aims of investigation are to determine the source of urinary loss and detect any underlying pathophysiological mechanism. The aim of treatment is to make the patient dry.

Classification

Incontinence may be classified according to the site of the abnormality or the clinical picture (Table 20.18).

Classification according to anatomical abnormality

Urethral incontinence

This is the most common form of incontinence in which there is an involuntary loss of urine through the urethra. This form of incontinence may be due to urethral, bladder or non-urinary causes.

- *Urethral abnormalities*: Urethral incompetence is a common condition in women, presenting as stress incontinence, i.e. urine loss via the urethra with increased intra-abdominal pressure in the absence of detrusor activity. Instances of increased intra-abdominal pressure are coughing, straining or lifting. Obesity, multiparity and difficult deliveries are predisposing factors. Urethral incompetence is less frequent in men, but may follow pelvic fractures or prostatectomy.
- *Bladder abnormalities*: Uninhibited detrusor contractions, which may be neuropathic (detrusor hyperreflexia) or non-neuropathic (detrusor instability) may cause incontinence. Frequency, urgency and urge incontinence are the usual symptoms. Sensory urgency due to infection, interstitial cystitis, bladder calculi and bladder tumours may also occur. In these patients frequency and urgency with urge incontinence may also be the presenting symptoms.

An overdistended bladder due to outflow obstruction (benign prostatic hyperplasia stricture) or an unobstructed atonic neuropathic bladder may present with outflow incontinence.

- *Non-urinary abnormalities*: Incontinence in elderly patients may be secondary to impaired mobility or impaired mental function. With impaired mental function the patient is unaware of bladder filling and voiding becomes a reflex action.
- *Non-urethral incontinence*: Loss of urine from an abnormal extraurethral orifice may indicate fistula or ectopic ureter.
- *Fistula*: Most urinary fistulae are vesicovaginal and most occur after hysterectomy, especially if there has been prior irradiation. Birth trauma during prolonged labour is a common cause in underdeveloped countries. Patients complain of constant urine leak.
- *Ureteral ectopia*: Ureteral ectopia is usually associated with a duplex collecting system and the ectopic ureter usually drains the upper moiety. Incontinence due to ureteral ectopia usually occurs in females due to the ureter draining via the urethra, vagina or perineum.

Classification according to clinical presentation

Stress incontinence

Stress incontinence is loss of urine via the urethra when intra-abdominal pressure rises due to coughing, straining or lifting in the absence of detrusor activity. Stress incontinence is usually due to urethral incompetence, but may also occur with overdistended bladders with normal sphincters.

Table 20.18 Classification of incontinence.

According to anatomical abnormality	According to clinical presentation
Urethral incontinence	Stress incontinence
Urethral abnormalities	Urge incontinence
Bladder abnormalities	Nocturnal enuresis
Non-urinary abnormalities	Constant urinary wetness
Non-urethral incontinence	
Fistula	
Ureteral ectopia	

Urge incontinence

Unstable detrusor contractions produce frequency, urgency and urge incontinence. This may be due to neuropathic bladder injury (detrusor hyperreflexia) or idiopathic unstable detrusor contractions. Increased sensory stimulation by stones, tumours or infection may also cause similar symptoms.

Nocturnal enuresis

Bed-wetting in older children is abnormal and may be associated with daytime voiding abnormalities such as frequency and urgency, consistent with unstable detrusor activity. In older men, bed-wetting may represent an overdistended bladder due to bladder outflow obstruction.

Constant urinary wetness

This may be due to urinary fistula or ectopic ureter.

Investigation

A detailed history to assess the pattern of voiding and incontinence will help in diagnosis. Symptoms of stress incontinence are both sensitive and specific for urethral incompetence, whereas symptoms of frequency and urgency are less reliable. Poor flow, hesitancy and postmicturition dribble suggest outflow obstruction and indicate that the incontinence may be overflow from an overdistended bladder. Dysuria may suggest infection, whilst haematuria should alert one to the possibility of tumour. Sexual function in males and bowel function in both sexes should be recorded, as abnormalities of these functions point towards a neurological cause. Assessment of mobility and mental status is particularly important in elderly patients. Past or present associated illness (e.g. diabetes) or surgery (abdominoperineal resection, hysterectomy) are also important.

Physical examination should include examination for a full bladder, digital rectal examination of the prostate in males and vaginal examination for cystourethrocele in women. A neurological assessment is also necessary. Laboratory investigation should include blood urea nitrogen estimation to assess renal function and urine microscopy and culture. In patients with symptoms of outflow obstruction, haematuria or a distended bladder, an IVU is important to assess the upper tracts and rule out stones and tumours.

Urodynamic assessment is necessary in all patients to define the exact form and cause of incontinence and to help in deciding the appropriate treatment. Uroflowmetry will show decreased flow rates in patients with bladder outflow obstruction. Cystometry will confirm the presence of unstable detrusor contractions in patients with urge incontinence and their absence in patients with stress incontinence. In addition, leakage on coughing can be demonstrated during cystometry to confirm a diagnosis of stress incontinence. Video screening during cystometry will show descent of the bladder neck with leakage during coughing in patients with stress incontinence. Cystoscopy is necessary where tumour, stone or fistula is suspected. In patients suspected of having a vesicovaginal fistula, vaginal speculum examination and a cystogram also aid diagnosis.

Treatment of incontinence

Urge incontinence

If urge incontinence is due to infection, stone or tumour, these causes must be treated respectively by appropriate antibiotic therapy, cystolithalopaxy or bladder tumour resection. If detrusor instability is due to bladder outflow obstruction the obstruction must be relieved. For patients with urge incontinence due to unstable bladder contractions, treatment is by pharmacological manipulation in the first instance with surgery for those patients who fail medical treatment.

Pharmacological therapy

Drugs with an anticholinergic and/or smooth-muscle relaxant effect may be used. Commonly used drugs are oxybutynin, emepromium carageenate and flavoxate hydrochloride. These drugs should be combined with bladder exercises where the patient gradually increases the intervals between voiding. Unpleasant side-effects such as dry mouth and blurring of vision are not uncommon with these agents.

Surgery

In its simplest form surgical treatment involves cystoscopy and bladder distension under general anaesthetic. This manoeuvre should be combined with a course of drug therapy and may give additional relief in a small number of patients. For those patients in whom drug therapy has failed and urge incontinence is severe, more extensive surgery is necessary. Partial bladder denervation by subtrigonal phenol injection or presacral neurectomy has been recommended but the results are poor and the significant complications may occur. More suitable alternatives are augmentation cystoplasty or substitution cystoplasty. In augmentation cystoplasty a detubularized segment of ileum is anastomosed to the bivalved bladder (clam cystoplasty), while in a substitution cystoplasty the supratrigonal portion of the bladder is removed and replaced with a caecal pouch.

Augmentation cystoplasty is associated with good functional results but an increased incidence of UTI can occur. Other potential complications include mucus production, atonic bladder (treated by clean intermittent self-catheterization; CISC) and a small potential risk of cancer in the bowel segment. Meticulous follow-up is required. Finally, for patients in whom these options fail, urinary diversion may be considered.

Stress incontinence

Stress incontinence requires surgical intervention in most instances. Minor degrees of stress incontinence may be treated with some success by pelvic floor exercises, oestrogen therapy for associated atrophic vaginitis and sympathomimetic agents such as ephedrine or α-adrenergic agonists, e.g. phenylpropanolamine, which improve bladder neck closure. However, most patients attending urology outpatients with incontinence will require surgical correction.

Surgery for female stress incontinence

The following procedures have been used in the treatment of female stress incontinence:
• *Retropubic urethropexy*: In these suprapubic repairs the bladder neck is hitched forwards and upwards by sutures attaching it to the pubis or pectineal ligament. This improves incontinence by lengthening the urethra and by supporting the bladder neck. There are a number of different types of operation which vary in respect to the site of placement of the sutures (Marshall–Marchetti–Krantz, Burch colposuspension, Lapides urethropexy). Success rates of over 90% can be anticipated.
• *Vaginal repairs*: Where stress incontinence is associated with a urethrocele or cystocele, a vaginal repair (anterior colporrhaphy) will repair the prolapse and prevent incontinence. Success rates, however, are lower (65%) than for retropubic repairs and this procedure should be reserved for patients with mild incontinence and prolapse.
• *Endoscopic urethropexy*: The Stamey–Raz urethropexy is a combined vaginal and suprapubic approach in which a long needle is passed from above through small suprapubic incisions to place nylon sutures on either side of the urethra. These sutures are then tied above the abdominal wall fascia, thus providing suspension of the urethra and bladder neck. Success rates of up to 90% have been reported. Periurethral injection of Teflon paste has also been advocated for patients with mild incontinence without prolapse. Success rates of 50% and greater have been reported. This technique is not widely used because of uncertainty about long-term side-effects such as foreign-body reaction and carcinogenesis.

• *Artificial urinary sphincter*: Failure of the above procedures may require the insertion of an artificial urinary sphincter. Success rates of 90% are reported but a reoperation rate of up to 30% to replace failed components is reported. Urinary diversion is the final option and is rarely required.

Surgery for male stress incontinence

Male stress incontinence is uncommon. It may complicate pelvic fracture or prostatectomy. Postprostatectomy incontinence should be treated medically using sympathomimetic or α-adrenergic agents initially. If this line of therapy fails, an artificial urinary sphincter may be necessary. Incontinence after pelvic fracture may be treated by sphincter insertion or very occasionally by urethral sphincter reconstruction.

Overflow incontinence

Overflow incontinence due to outflow obstruction from benign prostatic hyperplasia or urethral stricture is treated by TURP or urethrotomy respectively. Bladder emptying after surgery may be poor due to overstretching of the detrusor muscle, in which case catheter drainage followed by a trial of micturition 6 weeks later is the first line of treatment. If the patient is unable to void after the period of catheter drainage and there is no evidence of outflow obstruction (retrograde urethrogram or cystoscopy), then one may use pharmacological agents that stimulate detrusor contraction such as bethanechol or distigmine for a short period. If all else fails the patient may need to commence CISC or may be doomed to a long-term indwelling urethral catheter. Overflow incontinence secondary to a neuropathic atonic bladder is best managed by CISC.

Nocturnal enuresis

As children grow older an increasing number achieve continence. Daytime continence should be achieved by 2 years but nighttime continence takes a little longer and is more variable. About two-thirds of children are dry at night by the age of 3 years. At least half of the remainder will be dry by 10 years of age. By the age of 15 years only 2% of children are incontinent at night. Investigation of enuresis includes a detailed history and physical examination, urine microscopy and culture, an IVU and urodynamics.

Management consists of bladder training during the day, gradually increasing the interval between voiding, combined with voiding last thing at night. In younger children the parents should lift the child before they retire at night. Enuresis alarms which are triggered by small amounts of leakage may also be used. These alarms probably condition the patient to wake when the bladder becomes full. In addition, pharmacological manipulation using a variety of agents has met with good success.

The most commonly employed drug is imipramine (Tofranil), a tricyclic antidepressant, which acts by inhibiting detrusor contractions and reducing the depth of sleep so that bladder distension is appreciated and the patient wakes to void. Anticholinergic agents (Pro-Banthine, oxybutynin) may also be used to inhibit unstable detrusor contractions. Desmopressin is an ADH analogue which decreases urine output overnight and may help some patients. A daily diary should be kept to assess the success of treatment.

Failure of medical treatment with persistent bed-wetting is often associated with daytime frequency and urgency also. For these patients an augmentation cystoplasty may be the only solution.

Incontinence secondary to fistula

Surgical intervention is the only acceptable treatment for vesicovaginal fistula. There are a number of approaches. For simple fistula, a vaginal repair in two layers is recommended. For patients with recurrent or complex fistula a transabdominal transvesical repair with interposition of omentum is indicated.

Incontinence in the elderly

Approximately 15% of elderly patients experience incontinence. The percentage of nursing-home or hospital-dwelling elderly who suffer with incontinence is even higher. Treatment is determined by the cause. However, incontinence in the elderly is usually multifactorial, with decreased mobility and altered mental status having a significant impact on treatment options and outcomes. Regular toiletting is an important part of the treatment. Specific abnormalities are treated as indicated.

Summary

Incontinence is a common problem, especially in women. It is a physically and socially debilitating disease. A detailed history supplemented with urodynamic assessment will diagnose the underlying pathophysiology in most cases and indicate the correct treatment options. Cure can be expected in the vast majority of patients.

Neuropathic bladder disorders

The bladder and urethra act as a functional unit that allows storage of urine in the bladder without a change in the intraluminal pressure and voluntary evacuation (micturition) of the stored urine. As the bladder fills with urine the bladder muscle (detrusor) is stretched. There is an awareness of filling at a volume of 150–250 ml and a desire to void when normal bladder capacity (400–500 ml) is reached. Micturition is achieved by relaxation of the pelvic floor musculature, including the voluntary sphincter. The trigone contracts, opening the bladder neck and closing the ureteric orifices, thus preventing urine reflux during voiding. The detrusor then contracts, expelling the stored urine. These functions are dependent on an anatomically correct bladder and urethra with intact complex neurological pathways which involve the pelvic nerves, spinal cord, brainstem and cerebrum. The pelvic nerves supplying the bladder and urethra with afferent and efferent fibres synapse in the micturition centre located in the S2–4 segments of the spinal cord, which corresponds with the T2–L1 vertebral level. This centre is connected to centres in the pons and cerebrum which exert an inhibitory effect that is central to voluntary control. Disease or injury at any of these levels may result in abnormal bladder or urethra function.

Classification

Traditionally, neuropathic bladder disorders have been described according to the site of the neurological injury as upper or lower motor neuron injuries.
• Lesions above the micturition centre are characterized by detrusor overactivity, which is frequently associated with uncoordinated increased urethral sphincter activity.
• Lesions at the level of the micturition centre (S2–4) or lower are characterized by decreased activity of the detrusor and sphincter.

However, in individual patients a mixed pattern of injury is not uncommon and the clinical picture may not fit one or other neurological pattern exactly. For this reason the International Continence Society has classified neuropathic disorders according to urodynamic findings on assessment of detrusor and urethral function (Table 20.19).

This classification allows the assessment of the elements of neuropathic bladder in each individual case, thus enabling rational management decisions to be made.

Table 20.19 Classification of neuropathic disorders.

Detrusor activity	Urethral sphincter activity	Sensation
Normal	Normal	Normal
Overactive (hyperreflexic)	Overactive	Hypersensitive
Underactive (areflexic)	Incompetent	Hyposensitive

Table 20.20 Causes of neuropathic bladder.

Cerebral	Spinal	Peripheral nerves
Cerebrovascular accident	Trauma	Diabetes mellitus
Dementia	Multiple sclerosis	Surgical injury (pelvic surgery)
Frontal lobe tumours	Amyotrophic lateral sclerosis	
Parkinson's disease	Compression (tumour, abscess, disc prolapse)	
	Spina bifida	

Causes of neuropathic bladder

A large number of diseases which affect the nervous system from the cerebral cortex to the pelvic nerves may result in a neuropathic bladder (Table 20.20).

Investigation

Diagnosis of neuropathic bladder depends on a complete history and physical examination with an extensive neurological assessment. Investigation should include urinalysis to rule out infection and blood urea nitrogen estimation to assess renal function. An IVU is mandatory to document upper-tract (i.e. kidneys and ureter) status. Urodynamic assessment is the key to accurate diagnosis and essential in the follow-up of any treatment regimen.

Special features in the history are the voiding pattern, which should be described in detail with reference to frequency (day and night), urgency, incontinence, pain on urination, hesitancy, poor stream, straining to void, dribbling and incomplete emptying. In males sexual function should be documented with special attention to the presence or absence of erections and ejaculation. In both sexes any disturbance of bowel function should be noted. Associated medical disorders such as diabetes mellitus and present medication should also be noted. More generalized neurological symptoms such as disturbed cerebral function, weakness, sensory loss or altered co-ordination should also be enquired after. Visual disturbances may occur in patients with diabetic retinopathy or in patients with multiple sclerosis (retrobulbar neuritis).

Examination should include a full physical examination with special reference to urological and neurological examination. Urological examination involves examination of the kidneys for hydronephrosis, of the bladder for urine retention and the scrotum for epididymitis. Neurological examination involves assessment of cerebral function, sensory level, muscular tone, power and reflex activity.

An IVU is an invaluable examination. The preliminary plain film may show renal or bladder stones or spina bifida of the lower sacral vertebral. The contrast study may show pyelonephritic scarring of the kidneys or hydronephrosis. the ureters may be dilated from obstruction or reflux. The bladder may appear large, smooth-walled and overdistended or as a markedly trabeculated small-capacity bladder.

Urodynamics

Urodynamics is essential in the investigation of a patient with neurogenic bladder.

• *Uroflowmetry*: This is the study of the flow of urine from the urethra. The flow rate, volume voided, time of voiding, pattern on voiding and residual volume all give valuable information about lower urinary tract function. Low flow rates suggest outlet obstruction or a weak detrusor; higher flow rates suggest bladder spasticity whilst intermittent flow rates indicate spasticity of the sphincter or straining to overcome resistance in the urethra. The normal flow rates are 20–25 ml/s in males and 20–30 ml/s in females.

• *Cystometry*: This test evaluates the reservoir function of the lower urinary tract. Cystometry evaluates bladder capacity, intravesical pressure during filling, bladder pressure during voiding and the presence of premature unstable contractions. In addition, the patient's ability to perceive filling is tested. The first sensation of filling occurs at between 150 and 250 ml of urine and normal capacity is 400–500 ml. Normal voiding pressures are 30 cmH_2O.

• *Urethral pressure profilometry*: This technique involves measurement of urethral pressure with the bladder at rest and during voiding. This technique is reserved for difficult cases where a combination of uroflowmetry and cystometry has not produced a clear assessment of the neuropathic abnormality.

Management

The goals of treatment are to reverse the pathological abnormality where possible, alleviate the symptoms and preserve renal function. Treatment is dependent on the functional disorder produced by the disease or injury.

Management of incontinence

Incontinence may be due to detrusor overactivity or incompetent sphincter.

Detrusor overactivity

Detrusor hyperreflexia may be treated by drugs that have an anticholinergic and/or smooth-muscle relaxant effect, such as oxybutinin, flavoxate hydrochloride or emepromium carageenate. Side-effects such as dry mouth and blurred vision are common. Failure of pharmacological manipulation is an indication for surgical intervention. Phenol injection into the vesical nerves under the trigone and division of the anterior sacral nerve roots (presacral neurectomy) have been advocated but the results are poor. Augmentation of the bladder using a segment of bowel produces more reliable results. The most frequently used bowel segment is ileum (clam ileocystoplasty). Alternatively, the bulk of the bladder may be excised and replaced by bowel, usually caecum, in a substitution cystoplasty procedure.

Incompetent sphincter

Drugs with an α-adrenergic activity such as phenylpropanolamine and ephedrine increase bladder outflow resistance. If drug therapy fails, surgery is indicated in suitable patients. In women, the operation used for stress incontinence such as endoscopic urethropexy (Stamey–Raz procedure), retropubic urethropexy (Lapides urethorpexy) or colposuspension may be used. In men the options are more limited. Urinary condom catheters or urethral catheters may be used. In both sexes artificial urinary sphincters are suitable in carefully selected patients.

Management of retention

Urine retention is most commonly due to an underactive detrusor muscle but it may also occur in the presence of detrusor overactivity if the urethral sphincter is also overactive. This latter entity is called detrusor sphincter dyssynergia.

Underactive detrusor

It is important to establish proper bladder emptying to avoid infection, stone formation and renal impairment. Patients may empty their bladders simply by a combination of abdominal straining and manual pressure suprapubically (Credé manoeuvre). This is not a very efficient manoeuvre. Drugs which stimulate smooth-muscle contraction such as bethanechol or distigmine may also be used. It is important when using these drugs to ensure that there is no outflow obstruction, otherwise bladder rupture is a real possibility. A more widely applied alternative is the technique of CISC where the patient passes a 12F feeding tube into the bladder roughly every 4 h or as often as is required to maintain continence. Complications such as infections or stricture are surprisingly uncommon. For those patients unable to manage this technique, an indwelling catheter or a urinary diversion may be necessary.

Overactive urethral sphincter

In detrusor sphincter dyssynergia both the detrusor muscle and urethral sphincters are hyperactive. When the detrusor contracts the sphincter does not relax in the normal co-ordinated manner, resulting in a poor and intermittent stream with retention. Pharmacological agents which block the α-adrenergic nerve receptors such as phenoxybenzamine or prazosin may be used but side-effects are common. An alternative is sphincterotomy converting the patient from retention to incontinence which can then be managed with a urine collection device or catheter. The reason for treating retention in such a seemingly drastic manner is to avoid high vesical pressures which may cause renal impairment.

Progressive upper tract impairment or difficult incontinence may be managed by urinary diversion. Standard urinary diversion involves an ileal conduit with an abdominal stoma and urine collection bag. An alternative technique of continent urinary diversion using small or large bowel as a urinary reservoir with a continent abdominal stoma which the patient catheterizes at regular intervals is a more attractive option.

Management of specific causes of neuropathic bladder

Spinal cord injury

After the initial injury there is a period of spinal shock lasting on average 2–3 months. This results in paralysis of the detrusor muscle with retention of urine. It is important to avoid overdistension of the bladder to prevent permanent bladder dysfunction. A urethral catheter should be inserted when the patient presents with a spinal injury. To avoid the complications associated with long-term urethral catheterization (stricture), subsequent bladder emptying can be achieved by intermittent catheterization or a suprapubic catheter. When the period of spinal shock passes, bladder or urethral function is assessed by urodynamics and definitive therapy commenced based on the findings of this investigation. Regular follow-up with urinalysis, blood urea nitrogen, IVU and urodynamics is necessary.

Spina bifida

Spina bifida, which is due to failure of development of the posterior neural arches, takes two forms. Spina bifida occulta is a common X-ray finding with evidence of abnormal L5 or S1 vertebra without any neurological deficit. Spina bifida cystica may present as a meningeal sac protruding through a defect in the overlying skin (meningocele) or a meningeal sac with neural tissue (myelomeningocele). Bladder dysfunction is common in patients with spina bifida cystica. The first priority is to ensure adequate bladder emptying to prevent upper tract deterioration. In infants this may involve the parents in performing intermittent catheterization or alternatively a temporary vesicostomy may be formed. As the child grows older, control of incontinence becomes an important objective. Urodynamic assessment of bladder and urethral function will indicate the treatment options.

Diabetes mellitus

Peripheral neuropathy is a significant complication of diabetes mellitus involving both the sensory and motor nerves. Decreased detrusor activity leading to retention is the usual bladder abnormality. Clean intermittent self-catheterization is the most attractive treatment option.

Multiple sclerosis

Bladder dysfunction is a common complication of multiple sclerosis. Treatment is difficult because of the fluctuating nature of the disease. As the demyelination usually affects the spinal cord above the micturition centre (S2–4), an upper motor neuron-type lesion with detrusor hyperreflexia presenting as frequency, urgency and incontinence is the usual presentation. If the nerve supply to the sphincter is also involved, detrusor sphincter dyssynergia may result. Less commonly, the pelvic nerves are involved with an atonic detrusor and retention of urine. Urodynamic assessment will indicate the appropriate treatment. Where possible, a conservative approach is advocated as the bladder abnormality may change in nature as the disease progresses.

Cerebral disorders

Bladder dysfunction can occur with a variety of cerebral disorders such as stroke, Parkinson's disease, dementia and frontal lobe tumours. These disorders are characterized by a loss of cerebral inhibition of micturition leading to incontinence. Treatment is difficult and consists of regular toiletting and urine collection devices if necessary.

Complications of neuropathic bladder

The complications of neuropathic bladder are summarized in Table 20.21.

Infection should be treated rapidly and aggressively to prevent renal injury. Bladder stones are treated by crushing the stone (litholapaxy) and evacuating the fragments, whilst

Table 20.21 Complications of neuropathic bladder.

Recurrent urinary tract infection
Stone formation
Hydronephrosis secondary to obstruction or reflux
Renal dysfunction
Sexual dysfunction (impotence, lack of ejaculation)
Autonomic dysreflexia

renal stones may be treated by ESWL. Hydronephrosis due to reflux or obstruction is an emergency, as renal impairment leading ultimately to renal failure is a significant risk. Treatment is surgical and is determined by the urodynamic findings.

Impotence may be managed by pharmacological-induced erection or penile prostheses where appropriate. Autonomic dysreflexia occurs in patients with high spinal lesions in whom sweating, bradycardia and marked hypertension may occur with increased afferent input, as occurs with bladder distension or uncontrolled muscle spasms. Control of bladder emptying and muscle spasm will prevent this serious complication.

Prognosis

The greatest threat to the patient with a neuropathic bladder is progressive renal damage leading to renal failure, which may be caused by hydronephrosis (reflux or obstruction), infection or stone disease. Careful management of bladder function with regular follow-up has significantly improved long-term survival in these patients.

Disorders of the testis and scrotum, and impotence

Disorders of the testis and scrotum

Torsion of the testis

Torsion of the testis, or more correctly, torsion of the spermatic cord, may occur at any age but most commonly affects adolescent males. In most cases the underlying cause is a high insertion of the tunica vaginalis on the spermatic cord which allows the testis to rotate within the tunica. This

Urinary incontinence at a glance

DEFINITION

Urinary incontinence is defined as the involuntary loss of urine

PHYSIOLOGY

The normal bladder capacity is 350–400 ml. As the bladder fills with urine the detrusor muscle relaxes to accommodate the rise in volume without a rise in pressure (plasticity). When the bladder is full, stretch receptors in the bladder wall initiate a reflex contraction (via S3,4) of the detrusor muscle and relaxation of the urinary sphincter to empty the bladder. This spinal reflex is controlled by an inhibitory cortical mechanism which allows conscious control over micturition. Conscious control develops during early childhood

CLASSIFICATION

Anatomical abnormality	Predisposing factors
Urethral incontinence	
Urethral abnormalities	Obesity, multiparity, difficult delivery, pelvic fractures, postprostatectomy
Bladder abnormalities	Neuropathic or non-neuropathic detrusor abnormalities, infection, interstitial cystitis, bladder stones and tumours
Non-urinary abnormalities	Impaired mobility or mental function
Non-urethral incontinence	
Urinary fistula	Vesicovaginal
Ureteral ectopia	Ureter drains into urethra (usually a duplex ureter; Fig. 20.16)

PATHOPHYSIOLOGY

- Urine leakage occurs when intra-abdominal pressure exceeds urethral pressure (e.g. coughing, straining or lifting) — *stress incontinence*. This usually happens in the presence of urethral incompetence
- Loss of cortical control results in an uninhibited bladder with unstable detrusor contractions due to *detrusor hyperreflexia*. The bladder fills, the sacral reflex is initiated and the bladder empties spontaneously
- Damage to the efferent fibres of the sacral reflex causes bladder atonia. The bladder fills with urine and becomes grossly distended with constant dribbling of urine — *overflow incontinence*. Chronic bladder distension from obstruction produces a similar picture
- Idiopathic detrusor instability causes a rise in intravesical pressure and urine leakage — *urge incontinence*

CLINICAL FEATURES

- Stress incontinence: loss of urine during coughing, straining, etc. These symptoms are quite specific for stress incontinence
- Urge incontinence: inability to maintain urine continence in the presence of frequent and insistent urges to void
- Nocturnal enuresis: 10% of 5-year-olds and 5% of 10-year-olds are incontinent during sleep. Bed-wetting in older children is abnormal and may indicate the presence of an unstable bladder

- Symptoms of urinary infection (frequency, dysuria, nocturia), obstruction (poor stream, dribbling), trauma (including surgery, e.g. abdominoperineal resection), fistula (continuous dribbling), neurological disease (sexual or bowel dysfunction) or systemic disease (e.g. diabetes) may point to an underlying cause

INVESTIGATIONS

- Urine culture — to exclude infection
- IVU — to assess upper tracts and obstruction or fistula
- Urodynamics:
  (a) Uroflowmetry — measures flow rate
  (b) Cystometry — demonstrates detrusor contractures
  (c) Videocystometry — shows leakage of urine on straining in patients with stress incontinence
  (d) Urethral pressure flowmetry — measures urethral and bladder pressure at rest and during voiding
- Cystoscopy: if bladder stone or neoplasm is suspected
- Vaginal speculum examination ± cystogram if a vesicovaginal fistula is suspected

MANAGEMENT

- *Urge incontinence:*
  (a) Medical Rx: treat any underlying cause (infection, tumour, stone); bladder training — gradually increase intervals between voiding; anticholinergic/smooth-muscle relaxants — propantheline, flavoxate hydrochloride
  (b) Surgical Rx: cystoscopy and bladder distension, augmentation cystoplasty
- *Stress incontinence:*
  (a) Medical Rx: pelvic floor exercises, oestrogens for atrophic vaginitis, sympathomimetic agents (ephedrine) to enhance bladder neck closure
  (b) Surgical Rx: retropubic or endoscopic ureteropexy, vaginal repair, artificial sphincter
- *Overflow incontinence:*
  If obstruction present — treat cause of obstruction, e.g. by TURP
  If no obstruction — short period of catheter drainage to allow detrusor muscle to recover from overstretching — then short course of detrusor muscle stimulants (bethanechol, distigmine). If all else fails, clean intermittent self-catheterization — this is the treatment of choice for neurogenic overflow incontinence
- *Nocturnal enuresis:*
  Bladder training; 'lift' children around midnight; use of diary of dry nights; enuresis alarms; imipramine (inhibits detrusor contractions); anticholinergics
- *Urinary fistula:*
  Always requires surgical treatment

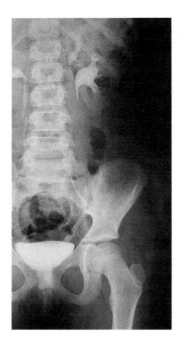

Figure 20.16 Duplex ureter on left side. Note the contrast in the vagina. The ectopic ureter drained into the vault of the vagina in this girl.

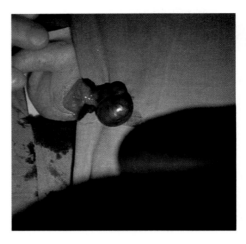

Figure 20.17 Torsion showing ischaemic testis and twisted spermatic cord.

abnormality is described as a 'clapper bell' deformity. Less commonly, a long mesentery may separate the epididymis and testis, allowing torsion of the testis on this long mesorchium. Undescended testes are more prone to torsion. In neonates torsion of the testis and the tunica vaginalis may occur. Torsion is more common at night.

The clinical features are a sudden onset of severe scrotal pain which may radiate to the lower abdomen. Nausea and vomiting may occur with the pain. In at least half such patients a preceding history of sudden-onset, short-duration scrotal pain can be elicited. These testes have twisted and untwisted (intermittent torsion). Patients with a history of intermittent torsion will be noted to have an abnormal horizontal lie of the testis when examined in the standing position. Because of the risk of acute torsion, urgent elective (i.e. the next operating list) fixation of the testes is recommended. Examination of the patient with acute torsion reveals a testis that lies higher in the scrotum than the opposite testis. This is due to shortening of the cord by twisting. The overlying skin is reddened and the testis is extremely tender. The spermatic cord is thickened and shorter.

The diagnosis is a clinical one and any difficulty in deciding whether the patient has torsion or not is best resolved at exploration. The diagnosis can be made accurately by colour Doppler ultrasonography or scintil-

lation scanning but these investigations are dilatory and a potentially viable testis may have infarcted by the time surgical exploration is undertaken. Therefore, patients with a suspected torsion require immediate exploration.

Exploration is carried out through a midline scrotal incision which will reveal a congested ischaemic testis with a twisted spermatic cord (Fig. 20.17). The cord is untwisted and testicular viability assessed. If operated on within 4 h of the onset of symptoms, normal function can be preserved in most cases. If the torsion is of greater than 6 h duration, future spermatogenesis is unlikely but testosterone production may still be maintained. Torsion of greater duration may produce a frankly infarcted testis or a testis of dubious viability that will almost certainly atrophy subsequently. If the testis is obviously infarcted, orchidectomy is advised. If the testis is viable, fixation of the testis at three points to the scrotal wall with non-absorbable sutures is the recommended technique. The tunica vaginalis should be excised or plicated. Because there is a 10% risk of torsion in the unaffected side it should also be fixed.

The differential diagnosis of torsion of the spermatic cord includes acute epididymitis and torsion of the testicular appendage (hydatid of Morgagni).
• Acute epididymitis may be bacterial or viral in nature and has similar presenting symptoms but signs of systemic upset such as pyrexia and rigors may be present. However, acute epididymitis is uncommon in adolescent males.
• Torsion of the testicular appendages, which are the vestigial remnants of the Müllerian duct, usually affects preadolescent males. The symptoms are those of acute torsion but differentiation may be possible at an early stage, when a normal testis is noted with an exquisitely tender upper pole and a blue dot visible through the scrotal skin. As the condition progresses, the tenderness becomes more

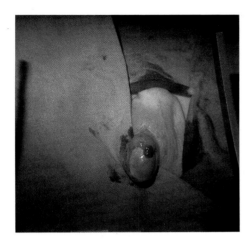

Figure 20.18 Torsion of the hydatid of Morgagni.

generalized and differentiation from acute torsion is impossible. The diagnosis is best made at exploration (Fig. 20.18). If the pain is due to torsion of the hydatid of Morgagni, the appendages should be excised.

Undescended testis

When a testis is missing from the scrotum several explanations are possible. The testis may be retractile, ectopic in position, undescended or absent (Fig. 20.19).

• A *retractile testis* can be coaxed to the bottom of the scrotum and does not require intervention. However, retractile testes should be monitored to ensure that they eventually achieve their correct position in the scrotum. If

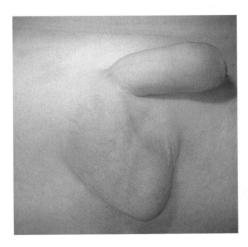

Figure 20.19 Underdeveloped right hemiscrotum secondary to an undescended testis. The testis was found lying at the superficial inguinal pouch.

the testis cannot be brought down to the bottom of the scrotum but only as far as mid or high scrotum, then it is not retractile. Approximately 5% of missing testes are truly absent but this diagnosis can only be made after ensuring by CT scan that the testis is not intra-abdominal.

• An *ectopic testis* is one which has strayed from the path of normal descent. Most commonly the testis lies in the superficial inguinal pouch. Other ectopic sites include the femoral triangle, perineum and the root of the penis. It is thought that ectopy results from an abnormal connection to the gubernaculum testis which leads the gonad to the abnormal position. Treatment is by orchidopexy to place the testis in the scrotum.

• An *undescended testis* is one which has stopped in the normal path of descent and may be intra-abdominal, inguinal, at the superficial ring or high in the scrotum. Several theories have been proposed to explain maldescent. These include an abnormality of the gubernaculum such as shortness or complete absence. The undescended testis may be intrinsically abnormal (dysgenetic) and thus insensitive to the gonadotrophins which stimulate descent. Equally, a deficiency of gonadotrophins which are produced in the last weeks of gestation may be responsible for maldescent. This latter explanation would explain the very high incidence of maldescent in premature infants. If a testis remains undescended the seminiferous tubules become progressively damaged with microscopic evidence of damage by 2 years of age and ultrastructural evidence of change at 1 year. Thus, early orchidopexy is mandatory to preserve spermatogenesis. However, as many as 10% of undescended testes are hypogonadal and may never attain normal spermatogenesis despite early orchidopexy.

Undescended testis is noted in 20% of premature boys but most descend to the scrotum within the first month of life. An incidence of roughly 4% is noted in full-term boys and half of these will have attained a normal scrotal position by the end of the first month of life. By the end of the first year of life 99% of testes should be descended and the remaining 1% require surgical correction (orchidopexy). Surgical correction should be undertaken at this time as delay serves no purpose. The reasons for surgical intervention are to preserve fertility, to deal with the coexistent hernial sac present in 90% of patients and to reduce the risk of torsion or traumatic injury. Orchidopexy may also decrease the risk of malignant change.

The risk of malignant change in an undescended testis is probably 30 times greater than in a normally descended testis. Seminoma is the most common tumour of undescended testes. Orchidopexy before the age of 8 years reduces the risk of malignant change but does not decrease it to the level of a normally descended testis. If a patient is aged 10 years or greater, orchidectomy is preferred to orchidopexy unless the maldescent is bilateral, in which case one testis is removed and the other brought down. Despite early orchidopexy, as many as 20% of patients with unilateral undescent will be infertile, whilst the remainder will produce sperm of poor quality. Bilateral undescent almost invariably results in infertility.

Scrotal masses

A mass in the scrotum may arise from the scrotum or its contents or may be due to an inguinoscrotal hernia. If one can get above the mass at the neck of the scrotum then it is scrotal in origin. Scrotal masses may be solid (tumour, chronic epididymo-orchitis) or cystic (hydrocele, epididymal cyst). Varicoceles may also present as a scrotal mass.

Hydrocele*

A hydrocele is a collection of fluid within the tunica vaginalis and may be congenital (infantile hydrocele) or acquired. Infantile hydrocele is due to a patent processus vaginalis which allows fluid from the abdominal cavity to collect in the scrotum. If the communication is wider, a hernia results. Most of these hydroceles will close spontaneously by the end of the first year of life. Persistent hydroceles require ligation of the patent processus vaginalis at the deep inguinal ring.

Adult hydroceles are non-communicating, i.e. there is no patent processus vaginalis. These hydroceles may be idiopathic or secondary to intrascrotal pathology such as tumour, torsion, trauma or infection. Hydroceles that are secondary to underlying disease tend to be acute whilst those that are idiopathic in nature are chronic. Hydroceles are fluctuant, unless very tense, and they transilluminate. The swelling lies anterior to the testis. However, the testes may be impalpable within a tense hydrocele. Hydroceles should not be tapped because of the risk of introducing infection or causing haemorrhage into the hydrocele by inadvertently stabbing a vein.

Hydroceles are dealt with by excision of the hydrocele sac or plication of the sac (Lord's procedure).

*A note on the etymology of -cele and -coele. There is some confusion as to the spelling of words such as hydrocele, varicocele, etc. Some think that the British English suffix is -coele and that the -cele version is American English. Not so. In fact both derive from Greek: κελε meaning 'tumour' and κοιλοσ meaning 'hollow'. The common usage therefore is -cele. It makes more sense to speak of a water tumour (hydrocele) than a water hollow (hydrocoele).

Epididymal cyst

Cystic swellings of the epididymis are located above and behind the testis and separate from it. If the cyst contains spermatozoa it is called a spermatocele. These cysts may be multilocular and/or multiple and may replace much of the epididymis. Epididymal cysts are usually asymptomatic but may cause discomfort. If symptoms are troublesome these cysts may be excised but the patient must be warned that the epididymis may also have to be excised if extensively involved. Bilateral cyst excision poses a very significant risk to fertility.

Varicocele

A varicocele is a scrotal mass due to varicosities of the pampiniform plexus of veins above the testis. It is present in 10% of men and is uncommon before adolescence. The majority of varicoceles (95%) are left-sided and are due to incompetence, or absence, of the valve at the termination of the left testicular vein before its insertion into the renal vein. On examination with the patient in the standing position it feels like a bag of worms. A varicocele of recent onset, especially one which does not empty on lying down, may be due to venous occlusion by a renal or retroperitoneal tumour and should be investigated by renal ultrasound. Varicoceles are believed to raise the temperature around the ipsilateral testis and some reports suggest that sperm count and motility are significantly decreased in 65–70% of patients. This is the usual indication for surgical intervention. The gonadal veins may be ligated within the inguinal canal (low tie) or in the retroperitoneum above the deep ring (high tie).

Disorders of the scrotal skin

Fournier's gangrene is an infection of the scrotal skin caused by the synergistic action of aerobic and anaerobic bacteria. It is predisposed to by diabetes mellitus, perianal sepsis or periurethral abscess. It causes gangrene of the scrotal and penile skin and may be life-threatening. Treatment is by intensive antibiotic therapy combined with extensive debridement of devitalized tissue with later plastic reconstruction. Idiopathic scrotal oedema is an acute oedematous swelling of the skin that occurs in young boys and may be infective in nature. Treatment is conservative.

Scrotal skin tumours are now rare (Fig. 20.20). In the past they arose from occupational exposure to soot (chimney sweeps' cancer was first described by Percival Pott in 1775), tars, oil and other petroleum products. Poor hygiene and chronic inflammation are predisposing factors today. Scrotal cancers are nearly always squamous carcinomas. Treatment is by wide excision and groin dissection if there is

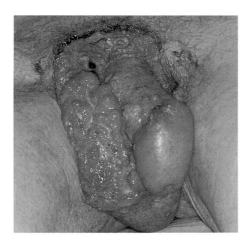

Figure 20.20 Carcinoma of the scrotum.

a suspicion of lymph node metastases. Prognosis is fairly good (60% cure) if the tumour is confined to the scrotum but poor (<25% cure) if metastases are present.

Benign disorders of the foreskin and penis

Balanitis

Balanitis is an infection of the foreskin (prepuce), usually seen in young boys and usually caused by staphylococci. The patient complains of a sore penis and on examination the foreskin is swollen and red with a purulent discharge. It is treated by bathing and penicillin and usually settles rapidly. If, when the infection settles, the foreskin is very adherent to the glands and cannot be retracted easily, then circumcision should be recommended (Table 20.22).

Phimosis

Phimosis is defined as a tightness of the foreskin of such a degree to prevent retraction. It may be congenital or

Table 20.22 Indications for circumcision.

Ritual
Moses
Mohammad
Social
Mummy
Money
Medical
Phimosis
Paraphimosis

secondary to infection. Ballooning of the foreskin may occur on micturition. On examination it will be possible to retract the foreskin and there may only be a small contracted orifice. Treatment is by circumcision.

Paraphimosis

Paraphimosis occurs when the foreskin retracts behind the corona of the glans penis producing a tourniquet effect. The foreskin and glands become oedematous, making it impossible to pull the foreskin forwards without great difficulty. As the oedema progresses the constriction becomes tighter and, if not treated, the foreskin will become ulcerated. Treatment consists of reduction of the paraphimosis under anaesthesia. Occasionally the constricting ring of foreskin has to be divided on the dorsal aspect to facilitate reduction. This is called a dorsal slit. Paraphimosis is an indication for circumcision, which may be undertaken as part of the emergency treatment if the tissues are not too oedematous. An iatrogenic cause of paraphimosis is failure to retract the foreskin following insertion of a urinary catheter.

Hypospadias

Hypospadias is a condition in which the urethral opening opens in an abnormal proximal position on the ventral surface of the penis or scrotum (Fig. 20.21). It occurs in about 1 in 800 live births. The majority (80%) are glandular with the urethral meatus lying at the base of the glans penis. In penile hypospadias the meatus is somewhere along the shaft of the penis and is always associated with ventral flexion deformity of the penis, referred to as chordee (Fig. 20.22). The most severe and rarest form of hypospadias is

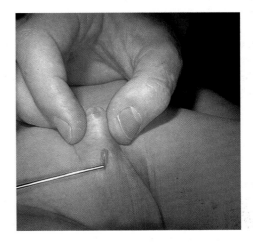

Figure 20.21 Hypospadias. The urethral orifice is on the ventral surface at the base of the shaft of the penis.

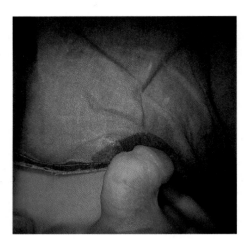

Figure 20.22 Chordee flexion deformity of the penis, always found in association with hypospadias.

perineal, in which the urinary meatus is found behind a cleft scrotum. It is important to differentiate this condition from an intersex problem.

Minor degrees of hypospadias require no treatment, while there are several complicated surgical procedures available for the management of more severe forms.

Epispadias

Epispadias is a condition in which the penile urethra opens on to the dorsum of the penile shaft (Fig. 20.23). It is very rare and in its extreme form may be associated with ectopia vesicae or exstrophy of the bladder (i.e. the bladder is

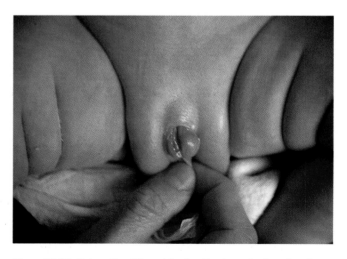

Figure 20.23 Epispadias. The urethral orifice is on the dorsal surface of the penis.

exposed on a poorly developed lower anterior abdominal wall). If epispadias is not associated with incontinence, surgical treatment is similar to that for hypospadias. The presence of incontinence makes management much more difficult.

Impotence

Introduction

Impotence or erectile dysfunction describes the persistent inability to obtain and sustain an erection sufficient for sexual intercourse. Primary impotence alludes to impotence throughout a patient's lifetime while secondary impotence refers to loss of previously normal erections. Psychogenic impotence is caused by psychiatric illness or emotional stress. This is in contrast to organic impotence which may result from physical causes such as vascular, neurological or endocrine dysfunction.

Erectile physiology

A thorough knowledge of the anatomy of the penis is important in understanding erectile function and dysfunction. The penis has paired erectile bodies called corpora cavernosa and the corpus spongiosum which surrounds the urethra. The tunica albuginea is the tough outer covering of the corpus cavernosum while the interior of the corporal bodies is made up of smooth muscle forming the walls of endothelial-lined vascular spaces.

The penis has a rich blood supply stemming from the pudendal artery and dividing into four branches, — the bulbous, urethral, deep penile and dorsal penile arteries. The deep penile or cavernosal artery further divides within the corpora to form helicine arteries and arterioles. The venous drainage of the penis is via the superficial dorsal, deep dorsal and cavernosal veins. These veins then drain into Santorini's vesicoprostatic plexus and the internal pudendal vein.

The erectile state is dictated by corporal smooth muscle. When the smooth muscle is contracted, blood is not able to enter the corporal cavernous spaces and thus blood is shunted to the venous side. When the muscle is in a relaxed state, blood can enter the corporal spaces and the penis becomes distended. This in turn causes compression of the venous channels and a reduction of venous outflow. The net effect is to cause rigidity of the penis. Detumescence results from increased smooth-muscle tone and corporal venous drainage.

The ability to develop an erection is also under the influence of specific neural pathways. The sensory or afferent limb of the erection is mediated by the dorsal penile nerve, a pudendal nerve branch. The efferent limb is mediated by the sacral outflow of the parasympathetic nervous system via the pelvic nerves. Pelvic nerve stimulation produces an increase in pudendal arterial flow into the cavernosal spaces. Detumescence is mediated by both sympathetic nerves and decreased parasympathetic outflow.

Aetiology of impotence

As noted, erectile dysfunction has both psychogenic and organic aetiologies. Although most cases (greater than 60%) have an organic basis, a large number of patients will have components of both contributing to the problem.

Vascular

Atherosclerosis is responsible for the majority of cases of erectile dysfunction in men over 60 years of age. Approximately half of men afflicted with peripheral vascular disease note some degree of impotence. Risk factors include diabetes mellitus, hypertension, cigarette smoking and hypercholesterolaemia. Impotence may also result from disruption of the venous mechanism involved with erection. Failure of corporal occlusion, known as corporal leak or venous leak, causes blood to drain from the cavernous spaces too fast or prematurely. Causes include atherosclerosis, trauma and Peyronie's disease.

Diabetes mellitus

Diabetes is the second most important cause of erectile dysfunction and impotence is known to occur 10–15 years prior to the general population and in up to 60% of men with the disease. Both vascular and neurological factors from small-vessel disease and peripheral neuropathic changes respectively contribute to the dysfunction.

Neurological

Men who have spinal cord lesions will have varying degrees of erectile dysfunction based on the level of the lesion. Approximately 50% of men with lumbar lesions will have erections while 70% of those with thoracic and 90% of men with cervical lesions are able to have erections. In addition to spinal cord trauma, other neurological causes of impotence include myelodysplasia, multiple sclerosis, tabes dorsalis and all peripheral neuropathies.

Endocrine

Endocrine disorders are a rare cause of impotence accounting for fewer than 5% of cases. Syndromes of hypogonadism are associated with erectile dysfunction, including hypogonadotrophic hypogonadism seen in Klinefelter's syndrome or surgical orchiectomy. Prolactin-producing tumours will lead to low testosterone levels and possible impotence. Isolated deficiencies of testosterone are uncommon.

Trauma

Traumatic rupture of the posterior urethra and perineal trauma, including straddle injuries, can lead to impotence. Pelvic fracture is also associated with impotence from arterial injury in up to one-third of patients.

Uraemic

Uraemic patients on chronic dialysis have a high incidence of impotence. However, half of these patients recover erectile ability after renal transplantation secondary to reversal of uraemic neuropathy.

Iatrogenic

Many surgical procedures may lead to vascular or neurological impairment and hence impotence. Radical prostatectomy or cystoprostatectomy were long associated with impotence. However, new techniques using an anatomical nerve-sparing approach have dramatically improved this. Aortic and peripheral vascular surgery may disrupt hypogastric arterial inflow. Neurological surgical procedures may produce impotence as a complication. Transurethral endoscopic procedures may cause thermal injuries leading to erectile dysfunction. Therapeutic measures such as pelvic irradiation are associated with an increased incidence of impotence.

Medications

Many commonly used drugs have long been known to cause impotence. Included in a patient's history, a thorough list of all medications used, both prescription and recreational, must be gathered. As is often the case, adjusting the dose or type of medication may correct a patient's erectile dysfunction. Table 20.23 lists potentially causative agents.

Diagnosis

Central to the diagnosis of impotence is a careful and detailed history. Questions related to onset, duration, degree and circumstances of erectile dysfunction are important. Past history should focus on those causes outlined in the section on aetiology. Psychological assessment

Table 20.23 Medications that may cause impotence.

Centrally acting agents	Hyperprolactinaemic agents
Phenothiazines	Oestrogens
Tricyclic antidepressants	Phenothiazines
Chronic ethanol abuse	Haloperidol
Narcotic abuse	Cimetidine
Marijuana abuse	Metoclopramide
Reserpine	Reserpine
	α-Methyldopa
Anticholinergic agents	Opiates
Tricyclic antidepressants	
Phenothiazines	Sympatholytic agents
Antimuscarinic agents (propantheline)	Clonidine
	Guanethidine
Antiandrogenic agents	Bretylium
Spironolactone	α-Methyldopa
Oestrogens	α-Blocking agents
Cyproterone	β-Blocking agents
Digoxin	
Ketoconazole	Agents with unknown mechanisms
Cimetidine	ε-Aminocaproic acid
Disopyramide	Naproxen
	Thiazide diuretics

From Siroky MB & Krane RJ (eds) (1990) *Manual of Urology Diagnosis and Therapy.* Boston: Little, Brown, 1990, with permission.

by trained professionals will allow identification and treatment of those patients with psychogenic impotence.

Physical examination should start with the evaluation of male secondary sexual characteristics. The penis is examined for length, plaques or deformity of the corporal bodies. Peripheral pulses must be evaluated, as absent pulse is indicative of peripheral vascular disease. The testes should be examined to assess presence or absence, size and consistency. Patients with androgen deficiency may have gynaecomastia. Neurological assessment should include sensory testing of the penile and perineal skin and the bulbocavernosus reflex to evaluate sacral reflexes.

Nocturnal penile tumescence testing will note changes in penis size during sleep. This test is based on the knowledge that, in normal postpubertal males, the stage of rapid eye movement (REM) sleep is associated with the development of erection. Several techniques are available to measure circumferential changes in penile size during sleep that would indicate the presence of erection. The penile brachial index is a technique used to assess penile blood pressure. Using a penile blood pressure cuff and Doppler signals, the systolic pressure of the dorsal and cavernosal arteries is determined and compared with systemic blood pressure measured at the brachial artery. Ratios of penile pressure less than 75% of systemic pressure are indicative of vascular impotence.

Biothesiometry is a method to test sensation of the penis by placing vibrations of differing intensity directly on the penis. Loss of vibratory sensation is an early sign of peripheral neuropathy.

Dynamic infusion cavernosometry and cavernosography is a technique used to assess the presence of venous leak or corporal leak as a contributing factor in impotence. Intracavernosal pressures are measured during infusion of saline after administration of intracavernosal papaverine. This agent produces arteriolar dilation and erection ensues. The inability to maintain normal intracavernosal pressures while infusing saline at a constant rate is indicative of venous leak impotence. Arteriography is reserved for cases of impotence felt to be secondary to arterial insufficiency but only when penile revascularization surgery is proposed.

Treatment

As discussed above, psychogenic impotence should be evaluated and treated by a trained psychotherapist or sex therapist.

Medical therapy

Medical therapy varies widely in both the proposed mechanism of action and effectiveness.
• Androgen replacement therapy with testosterone has been used with some efficacy in men with documented androgen deficiency. It is not indicated in patients with normal androgen levels and should not be given empirically. Parenteral testosterone enanthate or cyprinate is effective when given intramuscularly every 2–4 weeks. The oral form, methyltestosterone or fluoxymesterone, is available but is less effective than the parenteral form.
• Intracorporeal administration of vasoactive substances has proven efficacy. Papaverine hydrochloride is the mainstay of therapy and causes prolonged corporal arterial dilatation and venous compression. This drug may be combined with other vasodilators, including phentolamine. Prostaglandin E1 is also used extensively. Both helicine arteriolar and corporal smooth muscle relax in response to this therapy, causing corporeal occlusion. Patients will self-inject a solution containing a predetermined dose of these agents directly into the corporal space. Erections begin within 5 min of injection, with full erection being achieved within 15 min. Erections can last from 1 to 3 h.
• Another treatment alternative involves the use of a vacuum suction device that relies on negative pressure within the vacuum to allow the corpora to fill with blood, producing an erection. A constrictive band is placed at the base of the penis following removal of the vacuum cylinder

to reduce venous outflow. Many patients are able to achieve and maintain erections adequate for sexual intercourse.

Complications of intracorporal pharmacological therapy include local haematoma at the site of injection and induration from repeated injections. Priapism or prolonged painful erections can develop and potentially lead to permanent corporal fibrosis. Persistent erections from this therapy can be treated by corporal aspiration and infusion of α-adrenergic agents such as adrenaline to bring about detumescence. Complications following the use of vacuum suction include penile pain, ejaculatory difficulty and ecchymosis.

Surgical therapy

Surgical therapy for impotence includes the placement of intracorporal penile prostheses and, more recently, vascular surgical techniques in isolated cases of vasculogenic impotence.

• Penile prostheses are safe and effective, but it is a therapy that requires patient motivation. There are currently many devices available, including both non-inflatable and inflatable prostheses. Corporotomies are made in each corporal body, followed by dilation and measurement of the intracorporal space. An appropriately sized prosthesis can then be placed. The non-inflatable type can be rigid, semi-rigid or malleable, with a drawback being differing degrees of flaccidity. Inflatable prostheses consist of paired intracorporal cylinders attached to a reservoir and pump mechanism. The patient can inflate and deflate the device, which has excellent cosmetic and functional results.

• Vascular surgical techniques have met with varied success for arteriogenic impotence. Penile revascularization involves the microsurgical anastomosis of the inferior epigastric artery to the dorsal penile artery. When performed for patients with traumatic vascular occlusion, long-term restoration of function approaches 80%. However, in patients with atherosclerotic impotence, success is seen in only 50%. Venous leak impotence can be surgically treated by ligation of the dorsal vein. Success, however, is approximately 60% and may be short-lived as new venous channels develop.

21 Neurosurgical Disorders

The brain is a wonderful organ. It starts working the moment you get up in the morning and does not stop until you get to the office. (Robert Frost 1875–1963)

Introduction

Neurosurgery is concerned with disorders of the brain, spinal cord, peripheral nerves and their surrounding structures. Neurosurgical problems can be classified as follows:
- congenital anomalies — neural tube defects (spina bifida, meningoencephalocele), obstructive hydrocephalus, craniofacial anomalies;
- traumatic injuries — head injuries, spinal injuries, peripheral nerve injuries;
- tumours — primary malignant tumours (e.g. gliomas), secondary spinal and cerebral tumours (metastases from bronchial neoplasm), benign tumours (e.g. meningiomas);
- vascular disorders — subarachnoid haemorrhage, intracerebral haemorrhage, carotid artery disease;
- infection — cerebral abscess, meningitis;
- degenerative diseases — spinal degenerative diseases (e.g. disc prolapse), functional degenerative diseases (e.g. Parkinson's disease);
- hydrocephalus — congenital, acquired (e.g. postmeningitis);
- pain.

The management of head injury is probably the commonest neurosurgical problem encountered by most doctors and only a small percentage of these require specialist neurosurgical care.

Evaluation of patients with neurosurgical disorders

Clinical assessment

Symptoms

Careful, detailed chronological history-taking is essential for all neurosurgical patients. It needs to include a general history and family history and, when assessing paediatric neurosurgical problems, pregnancy and delivery history. History-taking will be difficult if the patient is confused or in a coma, but talking to relatives, friends, police and ambulance crews can be valuable. If the patient has come from another hospital, a close and critical review of the notes may be rewarding.

Neurological histories are:
- immediate, as in trauma or intracranial haemorrhage;
- progressive, as in tumours;
- intermittent, as in multiple sclerosis.

Sometimes an immediate event can be a feature of a progressive condition, for example a tumour can cause both a progressive deterioration and epilepsy.

Some important symptoms of neurosurgical disorders are given in Table 21.1.

Table 21.1 Symptoms of neurosurgical disorders.

Headache
Weakness
Numbness
Dizziness
Visual disturbance
Blackouts

• *Headache*: Headache may have extracranial or intracranial causes. *Stress or tension headache* arising from the muscles or fascia of the neck and scalp is probably the commonest extracranial headache encountered. It may be chronic and is usually helped by resting. A *migraine headache*, which is associated with prodromal visual symptoms, is severe and often unilateral and is accompanied by photophobia, nausea, vomiting and prostration. Unilateral headache may also occur with *giant cell arteritis* which is also accompanied by visual loss. Headache as a result of intracranial causes is usually due to *raised intracranial pressure*. Characteristically the headache is intermittent, severe on waking and disappears after an hour or two. Usually supratentorial lesions produce frontal headache while posterior fossa lesions induce occipital headache. Headache resulting from loss of cerebrospinal fluid, e.g. after spinal anaesthesia, is relieved by lying down and exacerbated by standing or sitting up.

• *Weakness*: Weakness may be described as general or specific. A general feeling of weakness may be indicative of a systemic disease, e.g. hypokalaemia, Parkinson's disease, but specific muscle group weakness is caused by upper or lower motor neuron lesions. With upper motor neuron lesions, e.g. following a stroke, the patient may complain of dragging or heaviness in a limb. With lower motor neuron lesions the patient will usually recognize loss of power in the muscle group supplied by the nerve, e.g. quadriceps weakness following femoral nerve injury.

• *Numbness*: Numbness means loss of cutaneous sensation and is seen with lesions of the peripheral nerves, e.g. the radial one-and-a-half fingers will be numb following transection of the ulnar nerve. Loss of sensation may also occur with cerebral pathology, e.g. during a transient ischaemic attack. Paraesthesiae or tingling may be encountered in patients with peripheral neuropathy (extremities), spinal cord lesions (from feet to waist), peripheral nerve lesion (unilateral), migraine, brainstem ischaemia, hypoglycaemia and hypocalcaemia (circumoral).

• *Dizziness and unsteadiness*: These symptoms can mean different things to different people. It is important to establish whether there are any precipitating factors, e.g. un-steadiness on standing up suddenly may indicate orthostatic hypotension, dizziness on looking upwards may signify cerebrobasilar vascular insufficiency. A rotational element in the description of dizziness usually indicates a vertigo. A history of continually veering to one side while walking may point to a cerebellar lesion.

• *Visual disturbances*: There are many visual symptoms which may occur and patients may have difficulty in describing them. Blurring or loss of vision in some or all of the fields of vision produces a confusing array of symptoms. It is very difficult for a patient who does not know the anatomy of the visual tracts to distinguish between hemianopia and monocular blindness. Therefore specific visual symptoms such as diplopia (seeing two of an object on moving the eye in one or more directions) or amaurosis fugax (transient blurring of vision in one eye) must be sought.

• *Blackouts*: A blackout is a spontaneous loss of consciousness. The common causes are epilepsy or syncope. A major epeliptic fit is characterized by aura, tongue biting, incontinence and convulsive movements, followed by headache and drowsiness. Syncope is produced when there is a reduced oxygen supply to the brain. The common causes of syncope are postural hypotension (the soldier who faints while standing rigidly to attention on a summer's day), Stokes–Adams attack (hypotension induced by heart block), and idiopathic orthostatic hypotension (caused by degeneration of the sympathetic autonomic nervous system or following drug treatment, e.g. antihypertensives). Unusual causes of syncope are micturition syncope and cough syncope.

Physical examination

Physical examination of a patient with a suspected neurosurgical disorder must include a thorough general examination, as the nervous system is commonly involved in cancer. For example, sciatica is often caused by a prolapsed lumbar disc, but can be the first manifestation of pelvic secondaries from rectal or gynaecological cancer. So always examine the abdomen of any patient with sciatica.

Neurological examination should be detailed and logical. One method is to assess higher mental function and level of consciousness while taking the history, and then to examine in order the cranial nerves from I to XII; the upper limbs, and then the lower limbs. When examining the limbs, test muscle tone and power first, then the reflexes, followed by coordination, sensation and gait (only for the lower limbs!). A useful mnemonic for the order of neurological examination is given in Table 21.2. Throughout the examination look carefully for any wasting, fasciculation or abnormal movement. In addition, compare right with left and upper

Table 21.2 Mnemonic for remembering the sequence of neurological examination of the limbs.

Member	Muscle tone and power
Royal	Reflexes
College	Coordination
Surgeons	Sensation
Glasgow	Gait

Table 21.3 Adult Glasgow Coma Scale.

	Score
Eye opening	
Spontaneous	4
To voice	3
To pain	2
No eye opening	1
Voice response	
Alert and oriented	5
Confused	4
Inappropriate	3
Incomprehensible	2
No voice response	1
Best motor response	
Obeys commands	6
Localizes pain	5
Flexes to pain	4
Abnormal flexion to pain	3
Extends to pain	2
No response to pain	1

limbs with lower limbs as differences can be important. For example, brisk lower limb reflexes in isolation suggest spinal cord pathology, but if accompanied by brisk upper limb reflexes and flexor plantars, they may be a feature of a nervous patient.

Examination of the unconscious patient

Unconscious patients need special care. Every effort must be made to obtain a history of events leading up to the coma. Occasionally, however, no helpful history is available. A low body temperature suggests that the coma is of at least 12 h duration, though this depends on the weather and where the patient is found. Before performing a detailed examination of any unconscious patient first check that the airway is protected, and that breathing, blood pressure and blood sugar do not need immediate attention. Look very closely at the whole body for signs of trauma and needle marks. At the same time someone else should look through the patient's possessions for drugs and relevant medical information. Such a search may reveal that the patient is a diabetic or has epilepsy.

The Glasgow Coma Scale

Terms such as 'semiconscious', 'very confused' or 'drowsy' give no meaningful information about a patient's state of consciousness as they can mean different things to different people. Therefore, reproducible scales based on objective criteria have been developed to record accurately the level of consciousness of a patient at any particular time. The most popular scale used today is the Glasgow Coma Scale. This scale is based on the measurement of three features that change with the level of consciousness: the stimulus needed to cause eye opening, the voice response and the best motor response (Table 21.3).

A fully conscious person will have a Glasgow Coma Scale score of 15, while the deepest level of coma will score 3. Although not absolutely defined, a score of 8 or less is generally considered to indicate coma. As this scale is reproducible, any changes in a patient's condition can be easily detected and communicated. The Glasgow Coma Scale must be used with some care and thought, however, as there are circumstances when responses can be wrongly interpreted. Such circumstances should be carefully noted and are as follows:

• Swollen eyelids: If a patient's eyelids are swollen, he or she will be unable to open the eyes.
• Intubation or tracheostomy: If a patient is intubated or has a tracheostomy, he or she will not be able to speak.
• Difficulty differentiating between a confused and inappropriate voice response: The difference between confused and inappropriate is a matter of degree — a patient may be confused about what hospital or city he or she is in or what day it is, but thinking he or she is at home, in a different country or year is inappropriate.
• Foreign language-speaker or aphasia: A patient may be alert and oriented in his or her own foreign tongue, but incomprehensible to the observer. Likewise, a patient may be fully conscious, yet aphasic and unable to speak.
• Best motor response in hemiplegia and paraplegia: For assessment of best motor response, the emphasis is on 'best'; a patient may be fully conscious and obeying commands, yet hemiplegic or paraplegic.

Some Glasgow Coma Scales omit the abnormal flexion category of the best motor response as there can be difficulty differentiating between a flexion withdrawal response and an abnormal spastic flexion. The maximum score a patient can reach is then 14, not 15. When recording the total Glasgow Coma Score the maximum total (i.e. 14 or 15) should be recorded and it should be split into its component parts, for example as follows:

Eyes open to voice	3
No voice response	1
Best motor response localizes to pain	5
Total	9/15

The pain stimulus should be sufficient to stimulate the patient and not leave unsightly bruises. The most appropriate pain stimulus is pressure on the nail beds with a pen.

Paediatric modifications   The language development of children under 5 years of age makes the use of the adult Glasgow Coma Score unreliable, but paediatric modifications are available, with rising levels of total score with increasing age.

Relevant neurological signs

Having assessed and recorded the level of consciousness it is essential to examine quickly for relevant neurological signs. In practice, for the patient in coma this means:
- checking that life-protecting cranial nerve reflexes are present (e.g. gag and cough reflexes);
- examining pupil size, equality and responses;
- looking for any localizing signs (e.g. conjugate or dysconjugate eye deviation, blink reflexes, facial palsy, hemiparesis, etc.).

This assessment should allow an estimate of the depth of the coma and its source, which may be general (i.e. metabolic or drug-induced), supratentorial, infratentorial or in the brainstem.

Investigations

The pace of investigation will depend on the clinical circumstances. There are situations, for example deteriorating undiagnosed coma, when the clinical team may have to take a history and examine at the same time as treating (i.e. securing an airway, raising blood pressure, giving anticonvulsants) and investigating (blood sugar) the patient. Whatever the situation, it is of no value to investigate to the detriment of a patient, for example subjecting a comatose patient to a computed tomographic (CT) scan before securing the airway and resuscitation. All too often, inadequately stabilized patients with a head injury or subarachnoid haemorrhage deteriorate during transit for a CT scan. Appropriate intubation, ventilation and transfusion would have saved them. The investigations commonly used in the management of neurosurgical patients are given in Table 21.4

General investigations

A decreased level of consciousness can be caused or compounded by abnormal serum levels of sodium, glucose, calcium, and urea, as well as by hypoxia and acid–base abnormalities. These must all be excluded. Haemoglobin and clotting screen should be routine. Because of the close association between the chest and intracranial problems a chest radiograph is essential, especially when an intracranial tumour is suspected as metastases are common.

Specific investigations

Lumbar puncture

Lumbar puncture is a useful investigation. It allows measurement of the cerebrospinal fluid (CSF) pressure in the cranial–spinal axis and examination of the CSF is important in diagnosing subarachnoid haemorrhage, meningitis, encephalitis, Guillain–Barré syndrome, multiple sclerosis and other less common conditions. In communicating hydrocephalus, a lumbar puncture allows therapeutic drainage of large volumes of CSF and lumbar puncture is essential for myelography.

Lumbar puncture is a dangerous investigation if the patient has an intracranial mass and must not be performed if there is:
- a history suggesting an intracranial mass (e.g. progressive morning headache, epilepsy, a combination of frontal sinusitis and headache that may be due to an abscess);
- a depressed level of consciousness;
- any focal neurological sign (e.g. hemiparesis, third cranial nerve palsy, nystagmus);
- papilloedema.

If any of these circumstances apply, obtain an urgent CT scan before performing a lumbar puncture even if meningitis is suspected. Lumbar puncture before scanning has no place in the diagnosis of coma.

Imaging

Plain radiography   With the development of more sophisticated radiological investigations such as CT and magnetic resonance (MR) scanning there is now little need for plain radiographs in the investigation of neurological disease. However, a plain skull radiograph still has a place in the management of trauma (see below), as it can help the doctor decide whether to discharge or admit a patient, or may indicate a need for urgent CT scanning.

In spinal disease plain radiographs are mandatory:
- in the management of suspected spinal trauma;

Table 21.4 Investigations available for assessment of patients with neurosurgical disease.

Investigation	Comment
General investigations	
Haematology	
FBC	Baseline investigation
Clotting screen	Promotes intracranial bleeding if abnormal
Biochemistry	
Urea, sodium, calcium	
Glucose	May cause or exacerbate coma if abnormal
Blood gas analysis	
Imaging	
Chest radiograph	Cerebral secondaries are frequent from a primary lung tumour
Specific investigations	
Lumbar puncture	Measure CSF pressure, useful in diagnosis of subarachnoid haemorrhage, meningitis, encephalitis, Guillain–Barré syndrome, multiple sclerosis
Imaging	
Skull radiograph	Diagnosis of skull fracture
CT scanning	Diagnosis of intracranial lesions, e.g. tumour, haemorrhage, infarct
MR scanning	More sensitive than CT. Imaging of choice for spinal cord pathology
Myelography	Invasive method of assessing spinal cord
Angiography	
MR angiography	Used to demonstrate intracerebral circulation and therapeutic embolization
Neurophysiological studies	
EEG	Used in diagnosis of epilepsy
SSEP	Assess sensory pathways
Nerve conduction studies	
EMG	Assess peripheral nerves

FBC, Full blood count; CSF, cerebrospinal fluid; CT, computed tomography; MR, magnetic resonance; EEG, electroencephalogram; SSEP, somatosensory evoked potential; EMG, electromyogram.

• in the management of cord compression from malignant disease;
• to assess spinal instability using flexion and extension views.

CT scanning   CT scanning has revolutionized neurosurgical practice in the last 15 years. Multiple X-rays generated on a rotating gantry that encircles the part of the patient being investigated show tissues of differing density on a screen or X-ray plate so that the image resembles a picture of the structures. CT scans are, however, only representations of X-ray density. It is due to computer graphics that the slices appear as if they are actual slices of the body. Skill and experience are therefore needed to interpret CT scans accurately, and appearances must be considered in conjunction with the clinical picture.

On a CT head scan denser tissues (e.g. blood, bone) appear white, water and CSF are black while the brain is a mottled grey. Intravenous contrast (Omnipaque, Niopam) will be taken up by a vascular tissue, tumours, and areas of blood–brain barrier breakdown, and contrast enhancement is therefore useful in the diagnosis of these conditions.

There is no standard system for printing the pictures — some scanners print the left side of the patient on the right side of the film and vice versa. Make sure you check which side is which. It is usually written somewhere on the scan, but may be in surprisingly small type. CT scans can be used for head and spinal scans. Reconstruction in coronal and sagittal planes, special views and three-dimensional effects can provide considerable information.

MR scanning   MR scanning is a more modern scanning system than CT scanning. MR scanning works on the basis that if a magnetic field is applied across a patient, different molecules have different rates of realignment if the field is altered. The energy released in these realignments can be detected and presented by computer graphics so that the image resembles a photograph of the tissue being scanned. MR scans tend to be more sensitive than CT scans.

However, the increased scanning time, cost and the claustrophobic nature of MR machines (the patient lies in a long tube) mean that MR scanning will not replace CT scanning at present. But MR scanning can complement CT scanning, especially in the investigation of pituitary, brainstem and spinal disorders (see Chapter 2).

Myelography   Myelography involves putting contrast, nowadays water-soluble contrast (e.g. Niopam, metrizamide), into the subarachnoid space by lumbar puncture or, rarely, cervical puncture. Allowing the contrast to float up and down the spine will demonstrate a partial or complete blockage, and there are typical appearances for disc prolapse, metastatic tumour and primary spinal tumour. Further information can be obtained by simultaneous CT scanning (CT myelogram) as the contrast clearly delineates the spinal cord. Myelography is, however, invasive, uncomfortable, and can be complicated by unpleasant headaches for a few days or arachnoiditis. As MR scanning becomes widely available, myelography is likely to follow air encephalography and ventriculography into the history books.

Angiography   Angiography is used to demonstrate the blood supply of the brain or spinal cord. This is usually achieved by direct injection of contrast into the blood vessels and the acquisition of multiplanar radiographs. Digital subtraction angiography is a technique whereby the soft-tissue images are subtracted from the angiogram, leaving a clear image of the blood vessels unobscured by the bones of the skull or vertebral column. Smaller amounts of contrast may be used with this technique. A newer technique is MR angiography, with which the direction and velocity of blood flow can be determined without need for any contrast injection. Duplex scanning is a useful screening investigation for extracranial vascular disease. Cerebral aneurysms, arteriovenous malformations (AVMs) and tumour circulations can currently only be accurately demonstrated by direct arterial puncture via a transfemoral catheter. Skilled neuroradiologists can extend these diagnostic pictures therapeutically by embolizing tumour vessels and AVMs, or occluding some aneurysms with balloons or platinum coils.

Neurophysiological investigations

Neurosurgeons rarely carry out neurophysiological investigations themselves. Instead they are performed by a neurophysiologist. Electroencephalograms (EEGs), somatosensory evoked potentials (SSEPs), nerve conduction studies and electromyograms (EMGs) all help locate the exact site of a lesion.

Most investigations used routinely in neurosurgery have been discussed above. However, a number of very specialized investigations may occasionally be used, often in a research setting. These include cerebral blood flow monitoring, positron emission tomography (PET) and single-photon emission computed tomography (SPECT) scanning, and cerebral metabolic studies.

Principles of management of neurosurgical patients

Having taken a history, examined the patient and performed the appropriate investigations, a plan of management can then be decided. As well as treating the condition, consider the effects the condition may have on the general well-being of the patient. Specifically for neurosurgery, this requires familiarity with the care of unconscious and paraplegic patients, whatever the underlying cause.

Care of the unconscious patient

In everyday life we protect ourselves without being aware of it — a cough clears our chest, a yawn opens up collapsed alveoli, a shuffle on our seats prevents a pressure sore, moving prevents contractures, and blinking protects our corneas from foreign bodies. We also take care of ourselves by deliberate actions, which include urination, defecation, feeding and washing. The unconscious patient is unable to do any of these things. The carers of an unconscious patient, therefore, need to anticipate and perform these activities of the patient on a regular basis. This requires much time and effort. Slapdash care, either through ignorance or overwork, can lead to secondary complications such as chest infections, pressure sores and corneal ulceration, all of which may ruin otherwise effective treatment (Fig. 21.1).

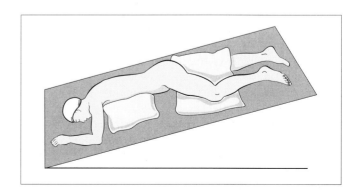

Figure 21.1 Position for nursing the unconscious patient. Note the feet-up, head-down position.

• *Chest care*: The airway must be protected at all times. Oral or nasal airway intubation or tracheostomy may be necessary depending on the depth of coma. The advantage of either intubation or tracheostomy is that they allow easy access to the bronchi with suction catheters to help clear secretions. Physiotherapists are a fundamental requirement for a neurosurgical unit, and chest physiotherapy takes priority over most things in the care of the comatose patient.

• *Pressure areas*: Lying on one area of skin for more than 2 h causes local ischaemia and breakdown of the skin. This can deteriorate to form a deep intractable ulcer, sometimes called a decubitus ulcer. The most common site is the buttock, but pressure sores are also common on the heels, elbow and occiput. Pressure sores reflect a failure of care and should never occur. They are prevented by regular turning and the use of sheepskins and water bags.

• *Hygiene and sphincters*: Scrupulous attention to hygiene, including mouth care, is essential. Urinary catheters should be used only if absolutely essential, though when the alternative is permanent wetness a catheter may be the only option. Regular laxatives or enemas are necessary to prevent constipation.

• *Eyes*: An exposed cornea will rapidly ulcerate and this may lead to blindness. The eyes of unconscious patient must always be closed, but also inspected regularly to exclude ulceration; any redness should be treated aggressively. Gelatin pads are the most effective compromise.

• *Feeding*: Most comatose patients, especially those with head injuries, have high calorific needs and if not fed adequately rapidly become malnourished. Feeding needs to be established as soon as possible, if necessary intravenously. When the gut is working nasogastric feeds should be introduced carefully. Reflux can readily occur and lead to aspiration into a poorly protected airway. The use of metoclopramide to improve gastric emptying and, if necessary, a percutaneous jejunostomy can reduce this risk. Diarrhoea is common with feeding, but usually resolves if the osmolarity of the feed is altered. Regular electrolyte checks are necessary and abnormalities should be corrected as they may prolong or worsen coma.

• *Movement*: Early, regular passive movement of the limbs is necessary to prevent contractures. Eventually, as the coma lightens, the patient will begin to move spontaneously and the movements may be powerful enough to result in falls from the bed or a chair. At this stage it is best to place the patient on the floor on a couple of mattresses or in a padded cot so that he or she can move around without injury.

• *General care*: Keep alert to other conditions that can occur when a patient is unconscious and unable to complain. Myocardial infarction, pulmonary embolus, meningitis and pneumonia may all present at first as an unexplained fever, tachycardia and tachypnoea in a comatose patient. Hyponatraemia may gradually develop and worsen the coma, and the use of steroids may predispose to gastric haemorrhage or silent perforation. Permanent vigilance is necessary, but when discussing the patient's condition at the bedside remember that the patient in coma may be able to hear every word that is said and behave accordingly.

• *Relatives*: Handling the relatives of comatose patients is usually difficult. As well as coming to terms with the illness and its implications, most relatives expect their loved one to wake up suddenly and say 'Where am I?' and be back to normal within minutes. When this does not happen they become frustrated and may take it out on the attendants — 5 min late with a turn becomes a major crisis. Frequent explanation is important and unhurried time set aside to answer questions is time well spent.

You may find it easiest to liken waking from a coma to the feelings we all have on waking in the morning, except that everything is in slow motion, lasting days or weeks rather than minutes. Many relatives, especially of children, like to become involved in the care by feeding, washing and turning. This is to be encouraged as it helps both relatives and hard-pressed nursing staff. Also encourage the relatives to talk to the patient. Nobody knows for certain whether a comatose patient is aware of voices — most who recover can't remember, and those who don't can't say — but it will not cause any harm.

• *Brain death*: Brain death exists when there is no demonstrable brainstem function in the presence of a diagnosis compatible with irreversible structural brain damage. On establishing brain death the patient may be considered for organ donation. If organ donation is not to be performed then the patient is disconnected from the ventilator (Table 21.5).

Care of the paraplegic and quadriplegic patient

Paraplegic and quadriplegic patients retain consciousness and higher mental functions. However, they have lost a large portion of their function and with it many everyday protective mechanisms. As with an unconscious patient, considerable time and effort coupled with psychological support are needed to care for these patients.

• *Chest*: The higher the level of spinal damage, the greater the extent of chest involvement; mid thoracic spinal lesions will result in paralysis of the intercostal muscles, cervical lesions may affect the diaphragm (remember C3, 4 and 5 keep the diaphragm alive) and higher lesions may involve the respiratory centres. Ventilation will be necessary if the respiratory centres or diaphragm are damaged. Good respiratory function can be maintained with a functioning

Table 21.5 Establishing brain death.

Tests for the absence of brainstem function
Do the pupils react to light?
Are there corneal reflexes?
Is there eye movement on caloric testing? (Ensure that the ears are clear of wax)
Are there motor responses in the cranial nerve distribution, in response to stimulation of face, limbs or trunk?
Is there a gag reflex?
Is there a cough reflex?
Is the patient apnoeic (in the presence of normocapnia)?

The following guidelines are important
There should be no doubt that severe irremediable structural brain damage has occurred. Reversible causes, including poisoning, prolonged response to drugs, hypothermia (<35°C), metabolic and chronic endocrinological disorders must have been excluded
Two doctors are needed to certify brain death. The first should be the consultant in charge of the patient or his or her deputy (who must have been registered for 5 years or more and be adequately experienced). The second doctor must be suitably experienced and clinically independent of the first. Neither doctor must be a member of the transplant team
The tests should be recorded on a suitable form
The diagnostic tests should be recorded on at least two occasions, separated by several hours. The exact time interval will depend on the patient's condition
The time of the patient's death is the time of completion of the second set of brain death tests. It is important that this is the time of death which is both recorded in the notes and written on the death certificate
If organ transplantation is not to be carried out, on completion of the second set of tests the patient may be left disconnected from the ventilator
Caring for the relatives at this time requires tact and understanding. If organ transplantation is not to take place, they may wish to remain in the room until the heart stops beating

---

diaphragm and paralysed intercostal muscles, but respiratory reserve will be less than normal and chest infections must be treated aggressively.

• *Homeostasis*: The higher the spinal injury the greater the dilatation of the blood vessels resulting from loss of sympathetic tone. Blood pressure falls and heat is lost, and both must be reversed in the acute phase. Never leave spinal patients lying around in casualty or the X-ray department uncovered. Space blankets and heating pads must be used.

• *Pressure areas*: The same attention to pressure areas must be given as for the unconscious patient (see above). In particular, watch the shoulder blades and occiput in those on cervical traction.

• *Hygiene and sphincters*: Most spinal patients will have disturbed bladder and bowel function. Before the availability of good spinal injury care the commonest cause of death in paraplegics was pyelonephritis. Early catheterization to prevent overflow incontinence is required, but as soon as possible the patient should be taught to express urine by suprapubic pressure or to self-catheterize intermittently. Urological evaluation to measure residual urine and other urodynamic parameters is advisable. Constipation must be prevented by laxative use and enemas.

• *Feeding*: Like comatose patients, paraplegic patients should be fed as soon as possible to prevent malnutrition and its complications. Paralytic ileus is common in the first few days after a spinal cord injury, and should be treated conservatively with a 'drip-and-suck' regimen, and intravenous feeding if necessary.

• *Movement*: Early mobilization is indicated if the spine is stable, though postural hypotension may delay this. The development of functioning muscle groups to compensate for non-functioning ones is a goal. Rapid learning of the use of any aids, for example a wheelchair or a computer for quadriplegics, is another goal and should not be delayed by unrealistic hopes for recovery, either on the part of the doctor or the patient.

Spasticity may be a problem and should be treated with an antispastic drug such as baclofen. Spinal patients are at considerable risk of developing deep venous thrombosis and pulmonary embolus. Prophylactic measures should therefore be taken for all patients. Some specialists of spinal injuries advocate full anticoagulation, while others use compression stockings (TED stockings) accompanied by low-dose subcutaneous heparin. Care of the paraplegic patient should be a standard practice in all units where neurosurgery is practised, but spinal injury units are so well-developed in this area that most patients should be transferred to one as soon as possible.

Common neurosurgical disorders

Head injury

More than 1 million patients present to UK casualty departments every year as a result of a head injury, which is one of the commonest conditions seen in hospital. The causes of head injury are many and varied, but it is common to see 'head injury' as the only description of the incident in hospital notes. Every effort must be made to discover its underlying cause, paying particular attention to:

• the likely speed of impact;

• any events which may have led to the injury (e.g. epilepsy, subarachnoid haemorrhage, alcohol consumption); and

• any events after its occurrence (e.g. vomiting, epilepsy, talking).

Pathology of head injury

The brain within the skull is liable to injury when deceleration occurs, i.e. when the neck flexes, extends or rotates. The brain moving within the cranial cavity may strike sharp objects such as the sphenoid wing and the frontal and occipital poles. In addition, points where the brain is tethered, such as the foramen magnum and the cranial nerves, are also potential sites of injury. Shaking of the brain when the skull moves at high speed therefore results in haemorrhage in the subarachnoid space and at the frontal temporal and occipital poles, and tearing of nerves and vessels. This damage can occur without the head being struck, for example in a high-speed car crash or in a fall from a height in which the body decelerates rapidly. It may also be associated with direct damage from a blow or a penetrating wound.

• *Primary damage*: The impact from a direct blow to the head is absorbed by the scalp and by the skull, which often fractures. The energy is then transmitted to the brain, damaging the tissue it strikes, and causing brain movement within the skull. This damage, which occurs at the time of impact, is called primary damage, or concussion. Survival depends on the energy reaching the brain which in turn depends on the velocity of impact (energy $= \frac{1}{2}$ mass $\times$ velocity^2). Therefore hitting a brick wall at 70 mph (110 km/h) will be fatal, but a kick to the head playing rugby will probably not be. Similarly, a shot from a high-velocity rifle will prove fatal, but a shot from an air rifle probably will not. The mechanism is the same, the degree is different. Severe primary damage is characterized by coma from impact. The ability to talk, even a few simple words, after injury indicates that, whatever else may happen, the primary injury was not severe and the injury is theoretically survivable.

• *Secondary damage*: Primary damage can be exacerbated by secondary damage (i.e. further insults to the damaged brain). These are important to understand as they can often be prevented and occasionally reversed, whereas nothing can be done about primary damage, except to avoid the accident. The main secondary effects are respiratory complications, perfusion failure, intracranial haematoma, cerebral swelling, epilepsy, infection and hydrocephalus.

  (a) *Respiratory complications*: Hypoxia, hypercarbia or obstruction to breathing will have disastrous effects on a damaged brain and can worsen the clinical picture dramatically. Head-injured patients are especially prone to respiratory problems because of lack of central drive, airway obstruction, haemo- or pneumothorax and/or aspiration pneumonia. It cannot be overemphasized that the most important aspect of head-injury care is care of the chest.

  (b) *Perfusion failure*: Perfusion failure will rapidly lead to cerebral ischaemia and a worsening of the clinical state. Head injury itself is rarely a cause of hypotension and other causes need to be looked for (e.g. ruptured spleen). Resuscitation must be rapid and patients with head injury accompanied by a systolic blood pressure of less than 60 mmHg for more than a few minutes rarely survive.

  (c) *Intracranial haematomas*: Intracerebral, subdural and extradural haematomas occur and can lead to deterioration following head injury. *Intracerebral* and *acute subdural* haematomas are usually associated with severe primary injury and carry a bad prognosis. In contrast, *subacute subdural* and *extradural* haematomas are often associated with little or no primary injury and bleed slowly over a few hours or days; removal before the intracranial pressure (ICP) is too high can lead to complete recovery.

  (d) *Cerebral swelling*: If you sprain your ankle it swells; if you sprain your brain, it also swells. As the brain is encased in a rigid box, cerebral swelling itself can cause damage by increasing ICP to levels at which cerebral perfusion fails. This leads to ischaemia which in turn leads to more brain swelling and a further increase in ICP. This vicious circle tends to be worse in those with severe primary damage.

  (e) *Epilepsy*: Fits are common in head injury and cause ischaemia while they are occurring. They must be stopped rapidly using intravenous diazepam in small doses, followed by phenytoin or valproate to prevent recurrence.

  (f) *Infection*: The development of meningitis or an abscess after injury can reverse a good recovery and must be watched for and treated vigorously.

  (g) *Hydrocephalus*: An absorptive hydrocephalus can occur during recovery and may slow or reverse recovery, but is relieved by shunting.

Classification of head injury

There are four types of head injury:
• *trivial*: little or no primary damage, no secondary effects;
• *apparently trivial, but potentially fatal*: little or no primary damage, but underlying secondary effect (e.g. extradural haematoma);
• *apparently hopeless, but potentially salvageable*: moderate to severe but recoverable primary damage and avoidable or reversible secondary effects;
• *hopeless*: overwhelming primary injury.

Management of head injury

The aims of management are:
• to recognize and treat those with apparently trivial but potentially fatal injuries at an early stage before brain damage occurs;

- to recognize those with hopeless injuries and to withdraw treatment at an early stage;
- to treat those with potentially salvageable severe injuries adequately and rapidly to minimize secondary effects and allow complete or partial recovery.

Trivial head injury

If the patient is conscious a history of the events leading up to the accident and subsequent to it is obtained. If the patient has sustained a period of unconsciousness it is helpful to obtain corroboration of this from witnesses. Retrograde amnesia for events leading up to the accident is a significant factor in the history. The duration of unconsciousness and retrograde amnesia are indicative of the severity of the injury and if very transient need not in the absence of other indications be a criterion for admission and further observation.

The questions to be asked are:
- Does this patient need a skull radiograph?
- Do I need to admit this patient to hospital?
- Do I need to refer this patient to a neurosurgeon?

These questions are easily answered by following guidelines laid down by a group of neurosurgeons under the aus-

Table 21.6 Kings Fund guidelines for managing a patient with a trivial head injury.

Criteria for skull radiography
Loss of consciousness or amnesia at any time
Neurological symptoms or signs
Cerebrospinal fluid or blood from the nose or ear
Suspected penetrating injury or scalp bruising or swelling
Alcohol intoxication
Difficulty in assessing the patient (e.g. the young, epilepsy)

Criteria for admission
Confusion or any other depression of the level of consciousness at the time of the examination
Skull fracture
Neurological signs or headache or vomiting
Difficulty assessing the patient (e.g. due to alcohol, young age, epilepsy)
Coexistence of other medical conditions (e.g. haemophilia)
Inadequate social conditions or lack of responsible adult or relative

Criteria for neurosurgical consultation
Fractured skull in combination with confusion or other depression of conscious level or focal neurological signs or fits
Confusion or other neurological disturbance persisting for more than 12 h even if there is no skull fracture
Coma continuing after resuscitation
Suspected open injury of the vault or the base of the skull
Depressed fracture of the skull
Deterioration

pices of the Kings Fund and published by the Royal College of Surgeons and the British Medical Journal. Their guidelines are shown in Table 21.6. The risk of a significant intracranial haematoma following head injury is 1 in 6000 among alert patients with no skull fracture, 1 in 120 among alert patients with a fracture and 1 in 4 among drowsy patients with a fracture.

An admitted patient needs regular neurological observation. Patients who suffered no loss of consciousness or who had no more than retrograde amnesia or brief loss of consciousness may be allowed home if they remain stable for 24 h. Simple fractures are not an indication for continued hospital stay. Compound fractures, i.e. associated with open scalp wounds or basal fractures with otorrhoea or rhinorrhoea, will need a more prolonged hospital stay and antibiotic therapy. Persistent rhinorrhoea requires surgical treatment to repair the ethmoidal defect.

Patients following head injury also need to be normally hydrated, not fluid-restricted. An intravenous infusion should be used if the patient is too sleepy to drink or is vomiting.

The only other aspect of care is to deal carefully with any scalp wounds, remembering to:
- shave hair for at least 2 cm around the wound;
- remove foreign bodies;
- debride the skin edges;
- suture the scalp in a single layer, leaving stitches in for at least 7 days; and
- use adrenaline with lignocaine to reduce bleeding.

Severe head injury

A person with a severe head injury will invariably arrive unconscious in the casualty department and the injury may be just one aspect of multiple trauma. The management is essentially the same whatever the cause and consists of intubation and ventilation, resuscitation, a thorough examination, radiography and deciding on treatment.

Intubation and ventilation An unconscious patient with a head injury should be intubated to protect his or her airway. This usually involves sedation and paralysis and so ventilation will be required. There is no reason not to intubate. Traditional reasons against it were that sedating the patient prevented neurological monitoring of any deterioration and that intubating put at risk an unstable cervical spine. Nowadays severe head injuries will have a CT scan so the first reason is less applicable and, although the cervical spine is also commonly involved in fatal head injuries, it is rarely injured in a survivable head injury. Having intubated and ventilated the patient, ensure the chest is moving properly, that there is no haemo- or pneumothorax, and check blood gases to ensure adequate oxygenation.

Resuscitation Insert one or more large-bore cannulae, a central venous pressure line if necessary, and a urinary catheter. Make sure that the patient's blood pressure and pulse are normal and that he or she has a good urine output. If there is bleeding find its source and stop it. Stop any fits with intravenous diazepam and phenytoin.

Assess the level of consciousness Once the airway has been established and cardiovascular stability achieved, the next priority is to assess the level of consciousness. Response to verbal and painful stimuli provides a simple evaluation but more objective analysis can be obtained by using the Glasgow Coma Scale. Any depression of consciousness is an indication for admission for observation. Confusion may arise if the patient has been taking alcohol or other drugs but this increases rather than diminishes the necessity for careful observation.

Thorough examination A full neurological and general examination is conducted to establish the presence or absence of focal neurological signs. Pupillary inequalities or abnormal response to light are indicative of intracranial haemorrhage. A falling pulse rate and rising blood pressure are also indicative of increasing intracranial pressure. In the conscious patient nausea and vomiting may suggest rising intracranial pressure from bleeding. In the unconscious or semicomatose patient vomiting may lead to aspiration into the air passage. Look at every part of the body. Pay particular attention to puncture wounds and the possibility of a spinal fracture.

Radiography Accompanied by competent staff the patient should be X-rayed thoroughly. Skull (see Table 21.6), cervical spine and chest films are mandatory, and if the patient has multiple injuries from a high-velocity injury, radiographs of the thoracic and lumbar spines, abdomen, pelvis and any suspected fractures should also be obtained.

Decide treatment plans There is no point in moving an unstable patient to another hospital for neurosurgery unless the instability is purely neurological. It is better to perform laparotomy or thoracotomy before transfer to stop bleeding and then to move the patient afterwards. Even if the patient is being transferred, spend a few minutes closing wounds and splinting fractures. Even if these procedures are crudely performed, it is better than not doing them at all, and they can be tidied up later.

Transferring a neurosurgical patient Unconscious patients do not travel well and care must be taken to ensure the safest journey. The patient must be stable before the journey starts as treatment of a deteriorating patient in a moving ambulance or helicopter is very difficult. The most experienced doctor available, preferably an anaesthetist and a nurse should travel with the patient. Lines and tubes must be well-secured before setting out and adequate supplies of paralysing agents, sedatives and fluids must be taken.

Neurosurgical management Invariably the first neurosurgical action, assuming the patient has been adequately resuscitated, is to perform a CT scan. This will show the presence of contusions, haematomas or hydrocephalus. If a haematoma or hydrocephalus is evident, treatment with craniotomy or drainage is necessary. If no clots are shown, or after surgery, a decision must be made whether or not to ventilate the patient. Views differ about who should be ventilated, but in the author's practice patients with respiratory problems or those at risk of developing them are ventilated to prevent hypoxia.

Ventilation is also used along with sedation and intermittent boluses of mannitol to control ICP. This treatment works by reducing Pco_2 which in turn reduces cerebral blood flow but this mechanism tends to be effective for only 48–72 h. ICP monitoring is essential in these circumstances, but is easily performed using a variety of methods. The simplest is to make a small twist drill hole in the skull, just penetrating the dura, screwing a tight-fitting metal bolt into the hole, filling it with saline and connecting it to a transducer. Normal ICP is less than 10 mmHg. If it is higher than 25 mmHg it is worrying and needs to be treated. If it is above 60 mmHg it is severe and is rarely associated with a survivable injury.

The patient is ventilated with full nursing care for periods decided on at the onset of ventilation (e.g. 48 or 72 h). After this period, if there are no problems and the ICP is low, sedation is stopped to allow the patient to waken. If the process runs smoothly, all is well and good, but if the patient becomes distressed or the ICP increases excessively, he or she should be reventilated for another set period. As the patient begins to wake he or she may be extubated as soon as the airway is secure. An active rehabilitation programme of physiotherapy, speech therapy and occupational therapy should be started to maximize recovery as soon as possible after recovery begins (see Chapter 30).

Special problems in head injury

• *Children*: Infants have a tendency to deteriorate dramatically after relatively minor injuries, becoming comatose and floppy, and then recovering again rapidly; this is the infant concussion syndrome. They also have a tendency to fit and may develop status epilepticus after minor trauma. Skull fracture and intracranial haematomas are less common in children than in adults. Non-accidental injury should always be borne in mind, especially when a child presents with acute subdural haematomas.

• *Depressed fracture*: In a depressed fracture bone is driven inwards and may penetrate the dura. CT scanning will show whether the dura is lacerated or not. Scalp lacerations over a depressed fracture must be closed urgently and the patient requires antibiotics. He or she may then be transferred at leisure to a neurosurgical unit where a decision can be made regarding wound exploration. If there is a suspicion that the dura is lacerated the fracture is always explored, but the indication for exploring a slightly depressed fracture is usually only cosmetic.

• *Missile injuries*: While high-velocity injuries are usually fatal, low-velocity injuries can be survivable. The patient should be resuscitated and transferred to neurosurgical care where the wound will invariably be explored to remove bone, skin and hair fragments. The missile itself however can often be left undisturbed.

• *Basal fractures* may be accompanied by rhinorrhoea, periorbital haematoma and subconjunctival haemorrhage if the anterior cranial fossa is involved or otorrhoea if the middle cranial fossa is the site. Subconjunctival haemorrhage in which the blood tracks forwards from behind so that there is no posterior margin to the haematoma is suggestive of anterior cranial fossa fracture. Direct injury to the eyeball produces a localized haematoma with visible margins. Periorbital bruising from direct injury is not confined by the orbicularis oculi, as is the case with intracranial (anterior fossa) injury.

• *CSF leak*: CSF leaks occur through the nose or ear, or silently down the back of the throat. Most clear up spontaneously within 2 weeks. Only a tiny percentage need surgical exploration to close the dural tear. Some neurosurgeons advocate no treatment for CSF leaks but it is probably safer to cover them with broad-spectrum antibiotics (e.g. ampicillin and flucloxacillin).

• *Cervical spine injury*: Injury to the cervical spine may accompany a head injury and fractures and dislocations in this area are common after road traffic accidents and falls. If a patient complains of neck pain or weakness and/or numbness in the limbs or if there is loss of sphincter control, an injury to the cervical spine should be suspected. Precautions should be taken to prevent further damage. Extension and rotation of the neck should be prevented, preferably by halter traction. Skull calliper may be applied later. Sandbags may help prevent movement in the emergency situation. Collars are of doubtful value. Lateral radiographs of the cervical spine, including all seven cervical vertebrae, are done as soon as possible. Movement of the patient is especially hazardous and five individuals are needed to move the patient, keeping the head and neck immobile. Unconscious patients following a head injury should be assumed to have

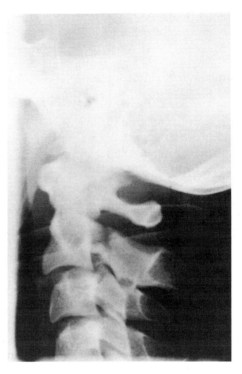

Figure 21.2 X-ray of cervical spine showing a fracture dislocation of the spine at C2–3 level — so-called hangman's fracture.

a cervical spine injury until proved otherwise by normal radiographs of the cervical spine (Fig. 21.2).

• *Other injuries*: Even relatively minor head trauma can be complicated by injuries to the eyes, facial skeleton, ears and cranial nerves. The cooperation of ophthalmic, ear, nose and throat, plastic and faciomaxillary surgeons is therefore needed. More serious head injury may also be complicated by cervical spine and carotid artery trauma, which may not be apparent at first.

Specific head injuries

Skull fractures

• *Skull vault fractures*, if linear and closed, do not of themselves require treatment and are more an indication of the severity of the trauma: attention is concentrated on the associated brain injury. Penetrating injuries may cause compound fractures with pieces of bone and foreign bodies penetrating the meninges or the brain itself. These obviously require careful exploration and wound toilet. Depressed skull fractures may lacerate meninges or brain and pressure from a depressed fracture may cause traumatic epilepsy.

- *Basal skull fractures* have already been mentioned. They are usually anterior or middle cranial fossa fractures and may communicate with the exterior with the risk of infection. Antibiotics should be given. Persistent rhinorrhoea in anterior cranial fossa fractures through the cribriform plate of the ethmoid may need formal repair.

Facial fractures

- *Nasal bone fractures* are common and are accompanied by swelling deformity and bleeding from the nose. Reduction is carried out to correct the deformity. If there is dislocation of the septum, reduction is necessary to relieve the obstructed nasal passage.
- *Fracture of the zygoma.* Direct injury such as a blow on the neck may produce a depressed fracture of the zygoma. There are three common fracture sites — the arch, the region of the infraorbital foramen and the frontomalar suture. On examination, circumorbital ecchymosis is evident with the bruising confined to an area within the orbital rim. Subconjunctival haemorrhage is also present without a posterior border. The cheek appears flattened and a bony step can be felt in the infraorbital rim with an area of paraesthesia below that in the distribution of the infraorbital nerve. Diplopia may occur and the patient may have unilateral epistaxis. Movement of the mandible may be restricted. Diplopia is usually temporary due to bruising of the inferior rectus and inferior oblique muscles. However, if there is entrapment of the muscles in the fracture, the diplopia may persist and an inability to elevate the affected eye can be demonstrated. Blowout fractures of the orbit are due to direct trauma to the eye with collapse of the orbital floor into the antrum. Entrapment of the inferior extraocular muscles may cause persistent diplopia. Zygomatic arch fracture should be elevated via a temporal incision within 10 days of the injury. An orbital blowout fracture requires elevation through the antrum or may need prosthetic replacement.

Fractures of the maxilla

Le Fort has separated fractures of the maxilla into three categories.

Le Fort I This fracture traverses the lower nasal septum and maxillary antrum, separating the dentoalveolar portion of the maxilla from the rest of the skull. The lower fragment is very mobile and dental occlusion is affected, giving an open bite.

Le Fort II In this higher-level fracture the line of the fracture extends through the nasal bones and medial portion of the orbit. Epistaxis and rhinorrhoea may occur. Perorbital bruising and subconjunctival haemorrhage are evident. Malocclusion is present with an anterior open bite.

Le Fort III This is a very high fracture above the level of the zygomatic arch and including the whole maxilla, which is pushed downwards and backwards. There is extensive facial oedema and periorbital ecchymoses with subconjunctival haemorrhage. Involvement of the cribriform frontal sinuses in the line of the fracture gives rise to escape of CSF as rhinorrhoea.

Fractures of the mandible

These fractures often occur in two places, sometimes involving identical sites on both sides, but sometimes involving quite different sites depending on the forces transmitted at the time of injury, e.g. a punch to the side of the jaw may cause a fracture through the premolar area on the side of the impact and a condylar fracture on the opposite side. The premolar area, angle of the jaw and the mandibular condyle are the common sites of fracture. The fracture is a compound fracture if it traverses a tooth socket and the patient should, accordingly, be treated with antibiotics.

Clinically a patient who sustains a mandibular fracture has a defective bite. Because of the upward pull of masseter and pterygoid muscles on the posterior fragment, posterior dental occlusion occurs prematurely and anterior dental occlusion cannot be achieved. The anterior fragment tends to be pulled downwards and backwards by the digastric muscles, thus further preventing occlusion. Damage to the inferior alveolar nerve may occur as it runs from mandibular to mental foramen, causing anaesthesia or paraesthesia in the area. A sublingual haematoma develops and a step may be felt in the line of the mandible.

Treatment is aimed at correcting the deranged dental occlusion and correcting the backward displacement of the horizontal ramus which can obstruct the airway. As in any fracture, reduction of the fracture with correct alignment of the fragments and immobilization achieves the desired result. Immobilization is achieved by fixing the upper and lower jaws together with cap splints or by direct wiring. Fixation for 4–6 weeks is usually required, except for unilateral condylar fractures where 10 days is deemed sufficient.

Intracranial haemorrhages

- *Extradural haemorrhage* occurs following a tear of the middle meningeal artery. The course of this vessel often runs through a bony canal in the temporal bone and a linear fracture in this area can cause a laceration of the artery.

Bleeding is rapid and an enlarging haematoma collects between the skull and the dura mater and compresses the underlying brain. The signs of increased intracranial pressure quickly develop with a rise in blood pressure, a fall in pulse rate, a dilated pupil and focal neurological signs, which include paresis or paralysis of the limbs on the opposite side and Jacksonian epilepsy. There is urgent need for intracranial decompression before coning and death occur. Evacuation of the haematoma via burrholes placed in the temporal region is a life-saving procedure and if necessary should be carried out on the spot as there may not be sufficient time for transfer to a neurosurgical unit. There may be time for CT scanning, particularly if there is a lucid interval and CT reveals the extradural haematoma compressing the brain.

• *Acute subdural haematoma*: This type of intracranial bleeding is more common than extradural haemorrhage and tends to occur in elderly patients who sustain a head injury because of the increased mobility of the brain within the skull cavity. It is accompanied by cerebral laceration or contusion and the patient tends to be in a confused or unconscious state from the time of the injury. The bleeding is the result of tearing of thin-walled veins traversing the space between the arachnoid and dura mater. The patient's neurological condition deteriorates progressively as the haematoma spreads. Even when the haematoma has been fully evacuated following craniotomy and incision of the dura mater, the patient may not fully recover because of the underlying brain injury or recovery may be slow.

• *Chronic subdural haematoma*: The condition develops over a period of days or weeks so that the initial head injury, often minor, which precipitated the bleeding is forgotten. The haematoma gradually enlarges, not as a result of continued bleeding, but because of absorption by osmosis of cerebrospinal fluid across the semipermeable membrane of the arachnoid into the clot. As the haematoma increases in size and the pressure rises, the patient exhibits drowsiness and confusion. Headache is not uncommon. Hemiplegia may develop. Pupillary changes develop late and are an indication of imminent cone formation. The symptoms may wax and wane depending on fluctuations in brain volume, which are dependent on changes in blood gases.

Identification depends on a high index of suspicion if symptoms such as headache or mental confusion persist after a head injury, even a minor one. Clinical diagnosis can be confirmed by CT scan. Treatment is by evacuation of the clot at operation. Burrholes are made and the dura, often stained greenish-blue by blood pigments from the underlying haematoma, is incised. The clot is sucked out and remaining thick blood is washed out with saline. Craniotomy may be needed to remove solid clot.

• *Intracerebral haemorrhage*: The patient is likely to be semicomatose or comatose on admission. The neurological deficit depends on the location and extent of the intracerebral bleeding. Much of the brain damage is irreversible but further damage from surrounding cerebral oedema and intracranial pressure can be minimized by ensuring adequate oxygenation. The period of unconsciousness may be very prolonged, requiring attention to nutritional requirements and other problems such as decubitus calculi, bladder function and bed sores.

Outcome from head injury

Mortality   Survival after head injury depends largely on the level of the consciousness on arrival in hospital, which reflects the severity of the primary injury. Those with a Glasgow Coma Score of 15/15 should have a mortality of no more than 1%; those scoring 8–12/15 have a mortality of 5%; those in actual coma on arrival with a score of 8–12/15 have a mortality of 5%; those in actual coma on arrival with a score of 8 or less have a mortality of 40% (Table 21.7).

Table 21.7 Outcome from head injury related to Glasgow Coma Scale (GCS) on admission.

GCS on admission (max. score = 15)	Mortality (%)
15	1
8–12	5
<8	40

Morbidity   Only 30% of those in coma on arrival (Glasgow Coma Score <8) will make a full recovery, while 20% will have some disability, but will be able to work and care for themselves. Ten per cent will require full care, being severely disabled or in a persistent vegetative state.

Postconcussion syndrome   Those recovering from even minor trauma may take a long time to get back to their old selves, suffering from the postconcussion syndrome. It is characterized by headaches, difficulty concentrating, dizziness and depression, and usually disappears after 3–6 months. Nothing can be offered except reassurance.

Other long-term effects   Survivors of more severe injuries often fail to return to their preinjury state as a result of personality change, memory impairment and depression, as well as any residual disability. Five per cent of people with a

Head injury at a glance

DEFINITION

- A *head injury* is the process whereby direct or decelerating trauma to the head results in skull and brain damage
- *Primary brain injury* is the damage that occurs to the brain immediately as the result of the trauma
- *Secondary brain injury* is the damage that develops later as a result of complications

EPIDEMIOLOGY

Head injury is very common. A million patients a year present to A&E departments in the UK with head injury and about 5000 patients die each year following head injuries

PATHOPHYSIOLOGY

- A direct blow to the head may cause damage to the brain at the site of the blow (*coup* injury) or to the side opposite the blow when the brain moves within the skull and hits the opposite wall (*contrecoup* injury). Similarly, deceleration of the head (e.g. with neck flexion, extension or rotation) results in the brain striking bony points within the skull (e.g. the wing of the sphenoid bone)
- The degree of primary brain injury is directly related to the amount of force applied to the head
- Secondary damage results from respiratory complications (*hypoxia, hypercarbia, airway obstruction*), hypovolaemic shock (head injury does not cause hypovolaemic shock: look for another cause), intracranial bleeding, cerebral oedema, epilepsy, infection, hydrocephalus

CLINICAL FEATURES

- History of direct trauma to head or deceleration
- Patient must be assessed fully for other injuries
- Level of consciousness determined by Glasgow Coma Scale (GCS)
  Fully conscious: GCS = 15; deep coma: GCS = 3

Eye opening		Voice response		Best motor response	
Spontaneous	4	Alert and oriented	5	Obeys commands	6
To voice	3	Confused	4	Localizes pain	5
To pain	2	Inappropriate	3	Flexes to pain	4
No eye opening	1	Incomprehensible	2	Abnormal flexion to pain	3
		No voice response	1	Extends to pain	2
				No response to pain	1

- Pupillary inequalities or abnormal light reflex indicate intracranial haemorrhage
- Headache, nausea, vomiting, a falling pulse rate and rising blood pressure indicate cerebral oedema

INVESTIGATIONS

- Skull X-ray (SXR) AP, lateral and Towne's views
- CT/MR scan Show contusions, haematomas, hydrocephalus, cerebral oedema

MANAGEMENT

Trivial head injury

- Patient is conscious, may be history of period of loss of consciousness (LOC). Retrograde amnesia for events prior to head injury is significant
- The indications for SXR, admission and referral to neurosurgeons are:

Indications for SXR	Indications for admission	Indications for neurosurgical referral
LOC or amnesia	Confusion or reduced GCS	Skull fracture + confusion/decreasing GCS
Neurological signs		
CSF leakage	Skull fracture	Focal neurological signs or fits
Suspected penetrating injury	Neurological signs or headache or vomiting	
Alcohol intoxication	Difficulty in assessing patient	Persistence of neurological signs or confusion for >12 h
Difficulty in assessing patient	Coexisting medical problem	Coma after resuscitation
	Inadequate social conditions or lack of responsible adult to observe patient	Suspected open injury to skull
		Depressed skull fracture
		Deterioration

Severe head injury

- Patient will arrive unconscious to A&E department. Head injury may be part of a multiple trauma
- ABC: Intubate and ventilate unconscious patients to protect airway and prevent secondary brain injury from hypoxia
- Resuscitate patient and look for other injuries, especially if the patient is in shock. Head injury may be accompanied by cervical spine injury and the neck must be protected by cervical collar in these patients
- Treat life-threatening problems (e.g. ruptured spleen) and stabilize patient before transfer to neurosurgical unit. When transferring, ensure adequate medical supervision (anaesthetist + nurse) during transfer

COMPLICATIONS

- Skull fractures: indicate severity of injury. No specific Rx required unless compound, depressed or associated with chronic CSF loss (e.g. anterior cranial fossa basal skull fracture)
- Intracranial haemorrhage:
  (a) *Extradural haemorrhage* — tear in *middle meningeal artery*. Haematoma between skull and dura. Often a lucid interval before signs of raised intracranial pressure ensue (falling pulse, rising BP, ipsilateral pupillary dilatation, contralateral paresis or paralysis). Rx is by evacuation of haematoma via craniotomy
  (b) *Acute subdural haemorrhage* — tearing of *veins* between arachnoid and dura mater. Usually seen in elderly. Progressive neurological deterioration. Rx is by evacuation but even then recovery may be incomplete
  (c) *Chronic subdural haematoma* — tear in vein leads to subdural haematoma which enlarges slowly by absorption of CSF. Often the precipitating injury is trivial. Drowsiness and confusion, headache, hemiplegia. Rx is by evacuation of the clot
  (d) *Intracerebral haemorrhage* — haemorrhage into brain substance causes irreversible damage. Efforts are made to avoid secondary injury by ensuring adequate oxygenation and nutrition

PROGNOSIS

Related to level of consciousness on arrival in hospital

GCS on admission	Mortality
15	1%
8–12	5%
<8	40%

closed head injury develop epilepsy, which may prevent return to work. Families are under great strain in these circumstances, but often little is done to help, except through self-help groups such as Headway.

Central nervous system tumours

Central nervous system (CNS) tumours arise from all tissues associated with the brain and spinal cord — bone, neurons, glia, meninges, pituitary and germ cells. In addition, metastatic disease commonly manifests itself in the CNS. Tumours usually present with epilepsy, raised intracranial pressure or a neurological deficit.
- Late-onset epilepsy is commonly caused by the presence of a tumour.
- Increased ICP: the presence of a tumour within the skull will cause ICP to rise. Early-morning headache made worse by coughing and straining is a typical symptom. Papilloedema may be evident, and may cause blindness. If untreated, the level of consciousness will fall, and lead to coma and death.
- A neurological deficit and its rate of progression will depend on the type and position of the tumour. A benign acoustic neuroma may cause deafness for many years before it begins to compress the brainstem, leading to ataxia and pressure effects from hydrocephalus. A malignant glioma in the motor strip may progress from mild contralateral weakness to hemiplegia within weeks. Pituitary tumours may have endocrine effects, and if growing upwards out of the pituitary fossa, may compress the optic nerves and lead to visual failure (classically, bitemporal hemianopia).

Classification of CNS tumours

While the terms primary, secondary, benign and malignant are relevant in the CNS, the tissue of origin and its anatomical position are more important. For example, a colloid cyst of the third ventricle is completely benign histologically but may present with sudden death because its position at the foramen of Munro can cause acute hydrocephalus.

Tumours found in the CNS are:
- gliomas: astrocytomas, oligodendrogliomas, ependymomas;
- meningiomas;
- lymphomas (previously known as microgliomas);
- neuromas;
- pituitary tumours;
- primitive tumours: primitive neuroectodermal tumours (PNETs), medulloblastomas;
- pineal tumours: pineocytomas, pineoblastomas;
- choroid plexus tumours;
- malformations: hamartomas, colloid cyst of the third ventricle, craniopharyngiomas, chordomas;
- metastatic tumours.

Specific CNS tumours

- *Glioma*: Gliomas are the commonest primary brain tumours arising from the supporting tissues of the CNS. They vary in their degree of malignancy, but are locally invasive and rarely metastasize outside the CNS. Gliomas are graded according to their histological appearance from grade 1 (slow-growing with a very good prognosis) to grade 4 (aggressive, with a survival that is usually less than 1 year after diagnosis, whatever treatment is given). Treatment includes surgery, radiotherapy and chemotherapy, either alone or in combination. As yet, nothing has been shown to be very effective. Most gliomas occur in the cerebral hemisphere in adults (Fig. 21.3). Grade 1 cystic astrocytomas occur in children and carry a good prognosis. Cerebral lymphoma used to be included with the gliomas and was called microglioma. It tends to be more radiosensitive, but its prognosis is still very poor, especially if associated with human immunodeficiency virus (HIV) infection.
- *Meningioma*: A meningioma is usually benign, but there are malignant variants. They arise from the dura and can occur anywhere within the skull or spinal canal but are

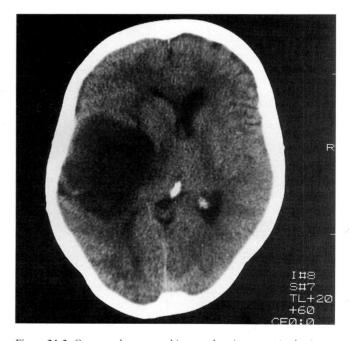

Figure 21.3 Computed tomographic scan showing extensive brain tumour in the left cerebral cortex.

most common in the cerebral hemispheres. If allowed by their anatomical position, removal is usually curative.

• *Neuroma*: A neuroma is a benign tumour arising from nerves. The most common is the eighth-nerve acoustic neuroma and the spinal neurofibroma. Removal is usually curative.

• *Pituitary tumours* (see also Chapter 15): A pituitary tumour can present with:

(a) pituitary over- or underactivity;

(b) visual failure due to chiasmatic compression (characteristically a bitemporal hemianopia);

(c) pituitary apoplexy.

Surgery is now less commonly performed for pituitary tumours than in the past because prolactin-secreting tumours can be controlled with bromocriptine. The transphenoidal route is the fashionable approach to the gland, but if the optic nerves are compressed, the transcranial route is still used (Fig. 21.4).

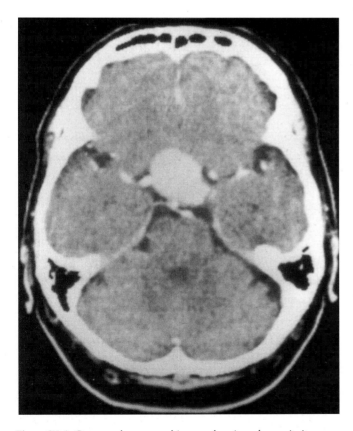

Figure 21.4 Computed tomographic scan showing a large pituitary adenoma. From Crockard A, Hayward R & Hoff JT (eds) *Neurosurgery, The Scientific Basis of Clinical Practice*, 2nd edn. Oxford: Blackwell Scientific Publications, 1992, p. 800, with permission.

• *Metastatic tumour*: Metastatic tumour (e.g. from a bronchial primary) is the commonest tumour in the CNS, but is uncommon in neurosurgical practice. Surgery is used where a diagnosis is in doubt or where there is a solitary secondary from a known, relatively slow-growing treated primary, e.g. the kidney. For certain types of chemosensitive tumour, such as trophoblastic tumours or testicular teratoma, a reduction of tumour bulk is essential for a cure; it is then worth being aggressive and removing all secondaries, even if multiple.

• *Other tumours*: Tumours other than those discussed above form only a small percentage of CNS tumours. In childhood, CNS tumours are the second commonest malignancy after leukaemia and are most common in the posterior fossa. The commonest childhood CNS tumours are cystic astrocytoma, which has a good prognosis, and medulloblastoma, which has a poor one.

Management of brain tumours

If a tumour is suspected, diagnostic tests need to be carried out urgently. Direct imaging is the investigation of choice. CT scanning is the mainstay of diagnosis, but MRI scanning will take over as it becomes more widely available; MRI is the first choice for posterior fossa, brainstem, pituitary and spinal lesions.

If the tumour is thought to be benign, surgical excision is the usual treatment. In certain situations, however, for example, if the patient is elderly and has no symptoms other than fits that are easily controlled by drugs, it may be safer to observe the tumour with serial CT scans rather than to attempt excision. If the tumour has the appearance of malignancy it is essential to establish the diagnosis. Rarely, such appearances may be mimicked by an abscess. If the tumour is easily accessible and not in a vital area such as the speech area or the motor strip, a craniotomy may be performed to debulk the lesion. If the tumour is deep or in a dangerous position, a needle biopsy under stereotaxic guidance is more appropriate. Further treatment of a malignant tumour usually involves neuro-oncologists and radiotherapists.

Intracranial haemorrhage

Haemorrhage can occur into any of the spaces (extradural, subdural or subarachnoid) within the skull, as well as into the brain itself.

Extradural haemorrhage (Fig. 21.5)

An extradural haemorrhage is almost invariably caused by trauma, the only other cause being postoperative. Usually the patient has a relatively minor blow that causes little

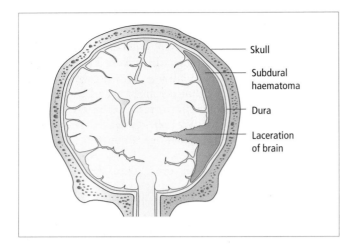

Figure 21.5 Extradural haematoma. From Ellis H & Calne R, *Lecture Notes in General Surgery*, 8th edn. Oxford: Blackwell Scientific Publications, 1993, p. 97, with permission.

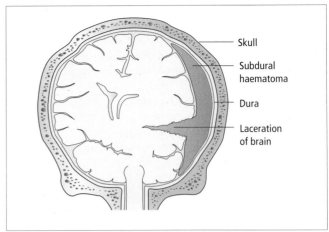

Figure 21.6 Subdural haematoma. From Ellis H & Calne R, *Lecture Notes in General Surgery*, 8th edn. Oxford: Blackwell Scientific Publications, 1993, p. 97, with permission.

primary brain damage, but which fractures the skull. Beneath the fracture a dural vessel, most commonly the middle meningeal artery, is torn and the bleeding strips away the dura from the inner table of skull. An expanding haematoma develops. The patient gradually sinks into a coma and will die from raised intracranial pressure if no action is taken. If, however, the haematoma is evacuated by craniotomy at an early stage, a full recovery is possible. The possibility of an extradural haematoma should be considered for any less than fully alert patient with a skull fracture and a CT scan should be performed before further deterioration occurs.

Subdural haemorrhage (Fig. 21.6)

A subdural haemorrhage may develop following a severe head injury, or chronically, following a minor head injury which is often unnoticed.

• Acute subdural haemorrhage carries a poor prognosis as it is usually associated with severe primary injury.

• Chronic subdural haemorrhage is seen in the elderly, alcoholics and infants who have been shaken. A small subdural bleed, often from a torn cortical vein, gradually enlarges over several days or weeks. The patient presents with a gradual deterioration in mental function accompanied by focal neurological abnormalities. CT scanning is diagnostic and evacuation of the haematoma is curative. In infants, chronic subdural haemorrhage usually presents with an enlarging head. The haematoma may be cured by aspiration, but if this fails, a subduroperitoneal shunt will be required.

Subarachnoid haemorrhage (SAH)

Acute haemorrhage into the subarachnoid space is caused by a ruptured aneurysm (usually a congenital berry aneurysm of the circle of Willis) in 70% of cases (Fig. 21.7),

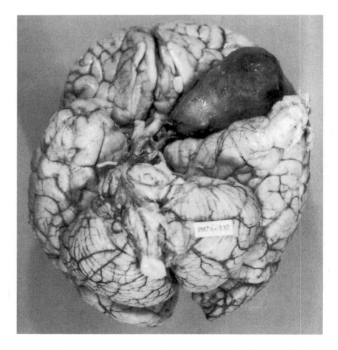

Figure 21.7 Cerebral aneurysm. From Crockard A, Hayward R & Hoff JT (eds) *Neurosurgery, The Scientific Basis of Clinical Practice*, 2nd edn. Oxford: Blackwell Scientific Publications, 1992, p. 617.

and an AVM in 10% of cases. No cause is ever found for 20% of patients. It is then presumed that a microaneurysm or AVM is the cause and destroys itself in the bleed.

• *Presentation*: SAH presents as sudden death (40% of cases) or as a severe sudden headache which may be associated with nausea, vomiting, coma or the development of focal neurology. Clinical examination will reveal an ill patient with neck stiffness and, possibly, neurological signs. A diagnosis of SAH (blood in the subarachnoid space) is made by CT scanning or lumbar puncture, which will reveal uniformally blood-stained CSF. The breakdown products of haemoglobin impart a yellow tinge to the supernatant (xanthochromia). SAH carries a poor prognosis – 30% of survivors of the initial event die within the next 6 weeks from the effects of the bleed, a further bleed or from delayed cerebral ischaemia in response to the initial bleed.

• *Delayed cerebral ischaemia* is related to the severity of the initial SAH. It develops about 5 days later and lasts for 7–10 days. It may be asymptomatic, mild or very severe, leading to infarction and death. Angiography shows diffuse spasm of the cerebral arteries and cerebral blood flow falls. No treatment is known to reverse delayed cerebral ischaemia, but its severity can be reduced by prophylactic treatment with the calcium channel blocker *nimodipine*. When cerebral ischaemia is established it is managed by nursing care, fluid loading to avoid a rise in blood viscosity and, if the source of bleeding has been secured, artificial hypertension using pressor agents to increase cerebral blood flow.

• *Rebleeding* is prevented by surgery to seal off the source of a SAH. Angiography will demonstrate the source and, if an aneurysm is seen, it is exposed by craniotomy and isolated from the circulation using a small metal clip. The timing of surgery is controversial. Many advocate early surgery, within the first 5 days of haemorrhage, to prevent rebleeding, and then to treat cerebral ischaemia if it arises. Others advocate surgery after 2 weeks (the main at-risk period for rebleeding and ischaemia). The risks of surgery are lower at that stage. Overall management mortality is the same whichever approach is used, but the individual who is likely to rebleed is better having an early operation, while the patient who will develop ischaemia should have delayed surgery. There is however no way of predicting which patients will do what with any accuracy.

If an AVM is found, the risks of a fatal rebleed are less and a more leisurely approach can be taken. If the lesion is near the surface it can be surgically excised, but if it is deep or in a dangerous position it is best treated by non-operative measures. Intravascular embolization or stereotactically guided radiotherapy are alternative treatment methods.

Intracerebral haemorrhage (Fig. 21.8)

Intracerebral haemorrhages occur spontaneously in elderly hypertensive patients and also in association with clotting defects or a pre-existing tumour. In young patients an AVM or aneurysm may be the underlying cause. An intracerebral haemorrhage presents with a sudden severe headache, which is followed by a rapidly progressive coma or focal neurological signs. Diagnosis is made by CT scanning, which is followed by angiography if an AVM or an aneurysm is suspected and surgery is contemplated.

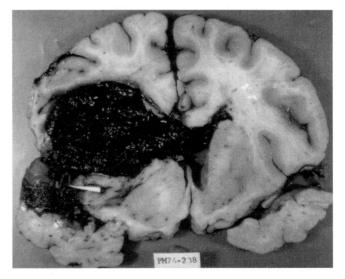

Figure 21.8 Intracerebral haemorrhage. From Crockard A, Hayward R & Hoff JT (eds) *Neurosurgery, The Scientific Basis of Clinical Practice*, 2nd edn. Oxford: Blackwell Scientific Publications, 1992, p. 619.

If a clot is seen it is tempting to remove it, but surgery is often not worthwhile except:
• when the clot is in the posterior fossa;
• when its removal can alter the outcome considerably;
• when a previously alert patient becomes progressively drowsier over a few hours due to the secondary effect of the size of the clot.

Comatose patients with a clot do badly and their outlook is not improved by its removal, while fully alert but hemiplegic patients with a clot usually improve, but their recovery is rarely accelerated by surgery.

Intracranial infection

Infection can involve the bones of the skull (osteomyelitis), the extradural or subdural spaces (empyema), the meninges

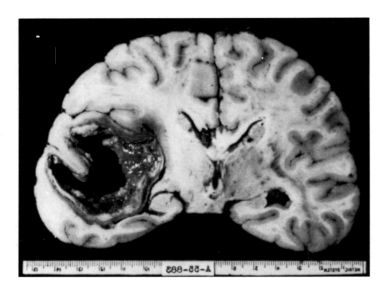

Figure 21.9 Postmortem specimen of pyogenic brain abscess. From Crockard A, Hayward R & Hoff JT (eds) *Neurosurgery, The Scientific Basis of Clinical Practice*, 2nd edn. Oxford: Blackwell Scientific Publications, 1992, p. 637.

(meningitis) or the brain itself, where an area of cerebritis can progress to abscess formation (Fig. 21.9). The source of an infection is either systemic (commonly associated with congenital heart disease, diabetes or septicaemia) or local (from middle-ear disease or sinusitis). Unless adequately treated, penetrating head trauma is a potent source of sepsis. A number of rare infections, especially toxoplasmosis, are now seen in association with HIV infection.

Diagnosis of an intracranial infection is often difficult until it is well-advanced. A history of a source of infection such as sinusitis followed by headaches often precedes a rapid deterioration accompanied by epilepsy, meningism and coma. CT scanning will reveal an empyema, area of cerebritis or abscess, and is the investigation of choice.

Treatment follows the usual lines of drainage of pus and antibiotics. Areas of cerebritis or small early abscesses may be cured by antibiotics alone, but close follow-up is needed with this regimen. If tuberculosis is suspected with reasonable certainty, surgery is best avoided, but if the lesions do not respond, biopsy is essential. Surgical drainage has the advantage of allowing an organism to be identified. It is important to treat the source of the infection at the same time as treating the intracranial problem. Appropriate antibiotics must be given in high doses for long periods — at least 3 months.

Hydrocephalus

Hydrocephalus is the accumulation of an excessive volume of CSF within the ventricular system and subarachnoid spaces. CSF is produced mainly by the choroid plexus of the lateral and fourth ventricles, although a small amount is produced by the whole neuraxis. Most is produced in the lateral ventricles at a rate of 0.3 ml/min. CSF then flows via the foramen of Munro to the third ventricle and thence down the aqueduct to the fourth ventricle, and out into the subarachnoid space. In this space it is absorbed by the arachnoid granulations over the surface of the hemispheres. The average adult CSF volume is 150 ml. CSF is therefore changed three times every 24 h.

Pathology

Hydrocephalus may result from overproduction of CSF, obstruction to its circulation or failure of its absorption. Whatever the cause, if CSF can leave the fourth ventricle and communicate with the subarachnoid space, it is called communicating hydrocephalus. When CSF is trapped within the ventricles and cannot reach this space, it is called a non-communicating hydrocephalus.

• *CSF overproduction*: Hydrocephalus due to CSF overproduction is the least common cause of hydrocephalus and is caused by a CSF-secreting tumour — a choroid plexus papilloma. These are usually benign tumours of childhood, and hydrocephalus is the presenting symptom. CSF production may be four times normal, and as the tumours tend to have minor haemorrhages, there is often an element of absorption failure as well. Fourth ventricular choroid plexus papillomas may block the fourth ventricle and also cause an obstructive hydrocephalus.

• *Obstruction to CSF flow*: Any obstruction to the flow of CSF within the ventricular system will cause an obstructive hydrocephalus. This results in non-communicating hydro-cephalus and usually occurs at the narrowest points of the CSF circulation, as follows:

(a) in the lateral ventricles, when an intraventricular haemorrhage fills the ventricles;

(b) at the foramen of Munro, which can be obstructed by intraventricular tumours — most commonly a colloid cyst, hypothalamic glioma, craniopharyngioma and, rarely, a pituitary adenoma;

(c) in the aqueduct if it is obstructed by a pineal region tumour, brainstem glioma, and congenital aqueduct stenosis or neonatal intraventricular haemorrhage, which commonly blocks the aqueduct;

(d) in the fourth ventricle, which can be blocked by a congenital fourth ventricular (Dandy–Walker) cyst, a fourth ventricular tumour (e.g. glioma, medulloblastoma, ependymoma), or any cause of cerebellar swelling (e.g. infarction, haemorrhage, tumour).

• *Failure of CSF absorption*: Any process that raises the protein content of the CSF in the subarachnoid space and blocks the arachnoid granulations will cause a communicating absorptive hydrocephalus. These are the commonest causes of hydrocephalus and include head injury, subarachnoid haemorrhage and meningitis. Likewise, any process that obliterates the subarachnoid space, for example, tuberculous meningitis, sarcoidosis and carcinomatous meningitis, will prevent CSF absorption.

Clinical manifestations

The symptoms and signs of hydrocephalus depend mainly on the speed of onset and age of the patient. Hydrocephalus should be confirmed or excluded in any patient with a head injury, haemorrhage or meningitis who reaches a plateau or deteriorates.

• *Infancy*: Before suture fusion at 18 months, a child's head is elastic. The main feature of hydrocephalus is therefore rapid head growth, as measured by the occipitofrontal circumference. This growth rate will exceed the rate of length and weight gain on a growth chart. If the rate of ventricular enlargement exceeds the ability of the head to expand, the anterior fontanelle will become tense and the sutures splayed — the scalp veins will distend and the baby will lose the ability to look upwards (the setting-sun sign). These signs indicate a sick baby who needs urgent intervention.

• *Childhood/adult*: Within a closed skull hydrocephalus causes the signs of raised ICP (headache and a falling level of consciousness). With very rapidly developing hydrocephalus, usually due to a colloid cyst completely occluding the foramen of Munro, the rise in ICP may be so fast that coma and death rapidly ensue.

• *Old age*: A syndrome that can affect the elderly is normal-pressure hydrocephalus (NPH), which is probably a variant of absorptive failure. The characteristic symptoms and signs are those of Adam's triad — dementia, ataxia and incontinence. There may be a history of head injury, meningitis or cerebral haemorrhage. It is difficult to differentiate NPH from senile dementia, and often they may coexist.

Investigations

• *Ultrasound*: In the infant with an open fontanelle an ultrasound probe can be used to measure ventricular size and plot the rate of growth.

• *CT scan*: The CT scan is the most useful investigation of hydrocephalus as it shows ventricular size and any underlying causes (Fig. 21.10).

• *Lumbar puncture*: Lumbar puncture must *not* be performed if there is a definite or a suspected non-communicating hydrocephalus. However, if it is clearly established that the hydrocephalus communicates with the subarachnoid

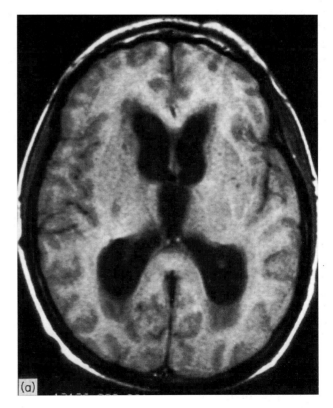

(a)

Figure 21.10 Computed tomography scan showing hydrocephalus. From Crockard A, Hayward R & Hoff JT (eds) *Neurosurgery, The Scientific Basis of Clinical Practice*, 2nd edn. Oxford: Blackwell Scientific Publications, 1992, p. 363.

space, lumbar puncture may be used to measure pressure and to test the effect of draining off a volume of CSF.

Treatment

At first, treatment must be aimed at removing the cause if possible, for example removing an underlying tumour. If this is not possible, treatment is directed at reducing the production of CSF, intermittently removing excess CSF or permanently diverting the CSF to a place where it can be absorbed.

• *Reduce production*: The carbonic anhydrase inhibitor *Diamox* and some diuretics can reduce CSF production. This tends to be a temporary effect and electrolyte balance must be carefully maintained. The choroid plexus can be destroyed either by open operation or by using an endoscope. This is popular with some neurosurgeons, but is not widely performed.

• *Remove excess CSF*: Ventricular tapping (in infants), ventricular drainage and lumbar puncture and lumbar drainage can all be used as temporary measures to remove excess CSF where appropriate. These methods are particularly useful after a haemorrhage or meningitis when high CSF protein makes shunting liable to failure.

Permanently divert CSF (shunt)

Permanently diverted CSF is drained via a silicone tube passing through a one-way pressure-regulated valve into the right atrium, pleura or, most commonly, the peritoneum, where it is absorbed back into the circulation. This is the most effective and permanent treatment of hydrocephalus. Once inserted, modern shunts are very reliable but are prone to complications arising from overdrainage, blockage or infections.

• Overdrainage in infants leads to overriding of the skull sutures and scaphycephaly and in adults causes subdural hygromas.

• Blockage usually occurs when the CSF is too thick because it contains too much protein. Hydrocephalus should be controlled by other means until the CSF protein content is reduced to prevent this complication. A late blockage arises when debris from the ventricles accumulates within the shunt, or when the choroid plexus or omentum occludes the shunt from the outside.

• Infected shunts can cause meningitis and chronic peritonitis, and if inserted into the right atrium, septicaemia, endocarditis, pulmonary hypertension and glomerulonephritis. Infected shunts need to be removed, and the CSF sterilized by antibiotics. The shunt can then be replaced.

Spinal surgery

Both neurosurgeons and orthopaedic surgeons who operate on the spine must have a thorough understanding of both the neurology and biomechanics of the spine, and be conversant with spinal stabilization techniques. The spinal surgeon must also be able to approach the spine from many directions, should be comfortable operating through the mouth, neck, chest and abdomen if necessary, and be able to use an operating microscope.

Special considerations

Radiography, myelography, CT and MR scanning and electrophysiology are used to answer the following fundamental questions:

• What is the diagnosis?
• What level of the spine is involved?
• Is the spine stable?
• Will treatment affect spine stability?
• What approach should be used?

Spine stability is maintained by the strength of the vertebral body, the lateral masses and the laminae. Destruction of one element does not usually affect stability, whereas loss of two is likely to cause instability, which is guaranteed if all three elements are destroyed. A typical example of this is malignant cord compression. If this is posterior and erodes the lamina, a laminectomy to decompress the spine will not affect stability. However, if the tumour is anterior and has eroded the vertebral body and lateral masses, a laminectomy will remove the only element giving stability, and the spine will become unstable with disastrous consequences. In these circumstances the operative approach has to be from the front, via the neck, chest or abdomen. The vertebral body is removed and replaced by a bone graft, metal or cement.

Spine stabilization

The spine can be stabilized either externally or internally.

External stabilization

External stabilization is most effective for the neck, either by traction or a halo device.

• Traction is applied by callipers fixed to the skull. Weights are applied until the cervical vertebrae are correctly aligned and the alignment is then held by the weight of the traction. This is the first treatment used for neck fractures, and may be used for 6–8 weeks until fusion has occurred.

• A halo is a metal ring fixed to the skull from which four metal rods pass to a strong plastic or plaster jacket worn over the chest and abdomen. It holds the neck rigid until fusion occurs, which usually takes 3 months.

Internal stabilization

Internal stabilization is performed at operation and a wide variety of techniques are used, sometimes in combination or along with external fixation. There are three broad categories: bone grafting, cement and prosthetics.

• *Bone grafting*: Bone grafts can be used to stabilize the spine using either the patient's bone, usually from the iliac crest, or a commercial preparation of dried animal bone. Bone grafts are rarely sufficient by themselves for immediate stabilization, but when incorporated are the most effective method of giving long-term stability.

• *Cement*: Biological cement is useful for replacing vertebral bodies, but there are risks, particularly of infection. It is most useful when long-term survival is unlikely, for example for malignant cord compression.

• *Prosthetics*: Replacing or supporting bone with prosthetic material is a common technique, and can be accompanied by bone grafting or cement. Techniques vary from a simple wiring together of two spinous processes to the replacement of a number of vertebral bodies with a tailor-made metal or porcelain prosthetic body.

Most parts of the spine from the odontoid to the sacrum can now be stabilized from one direction or another.

Spinal disorders

Care of the paraplegic patient is discussed on pp. 429–430. Other common spinal conditions are spinal injury, spinal tumours and malignant cord compression, disc prolapse, spondylosis, rheumatoid arthritis, infection and haemorrhage.

Spinal injury

Spinal injury is about one-tenth as common as head injury, but the basic pathology is the same. Such an injury may be complete (rendering the patient functionless below the level of the lesion) or incomplete (some function is preserved). Secondary effects, including hypoxia and perfusion failure, can also occur. Compression of the cord, however, is less common than compression of the brain following head injury. The causes of cord compression are bone fragments, haematomas and acute disc prolapses.

Management of spinal injury

Three fundamental questions must be answered when managing a spinal injury:

• At what level is the injury?
• Is the cord lesion complete or incomplete?
• Is the bony architecture stable or unstable?

Flaccid paraplegia with no preservation of sensation usually indicates a complete lesion. The sacral dermatomes are the most resistant to injury and sacral sparing is a cause for optimism. If the lesion is incomplete, every effort must be made to prevent deterioration. Thus the spine must be held in a stable position, hypoxia prevented and hypotension corrected. Early investigation with CT myelography or MRI scanning will exclude cord compression.

If the bony architecture is displaced or thought to be unstable it should be reduced and stabilized. When the cervical spine is injured this can be done with traction only, but if the thoracic and lumbar spines are involved, open reduction may be required. It is now common to perform an early operative fixation with bone grafts and metal for both incomplete and complete lesions. This allows early mobilization which in turn reduces the risk of chest complications and deep vein thrombosis. At the earliest opportunity the patient should be transferred to a spinal injuries unit.

Spinal tumours

Primary spinal tumours are much less common than brain tumours, but cord compression due to metastases is common. There is an increasing tendency to give radiotherapy as the treatment of choice for malignant cord compression, reserving surgery for when the diagnosis is uncertain or radiation has failed. Care must be taken to avoid destabilizing the spine; major surgery involving vertebral body excision, bone grafting and metal support may be required. Any treatment of malignant cord compression is pointless if the patient is already paraplegic. Therefore, if a patient who is known to have cancer complains of girdle pain, leg weakness or difficulty in passing urine, he or she should be investigated (and treated) urgently.

Primary spinal tumours

Primary spinal tumours are either extramedullary, i.e. within the dura, but outside the cord, for example a meningioma, or a neurofibroma, or intramedullary, i.e. within the spinal cord, for example an astrocytoma, or an ependymoma.

Extramedullary tumours are benign and should be removed when discovered. They usually cause pain or neurological deficit. Intramedullary tumours tend to be slow-growing but invasive. Sometimes they can be removed, but commonly they can only be biopsied and debulked and then treated with radiotherapy. Survival is usually good, but progressive neurological impairment is common.

Malignant cord compression

Pathology

Metastatic compression of the spinal cord is common in advanced cancer, particularly with tumours of the bronchus, breast, prostate and kidney and myeloproliferative disorders. The spread is usually haematogenous, but can result from direct extension from a bronchial carcinoma. Malignant cord compression is usually extradural, though intradural compression does occur, and destruction of surrounding bone is common. The thoracic spine is the commonest site, but any level of the spine can be involved. Although metastatic spread often involves multiple levels of the spine, usually only one is symptomatic at any one time.

Clinical features

Malignant cord compression presents with pain in the affected dermatome, and this is followed by progressive spastic paraparesis below the level of the lesion. The rate of deterioration depends on the rate of compression, but sudden deterioration is commonly precipitated by bony collapse. Cord compression must be considered in any patient with known or suspected cancer who develops pain, especially girdle pain, followed by leg stiffness or difficulty walking. If compression develops to the point of paraplegia the patient will never walk again, but if dealt with when there is only pain or slight weakness, full recovery is possible. It is not uncommon for patients in bed gradually to deteriorate without their doctors realizing it, the diagnosis only being considered when urinary retention develops. This should not happen and the patient's complaints must be taken seriously. Investigation of malignant compression is by plain radiography to reveal any bony erosion or collapse, followed by myelography, preferably with CT or MR scanning. These investigations confirm cord compression, establish single- or multiple-level involvement and allow for planning of appropriate treatment.

Management

Treatment should start as soon as the diagnosis of malignant compression is suspected. Dexamethasone is commenced to slow further deterioration and the patient should be transferred rapidly to neurosurgical care for investigation. Further treatment will be either surgery or radiotherapy or both. If there is no established diagnosis, histology must be obtained either by open operation or needle biopsy. If the diagnosis is known the first line of treatment is radiotherapy as this is as effective as an operation without the risks of surgery.

Surgery is reserved for those patients in whom the diagnosis is not established and needle biopsy is impractical or fails, and for those who do not respond to radiotherapy. The aim of surgery is to decompress the spine without making it unstable. If the compression is purely posterior and there is no destruction of the vertebral bodies, laminectomy is appropriate. If the vertebral bodies are involved, the anterior approach is required; this is more demanding for both patient and surgeon. The patient's expected survival from cancer must be considered before embarking on major surgery.

Disc prolapse (see also Chapter 22)

Pathology

The intervertebral discs are the shock absorbers between the vertebral bodies. They consist of a tough outer ring, the annulus fibrosis, which surrounds a gelatinous centre, the nucleus pulposus. With ageing the disc dehydrates and the collagen weakens. This can lead to rupture of the annulus fibrosis and extrusion of the nucleus pulposus into the spinal canal, where it sets up an inflammatory response and hardens. The hardened extrusion causes pain both by inflammation and by stretching the spinal nerves. Large prolapses may stretch the spinal nerves, causing numbness and weakness in their distribution, and if large enough may even cause spinal cord or cauda equina compression.

Disc prolapses usually occur spontaneously, either acutely or gradually, but may also be precipitated by trauma and complicate spinal cord injury. The commonest sites of disc prolapse are the lower lumbar region, especially L4/5 and L5/S1, and the lower cervical region, especially C5/6 and C6/7, probably because these are the most mobile areas of the spine. Less mobile segments are less often involved; the relatively immobile thoracic spine is rarely affected. However, because of the narrowness of the thoracic spinal canal, disc prolapse in this region may have serious consequences.

Clinical features

Disc prolapse usually presents with pain in the affected dermatome and area of the spine; lumbosacral prolapses present with low back pain associated with pain in the leg (sciatica), while cervical prolapses cause neck pain and pain in the affected arm (brachialgia). There may be signs of root tension such as limited straight leg raising, and neurological signs, including weakness in the affected myotome and reflex changes (e.g. footdrop and an absent ankle jerk and an L4/5 prolapse). Sensory changes may occur, but are often inconsistent. A large central lumbar disc prolapse may cause bilateral sciatica, saddle anaesthesia and urinary retention. This is an emergency and warrants immediate referral to a neurosurgical unit as delay may lead to persisting urinary problems. A central cervical prolapse may cause quadriparesis or quadriplegia and is also a major emergency.

Management

At first a disc prolapse is treated with rest, adequate analgesia and sedation. A patient with lumbar prolapse requires strict bedrest, rising only to go to the toilet, whereas a cervical collar is necessary for cervical prolapse: a firm collar is more useful than a soft one. On these regimens 95% of prolapses settle spontaneously within 2 weeks.

Surgical intervention is required only if:
- the prolapse does not settle acutely;
- the symptoms relapse within a short time;
- the symptoms improve but never settle completely and become chronic; or
- there is an associated neurological deficit, such as footdrop.

Surgery is usually undertaken after appropriate investigation to confirm the clinical level. Plain CT, myelography, CT myelography or MR scanning may all be used, although in years to come MR scanning will probably be the investigation of choice. The surgical options include percutaneous discectomy under radiological control, chymopapain injection into the disc prolapse to dissolve it, or open discectomy. The first two options have not gained widespread popularity and can only be used in the lumbar region. Open discectomy is the most widely used surgical procedure. Only the prolapse is excised and the centre of the disc is cleared of as much of the nucleus pulposus as possible to reduce pressure within it and allow healing of the tear in the annulus fibrosis. The disc itself is not removed. It is now common practice to make the incision as small as possible and to use a microscope to cause minimal disturbance to the normal tissues (microdiscectomy). Early mobilization is encouraged to prevent back stiffness.

Spondylosis

Pathology

Spondylosis is the response of the spine to ageing, although some individuals may develop it prematurely, especially if they have a history of trauma. Wear and tear of the spine causes bulging of the intervertebral discs, new bone formation (osteophyte formation) within the spinal canal, usually at the intervertebral joints and calcification of the ligaments, especially the ligamentum flavum. As a result the spinal canal and the root-exit foramina gradually narrow.

This may cause progressive spinal ischaemia (the blood supply of the spinal cord is via radicular arteries passing through the root-exit foramina) and direct compression of the spinal cord and its roots. As with disc prolapse, the more mobile areas of the spine are most commonly affected, and the disease is most prominent in lumbar and cervical regions.

Clinical features

The symptoms of spondylosis are usually progressive and are most common in old age. They include pain in the affected part of the spine, and radicular pain due to root irritation. Interference with the blood supply and direct cord compression due to cervical spondylosis may result in spastic quadriparesis, while a syndrome of leg numbness and weakness on exercise, which is relieved by rest, results from cauda equina ischaemia due to lumbar canal stenosis. An acute event such as a fall may cause an acute deterioration against a background of chronic spondylosis, particularly if it involves the cervical spine.

Management

Spondylosis is very common in the population, but only a few people require treatment. The indications for surgery are not clearcut and good clinical judgement is necessary. Essentially severe symptoms or a progressive neurological deficit are the main reasons for surgery. Operations for spondylosis prevent further deterioration rather than reverse changes that have already occurred. Surgery may not be indicated for mild numbness of the fingers in cervical spondylosis, but waiting for the symptoms to progress to a stage where the hands are too weak to be of any use is too late. Age is no bar to surgery if the patient's general health is good. At operation the area of entrapment is released. As spondylosis is usually diffuse, long cervical or lumbar laminectomies are often necessary, although in the neck single- or two-level anterior decompressions may be appropriate.

Rheumatoid arthritis

Although the spine may be affected by rheumatoid arthritis at any level, the atlantoaxial junction is most commonly involved. Atlantoaxial subluxation may result and may be asymptomatic or may be associated with pain, especially occipital pain, or cord compression from a translocated odontoid peg. Atlantoaxial subluxation makes endotracheal intubation of patients with rheumatoid arthritis very hazardous. The atlantoaxial junction may be fixed to the occiput using wires, but if there is anterior compression it may be necessary to remove the odontoid peg via the mouth, and carry out posterior wiring at the same time.

Infection

The spine may be affected by metastatic pyogenic infection or tuberculosis, which usually presents with spinal cord compression (Pott's spine). Severe local pain and tenderness are features of pyogenic infection. To exclude infection, histological confirmation of the cause of a compression is mandatory before any treatment is undertaken. If pyogenic infection is suspected, open drainage, usually by laminectomy, and high-dose antibiotic treatment is given. If a diagnosis of tuberculosis is certain, antituberculous chemotherapy without surgery is acceptable, but if there is doubt about the nature of the compression or a deterioration in the patient's condition despite adequate treatment, surgical exploration is necessary.

Haemorrhage

Spinal haemorrhage is relatively rare and when it does occur it is commonly missed. Haemorrhage may occur within the cord, or in the subarachnoid or extradural space. Spontaneous cord or extradural haemorrhage is most common in anticoagulated patients, while SAH is usually associated with a spinal AVM. Spinal haemorrhage should be suspected if there is a sudden onset of spinal pain associated with a spinal cord syndrome. Such a suspicion warrants urgent investigation by myelography or MR scanning. Cord haemorrhages are not usually helped by surgery, but early evacuation of an extradural haemorrhage can lead to recovery, even when severe. Spinal AVMs can be treated by embolization or surgery.

Peripheral nerve disorders

Like spinal surgery, peripheral nerve surgery may be performed by neurosurgeons, orthopaedic surgeons and plastic surgeons. Peripheral nerve problems tend to be due to trauma, tumour or entrapment.

Trauma

Traumatic nerve injuries usually result from penetrating wounds (often caused by a knife or bullet), or from fractures. The commonest example of a fracture-induced nerve injury is a radial nerve palsy following a humeral shaft fracture. Another common injury is trauma to the brachial plexus after a fall on to the shoulder. When peripheral nerve trauma is suspected, the wound should be explored. If possible the nerve ends are sutured together by the perineurium. If there is infection or a loss of length preventing tension-free apposition of the divided nerve ends, the nerve ends should be marked and a delayed repair is performed. The nerves recover by regrowing down the neural tube, but this is slow, and often associated with aberrant reinnervation. Specific nerve injuries are discussed in Chapter 11.

Tumour

Significant peripheral neurofibromas are common in von Recklinghausen's syndrome, but rarely cause a serious neurological deficit, any problem being cosmetic. Brachial plexus neurofibromas can affect upper limb function and should be excised.

Peripheral neuromas are a rare cause of severe pain.

Entrapment neuropathies

Peripheral nerves can be compressed by anatomical variants, the commonest being:
* cervical rib, causing weakness and wasting of small hand muscles;
* ulnar nerve entrapment at the elbow, causing numbness of the little and ring fingers;
* median nerve entrapment in the carpal tunnel at the wrist, causing numbness of the radial three fingers.

Diagnosis of an entrapment neuropathy is confirmed by EMG studies. It is treated by surgical exploration of the nerve and decompression.

Miscellaneous neurosurgical problems

Congenital anomalies

There is a wide range of development anomalies of the CNS, some of which are amenable to surgery. Often the abnormalities are complex, particularly with some craniofacial anomalies. Surgical correction of such complex abnormalities requires a multidisciplinary approach involving neurosurgeons, plastic surgeons, faciomaxillary surgeons, orthodontists, ear, nose and throat surgeons, ophthalmic surgeons, paediatricians, anaesthetists and psychologists, as well as dedicated nurses and physiotherapists. Care of these children may continue into adult life and the neurosurgeon undertaking this work should have a special interest and expertise in the type of surgery required and appropriate back-up facilities.

Pain

Neurosurgery may be of value in the treatment of pain in conjunction with a pain clinic. Surgery may cure pain caused by a mechanical problem, such as a disc prolapse, spinal instability or trigeminal neuralgia. When the disease cannot be cured, pain control may be achieved by implanting electrical stimulators or injection catheters into appropriate areas of the CNS. As a final option, when all else fails and life expectancy is limited, destructive operations such as rhizotomy or cordotomy may be appropriate.

22 Musculoskeletal Disorders

Where water, warm or cool is
Good for gout — at Aquae Sulis.   (Graffito in the Pump Room, Bath, *c*. 1760)

Introduction

The word 'orthopaedics', which comes from Greek and literally means 'straight child' ($o\rho\vartheta o\sigma$ = straight and $\pi\alpha\iota\sigma$ = child), reflects the history of the subject, which was based around developmental musculoskeletal conditions in childhood. The subject now spans all musculoskeletal disorders throughout life. With few exceptions, these disorders are non-fatal and cause pain and disturbance or loss of function. Dealing with non-fatal conditions requires a special kind of balanced clinical judgement to ensure that the potential benefits of a particular treatment will outweigh inevitable risks from surgery. In order to reach such a judgement we must know our patients well as individuals and understand their goals of treatment. If the patient's perceptions of outcome differ significantly from the clinician's then a satisfactory result is unlikely. The making of a diagnosis in the musculoskeletal system generally is not difficult, although where there are exceptions to this observation, then it will be pointed out where appropriate. The real difficulty is not in diagnosis but in management and for good management we must have accurate assessment.

Evaluation of the patient with orthopaedic disorders

Clinical assessment

Symptoms

The general principles of history-taking have already been discussed, but there are a number of points worthy of particular attention when considering orthopaedics.

Pain

Assessment of pain concentrates on severity rather than location. With a few exceptions, musculoskeletal disorders are easy to localize. Pain is generally related to the activities being carried out by the subject and so a pain–function relationship should be established. This may be summarized in a spectrum:

No pain—Pain on—Pain at—Pain — Pain — Pain—Night
  vigorous work walking walking at rest pain
  activity outside inside

In general terms, pain occurring at night is an absolute indication to do something for the patient, although one's threshold will vary from individual to individual. For example, a 45-year-old man who gets knee pain playing football for his pub team may well be relieved by retiring from the game, but a young and otherwise fit man who plays for his county will have different priorities.

Drugs

The above system works extremely well in practice but it is useful to have other information and much can be learnt from finding out what drugs the patient takes for the pain. The type, dose, frequency and efficacy of analgesics give the clinician a valuable insight into the level of a person's discomfort. The severity of the pain in practice is roughly reflected in the potency of analgesics, as shown below:

No drugs—Proprietary—Non- ——— Non-opiate—Opiates
over-the- steroidal central-
counter anti- acting
agents inflammatory agents
agents

This spectrum is not designed to decry simple analgesia, which includes aspirin, as such drugs can be very effective in the treatment of inflammatory conditions and this should be borne in mind.

How does the patient function?

Having established the level of pain and loss of function or disability, then this must be offset against the lifestyle, age and outlook of the patient. The general physical and medical state of the patient will also need assessment, particularly if a surgical solution is contemplated.

The risk balance

With all this information it is possible to construct a risk–benefit balance, such as is outlined below. Essentially the benefits must outweigh the risk before embarking on treatment.

Physical examination

It is important to examine the bones, soft tissues and skin, and an assessment of peripheral neurological and circulatory function should also be made. The examination of patients with orthopaedic problems is largely concerned with the examination of *joints*. Remember that the spine is a collection of segments joined by joints! Alan Apley was the doyen of teachers in orthopaedics and it was he who coined the notion that joints should be examined in three stages:

1 look;
2 feel;
3 move.

Looking

We should inspect the joint to exclude scars, muscle wasting and obvious swelling. The general posture will give us insight and any obvious deformity or shortening is noted.

Feeling

The key is to know what you are feeling and to ask oneself: 'what is happening underneath?' Lumps, bony or otherwise, swellings and joint effusions can well be appreciated in certain joints, but not so easily in other situations. For example, the hip is covered by thick muscle and so is not easy to feel, but the knee is largely crossed by tendons, especially at the front and sides, and so a more direct examination of the joint may be made.

Move

Start by obeying some simple rules:
• Know what movements the joint can do.
• Appreciate that loss of certain movements is more significant than others.
• Place the joint in its anatomically neutral position.
• Break the movements into their simple anatomical components (for example, see Box 22.1).

Investigations

The investigations frequently performed in assessment of musculoskeletal disorders are given in Table 22.1.

Problems with joints

Introduction

Of all the conditions treated by orthopaedic surgeons, arthritis takes up much of the clinic and operating theatre time. This reflects the high prevalence of arthritis in the western world and it is, therefore, important to understand this orthopaedic condition above all others. In general terms, arthritis is a painful and distressing disorder which has profound effects on how well people live. There is no specific treatment and all our strategies are based around symptom relief.

Assessment of movement of the hip joint

Know what movements the joint can do

The movements of the hip joint are:
- Flexion and extention
- Abduction and adduction
- Internal and external rotation
- Circumduction

Appreciate that loss of certain movements is more significant than others

Losses of major functional significance to the hip are extension, rotation in extension and abduction. Of course loss of any movement may matter but movements are relative and in day to day activity loss of key movements in walking are of most significance.
- Loss of extension

When we walk we do so in a way that minimizes energy consumption. Loss of energy conserving movements makes walking literally hard work. To go forward we shift our centre of gravity in front of our feet so that we must fall forwards. To stop ourselves falling we put out the leading leg, leaving the trailing leg behind. In this manoeuvre we flex the leading leg a little and also extend the trailing leg. In relative terms we would have to lose an awful lot of our range of flexion before this affected walking, but the loss of only some of our rather limited extending ability would be highly significant. Loss of the ability to leave the trailing leg behind, through loss of extension is an early feature in hip disease.
- Loss of rotation

Another mechanism we use to conserve energy in walking is to make maximum use of our bodies in generating forward momentum through twisting. We are all familiar with soldiers who swing their arms as they march and all of us when our hands are free and we are in a hurry tend to do the same subconsciously. Arm swinging and twisting of the upper limb girdle travels down the trunk and into the pelvis and lower limbs. The twisting is converted into forward movement as the legs swing. Most of the swinging occurs as the legs are in neutral or extended as the centre of gravity passes from one leg to the next, with the weight just on the extended trailing leg. Loss of rotation of the hips in the neutral or extended position is therefore very important. Loss of this ability again makes walking difficult and hard work. Loss of rotation in extension is not uncommon in early hip disease, particularly degenerative disease.

Place the joint in its anatomically neutral position

When a patient lies on an examination couch the hip joints are not in the anatomically neutral position. Because the lumbar spine is lordotic, then the pelvis is tilted as it rests on the couch. The hip is flexed, as are the knees, such that the calves make contact with the couch. In order to get rid of this overt hip flexion the contralateral hip should be fully flexed, so tilting the pelvis backwards and straightening the lordosis. The manoeuvre is known as Thomas' test, after Hugh Owen Thomas who devised it. The significance is that it puts the pelvis in the neutral position and so any fixed flexion deformity will be revealed. The importance of showing fixed flexion is that it means there must be loss of extension which we now understand is highly significant in assessing the hip. Loss of extension means profound disturbance of walking.

Break the movements into their simple anatomical components

Some of the movements that take place in the hip also take place in adjacent joints, particularly in the lumbar spine which results in pelvic tilt and twist. If Thomas' test is taken too far the lumbar spine and the pelvis flexes and equally if abduction is taken too far the pelvis tilts laterally due to spinal movement. It is therefore important not only to neutralize the joint but to fix the pelvis to ensure only pure hip movement is being measured.

Box 22.1

Osteoarthritis

Osteoarthritis is a syndrome of pain and limitation of movement associated with a breakdown of the balance between the wear and repair processes in the joint. It occurs with increasing age, although it would be misleading to suggest that osteoarthritis is an inevitable accompaniment of old age.

Aetiology

It is convenient to classify osteoarthritis according to aetiology. The classification starts by grouping patients into those who have a known cause — secondary osteoarthritis — and those where the cause remains unknown — primary osteoarthritis. It is important to appreciate that the vast majority of patients fall into the primary category.

Primary osteoarthritis

This is a term of convenience and, despite much effort, there remains little insight into the cause of this very common condition.
- It is probably true that many cases of arthritis are in reality secondary to *mechanical stress*, e.g. congenital deformity, previous joint or bone injury, obesity. However, in the vast majority of patients with osteoarthritis the cause is obscure. It must be assumed that the primary cause is localized to the affected joints as a systemic disorder would be expected to affect most joints. There are a few cases who do appear to have generalized osteoarthritis but these are rare.
- One possible aetiological factor is that the mechanism of *cartilage nutrition*, which is mediated largely via the synovial fluid, is in some way abnormal.
- *Cartilage fragments* are found in worn joints and such minute fragments are known to initiate intense inflammatory reactions which then lead to further cartilage damage. An initial event (such as trauma) might

Table 22.1 Investigations for assessment of musculoskeletal disorders.

Investigation	Comment
Blood investigations	
Haematology	
FBC	Baseline investigation, may be anaemia in arthritis
ESR	Simple test to perform, may be elevated in rheumatoid arthritis, osteomyelitis, multiple myeloma
Biochemistry	
Calcium phosphate	Will be abnormal in metabolic bone disease (e.g. hyperparathyroidism, rickets and osteomalacia)
Enzymes	
Alkaline phosphatase	Marker of bone turnover, raised in Paget's disease
Immunology	
Rheumatoid factors	Autoantibodies which react with the patient's own IgG are present in patients with rheumatoid arthritis
Imaging	
Plain radiography	
Look at:	• The bones in general for shape (deformity) and density
	• The cortex of the bone for breaks in continuity
	• The medulla of the bone for destruction or sclerosis (secondary deposits)
	• The joints for narrowing of the joint space, erosion, irregularity or new bone formation (osteophytes)
	• The soft tissues for calcification, foreign body or gas
Contrast radiology	Myelography or radiculography is used to assess the spinal canal
Tomography	By moving the X-ray plate and tube in opposite directions a structure in the long axis of the movement can be kept in focus while the surrounding tissues are blurred. Useful in exposing the spine but has been superseded by CT and MR scanning
CT and MR scanning	Very useful for detecting subtle changes in bone and (especially MR) in soft tissues
Radioisotope scanning	Used for detecting skeletal metastases, primary bone tumours, bone and joint infections and stress fractures
Endoscopy	
Arthroscopy (Fig. 22.1)	Used mostly for assessment of pathology in the knee and shoulder joints

FBC, Full blood count; ESR, erythrocyte sedimentation rate; IgG, immunoglobulin G; CT, computed tomography; MR, magnetic resonance.

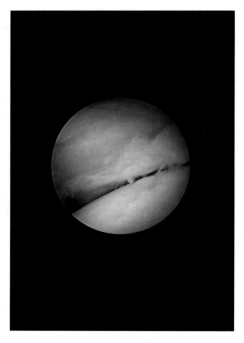

Figure 22.1 Arthroscopic view of a knee joint.

release a cartilage fragment into the joint, initiating a self-perpetuating cycle which leads ultimately to joint destruction.

Secondary osteoarthritis

In this minority group we see obvious causative factors which quite reasonably may be assumed to be responsible for the development of osteoarthritis. These are listed in Table 22.2 and are discussed elsewhere in this chapter.

Table 22.2 Conditions which predispose to the development of secondary osteoarthritis.

Congenital	Congenital dislocation of the hip
Childhood	Perthes disease, infection
Trauma	Fracture into a joint, cartilage tear
Metabolic	Gout, crystal arthropathy
Infection	Tuberculosis
Chronic inflammation	Rheumatoid arthritis

Clinical presentation

Osteoarthritis can present at any age but becomes increasingly common in later decades. In the younger patient there is more likely to be a recognizable predisposing cause, but not always so. Both in history and examination it is essential to gain an overview of the patient's general health as not only is a diagnosis being reached but a plan of management which may include surgery is being assembled.

History

The patient presents with *pain* and associated *loss of function*. *Stiffness* is a feature but is nearly always secondary to pain. The onset may be insidious but occasionally the presentation can be quite dramatic and relatively short, making the diagnosis difficult. Initially pain is associated with activity and if a lower limb joint is affected the patient is often left with an *indiscernible tiredness* towards the end of the day. This latter feature is often caused by the gait modifications discussed above.

Help is sought when simple analgesia no longer relieves pain and specialist help is demanded by the primary carer when sleep is disturbed. The threshold for referral varies from patient to patient but in general, younger patients tend to present earlier than the elderly who expect a degree of arthritis as they get older.

Management is heavily dependent on the clinician's ability to distinguish between many individuals and treat and offer surgery appropriately. It is important at this stage to have a clear concept of one's aim in treatment, which is to relieve pain.

Examination

The striking feature on physical examination is the limitation of movement by pain. It is important to appreciate that the perceived limitation of movement on routine examination is greater than any limitation observed during an examination under anaesthetic. Once this is appreciated then the clinician will soon come to realize that results of surgery are related to pain relief rather than improvements in stiffness of the joint caused by the disease.

Investigations

In general, a *plain anteroposterior* and *lateral radiograph* is all that will be required (Fig. 22.2). Occasionally in a very acute presentation a *bone scan* may be useful in order to isolate the occasional patient presenting with a metastatic deposit.

The typical radiographic findings are:
• joint space narrowing: this indicates a loss of articular cartilage.

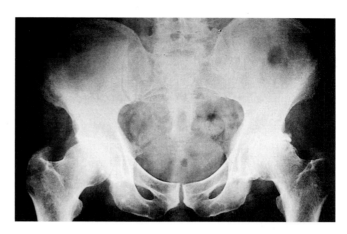

Figure 22.2 Osteoarthritis of the hips showing joint space narrowing, osteophyte formation and subchondral sclerosis.

• osteophyte formation: bony outgrowths at the joint margin, of obscure significance.
• cyst formation: around the subchondral region.
• subchondral sclerosis: a thickening of bone induced by the loss of shock-absorbing cartilage.

Management

The key to management is to realize that there is no cure for osteoarthritis and that the clinical course is erratic. All management is aimed at pain relief and, through this, return of function. The ultimate way of relieving pain is surgery, although there are general measures which will alleviate symptoms and postpone the need for operation.

Non-surgical options

These include weight loss, use of a stick, rest and physiotherapy. Analgesia may be used subsequently or in parallel with these measures.

Weight loss

Lower limb joints in particular are subject to large loads which are the result of the leverage effects of muscles sited to good mechanical advantage. For example, the hip abductors arising from the pelvis are inserted on the trochanters well away from the centres of rotation of the hip joint. These leverage effects mean that quite modest changes in body weight will have useful effects on the total loads being borne by the joint. Weight loss is usually accompanied by a general improvement in well-being which often affects the overall pain perception.

Walking stick

In lower limb joint disease, particularly in the hip, the use of a stick in the *contralateral hand* means that the shoulder girdle can help in tilting the pelvis and so assist in weight-bearing. This has the effect of reducing the work required of the weight-bearing abductors, which dramatically reduces the muscle-induced loads on the hip.

Physiotherapy

The role of physiotherapy and rest remains controversial and a balance is required. Overexercise cannot in the long term be beneficial but some exercise does relieve stiffness and spasm and pain. Young sufferers should be advised against excessive unnecessary activity and a change to a light job is useful, if practicable. Total rest is however equally counterproductive, especially in the elderly where maintenance of the activities of daily living is essential. Local heat and muscle-strengthening exercises are also useful, e.g. 'quad' exercises in osteoarthritis of the knee.

Drug therapy

Drugs do not alter the course of osteoarthritis and there is no place for drug therapy in the absence of pain. However, in the presence of pain non-steroidal anti-inflammatory drugs (NSAIDs) and occasionally local corticosteroid injections may provide useful relief.

Several different NSAIDs are available (Table 22.3) and individual patients respond differently to different agents. Thus a therapeutic trial is often necessary to find the drug that is most suited to the patient.

Local steroid injection is useful for acute exacerbations or persistent pain and swelling in one or two joints. Steroid injections should be administered under aseptic techniques and should not be given if there is any suspicion of infection.

Surgical options

For most forms of arthritis there remain four options: nothing, arthroplasty, arthrodesis and osteotomy.
- *Nothing* should always be borne in mind and the patient must appreciate that the benefits must outweigh the risks when surgery is being considered. Equally, for very disabled patients in a great deal of pain, the option to take risks must be considered. Provided patients have a good grasp of the risk–benefit equation as it affects them, then they may take the lion's share in the decision to have surgery. Patients should also understand the limitations of surgery — it can relieve pain but is not likely to alleviate disability due to intrinsic stiffness.
- *Arthroplasty* or joint replacement is probably one of the most successful surgical treatments ever devised. Hip and knee arthroplasties are now performed routinely with excellent results. However, there are some principles to be followed in selecting patients for arthroplasty and the procedures are not without complications. Arthroplasty is discussed more fully below.
- *Arthrodesis* or surgical fusion in a position of function is an appropriate operation in a young person with a painful and limited range of motion. In the hip, for example, fusion in 30° of flexion and some abduction produces painfree and functional gait, whilst permitting sitting. It is more acceptable to the male than the female as any hip fusion is likely to interfere with female sexual activity.

Table 22.3 Non-steroidal inflammatory drugs available for treatment of arthritis.

Drug group	Name	Dose	Side-effects
Salicylates	Aspirin	up to 4 g/day	GI upset*, tinnitus and deafness, bruising and bleeding, hypersensitivity reaction†, drug interactions
Propionic acid derivatives	Ibuprofen	400 mg t.d.s.	GI upset*, hypersensitivity reactions
	Naproxen	250–500 mg b.d.	
	Fenprofen	300–600 mg q.d.s.	
Indole acetic acid derivatives	Indomethacin	25 mg b.d.-q.d.s. 50 mg nocte	GI upset*, CNS symptoms (headache, vertigo, dizziness, depression, nightmares), hypersensitivity reactions
Enolic acid derivatives	Phenylbutazone	100–400 mg/day	GI upset*, hypersensitivity reactions, aplastic anaemia, neutropenia, thrombocytopenia, agranulocytosis, salt and water retention, drug interactions (e.g. potentiate oral anticoagulants and hypoglycaemics)

*Gastrointestinal (GI) upset includes dyspepsia, nausea and vomiting, gastric erosions and bleeding and peptic ulceration.
†Hypersensitivity reactions are not uncommon and care should be taken in prescribing these drugs to patients with asthma.

Fusion is not a technically easy procedure and requires a prolonged recovery period of up to 6 months, often in a plaster splint. The long-term disadvantage of arthrodesis is that it puts stress on the adjacent joints. For example, in the hip this means extra stress on the lumbar spine and knee as well as the opposite hip. However, this problem may be anticipated by electing to fuse until the fifth decade and then performing a second operation to 'unpick' the arthrodesis and convert it to an arthroplasty. This latter operation has proved to be surprisingly effective for the hip with good return to function of the temporarily defunct abductor muscles. Fusion is however still a difficult option to 'sell' to patients, however logical the procedure.

Joints that are usefully fused are the ankle and the wrist. These are joints which are at present difficult to replace and which have a relatively limited range of functional movement in any case.

• *Osteotomy* or surgical realignment of the joint is an option used widely in Europe and with varying degrees of popularity in the UK and the USA. This difference of attitude is traditional and otherwise impossible to explain. Accurate surgical realignment is technically difficult and very time-consuming. Perhaps the most likely reason for its varying popularity is the widely differing results of effectiveness and long-term outcome. Even in the best hands, osteotomy can only be viewed as a temporary measure lasting from 1 or 2 years to around 10 years.

Osteotomy may be used to realign any deformity in any bone. When used to treat arthritis, osteotomy is valuable in young patients who have maintained a good range of movement, despite pain. The hip and the knee are suitable for osteotomy and we may use the hip joint as our example again. Osteotomy may be performed on the pelvic side, either by forming a shelf or by total acetabular realignment. It may be performed on the femoral side by altering the angle of the femoral neck so as to change the attitude of the femoral head relative to the acetabulum.

In general, the effects of osteotomy are threefold:

(a) to alter the angle and so mechanical advantage of the muscles. For example, at the hip the action of the abductors may be modified. It may also be used to get rid of flexion deformity — the so-called extension osteotomy;

(b) to alter the contact area between surfaces. This may be particularly useful following a deformity leading to secondary osteoarthritis;

(c) to alter the dynamics of blood supply to the joint. It has been proposed that the pain of arthritis is due to subchondral venous tension and so osteotomy in crude terms may decompress the femoral head. This is very much a speculative idea but would at least in part explain dramatic pain relief following this sort of surgery.

In general terms, osteotomy may be said to be a good operation in young people who retain in the main part a good range of motion and have a reasonable preservation of articular cartilage.

Joint replacement (arthroplasty)

Strictly, the term arthroplasty means the surgical reshaping of a joint but it has come to be synonymous with joint replacement and will be used in this accepted way here.

The principles of joint replacement

The same basic rules apply to all joints and, provided that they can be obeyed, then arthroplasty may be performed.

Lower limb

Hip and knee arthroplasty are now very successful operations. The reason why arthroplasty of the hip is held in such high regard is due to the success of the operation, which achieved its current level of 80 000 cases per annum in the UK, largely through the work of Sir John Charnley. For the majority, artificial joints work very well indeed, and well in excess of 90% will still be *in situ* after 10 years. However, most hip arthroplasties are carried out in older patients with a lower functional demand. Knee arthroplasty is also better carried out on older patients. In the UK osteoarthritis of the knee is the most common disabling form of the disease and the emergence of a successful prosthetic joint is very encouraging (Fig. 22.3).

Upper limb

In the upper limb the relationship between pain relief and function is quite different to that observed in the lower limb. In the case of the arm the loads involved are quite low but the available range of motion required for normal function is large. Despite the low loads, the demanding range of movement seems to lead to early failure in many upper limb joint replacements through loosening. Remember that arthroplasty in particular tends to improve pain-related loss of function but does relatively little for intrinsic stiffness. In the upper limb this poses a problem if arthroplasty is contemplated. For example, the elbow must flex to 90° to permit eating (try reaching your mouth with an arm fixed at a greater angle!) and must extend more or less fully to reach the anus for cleansing. Therefore, any surgery must cater for these two fundamental activities of daily living. Slowly elbow and shoulder replacements are approaching such high levels of function. Not so the fingers, and to a much lesser degree the wrist. Therefore for the moment upper

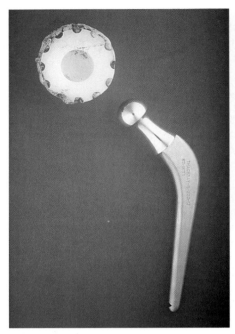

(a)

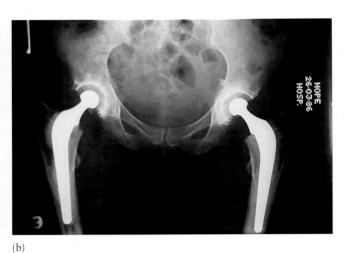

(b)

Figure 22.3 (a) Components of an artificial hip joint. (b) Radiograph of the hips following bilateral total hip replacement.

limb replacement cannot be regarded as routine but rather a highly specialized, and gradually emerging specialty. Much progress is still to be made in this area.

Requirements of an artificial joint

The key to understanding joint arthroplasty is to appreciate the requirements of an artificial joint. The new joint must:
- be capable of a functional painfree range of movement;
- be able to withstand the forces placed upon it without undue wear and without working loose.

It must achieve all this whilst remaining stable.

Lower limb

On first reflection it is perhaps surprising that the hip joint proved to be the first really successful replacement as this joint has tremendous demands placed upon it. Against the large loads is offset the generally stable configuration of a ball and socket and the fact that the functional range of hip motion is in practice fairly limited. In practical terms, if we retain 10 or 15° of extension and 30–50° of flexion with a few degrees of abduction and rotation, particularly in extension, then useful hip function for daily living is maintained.

In the case of the knee the functional range of movement is surprisingly limited, although ideally 90° of flexion must be achieved in order to get up and down stairs. In the knee, stability in extension is essential and to achieve this the

surgery must achieve an accurate soft-tissue balance through resection of the capsule and the ligaments.

Upper limb

In the upper limb, progress has been made in developing elbow and shoulder arthroplasty. Elbow replacement has been limited by difficulties in anchoring the prosthesis to the bone. The principal problems in the shoulder centre around the need to maintain good muscular function of the rotator cuff.

Complications of arthroplasty

Complications of arthroplasty may be divided into those general for any major surgery and those specific to the operation.

General complications

One must bear in mind that most patients undergoing surgery for arthritis are older: this is not to say that age *per se* is a risk factor. It is true that older people are more likely to have medical conditions predisposing to risk and if these are not recognized then problems may arise.

Patients undergoing major surgery are prone to problems such as respiratory and urinary tract infections. They may also develop pressure sores if they are not nursed adequately. Deep vein thrombosis and pulmonary embolism may follow any surgical procedure, but patients undergoing hip surgery are especially at risk, as are patients who require any surgery in and around the pelvis.

Specific complications

These may be further classified into early and late.

Early complications

• *Dislocation*: In the immediate postoperative period the prosthesis will not be fully supported by the surrounding soft tissues. The muscles and their proprioceptors may be temporarily out of action because of surgical trauma and anaesthesia or analgesia and a secondary fibrotic capsule will not yet have formed around the prosthesis. The hip in this period is at risk from dislocation, particularly before the effects of anaesthesia wear off. The risk of dislocation is reduced as time passes but even after a long time an injudicious move (e.g. extreme flexion with adduction and internal rotation in the case of the hip) may result in a painful dislocation. For this reason the patient will need advice about dressing and may need aids to help in fitting stockings and also benefit from having a raised toilet seat.

• *Deep vein thrombosis*: As stated above, patients undergoing arthroplasty are at risk from deep vein thrombosis and some sort of prophylaxis is probably justified. It must be accepted, however, that this is by no means a clearcut argument and even if prophylaxis is thought advisable, the best agent or technique is by no means universally agreed. The best prophylaxis is to keep both pre- and postoperative immobilization to a minimum.

• *Infection*: Infection is always a risk following implantation of foreign material into the body. Infection may develop soon after surgery (early) or may be delayed for months or years (late). Many factors make an artificial agent prone to infection, not only from recognized hospital pathogens such as *Staphylococcus aureus* but also from organisms normally regarded as commensals, such as *Staph epidermidis*, universally found in skin flora. It would appear that the presence of foreign material inhibits normal immune defences.

Infection of a prosthesis is such a disaster (see below) that every effort, including antibiotic prophylaxis and the provision of an ultraclean air environment, must be made to avoid this complication. If these precautions are taken then immediate infections should be eliminated and long-term infections reduced to less than 0.1%. Unfortunately in the UK this figure is often exceeded, with rates of 1–3% being not uncommon. Certainly anything greater than this is entirely unacceptable.

Late complications

Problems with joint replacement may occur as late as 10 years or longer following surgery. The principal problems are late infection, loosening and wear.

• *Infection*: The causes of infection have already been discussed and it is probable that most cases of infection are caused at the time of insertion of the prosthesis. Why late infections occur is not fully understood. One suggestion is that infection may occur by other routes, e.g. blood-borne infection as a consequence of 'normal' bacteraemias. There is circumstantial evidence that some infections may follow tooth extraction, which is known to cause significant bacteraemias and may be a cause of endocarditis.

• *Loosening and wear*: Loosening is to some degree probably inevitable, though efforts are made to delay it as long as possible. The incidence of loosening increases with the age of the prosthesis. Loosening and wear are the factors in the life of an implant that mean that replacement is best delayed as long as possible, so that the joint may outlast the patient. Of course this is not always possible in the young. It is for this reason that we still need the alternative procedures described above and why research must continue to find better materials and methods of prosthetic fixation.

The limitations of joint replacement

In the modern era of orthopaedics the treatment of osteoarthritis is almost synonymous with joint replacement and in the hip joint this is very much the rule. However, it should not be regarded as the only treatment, although clinicians often come under strong pressure from patients, whatever their age, to offer the patient 'a new joint'.

It is not always appreciated that the consequences of early prosthetic failure can be devastating. It is important to appreciate that a hip replacement is an artificial joint, not a new transplant, and that from the moment it is put in it begins to wear out. The strategy of replacement should be to provide a joint which outlasts the likely lifespan of the patient, and at our current level of knowledge this cannot be guaranteed for the younger patient, and so alternatives (e.g. arthrodesis, osteotomy) are still required.

Rheumatoid arthritis

Aetiology

Rheumatoid arthritis (RA) is a multisystem disorder of unknown cause. It is a chronic inflammatory disease which predominantly affects synovium. It has some clear links with abnormalities of the immune system (autoantibodies which react with the patient's own immunoglobulin G are

Osteoarthritis at a glance

DEFINITION

Osteoarthritis is a degenerative joint disease involving damage to the cartilage-bearing surfaces of the involved joint, characterized by pain and limitation of movement

EPIDEMIOLOGY

F>M   Age: 40s and 50s onwards

AETIOLOGY

Primary osteoarthritis
Increased mechanical stress to the joint
Poor cartilage nutrition
Cartilage fragments

Secondary osteoarthritis	*Predisposing causes*
Congenital	Congenital dislocation of the hip
Childhood	Perthes disease, infection
Trauma	Fracture into a joint, cartilage tear
Metabolic	Gout, crystal arthropathy
Infection	Tuberculosis
Chronic inflammation	Rheumatoid arthritis

PATHOLOGY

Progressive degradation of articular cartilage leads to joint narrowing, subchondral bone thickening, bone cysts and peripheral bone nodules (osteophytes). Altered proteoglycan metabolism in the joint may be the biochemical stimulus to cartilage degeneration

Clinical
- Joint pain and loss of function
- Stiffness
- Tiredness, especially towards the end of the day
- Limitation of joint movement because of pain

Investigations
- Anteroposterior and lateral X-ray of the affected joint — joint space narrowing, osteophytes, bone cysts, subchondral sclerosis

MANAGEMENT

- The aim of management is pain relief and return of function. The degree of pain the patient is suffering is the deciding factor in how aggressive the treatment should be
- Non-surgical management
  - (a) Weight loss
  - (b) Physiotherapy
  - (c) Drug therapy: non-steroidal anti-inflammatory drugs (NSAIDs); local steroid injection
- Surgery
  - (a) Arthroplasty: joint replacement is very successful and is the surgical option of choice for osteoarthritis of the hip and knee joints in the elderly
  - (b) Arthrodesis: fusion of a joint in a position of function may provide useful relief in a young person with severe wrist or ankle disease
  - (c) Osteotomy: realigns the joint and may have a role in young patients with a good range of movement. Not often performed

PROGNOSIS

At present there is no treatment available which stops the progress of cartilage degeneration. All therapy can therefore be considered palliative, although this is very effective, especially in relation to arthroplasty

---

found in the serum of patients with RA) and there is growing evidence that there may be a genetic abnormality which causes an idiosyncratic reaction to certain infective agents, which is expressed as RA.

Clinical presentation

The most obvious clinical presentation of RA is severe pain, swelling and deformity of the joints (Table 22.4). The principal joints affected are the small joints of the hands and feet and in a minority the larger joints are affected. The small joints are affected symmetrically but the larger joints are involved haphazardly. There is no known reason for this. RA may strike at any age and women are more affected than men. Classically it first presents with morning stiffness, improving through the day, in contrast to osteoarthritis.

The disease may also affect the cardiovascular system and can cause myopathies and small-vessel disease. It can also cause pulmonary fibrosis and treatment with steroids can make the skin thin and delicate.

The role of surgery in rheumatoid arthritis

The role of the surgeon is to make the patient as comfortable as possible whilst retaining function. Patients with RA are best seen in conjunction with a rheumatologist who will be responsible for therapeutic care. This is a disease to be tackled by a team.

Soft tissues

The rheumatoid process may result in pannus tissue invading tendon sheaths and the tendons themselves. Damage

Table 22.4 Clinical features of rheumatoid arthritis.

Symptoms
Stiffness, early-morning and after inactivity
Pain, tenderness and swelling of joints
Functional impairment, e.g. loss of hand grip strength
Constitutional symptoms, e.g. malaise, tiredness and depression

Physical signs
General
   Symmetrical joint involvement
   Joint swelling and deformity
   Muscle wasting around involved joints

Hands (Fig. 22.5)
   MCP joint swelling and subluxation
   PIP joint swelling 'spindling'
   'Buttonhole' and 'swan neck' deformities of the fingers
   Extensor tendon rupture, finger drop
   Ulnar deviation of the fingers and hand
   Carpal tunnel syndrome

Other joints
   Wrists, knees, temporomandibular joint and cervical spine
   Atlantoaxial subluxation is a potentially lethal problem

Non-articular manifestations
   Skin: rheumatoid nodules
   Cardiac: myocarditis, pericarditis
   Vascular: vasculitis
   Haemopoietic: anaemia, splenomegaly
   Pulmonary: fibrosing alveolitis, pleural effusion
   Neurological: entrapment neuropathy, e.g. carpal tunnel syndrome
   Eye: keratoconjunctivitis, episcleritis

MCP, Metacarpophalangeal; PIP, proximal interphalangeal.

may be limited by removing excessive synovial swelling by synovectomy. This is a good operation at the wrist for extensor tendons. Sometimes tendons about the wrist actually rupture and some sort of repair is needed.

Joints

In early disease it is sometimes possible to reduce pain and stiffness by removing the joint synovium — synovectomy. This is of value in the younger patient who retains movement, but who has pain. It is useful at the elbow and wrist where it may be combined with a limited excision of the joint — excision arthroplasty. This relieves pain but because some joint has been removed there can never be a full return of function.

The surgeon's main role in the management of RA is salvaging function. The goals of surgery are pain relief and return of function. The surgeon must be sure that the chemotherapeutic control of the rheumatoid process is adequate or otherwise doctor and patient may be disappointed. The surgeon should also be sure that the aim of improvement is function and not deformity. This is particularly true in the hands, where even impossibly distorted hands often belie excellent function.

Avascular necrosis

Aetiology

Bone tissue death through loss of blood supply is found in certain circumstances throughout the body. In some cases the cause is clearly traceable to an anatomical source on

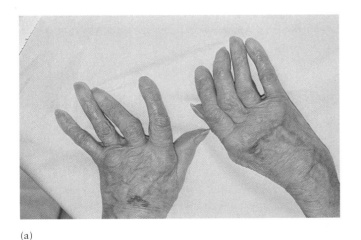
(a)

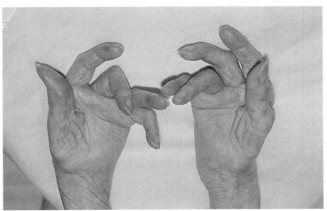
(b)

Figure 22.4 Severe rheumatoid arthritis of the hands showing (a) swelling and subluxation of the metacarpophalangeal joints, spindling of the proximal interphalangeal joint and ulnar deviation; (b) joint swelling, muscle wasting and finger deformity.

Rheumatoid arthritis at a glance

DEFINITION

Rheumatoid arthritis is a generalized (autoimmune) disease characterized by inflammation of the synovium with progressive peripheral joint erosion, destruction and deformity and systemic manifestations in 30% of patients

EPIDEMIOLOGY

F/M = 1:3   Age: young and middle-aged adults. Occurs in about 1–3% of the population

AETIOLOGY

- Genetic — associated with HLA-DRW4
- Hormonal — commoner in females, onset between menarche and menopause, improves with pregnancy
- Immune mechanism — immune complexes (IgG, IgM and complement) are found in the joints and serum of patients. IgG production is stimulated and in turn acts as an antigen triggering the production of antibodies, IgM (rheumatoid factor)
- Infection — autoimmunity may be triggered by an infection

PATHOLOGY

- In response to an unknown stimulus (?virus) the synovial membrane thickens and folds into a pannus which erodes the articular cartilage and adjacent bone
- There is an increase in volume of synovial fluid which contains protein (IgG) and polymorphonuclear neutrophils (PMNs)
- Immune complexes are phagocytosed by PMNs with release of lysozymes and further destruction
- T lymphocytes may also play a role

CLINICAL

- Pain, swelling and symmetrical deformity of the small joints of the hand. Large joints may be affected, but not symmetrically
- Early-morning stiffness
- Functional impairment (loss of handgrip strength)
- Constitutional symptoms: malaise, tiredness

Hands

- MCP joint swelling and subluxation
- PIP joint swelling, 'spindling'
- 'Buttonhole' and 'swan neck' deformity
- Extensor tendon rupture, finger drop
- Ulnar deviation of the fingers and hand
- Carpal tunnel syndrome

Non-articular manifestations

- Skin: rheumatoid nodules
- Cardiac: myocarditis, pericarditis
- Vascular: vasculitis
- Haemopoietic: anaemia, splenomegaly
- Pulmonary: fibrosing alveolitis/pleural effusion
- Neurological: entrapment neuropathy
- Eye: keratoconjunctivitis, episcleritis

INVESTIGATIONS

- FBC: anaemia common
- Rheumatoid factor: positive in 75% of patients
- X-ray joints: soft-tissue thickening; juxta-articular; loss of joint space; subluxation

MANAGEMENT

- The aim of management is pain relief and return of function
- Medical management
  - (a) Physiotherapy and occupational therapy for exercise/splintage and provision of aids for activities of daily living
  - (b) Drug therapy: non-steroidal anti-inflammatory drugs (NSAIDs); local steroid injections; gold, penicillamine, sulphasalazine, chloroquine, azathioprine, methotrexate
- Surgery to improve function, not deformity
  - (a) Synovectomy is useful at wrist to remove pannus
  - (b) Ruptured tendons should be repaired early
  - (c) Arthrodesis and arthroplasty

PROGNOSIS

Rheumatoid arthritis is a chronic disease but 60% of patients have only moderate impairment of activities. 40% become severely disabled

---

which a secondary event is superimposed. Quite often avascular necrosis occurs spontaneously for no apparent reason.

Posttraumatic avascular necrosis

Certain sites where the anatomical blood supply is unusual are at risk following trauma. These include the *femoral head*, the *proximal part of the scaphoid* in the wrist and the *proximal part of the talus*. In these situations trauma cuts an otherwise good, if rather awkward blood supply. In femoral neck fractures the damage to the capsular blood vessels puts the head at risk and in the other two sites a

distal blood supply is severed from the proximal part of the bone.

Idiopathic avascular necrosis

In other areas such as the lunate, avascular necrosis occurs in less obvious circumstances. Avascular necrosis of the head of the femur is seen following chronic alcohol abuse, high-dose steroid therapy and in deep-sea divers (Caisson's disease). The cause and effect in these diverse associations remain a mystery. The patient presents with acute and often severe joint pain which is exacerbated by movement and to some degree relieved by rest. With the passage of time, symptoms become indistinguishable from osteoarthritis.

Investigations

Avascular necrosis may be reversed if a blood supply can be re-established. However, in the revascularizing phase the bone is very soft and prone to distortion, with secondary arthritic changes. Diagnosis can be very difficult. Initially there are no radiological changes. However, later the bone appears dense, reflecting the absence of blood vessels. Technetium bone scanning shows a reduction in uptake of isotope.

Management

Treatment is non-specific. If possible, the affected joint should be rested. Surgery is of no value in treating the underlying condition and often the surgeon is left to salvage the situation with a joint replacement. As such patients are usually very young this is, as explained above, highly problematical.

Crystal arthropathies

In these conditions crystals of body products are deposited in the joints on the surface of the articular cartilage and within the synovial fluid. They cause a chronic degenerative change in the joint and may be a cause of secondary arthritis. They also cause acute inflammatory episodes which are generally self-limiting.

Gout

Gout is caused by urate crystal deposition. Urate is a product of nucleic acid metabolism. It becomes deposited in circumstances such as dehydration (particularly post-surgery), and after chemotherapy with antimetabolites for malignancy. Probably the commonest cause in western societies is the injudicious overuse of diuretics.

Gout presents with a hot, tender and swollen joint. Any joint can be affected but it is seen commonly in the knee and in the hallux. It is important to exclude infection early in the differential diagnosis. Diagnosis is made by the presence of a high *uric acid* in the blood and more accurately by the presence of birefringent urate crystals in joint fluid aspirated on admission. It may be treated using *indomethacin* in the relatively high dose of 50 mg three times a day. Chronic gout may be controlled with *allopurinol*.

Pseudogout

Pseudogout may mimic gout but usually has a less acute presentation. In this case the cause is the deposition of *py-rophosphate*, the origin of which is obscure. Chronic crystal arthropathy of this kind classically causes calcification of joint surfaces and the menisci in the knee. Symptoms may be controlled with anti-inflammatory drugs but long-term degeneration is likely.

Septic arthritis

Acute septic arthritis

Aetiology

Acute septic arthritis is usually blood-borne in origin, often originating from a distal site of trivial infection. It may come from an adjacent infected bone, especially in children where a metaphyseal site may be within a joint capsule — this is notably so at the hip. Very rarely it may occur from a direct penetration of the joint. Three groups are at risk:
- children;
- immunosuppressed adults;
- anyone with chronic degenerative joint disorders.

Clinical presentation

In children septic arthritis usually presents with a nasty acute illness and the child is unwell with a high fever. The affected joint is held stiff and is hot and tender. The most frequent causative organism in this group is *Staphylococcus aureus*. In contrast, the other patient groups often present with a much less florid picture. The immunosuppressed or the chronically abnormal joint may give a false impression of a minor upset. The patient remains unwell for many days before presenting with a septicaemia, which is often difficult to ascribe to any source. Many of these patients die because of the delay in recognizing the condition. Beware also of the child on an intercurrent antibiotic as symptoms may also be blunted. In the relatively rare instance of a young adult presenting with a septic arthritis, often with little constitutional upset, then the most likely cause is gonococcus.

Management

Treatment consists of surgery and intravenous antibiotics. The joint should be opened and all loculated compartments broken down and irrigated. Antibiotics should be given according to culture. The first-guess antibiotic should be an antistaphylococcal agent in children as this is still overall the most likely infecting organism. In adults penicillin should be given intravenously to cover the risk of gonococcal infection. If treatment is not instigated then, apart from the risk of septicaemia, the articular cartilage is at great risk and may undergo lysis, leading to fibrous or even bony fusion of the joint.

Chronic septic arthritis

Aetiology

Tuberculosis is still an important cause of joint infection worldwide and has seen a resurgence in patients with acquired immune deficiency syndrome (AIDS) recently. Joint tuberculosis is acquired from blood-borne spread and there is a strong relationship between urinary and joint tuberculosis.

Clinical presentation

The clinical picture is of chronic malaise, weight loss and marked muscle wasting around the affected joint. The radiographs show highly characteristic loss of bone density.

Management

Treatment is by chemotherapy and only rarely is surgery necessary. Combinations of drugs such as ethambutol and rifampicin are given for many months.

Knee problems

Clinical presentation

Knee problems may present as chronic discomfort, or as acute lesions, which commonly have a background of chronic trouble or a previous injury. The cardinal symptoms of knee pathology are:
- swelling;
- locking;
- giving way;
- pain.

Swelling

Information regarding the onset of swelling relative to an episode of pain or an accident is valuable. A rapid accumulation of fluid suggests bleeding while a less dramatic and slower build-up of fluid (over hours or days) suggests an effusion of synovial fluid. A chronic and boggy swelling which never changes indicates a synovitis.

Locking

This is a symptom which must always be probed. Most patients use the term when they mean painful stiffness, often occurring on movement after rest in a sitting position. True locking is an inability to extend the knee fully due to a painful mechanical block commonly caused by a torn meniscus, a loose body or, more rarely, by a torn cruciate ligament. In contrast to painful stiffness, flexion is nearly always possible without pain in the locked knee.

Giving way

This means that the patient is unable to maintain the knee in extension and when weight is applied to the leg the knee simply flexes and the patient may fall. This is similar to locking in that it suggests a painful block to movement which causes a reciprocal quadriceps inhibition and so loss of active extension in the flexed knee. A slight jerk on descending stairs is suggestive of an internal ligamentous injury to the cruciates.

Pain

Pain may be linked to any of the above symptoms. Unremitting pain, worse on exercise and eventually causing loss of sleep, may indicate a degenerative knee disorder.

All the above features may also be elicited as physical signs. A useful sign of significant knee pathology is wasting of the quadriceps muscle, which may be seen easily if the patient is asked to actively extend the leg.

Meniscal lesions

Aetiology and patterns

The medial meniscus is generally more frequently torn than the lateral. The meniscus may be torn at its peripheral attachment to the joint capsule or within its substance. The meniscus may split horizontally — a so-called cleavage lesion — this is very common in old age and may not generally be important. Occasionally these cleavage lesions act like flap valves and allow a build-up of synovial fluid within the meniscus; this forms a cyst. Common pathological tears within the substance of the meniscus are in the vertical plane and can either be a split off one end of the meniscus (the parrot beak) or a vertical split which is anchored at both ends (the bucket handle).

Clinical presentation

Although seen in both sexes, meniscal lesions are relatively rare in women. Although not common it is well to remember that they can occur in adolescents. Occasionally children are born with an abnormal, discoid lateral meniscus. They present with pain, effusion, sometimes with locking and/or giving way. Their tenderness is poorly localized on examination, although generalized discomfort may be elicited by gently but forcibly extending the knee.

Management

The meniscus is an important structure and as much of it as possible should be preserved to help in distributing the load between femur and tibia. Peripheral tears can be re-attached with sutures. Substance tears have no apparent capacity to repair and so the torn peripheral part should be removed, usually by arthroscopy. Once there is a clinical suspicion of a meniscal tear the patient should undergo arthroscopy.

Most meniscal lesions can now be removed via an arthroscope, although some require a small arthrotomy. The principal advantage of arthroscopic meniscectomy is that most patients recover from it within a few days or weeks. Open meniscectomy has a much more prolonged period of rehabilitation.

Loose bodies

Aetiology

In a knee injury small fragments of cartilage and bone (osteochondral fragments) may be sheared off into the joint space to become loose bodies. The original injury may be remembered by the patient as the knee probably became swollen from associated bleeding (haemarthrosis). The osteochondral fragment is often not resorbed but survives floating free in the joint, getting its nutrition from the synovial fluid. The bulk of the loose body, if not all of it, is cartilage and so it may be radiolucent.

Clinical presentation

Months or years after a knee injury the patient presents with locking, pain and giving way. Often there is a knee effusion.

Management

Loose bodies are a nuisance and should be removed, preferably via the arthroscope. Very rarely in adolescents osteochondral fragments occur spontaneously: this condition is known as *osteochondritis dissecans*. Such a condition tends to settle spontaneously but loose bodies may require removal.

Cruciate ligament injury

Aetiology

The cruciate ligaments are not capable of spontaneous healing and, if torn, they are lost, except in the rare circumstances when they are pulled off with a fragment of bone. Even then the fragment must be replaced surgically. The cruciate ligament is commonly injured by either hyperextension or a twist, often in association with a foot being anchored by a studded boot or a ski.

Clinical presentation

In the acute injury the knee swells quickly, indicating a haemarthrosis brought on by active bleeding from the end-artery in the cruciate ligament. Sometimes the patient reports feeling a 'pop', which is the ligament tearing. The swelling eventually resolves and it is only after a few weeks that the chronic problems arise. Loss of a cruciate leads to loss of anteroposterior stability, particularly in flexion. Thus, difficulty in going up or coming down stairs is a common symptom. There is also a loss of rotatory stability when twisting and turning, making cruciate injury particularly disabling for athletes. Interestingly, however, not all patients get symptoms, a fact for which there is no explanation at present. Many patients only experience symptoms when involved in the sort of activities described above.

Management

In general, cruciate ligament injuries should be left untreated for a while and the knee muscles rehabilitated. Only if symptoms interfere with daily life or if the patient demands it, should treatment be offered. This consists of replacement of the torn ligament with a prosthesis. These prosthetic ligaments are new and have a dubious life span. Certainly, if patients persist in vigorous activity the insensitive prosthetic ligament is likely to fail.

Soft-tissue injuries to the collateral ligaments of the knee heal spontaneously.

Dislocation of the patella

Aetiology

This condition is usually associated with a malformation of either the patella or the lateral femoral condyle. This leads to lateral maltracking which in itself is painful.

Clinical presentation

In some patients spontaneous dislocation of the patella and failure of the extensor apparatus occur. The net result is that the patient falls to the ground.

Management

Minor degrees of maltracking are dealt with by lateral release of the vastus lateralis aponeuroses. If it is recurrent and severe then a medial refining of the vastus medialis may be required and, once growth has ceased, the patellar tendon may be resited more medially on the tibia. This condition should not be confused with anterior knee pain often seen in adolescence, particularly in girls. This condition is a poorly understood condition and best left alone, as most settle spontaneously.

Backache and neckache

Introduction

It is no exaggeration to suggest that everyone will get backache or neckache at some time during their lives. This is often attributed to the fact that humans walk upright. However, we know that quadripeds also get backache and so we must look elsewhere for an explanation. Although common, most backache is usually self-limiting, and so in that sense is not serious. Unfortunately, it is difficult to tell the small number of patients with serious back problems from the majority of minor aches and sprains; the result is that all are often extensively investigated to pick out the minority with serious pathology.

Inappropriate investigation and management of back pain may create a new category of back sufferer — those who think they have a serious problem. Consider the scenario in which a patient presents with backache which lasts for a few weeks. The patient is referred to a hospital, thus reinforcing in his or her mind the possibility that the condition may be serious. The hospital doctor arranges a whole gamut of investigations, confirming the patient's worse fears. On a return visit the patient sees another doctor who orders more tests or even institutes empirical treatment. Now the cycle is almost complete: pain, some tests, treatment, more tests, more treatment and so on. In this situation the patient concludes that the pain must be significant and it grows in importance; as the patient does not 'respond to treatment', all is reinforced and unwittingly doctor and patient collude in what is known as illness behaviour. This section is about learning to distinguish significant from insignificant back pain and so prevent the onset of illness behaviour.

Anatomical considerations

The vertebral column consists of bony, muscular and ligamentous elements and neurological tissue which takes advantage of the bony protection afforded by the vertebrae. The non-neurological tissues are termed the spondylitides and abnormalities of these tissues are rather crudely termed spondylitis. Abnormalities can occur only in the spondylitides or, very rarely, only in the nerve tissue. Not uncommonly, structural abnormalities may lead to abnormalities in the nerve tissue due to compression, which may affect the spinal cord itself, or more commonly, the nerve roots.

Pain in spinal disorders

Pain may occur locally or be referred, or may occur along the distribution of nerves.

Local pain

In general, pain is fairly poorly localized in the back. It tends to be related to a whole region, such as the lumbar or dorsal regions, and it is unusual to be any more specific.

Referred pain

The picture may be further complicated by referred pain from the back to the buttock and leg, or from the neck to the shoulder and arm. Elsewhere we have learnt that abdominal pain can represent referred pain from other parts of the body and this is of use in helping us reach a diagnosis. In contrast, when considering pain in the vertebral column, referred pain can be confusing and difficult to discern from root pain (see below). Leg pain occurring in the buttock and thigh and descending to the mid-calf is usually referred pain and is associated with a mechanical and poorly localized spondylitic disorder. Neck pain that radiates to the shoulder and upper arm is usually referred in a similar way, although this feature is less specific in the neck compared with the lumbar spine.

Nerve root pain

The nerve roots emerge from the vertebral foramina, which are in part bordered by the facet joints behind and the disc in front. Diseases of these structures may affect the nerve roots by direct pressure, inflammation or oedema. The brain interprets such disturbances as pain in the distribution of the affected spinal nerve. This commonly happens in lower lumbar foramina and so the nerve distribution of pain perception follows the sciatic nerve and hence gives origin to the term sciatica. Sciatica is characterized by pain in the leg, mainly down the back but almost always into the foot. It may be exacerbated by coughing as this activity increases intrathecal pressure.

In the cervical spine the mid to lower foramina are commonly affected and so hand and forearm pain, often associated with tingling, is characteristic. Both in the lumbar and cervical spines it is easy to see how referred pain and root pain may be confused. It should be noted that in general, root pain is much rarer than referred pain. If the nerve root is significantly compromised, then localizing signs may be elicited and these may be sensory or motor.

Cauda equina syndrome

Cauda equina syndrome is rare but very important. It is due to central pressure on the cauda equina. This is commonly associated with a prolapsed disc, although tumours, particularly secondary neoplasms, may also cause this problem. The pressure on the cauda causes bowel and bladder disturbances, usually urinary retention, often with overflow incontinence. These symptoms should be positively excluded by direct questioning and whenever root entrapment is suspected a rectal examination should be routine in order to test anal tone. This condition is a real emergency and urgent investigation and surgery are mandatory if these important visceral functions are to be preserved.

Common causes of back pain

The common causes of back pain are listed in Table 22.5. Many of the visceral disorders should be excluded by taking a good history and by examining the patient. Some of the rarer pathologies, particularly tumours, are relatively easy to miss, often because they are not thought about. Progressive signs and unremitting symptoms should alert the clinician to a neoplastic pathology.

Back sprains

Aetiology

As mentioned above, almost everyone will suffer from an episode of back pain at some time in their lives. Most causes are associated with ill-advised manoeuvres or poor lifting, which cause muscle or ligament injuries. These conditions should be separated from neurological causes by the absence of signs of nerve tension or compression.

Management

Back sprains require a brief period of rest followed by a gradual return to normal activities. Non-steroidal drugs aid

Table 22.5 Common causes of back pain.

Related to the spondylitides
Aches and sprains
Mechanical back pain
Spondylolisthesis
Ankylosing spondylitis

Entrapment neuropathies
Discogenic
Bony root entrapment

Neurological and support tissues

Tumours and space-occupying lesions

Arachnoiditis

Other visceral causes
Urinary tract infection
Leaking aortic aneurysm
Duodenal ulcers
Pancreatic lesions

in the relief of symptoms, although simple analgesia is usually sufficient. These conditions are common but must not be taken lightly should the doctor be consulted. A careful exclusion of significant pathology should be followed by a proper explanation in order to prevent the development of an illness cycle. Only one or at the most two visits to a clinic should be encouraged.

Mechanical backache

This is often difficult to discern from acute sprain episodes, except that mechanical backache is chronic or often consists of a series of acute exacerbations against a background of less significant chronic discomfort.

Aetiology

The cause of mechanical back problems is unknown, although, as the name implies, it is a non-neurological entity. Confusion may arise if referred leg pain is one of the presenting symptoms; difficulty may also arise in middle-aged patients, a minority of whom develop genuine root signs. Suggested causes include disc degeneration which leads to increased loading and secondary osteoarthritis of facet joints. Primary arthritis of the facet joints has been implicated but there are probably many other factors such as ligament or muscle pathology which have yet to be determined.

Management

Recurring episodes of back pain are the norm for this condition. It is important to explain this to patients and reassure them that, while the condition is chronic, it does not deteriorate. There is no known cure for mechanical back pain and judicious use of rest, physiotherapy and medication will help the patient through a bad episode.

Most patients learn to live with their bad back and how to prevent recurrences. Support should be provided by general practitioners with occasional interjections by specialists. Regular hospital review is to be discouraged, provided the general practitioner has access to support services. Physiotherapists may be of great value in providing such support. Alternative medical practitioners such as osteopaths and chiropractors can provide both time to listen and some ease by manipulation. It is important, however, that everyone concerned, including the patient, is clear on the pathology and the uncertain nature of the condition is kept in perspective.

Spondylolisthesis

This is a not uncommon finding on radiographs of patients presenting with back pain. The term refers to the slippage of one vertebra relative to another and is commonly seen in the lumbar spine. It is caused by an abnormality in the posterior complex of the spine which interferes with the stability of the facet joints and their associated bony and ligamentous elements.

Aetiology

Spondylolisthesis may be congenital or acquired and it is important to realize that it may present at any age, including infancy. Adult spondylolisthesis is thought to be acquired, although some may be late-presenting and mild congenital abnormalities. The mechanism of acquisition appears to be an acute, or more likely a fatigue, fracture of the pars interarticularis, which is that part of the neural arch linking the superior and inferior facets of any vertebrae.

Clinical presentation

The patient presents with low back pain, which is almost identical to mechanical back pain. Diagnosis is nearly always made on X-ray, although in severe slippage a step may be felt at the affected level. Oblique films should be requested if spondylolisthesis is suspected, as these more clearly show the facets and their connecting bony bridges. Very rarely will the patient present with neurological deficit. Congenital spondylolisthesis is an exception and the

stability may be so insecure as to threaten neurological structures.

Management

Most patients, surprisingly, do not require surgery and decisions to operate depend almost entirely on the severity of the symptoms. A spinal support which offloads the spine by increasing intra-abdominal pressure may help. Otherwise the patient may be managed conservatively, rather like the mechanical back pain sufferer.

The pars defect described above may be seen on X-ray without a slip. This is known as *spondylolysis*. The significance of this finding should be viewed with caution as it may not be the cause of the pain. Such patients usually will respond to conservative measures, but severe pain may require spinal fusion.

Ankylosing spondylitis

This is a rare disease affecting men in early adulthood and usually presenting before 30. The spine is predominantly affected but major joints, particularly the hips, may also be affected. The patient presents with general back pain, tiredness and malaise. Early-morning stiffness is common. Investigations show a high erythrocyte sedimentation rate and the presence of the human leukocyte antigen (HLA)-B27 antigen in most patients. The natural history is of progressive stiffness and ultimately bony fusion of the whole of the spine. Patients need to be kept mobile and with good posture. Symptoms respond to NSAIDs. The major joints may require replacement.

Entrapment neuropathies

Prolapsed intervertebral disc (Fig. 22.5)

It is essential from the outset to allay the commonly held view in the general population that most back and leg ache is caused by 'a slipped disc'. This is a relatively rare condition and in any case the disc does not 'slip', but rather the disc contents prolapse.

Disc prolapse was first described in the late 1940s but first became a popular diagnosis in the early 1960s. It is true to say that since then the diagnosis has become somewhat overused. Disc prolapse may occur in the lumbar or cervical spine but the description below assumes that the condition is in the lumbar spine.

Aetiology The cause of symptoms is an abnormality in the intervertebral disc which leads to prolapse of the nucleus

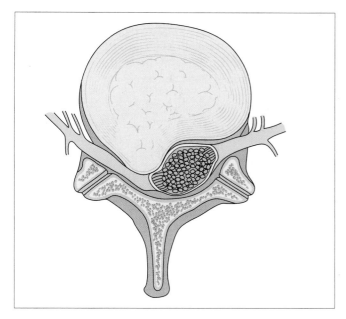

Figure 22.5 Schematic drawing illustrating disc tissue displacement (protrusion) resulting in nerve root compression and displacement of the spinal cord. From Crockard A, Hayward R & Hoff JT (eds) *Neurosurgery, The Scientific Basis of Clinical Practice*, 2nd edn. Oxford: Blackwell Scientific Publications, 1992, p. 705, with permission.

pulposus material through the surrounding annulus fibrosus with impingement on the spinal contents. If the material passes backwards and laterally it impinges on the nerve roots while posterior prolapse results in cord or cauda equina compression. The discs between the sacrum and the fifth lumbar vertebra are most commonly affected and the condition occurs with decreasing frequency further up the lumbar spine. Disc prolapse often presents with 'sciatica' as the nerve roots most frequently compressed are those forming the sciatic nerve. However, prolapse may occur at higher lumbar levels and may be perceived as pain in the distribution of the femoral nerve. Large centrally prolapsing discs can lead to the cauda equina syndrome (see above) and the patient may present with bowel or bladder incontinence.

Clinical presentation The classical symptoms occur in people under 40, in either sex. The condition presents acutely with backache and leg ache or sometimes with leg ache alone, with backache developing later. Patients may describe a single event of lifting or strain, but there is no known correlation between cause and condition; it may arise spontaneously. The characteristic symptom is of leg ache passing down the back of the thigh and leg to the foot. This is in contrast to referred backache which usually goes no further than the knee or upper calf.

On examination, the features of nerve root irritation may be present; straight leg raising will be restricted and there may be tenderness on compressing the nerve (see Fig. 22.5). There may or may not be localizing signs. A rectal examination is essential to assess sphincter tone if there is any history of bowel or bladder abnormalities.

Management First central disc compression has to be excluded. The patient may then be treated by a combination of rest and gentle, progressive mobilization. Analgesics and anti-inflammatory drugs may aid in symptom relief. Bedrest should be for a minimum period and traction only used to enforce rest — it will not materially alter the condition. It should be emphasized that with time most disc prolapses will resolve spontaneously. If symptoms do not relapse after about 6 weeks, or if pain is uncontrolled, or if localizing neurological signs progress, then the patient should be investigated with a view to surgery. A radiculogram is a contrast study where radiopaque contrast medium is injected into the thecal space and any occupying lesion will be highlighted. A computed tomographic (CT) scan at the same time also gives useful information. However, magnetic resonance imaging (MRI) scans will probably replace CT scanning and radiculography in future.

Bony root entrapment neuropathy

In contrast to disc prolapse, this condition has been ignored until fairly recently. It has come to significance through the improved imaging techniques described above.

Aetiology The cause of the condition is commonly due to bony overgrowth around the vertebral foramina where the nerve roots emerge. The cause of the bony overgrowth would appear to be secondary to degenerative changes in the adjacent facet joints. These may degenerate from primary osteoarthritis or secondarily subsequent to disc degeneration (not prolapse!).

Clinical presentation The clinical syndrome consists of a previous history of backache of a mechanical type occurring in a person of either sex, usually aged over 40. These patients are usually known back sufferers but they develop new symptoms of leg pain radiating to the foot, usually exacerbated by exercise. Such a syndrome is rather poorly named as spinal claudication, although it may indeed be confused with vascular disease. Episodes are usually acute and recurrent against a chronic history of back pain. The episodes may remain mild or may progress to affect the patient's lifestyle. Remedial therapy is unlikely to help and, should symptoms be severe, they should then be referred for surgery.

Management Removal of the disc in such patients may make the condition worse and a removal of bone is needed to free trapped nerve roots. This may destabilize the spine and lead to a need to fuse it. The decision to operate is entirely determined by the severity of the patient's symptoms.

Cervical spine disorders

The cervical spine is a very mobile part of the vertebral column and it is no surprise to find it prone to disease and injury. Most conditions are exactly analogous to those found in the lumbar spine.

Cervical spondylosis

This is very like the degenerative disc and joint disease seen in the lumbar spine and the aetiology, as far as any is understood, is the same.

Clinical presentation

The patient is usually over 40 and is more frequently female than male. The patient presents with dull neckache and this is often referred to the shoulders and upper arms. The tingling in the arms is often assumed to be an entrapment of nerve roots but this is not always confirmed on investigation. The spondylitic process can however be progressive and bony root entrapment may occur, with localizing neurological signs. These signs may be confused with local nerve entrapments. Nerve conduction studies or even cervical myelography may be useful in making the diagnosis.

Management

Without localizing nerve signs the patient simply needs NSAIDs, a soft collar and physiotherapy, which helps spasm. Patients need counselling and a good explanation of the condition. They need to be warned that the natural history, as in the lumbar spine, is for acute episodic recurrence. If root entrapment is confirmed then surgical intervention with anterior fusion and decompression may be indicated if symptoms cannot otherwise be controlled.

Cervical disc prolapse

Although not as frequent, cervical disc disease presents with a similar pattern to that of the lumbar spine. The lower cervical discs are most likely to cause the problem. Pain and referral are similar to spondylitic pain. The differential diagnosis can be difficult, although disc sufferers tend to have no previous history of neck trouble and characteristi-

cally the neck muscles are in more spasm following disc prolapse and the associated stiffness is severe. Most patients recover with a cervical collar or with gentle traction. If localizing signs are marked or symptoms do not regress then surgery and fusion of the affected segment may be necessary.

Minor adult disorders

Introduction

In many ways the term 'minor' does some injustice to the conditions discussed below. It is important to appreciate that these conditions are common and will be of sufficient severity to cause considerable inconvenience and discomfort to the patient and may have important social and economic consequences. They are minor in the sense that many are self-limiting in their natural history and many have non-surgical solutions. They all need care in assessment and in management, as it is possible to make people worse by casual or inaccurate management.

Enthesopathies

The enthesis is the term given to the short fibrous origin of a muscle and so an enthesopathy refers to an inflammation of a muscle origin. Common sites of enthesopathies include:
- the common flexor muscle origin of the forearm: *golfer's elbow*;
- the common extensor origin of the forearm: *tennis elbow*.

The patient often complains of quite severe discomfort on using the affected muscle. It is possible that many entheses may be inflamed at one time, giving rise to many aches and pains. The common enthesopathies around the elbow may arise spontaneously, although they are commonly associated with repetitive movements or overuse. The prognosis is generally favourable, especially if there is a clear cause and rest will result in a spontaneous recovery.

Occasionally the condition may become chronic, or be severe enough to warrant intervention. Recovery may be speeded up with a course of anti-inflammatory agents. Local steroid injections into the point of maximum tenderness can also be of value. Care must be taken to ensure that the steroid is injected into the enthesis with no leakage into the subcutaneous fat or skin as otherwise the pain may be exacerbated and the patient left with an unsightly atrophic dimple. A very small number of patients require surgery which consists of a scraping of the origin of the muscle from the bone, permitting it to slide distally and so decompress the area. If possible, patients should be encouraged to wait, as the long-term chance of spontaneous recovery is high.

Nerve entrapment syndromes

All nerves are sensitive to compression. Continued pressure will lead to *neuropraxia* and, if not relieved, atrophy of the nerve. At best such injury takes a very long time to recover and usually recovery is not complete. Therefore early diagnosis and management are likely to give the best results.

Nerve entrapments may be extrinsic to the body or intrinsic. Extrinsic causes include accidents where consciousness is lost and the victim inadvertently presses on a nerve (e.g. compression of the radial nerve between the humerus and the arm or back of a chair during inebriated sleep). Patients in bed, on the operating table and in plaster casts are at risk from pressure on nerves in exposed sites. The most common site at risk is the common peroneal nerve as it winds around the fibula head.

Most nerve entrapments, however, are intrinsic and common sites are:
- the median nerve at the wrist (carpal tunnel syndrome);
- the ulnar nerve at the elbow (ulnar neuritis);
- the ulnar nerve at the wrist;
- the posterior tibial nerve at the ankle (tarsal tunnel syndrome).

Carpal tunnel syndrome (median nerve entrapment at the wrist)

Aetiology

The median nerve supplies the intrinsic muscles of the thumb and sensory fibres to the volar surface of the hand and radial three-and-a-half fingers. The sensation to the palm is provided by a small branch passing over the flexor retinaculum at the wrist but the bulk of the nerve passes under the retinaculum through the carpal tunnel. Anything that limits the space in the carpal tunnel will compress the nerve and give rise to symptoms. Most causes of carpal tunnel syndrome remain obscure but a number of specific aetiologies are recognized:
- trauma: following wrist fractures and dislocations;
- pregnancy: associated with fluid retention;
- rheumatoid arthritis: linked to the space occupation by granulation tissue.

Clinical presentation

Classical symptoms include numbness and tingling in the sensory distribution of the nerve, associated with certain positions of the wrist, worse at night. Patients are often woken and have to dangle the wrist and shake it to relieve the discomfort. The cause of this classical symptom is unknown. In later stages patients also complain of weakness of grip, clumsiness and a tendency to drop objects. Examination can be normal, although the symptoms may be reproduced by flexing the wrist and holding it for a few seconds. In 25% of cases the reverse manoeuvre may be required to reproduce the phenomenon. In more advanced cases the thenar eminence may be seen to be wasted and sensory changes associated with dry skin may be observed. Remember that the sensation to the palmar branch will be preserved and this will distinguish compression at the wrist from compression from a more proximal source.

Nerve conduction studies

Generally, investigations are not necessary; however, occasionally the clinician may be confused by symptoms of discomfort more proximal to the wrist that occur for obscure reasons. In these cases nerve conduction studies tend to be unequivocal and will distinguish between nerve root and peripheral nerve problems.

Management

Management will depend on the cause. In the case of trauma, fractures require reduction, but the nerve may still have to be decompressed by dividing the flexor retinaculum. In the case of pregnancy this is a self-limiting condition which may be relieved temporarily by conservative measures, described below. In RA the compression of the nerve is but one feature of a complex problem which may need a radical solution, including synovectomy and wrist joint fusion.

In most cases where a cause is not apparent, surgery will be the treatment of choice if there are signs of nerve dysfunction. Surgery consists of decompressing the nerve by dividing the flexor retinaculum at the wrist and into the palm. In less severe cases, temporary splintage of the wrist in a 'cock-up' position is often adequate and certainly helps confirm the diagnosis. Some advocate steroid injections, although the results are mixed. Surgery consists of division of the flexor retinaculum but one should be aware that a significant percentage are not completely relieved and patients should be warned of this possibility.

Ulnar neuritis (ulnar nerve entrapment at the elbow)

Aetiology

The nerve is compromised by stretching and/or compression for a number of reasons. The nerve may be irritated by repeated trauma, as is sometimes seen in those using crutches. It may be stretched by abnormal growth or malunion following elbow fractures. The nerve can be entrapped by a tough fibrous band as it passes between the two origins of flexor carpi ulnaris. Generally, however, most cases are of unknown cause.

Clinical presentation

Symptoms reflect the course and function of the ulnar nerve distally. Tingling in the little finger is common and loss of intrinsic muscle function in the hand, with consequent lack of fine finger movement, ensues. Examination reveals tenderness of the nerve on the medial side of the elbow, which is often quite exquisite. Dryness of the skin on the medial (ulnar) border of the hand and sensory changes are early features. Small muscle wasting is a serious sign and is indicative of a poor prognosis. Once present, this condition tends to persist and once signs are elicited it is unlikely that they will be completely reversed, even with treatment. Decompression transposition of the nerve to the front of the elbow is always recommended as this will usually halt the progress but, as implied above, rarely reverses it. It is important to distinguish ulnar neuritis from an enthesopathy and, although this is usually easy with a proper history and examination, nerve conduction studies will be definitive.

Ulnar entrapment at the wrist

Although less common than median nerve compression, this condition may occur, often in combination with median nerve entrapment. This is particularly so in RA and trauma. The nerve passes through its own tunnel at the wrist and so will require particular attention at surgery.

Tarsal tunnel syndrome (posterior tibial nerve entrapment at the ankle)

This is a rare condition, and generally overdiagnosed. The posterior tibial nerve becomes entrapped as it passes beneath the retinaculum behind the medial malleolus. This causes foot pain, particularly at the heel, and can be confused with plantar fasciitis. It may be differentiated by testing sensation of the heel and commonly is accompanied by fasciculation of the medial plantar muscles. Nerve conduction studies are not reliable and surgery should be reversed for patients with the clinical signs described above.

Tenosynovitis

Inflammation of tendons and their associated synovial sheaths is a common problem. It is of course associated with RA where it is part of a multisystem disease. In other situations it may arise spontaneously, often with no known cause, but usually it is precipitated by unusual levels of ac-

tivity, or overuse. It is an important condition to be aware of, as it is often associated with worker compensation and litigation.

Bursitis

Bursae are synovial-lined structures adjacent to joints which act as a natural form of bearing aimed at improving muscle and joint function. They are prone to inflammation through repetitive movement or strain, or due to them being subject to abnormal loads. Bursae around the shoulder are commonly affected and these are dealt with in a separate section on shoulder discomfort. The common sites of bursitis are around the knee and the elbow, although the greater trochanter is not uncommonly affected at the hip.

The patients generally complain of chronic discomfort over the bursa, usually associated with the causative element, such as movement or pressure. They may present because of swelling of the bursa, such as is seen in *housemaid's knee*, when the prepatellar bursa swells. Occasionally a bursa becomes infected, resulting in a tense swelling associated with cellulitis and general malaise. Infected bursae should be incised and drained and often this leads to a spontaneous recovery through scarring and fibrosis.

Chronic bursal swelling with no symptoms is benign and needs no treatment unless the patient demands it either for convenience or cosmesis. If tender, bursae may be excised, although the patient should be encouraged to address the underlying cause (e.g. by using a kneeling mat). Bursae are sometimes seen in children around the hamstrings at the knee — the so called semimembranosus bursa. This is naturally a cause of parental anxiety but most disappear as the child develops.

Shoulder discomfort

Introduction

The shoulder girdle consists of an articulation between scapula and chest wall as well as between scapula and humerus. There are of course other joints to consider, particularly the acromioclavicular joint. Good shoulder function relies on healthy ligaments, muscles and tendons. All of these structures are frequently injured, particularly those involved in heavy, repetitive work and contact sports.

Clinical presentation

Symptoms include pain, particularly on movement, and the pain may be limited to a particular range of movement. Symptoms quite frequently are associated with a recent incident such as a pull or a period of unusual activity such as DIY.

The following structures are commonly involved in pathological conditions causing shoulder discomfort:
- the subacromial bursa;
- the supraspinatus tendon;
- the acromioclavicular joint;
- the biceps tendon;
- the rotator cuff.

Unfortunately it may be difficult or impossible to localize which of these structures gives rise to the symptoms. Fortunately, most of the minor conditions settle with rest and time. To resolve, the differential diagnosis may require specialist examination, including arthrography or arthroscopy.

Management

If rest, gentle exercise and anti-inflammatory drugs do not help, then a careful examination may reveal a point of tenderness. Tenderness under active movement within a painful arc is suggestive of a supraspinatus tendon inflammation or a subacromial bursitis. Injection of steroid into the bursa or around the tendon, but not into it, can be very effective. It remains controversial whether this is reasonable and certainly should only be done with care. Occasionally the patient may present with very severe pain and a radiograph will show calcific material within the supraspinatus tendon. Injection or even surgery in this case is well-justified for the pain relief achieved.

Unfortunately, many patients only respond temporarily to the injection. Repetitive injection is not indicated and further investigation often shows degenerative change in the acromioclavicular joint with osteophytic impingement on the supraspinatus tendon. This may lead to attrition rupture of the supraspinatus, which is part of the rotator cuff. Such rotator cuff tears can become large rents and even small ones cause a lot of discomfort and pain. Surgery to relieve the cause and repair the cuff will bring effective pain relief and some return of function. Repetitive injections in such patients can result in further degeneration of the cuff and should not be practised.

Frozen shoulder

Most so-called frozen shoulders are sore shoulders and fit into the collection of conditions outlined above. True frozen shoulder is a condition where there is little or no glenohumeral movement. It occurs rarely, often in those who have had a specific trauma incident, particularly an epileptic fit or an electric shock. Often the cause is obscure. Such patients eventually recover in 18 months to 2 years. They require a lot of psychological and physiotherapy support. The condition may be helped by manipulation under anaesthetic.

Adult foot disorders

Introduction

Abnormalities of the feet are relatively common in the western world and this must relate in many ways to our shodden state. Also our perception of abnormality is very varied — as varied, in fact, as our feet. The only foot abnormalities that matter are those which cause symptoms and usually pain is the principal problem. Treatment or surgery is seldom if ever justified in the absence of functional abnormality and disaster will likely follow if operations are done to get people into their preferred footwear. Foot-shaped shoes are the order of the day — not shoe-shaped feet.

Flat foot

The painful flat foot is a rare entity. Symptom-free flat feet are a variation on normal and are very common in certain races. The problem usually presents in childhood (see below) or in adolescence around the final growth spurt. Rarely, a very painful spasmodic flat foot may be associated with infection or chronic inflammatory disease. Occasionally it may present acutely in middle age and examination reveals a painful and tender swelling over the insertion of tibialis posterior. This may indicate acute or impending degenerative rupture and warrants early intervention. Mostly the condition is benign and, if painfree, should be ignored. If associated with pain a medial heel lift will correct the deformity of the hind part of the foot and stabilize the medial arch. If pain is a persistent problem, fusion of the subtalar joint will help, although this is not something to contemplate lightly as it disturbs foot and ankle function profoundly.

Bunions and corns

Bunions are fluid-filled bursae which are found around bony prominences, commonly over the distal part of the first metatarsal and occasionally over the fifth (Fig. 22.6a). They are a natural response to pressure and indicate an underlying abnormality which should be treated rather than the bunion. Occasionally they become infected and need drainage, followed a few weeks later by treatment of the cause or a review of the footwear.

Corns are another way in which the body reacts to areas of high pressure. The painful excessive corny skin may be superficially removed but in the long term it will recur unless the underlying abnormality causing the high pressure is removed.

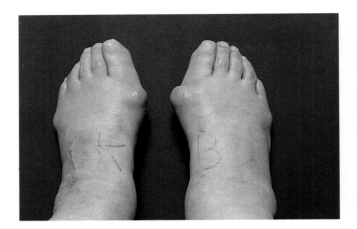

(a)

Figure 22.6 (a) Bunions are fluid-filled bursae which are found around bony prominences, commonly over the distal part of the first metatarsal. Occasionally they become infected and need drainage, followed a few weeks later by treatment of the cause or a review of the footwear.

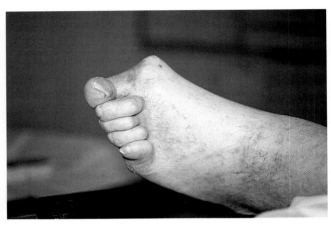

(b)

(b) Hallux valgus is a deformity of the big toe with turning away of the phalanges from the midline, usually because of a deformity at the joint line. It is usually associated with an exostosis of the head of the first metatarsal and an overlying bursa may be present.

Hallux valgus and hallux rigidus

The hallux refers to the big toe and really these conditions are disorders of the first metatarsophalangeal joint. *Hallux valgus* is a deformity of the big toe with turning away of the phalanges from the midline, usually because of a deformity at the joint line. It is usually associated with an exostosis of the head of the first metatarsal and an overlying bursa may be present (Fig. 22.6b). *Hallux rigidus* is a poor term indicating osteoarthritis of the metatarsophalangeal joint. The two conditions may occur separately or together and treatment depends upon that and the age of the patient.

Hallux rigidus alone

Hallux rigidus in isolation can occur in adolescents and adults. In adolescents it is said to be as a result of osteochondral fracture, although this is not always easy to prove. Conservative treatment includes the use of a metatarsal bar to provide a rocker at the front of the foot so that the toe need not bend in normal walking. This usually fails because youngsters do not accept the cosmetic consequences on their shoes and so the same surgery as practised in adults is required. In adults the condition may present at any age, although in the elderly it rarely occurs without hallux valgus. Conservative measures are rarely sufficient and surgery is required. Removal of osteophytes with an osteotomy of the proximal phalanx for minor cases is often sufficient. Fusion is most reliable in a neutral position. Despite much folklore,

this rarely gives women problems over the heel height. Interposition arthroplasty with a Silastic spacer is an alternative which gives mixed results.

Hallux valgus alone

Hallux valgus alone may occur at any age. It gives more problems in women than men because of fashion in shoes. There is no evidence that shoes cause the condition. Many, but not all, sufferers have a short, often varus, first metatarsal. The cause of this common and troublesome condition is unknown. Management depends on age. Realignment of the first metatarsal to a more lateral position and excision of the exostosis over the first metatarsal head give satisfactory results at almost any age. Excision of the metatarsophalangeal joint (*Keller's operation*) is to be avoided in the young and is probably unnecessary if the joint is not painful.

Hallux valgus with hallux rigidus

This combination is seen in older patients where joint degeneration is usually secondary to the valgus deformity. These older patients may well be satisfied by having their pain relieved by well-fitting, extra-depth shoes. If this fails, then Keller's arthroplasty is a safe and rapid way of giving some relief. This operation is not benign, however, and severely disrupts normal foot mechanics and so should be reserved for the older, less active patient.

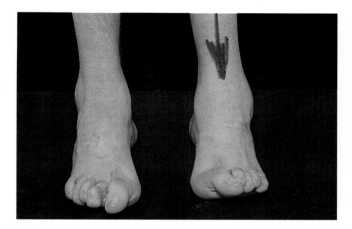

Figure 22.7 Claw and hammer toes.

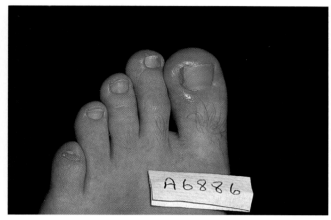

Figure 22.8 An infected ingrowing toenail.

Claw and hammer toes

These common abnormalities are almost a normal variant (Fig. 22.7). Clawing suggests intrinsic muscle weakness or deficiency. Indeed, on close analysis, many of these patients do indeed have weak or denervated small muscles of the feet. This is often associated with minor spinal abnormality such as spina bifida occulta. This means that claw toes should be approached with caution as far as surgery is concerned and only limited goals sought. Hammer toes are secondary to disruption of the metatarsophalangeal joints. Abnormalities of the foot leading to prolapse of metatarsal heads and joint disruption are not understood. The patients may present with generally sore forefeet — often called, rather grandly, metatarsalgia. The cause of the primary lesion is unknown and treatment is often unsatisfactory. Surgery to the secondary hammering of the toes includes fusion of the interphalangeal joints in a straight position, so that they do not rub on the shoes. Often a good pair of soft and comfortable shoes is all that is required.

Neuromas

The cutaneous nerves to the toes may become trapped or irritated between the metatarsal heads, giving rise to a neuroma (*Morton's neuroma*). The cause is uncertain, except that it is almost certainly secondary to repetitive trauma and may therefore be associated with metatarsal head prolapse, as described above. The condition is difficult to diagnose with certainty, although the pain is characteristically dull and throbbing, often with sharp exacerbations which are accompanied by tingling of the toes. It is equally difficult to localize, although it is most frequently seen in the lateral two spaces. Classically, sideways compression of the foot produces a palpable click, reproducing the symp-

toms. Treatment by excision may be accompanied by subsequent sensory disturbance to the affected toes. Recurrence is common even with care, and patients should be warned about this.

Ingrowing toenails (see Chapter 17; Fig. 22.8)

Plantar fasciitis

This term often includes a number of vague, but nevertheless very incapacitating painful disorders of the foot. Its cause is entirely obscure and it originates spontaneously with a fairly sudden onset. Patients characteristically complain of a soreness of the instep, often worse first thing on rising, or after sitting for a few hours. The symptoms are minimally relieved by walking but then persist as a debilitating ache, often exacerbated by a change of direction or rough ground. Most cases are self-limiting, although the symptoms may last a few months and some go on for years. On examination point tenderness may be elicited on the hindfoot at the origin of the plantar fascia medially. Discomfort is often more diffuse and care must be taken to exclude a tarsal tunnel syndrome, as described above.

There is no specific cure and methods of relieving symptoms are various and less than satisfactory. Patients should be reassured that the tendency will be for the condition to get better. Insoles that are hollowed out over the tender area may help, but may cause discomfort around the edge of the hollow. Soft shoes and insoles, particularly modern sports trainers, can be of considerable value. If there is marked point tenderness then a local injection of steroids and long-acting local anaesthetic can be very effective, albeit rather painful to administer. Some demand a surgical solution and stripping of the fascia from the os calcis is practised. Results are entirely unpredictable, illustrating the highly uncertain nature of this otherwise self-limiting condition.

Neuropathic feet

Feet without sensation (i.e. a sensory neuropathy) are prone to developing sores caused by the inability to perceive minor trauma from rubbing or treading on objects. Such problems are seen most commonly in the world where *leprosy* is endemic, particularly in the Far East. In the western world the commonest cause of neuropathy is *diabetes mellitus* and all diabetics need to be aware of the potential risk which may creep up on them gradually (Chapter 18; Fig. 22.9). Such patients should regularly inspect their feet and be sure the nails are tidy. Footwear must be chosen with care and, if necessary, extra-depth shoes which are very soft on the uppers may be prescribed. Once established, ulcers are difficult to heal and secondary infection may lead to amputation.

Achilles tendinitis and rupture

Pain around the tendo Achilles where it inserts into the os calcis is seen in two groups. In the younger athlete it may signify overuse. The area may be tender or even swollen. Rest is usually adequate. If it is recurrent, then surgical decompression of the paratenon tissue will often eradicate

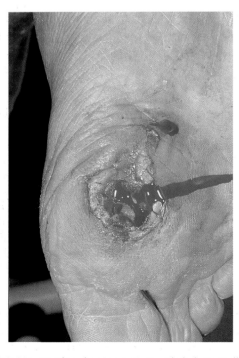

Figure 22.9 Neuropathic ulcer in a patient with diabetes mellitus.

symptoms. Steroidal injection is to be avoided as penetration of the tendon may lead to rupture.

In the middle-aged man a phase of discomfort may precede rupture of the tendo Achilles and this indicates degeneration within the tendon tissue. The cause is little understood, although we know that the lower part of the tendo Achilles has a poor blood supply and is often a point of weakness in some people who keep particularly active into middle age.

If the tendon ruptures it will heal without surgery if the ankle is kept in an equinus plaster for a minimum of 8 weeks. The tendon can be sutured either by a closed technique or by open suture. The latter technique has a high risk of complication.

Whatever method is chosen, there is a significant risk of rerupture which decreases with time. Patients would be encouraged to wear a felt raise inside the heel of their shoes for as long as they will tolerate it.

Orthopaedic conditions of childhood

Introduction

Some childhood musculoskeletal problems are common and minor, while others are rare and important and have major consequences for the child and the family. It is important to understand the nature of the minor conditions and treat them appropriately and have a more general understanding of the rarer major ones which need specialist, often multidisciplinary care. The orthopaedic conditions of childhood are summarized in Table 22.6

Minor conditions

Walking and posture problems

Children are often sent to an orthopaedic clinic because of parental anxiety about how or when children walk and stand. Normally children reach developmental milestones at certain times; children normally sit independently at 6 months, stand at a year and walk at about 18 months. These are averages and parents should be reassured that failure to achieve these goals by the specified age is not a sinister sign. When children start to walk their gait takes many months to mature and so minor variations are to be expected. Very occasionally failure to achieve milestones will portend a serious problem but these are rare cases and will be found in our serious category.

All children referred should be examined carefully to exclude serious pathology. Ask the parents or grandparents

Table 22.6 Common orthopaedic conditions of childhood.

MINOR CONDITIONS
Walking and posture problems
Knee deformities
    Knock knees (genu valgum)
    Bow legs (genu varum)
Intoeing
    Femoral neck angle variation
    Tibial torsion
    Abnormal forefeet
Flat feet
Curly toes

Pain around the knee
Osgood–Schlatter disease
Adolescent knee pain

MAJOR CONDITIONS
Congenital dislocation of the hip (CDH)

Club foot (talipes equinovarus)

Neurological conditions
Spina bifida
    Spina bifida occulta
    Spina bifida cystica (meningocele, meningomyelocele, Arnold–Chiari lesion)
Cerebral palsy

Scoliosis

Limp in childhood

From birth	CDH
	Infection of the hip
1–4 years	Infection of the hip
4–10 years	Perthes disease
10–15 years	Slipped upper femoral epiphysis

Table 22.7 Common causes of poor standing or walking in children.

Knee deformity
    Knock knees (genu valgum)
    Bow legs (genu varum)
Intoeing
    Femoral neck angle variation
    Tibial torsion
    Abnormal forefeet
Flat feet
Curly toes

about their own milestones, which is often reassuring as these tend to be strongly familial in pattern. Common minor problems associated with gait and stance are given in Table 22.7.

Knock knees (or genu valgum; Fig. 22.10a) and *bow legs* (or genu varum; Fig. 22.10b) are frequently seen. These conditions are rarely, if ever, serious. The normal alignment of the knee is in valgus and when a child stands to attention there is normally a gap of 4 cm or so between the feet. If the gap is diminished the knees are in varus and if is increased they are in valgus. If the children are followed until 7 years nearly all will have normal knee alignment.

Very rare serious causes of knee deformity are rickets, and epiphyseal growth disorders. The child should not require an X-ray initially to exclude these conditions but should be seen again on one or two occasions and only investigated further if the condition gets worse or does not correct with the passage of time.

Intoeing

This is a frequent cause of parental anxiety where a child stands pigeon-toed and this is often exaggerated when they run. The child is often referred with clumsiness but a careful enquiry suggests that the child is no more prone to falling than other children. Parents also often complain bitterly about shoe wear.

Femoral neck angle variation In the normal development of the fetus in its later stages, the leg rotates on the pelvis so that the acetabulum points almost backwards and the femoral head on the neck is oriented forwards. Sometimes the rotatory process is not completed by birth and so the femoral neck is more anteriorly orientated, i.e. it is anteverted. This means children born like this can internally rotate their femur a lot and externally rotate a little. This is reflected in their posture and they have an intoed gait. All will correct this delayed development by the time they are 10, although some are left with residual deformity. This is seldom, if ever, severe enough to warrant surgery.

Tibial torsion Tibial torsion is a normal variation of normal and should be ignored.

Abnormal forefeet Abnormal feet, particularly the hooked or adducted forefoot, are commonly seen. They are a variation on normal. It is dubious whether surgery is ever justified and certainly should not be considered before 7 years. The vast majority correct spontaneously by then and any residual hooking rarely causes functional difficulties. There is no evidence that special shoes make any difference.

Flat feet

Flat feet is an abnormality in the minds of the public of the western world. In some races a flat foot is normal and indeed universally a flat foot is a normal variation which very rarely causes functional abnormalities apart from

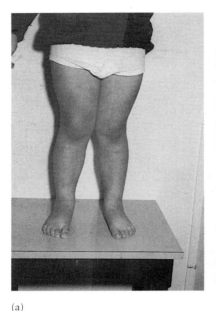

(a)

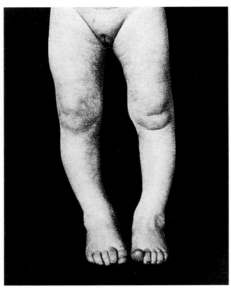

(b)

Figure 22.10 (a) Knock knees and (b) bow legs.

uneven shoe wear. There are two kinds of flat foot — rigid and mobile. The vast majority are *mobile* and entirely innocuous. All children's feet are flat at birth and indeed the normal arch may not form until the child is 7. In the infant the flatness of the medial arch is often exaggerated by a fat pad in the vicinity which is normal. The essence of any child's deformity is that if it may be corrected passively it will correct spontaneously.

Reassurance is required and all pressure to intervene should be resisted. Referral to hospital for mobile flat foot is not really required.

A *rigid* flat foot is rare in any age. It may be due to a tarsal coalition which can be bony or fibrous. Even a tarsal coalition rarely needs surgery unless the foot remains stiff and painful.

A note on shoes Children should be kept out of shoes until walking is established. Then they require well-fitting shoes which leave room for growth. They also need well-fitting socks which do not constrict the foot. There are no other rules and certainly young and healthy feet need no extra support from shoes or manufacturers. If the feet are more valgus than normal, then a heel seat may prevent excessive wear on the sole, but you must be clear you are treating the shoes and the parents' purse, not the child's foot.

Curly toes

Minor overlapping, excess webbing or hooking, particularly of the fifth toe, are common. Most correct passively and should be left. Occasionally the fixed and hooked fifth toe causes discomfort in shoes. If fixed it requires surgical correction. Surgery on other curly toes should be discouraged despite often heavy parental pressure.

Pain around the knee

A very common cause of children's referral is pain around the knee. This is seen in both sexes from about 10–12 years and then far more commonly in older girls as they develop secondary sexual characteristics.

Osgood–Schlatter disease

Osgood–Schlatter disease is a traction epiphysitis of the patellar tendon insertion in the tibia. It accounts for the younger age of referral in both sexes. The cause is unknown but it is commoner in very active children, often associated with organized sport, and so may be an overuse injury. The condition causes localized tenderness and discomfort, worse after exercise. It may be associated with a swelling and radiographs are characteristic.

The condition is episodic and usually can be treated by rest. Rarely it is necessary to enforce rest with a plaster cast and occasionally in late adolescence sequestrated calcific bumps may be so uncomfortable as to require excision. Most important is to explain that the condition will settle with rest and the child will cease to have symptoms in middle adolescence when the epiphysis fuses.

Adolescent knee pain and chondromalacia

Adolescent knee pain is seen mostly in girls and is of unknown cause. It is not the same as dislocation of the patella. Rarely on arthroscopy an area of patellar cartilage is seen to be eroded — chondromalacia patellae. Most, but not all, girls grow out of the condition and a watching brief should be kept. Only if symptoms persist should arthroscopy be offered. Speculative surgery is to be avoided and often is psychologically harmful, reinforcing the condition and leaving scars which are often resented later.

Major conditions

Congenital dislocation of the hip (CDH)

Introduction

CDH occurs in 1 or 2 live births per 1000. It is a badly namely condition because the hip is rarely completely dislocated at birth, but it is abnormal and is likely to become troublesome if ignored. A better name would be congenital hip dysplasia, reflecting the underlying abnormality of the femoral head, the acetabulum or both (Fig. 22.11). The condition is more frequent in girls than boys, there are familial and racial tendencies and a significant number are bilateral.

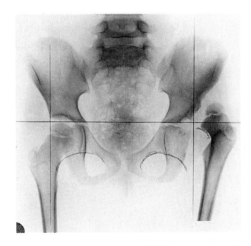

Figure 22.11 Congenital dislocation of the hip (CDH) can be diagnosed radiologically by drawing Perkins' lines on the radiograph. The normally sited head of the femur lies below a line drawn horizontally through the triradiate cartilages and medial to a vertical line drawn from the outer edge of the acetabulum. In the illustration the right femoral head is normal but the left is congenitally dislocated.

Clinical presentation

All children should be screened for CDH at birth and rechecked at 3, 6 months and a year. At birth it is diagnosed using a technique either to try and dislocate the hip or relocate it if dislocated. The test often produces a slight click or, more seriously, a 'clunk' as the hip dislocates or relocates. Occasionally the test will fail to detect a dislocation if the hip cannot be reduced. The hip is often stiff and abduction is limited. Occasionally CDH goes unrecognized at birth and then it presents either late, either before weight-bearing, i.e. sitting, or after weight-bearing, i.e. standing or even when walking has been established. In the later cases clinical signs include shortening, asymmetrical skin creases, limited abduction and later a limp.

Management

All infants with hips that click should be re-examined in a specialist clinic at 3 months and a radiograph is usually then justified. All 'clunks' should be treated from birth. If the head is reduced and maintained in the acetabulum then the vast majority will then settle and give no further trouble as the hip starts to develop normally.

The position of reduction at birth is in abduction at 45°, flexion at 90° and slight internal rotation. This is held using a metal splint or harness. A radiograph in the splint is essential to ensure that the hip is being held in reduction. If there is any doubt, an arthrogram should be taken in the operating theatre. Reduction may be prevented by an infolding of the capsule into the joint — the limbus — or by a tight psoas tendon.

If discovered late but before weight-bearing, the hip may be reduced by a period of gentle traction followed by open or closed manipulation. It is then splinted in plaster for 3 months. If discovered late and walking has commenced, then major surgery is required to deepen the developed acetabulum and re-angulate the femoral neck to stabilize the hip. The results of this are at best moderate and secondary arthritis is highly likely. This is why early diagnosis is so important.

Club foot (talipes equinovarus)

Introduction

Talipes equinovarus is a deformity of the foot which makes it look like a golf club. It is important to recognize because, if treated early, mild cases can be fully corrected and major cases much improved to give an acceptably functioning foot (Fig. 22.12)

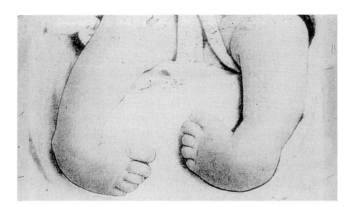

Figure 22.12 Bilateral talipes equinovarus or club feet.

Aetiology

The condition is common and is seen in a mild, postural form and a fixed form. The milder forms are often seen after breech presentation and are probably related to intrauterine posture and the severe forms are associated with development abnormalities of nerves and muscles of the leg and back.

Management

The mild form is usually easily corrected at birth. The severe forms can also be corrected at birth, but with great difficulty; there are usually fixed skin creases, and the whole leg seems smaller then the unaffected side. In both cases the condition can be bilateral. Initial treatment is gentle stretching which should consist of two phases. First, correct the hindfoot equinus and second, correct the mid and forefoot varus. In the mild cases 6 weeks of stretching and strapping in a corrected or overcorrected position is all that is required. In severe cases after 6 weeks the deformity should be reassessed and if correction is incomplete or cannot be maintained, then surgery is necessary. The children all need follow-up and special firm shoes until the feet stop growing at age 14 as late relapse requiring further surgery is possible. The affected foot is often always significantly smaller than the normal one, which can give difficulties in shoe fitting.

Neurological conditions

Conditions affecting the neurological structures at birth lead to abnormalities of the muscular and skeletal system with growth and development.

Spina bifida and meningomyelocele

Abnormal developments of the neural plate during the first 3 months may result in failure of closure of the spinal cord and vertebrae.

Spina bifida occulta This is a minor bony abnormality with failure of formation of vertebral spines which affects 2% of the population. This is usually of no significance, although some go on to get mechanical backache and a very small number may get spinal cord tethering during growth — diastematomyelia.

Spina bifida cystica A small and decreasing number of babies are born with the neural plate tissues open and little or no skin or bony cover. This is spina bifida cystica. The condition can be recognized during prenatal routine blood screening for α-fetoprotein. The nerve tissue may be covered by a cyst (*meningocele*; Fig. 22.13) or the nerve tissue may be incorporated in the cyst wall (a meningomyelocele). Many children also have a malformation of the brain, leading to hydrocephalus (the *Arnold–Chiari lesion*).

Many children die at or soon after birth. Some survive and have surgery to close the lesion on their back. Many of these children have formidable problems, including paralysis which may be flaccid or spastic, flexion contractures of their knees and dislocation of the hips, secondary growth deformities through muscle imbalance and incontinence. Many, but by no means all, are mentally retarded. All this is a major burden for the child and the family who need support from a team consisting of surgeons, therapists and social workers. Many children with spina bifida need early surgery to their feet to maintain a reasonable shape.

Every effort should be made to keep the child mobile until adolescence so that they grow to a reasonable size.

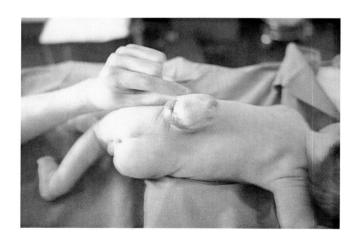

Figure 22.13 Spina bifida and meningocele.

Many children manage to walk aided by splints and hand-held aids until then. As they reach adolescence many go into a wheelchair as they find this socially and cosmetically easier for themselves. The care of such children and adults is a specialized area with an ability to work with other team members who often have much more to contribute than the doctor. All must support the family as a whole.

Cerebral palsy

Cerebral palsy consists of a birth abnormality of the brain which results in delayed or arrested neuromuscular development. The spinal tissue develops normally and so such children have uninhibited spinal reflexes but lack higher-centre control and purpose. This results in a spastic type of paralysis. Some muscles are very spastic, whilst others are very weak and flaccid and this imbalance leads to abnormal muscle and bone growth with secondary deformities of joints. Some patterns are common, such as one arm and ipsilateral leg (hemiparesis). Two legs are often affected (paraparesis) and not uncommonly all limbs are affected (quadriparesis). Most, but not all, spastic children are mentally retarded and often are blind and/or deaf as well. Occasionally children are spared mental and sensory impairment and such tragic cases are often unrecognized, to the utter frustration of the individual.

It is important to recognize that some people have very minor degrees of spasticity which may only affect one muscle group. These people commonly present with toe walking in adolescence. Examination reveals calf muscle spasticity and some may need tendo Achilles lengthening before growth ceases. Orthopaedic problems with growth are similar to those found in spina bifida but often much more severe. Deformities can be minimized by careful physiotherapy. Splintage should be used with caution as overzealous splintage can lead to increased spasm and ultimately deformity. Careful use of surgery to lengthen tight muscles, denervate them or occasionally to move them may maintain acceptable posture and help maintain some function. There is a need to recognize the importance of being part of a much wider supportive team who will provide regular day-to-day contact.

Scoliosis

Curvature of the spine with a rotatory abnormality of the vertebrae is known as scoliosis. It is a three-dimensional deformity based on an abnormal lordosis of the spine which leads to buckling and twisting of the vertebral column through muscle action and gravity (Fig. 22.14).

Aetiology

Scoliosis may be caused by congenital abnormalities of the vertebrae or neuromuscular imbalance but most cases have no known cause. Idiopathic scoliosis occurs in adolescence,

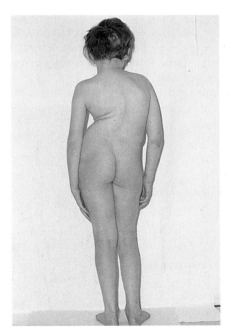 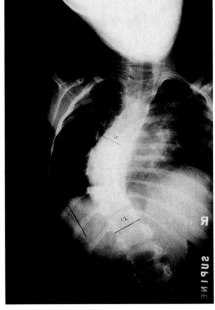

Figure 22.14 (a) Clinical and (b) radiographic appearances of severe scoliosis.

(a)　　　　(b)

although it may occur in infants and, rarely, in adults. It is far commoner in girls than boys. Its principal effects are cosmetic, which is not to be underrated as a cause of distress. It rarely causes physiological disturbances in the common idiopathic group.

Clinical presentation

The child usually presents because of twisting of the ribs which causes a hump at the shoulder on one side. Girls also complain that their skirts hang crookedly. It may be painful but this is usually secondary to the anxiety and distress of what is commonly known as a sinister condition.

Management

Treatment is dictated by cosmetic problems. Not all curves progress and this should be emphasized to parents. If the curve is progressive or is causing distress, treatment should be offered early. Braces have no benefit and should not be used as they add to the stigma of the disease. If treatment is demanded due to distress or progress, then surgical correction is essential. The rotatory element of the deformity must be corrected as otherwise the hump remains, which is what distresses the patient. This is very complex surgery which is only carried out in a handful of regional spinal centres. All children with scoliosis should be referred for a specialist opinion if treatment is demanded or the curve is progressive. The earlier the referral the better.

Limp in childhood

A limp at any age must be taken seriously. Quite often the cause will be obscure and the condition will settle. However, when there is a serious cause it demands treatment and so the conditions listed in Table 22.8, which occur within characteristic age bands, must be excluded.

Table 22.8 Serious causes of limp in childhood.

Age	Cause
From birth	Congenital dislocation of the hip Infection of the hip
In infancy	Infection of the hip
4–10 years	Perthes disease
10–15 years	Slipped upper femoral epiphysis

Perthes disease

This is an osteochondritis of the femoral head epiphysis. It is commoner in boys than girls and in 20% is bilateral. The cause is unknown but it has an incidence of up to 5 per 1000 children.

Clinical presentation

The natural history is for the child to present with a painful limp which is followed by a slow recovery. Radiologically the femoral head may be normal on first presentation but it later fragments to a greater or lesser degree. The condition is felt to have a vascular component and the condition is an avascular necrosis of the growing femoral head (Fig. 22.15). Nevertheless, the cause is obscure. Eventually the head will revascularize and reossify but the head may be enlarged and deformed.

Diagnosis is made from a high index of suspicion. Radiographs repeated at a month may show previously unrecorded changes. Ultrasound reveals fluid in the hip joint and a bone scan is positive.

Management

The strategy of treatment is to maintain the head concentrically within the acetabulum until the natural process of the disease run its course. Minor degrees (up to half of the head involvement) need no treatment as the prognosis in such children is good. In older children with full head involvement the prognosis is less good, although the child will return to normal in the short term, but will be prone to secondary osteoarthritis in early middle age. In these severe cases splintage to achieve containment may help and some

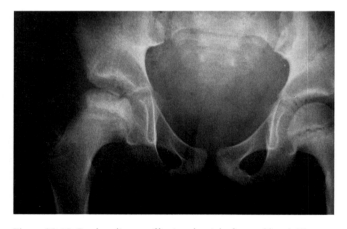

Figure 22.15 Perthes disease affecting the right femoral head. Note the increase in the joint space on the affected side.

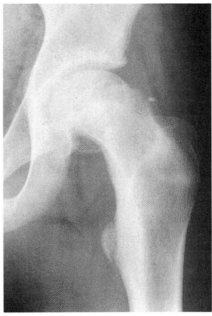 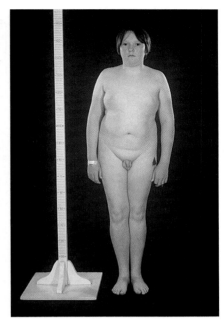

Figure 22.16 (a) Radiological and (b) clinical appearances in a patient with a left slipped upper femoral epiphysis.

(a)   (b)

believe that osteotomy either to enlarge the acetabulum or to redirect the femoral head helps. All these treatments are of dubious value and careful follow-up with periods on traction to alleviate symptoms is probably all we can do to help these patients.

Slipped upper femoral epiphysis (SUFE)

This is a condition seen in boys in their early teens who are sexually immature for their age (Fig. 22.16) and in girls who are a little older and who have recently undergone an adolescent growth spurt. It consists of a slippage of the capital femoral epiphysis on the neck. The neck comes to lie anteriorly and the head is tilted off behind. The cause is unclear but affected children appear to have an abnormal hormonal balance which must be associated in some way.

Clinical presentation

The child presents with a limp which may not be particularly uncomfortable or may include pain which sometimes radiates to the knee in the sensory distribution of the obturator nerve. Any child with knee pain must have the hip examined. The slip may occur acutely or it may be preceded by many months of discomfort without clinical or radiological signs. All young adolescents with a painful hip must be regarded as having this condition until it is clinically and radiologically excluded. On examination there is limitation of abduction in flexion with loss of internal rotation because of the distorted femoral head on the neck. A radiograph must include a lateral view or minor degrees of slippage may be missed.

Management

Treatment is surgical. If the slippage is minor or moderate, the hip should be pinned in its new deformed position. If the slippage is major a gentle reduction may be attempted, although the risk of avascular necrosis is high. The other side should be watched radiologically and pinned if any suspicion of slippage arises. The pins are best removed at fusion of the epiphysis around the age of 18 years.

You can put anything you like on a pressure sore as long as it's not the patient. (David Bouchier Hayes)

Introduction

The skin is the largest organ in (or on!) the body and a major part of plastic surgery is the adjustment and movement of tissues, mainly skin, within local areas and between distant sites. The word plastic comes from the Greek word πλαστιχοσ, meaning to mould or form, and has been in use in English since the 16th century. The scope of modern plastic surgery is outlined in Table 23.1.

Fundamental techniques in plastic surgery

The fundamental techniques of plastic surgery include simple wound closure, partial and full-thickness skin grafting and flap reconstruction ranging from simple local flaps to complex free-tissue transfers.

Wound closure

• *Primary wound closure* means that a wound is approximated by sutures or staples which are retained until the wound has healed. This technique is used to close surgical incisions and clean wounds caused by trauma. In certain circumstances it may be appropriate to close a wound primarily where there has been loss of tissue (e.g. wide excision of a skin tumour) with either a skin graft or a flap repair.

• *Delayed primary closure* is always used for contaminated wounds and often following debridement of devitalized

Table 23.1 The scope of plastic and reconstructive surgery.

Congenital conditions	Acquired conditions
Head and neck	*Trauma*
Cleft lip and palate	Faciomaxillary
Prominent ears	Hands
Accessory auricles	Soft tissues (tendons, nerves,
Dermoid cysts	muscles)
	lower limb
Congenital ptosis	
Branchial cyst and sinus	*Reconstructive surgery*
Thyroglossal cyst	Breast
	Chest wall
Vascular malformations	*Aesthetic surgery*
Strawberry naevus	Facial rejuvenation
Capillary haemangioma	Breast augmentation and
(portwine stain)	reduction
Cavernous haemangioma	Liposculpture
Lymphangioma	Abdominoplasty
Pigmented naevi	*Neoplasia*
Abnormalities of	Skin cancer
the genitourinary system	Basal cell carcinoma
Hypospadias	Squamous cell carcinoma
Epispadias	Malignant melanoma
	Head and neck cancers
Congenital hand deformities	
Polydactyly	*Miscellaneous*
Syndactyly	Pressure sores
	Facial palsy

tissues. The wound is left open and packed with a suitable dressing such as Jelonet or proflavine-soaked gauze. Wound

485

closure is undertaken 2–3 days later with sutures or staples providing the wound is clean.

Grafts and flaps

Tissue transfer can be achieved in two ways:
• as a *graft* — a term signifying total detachment of the grafted tissue from the body at some stage of its transfer;
• as a *flap* — the tissue is attached at all times to the body. The attachment of the flap to the body supplies the blood to the flap and is called the *pedicle*.

Grafts consist of pieces of tissue which are sufficiently small (in volume terms) for cell viability to be sustained by diffusion alone until such time as vascular link-up can occur to perfuse the tissue (about 5 days). Various forms of tissue may be grafted (skin, muscle, bone, nerve) but the majority are skin grafts — either *split-skin grafts* or *full-thickness skin grafts* (Fig. 23.1). Another type of graft is the microvascular graft (also called a *free flap*) where a large volume of tissue is totally detached and then reattached at another site, with microsurgical techniques being used to reconnect the arteries and veins to vessels in the recipient site.

Skin grafting

Split-skin grafting

A partial-thickness or Tiersch graft is taken with a hand-held graft knife (Humby knife) (Fig. 23.2) or mechanical dermatome, usually from the arm or thigh. The skin is shaved off by setting the knife blade to an appropriate thickness so that only part of the dermis is removed. Only those tissues that produce granulations will take a split-skin graft. Thus *inappropriate* sites for skin grafting include cortical bone, cartilage, bare tendons and cavities.

The skin graft may be applied as a sheet or as a meshed graft (Fig. 23.3). The latter enables the graft to be expanded

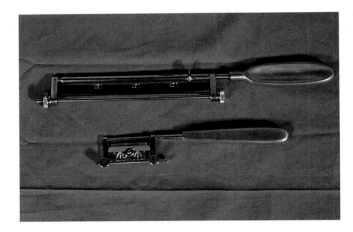

Figure 23.2 Hand-held skin graft knives.

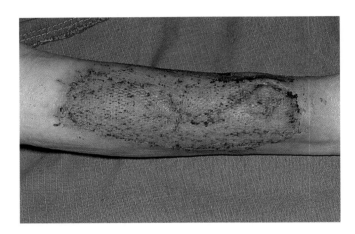

Figure 23.3 Meshed split-skin graft.

after it has been put through a mesher (Fig. 23.4). Meshed grafts are used in the following circumstances:

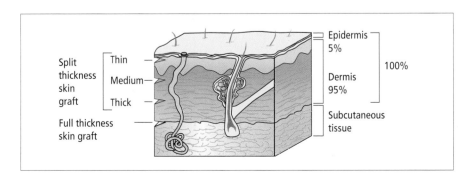

Figure 23.1 Thickness of skin grafts relative to thickness of skin.

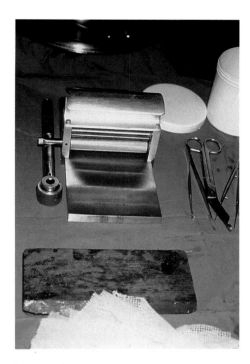

Figure 23.4 Skin graft mesher.

Some characteristics of split skin grafts

• Split skin grafts are **hairless and dry** because the sweat glands and hair follicles which lie in the deepest part of the skin are not taken with a split skin graft

• **Primary contraction** of the graft occurs due to the elasticity of the skin and subcutaneous tissues. Once a graft has been taken from the donor site it will immediately contract. This contraction has to be taken into account in measuring a graft for a particular defect

• **Secondary graft contracture** occurs over a period of months or years and is inversely proportional to the thickness of the graft, i.e. thin grafts tend to contract more than thick grafts

• Skin from different parts of the body have **different colours**. For the best cosmetic results the donor skin should match the colour of the recipient area. For example, skin taken from the abdomen or leg applied to the face has an unattractive yellowish hue. On the other hand, graft taken from the upper inner thigh which is pigmented may be adequately used for reconstruction of the areola of the nipple in breast reconstruction

Box 23.1

• for expansion, e.g. in a burn where there may be limited donor skin available;
• on relatively dirty wounds, e.g. a leg ulcer; and
• on muscle, which tends to produce a quantity of serous fluid causing grafts to float free.

Graft take depends upon the following factors:
• close approximation of the graft to the bed;
• immobility;
• capillary ingrowth; and
• absence of specific infections.

Close approximation (which prevents haematoma or seroma formation beneath the graft) and immobility are achieved by application of appropriate dressings. Once a graft has been applied to an appropriate bed, diffusion of plasma sustains it until blood flow is established by ingrowth of capillaries into the graft at about 5 days. Dressings should be left in place for 5 days when they should be carefully removed by the surgeon who performed the grafting. β-Haemolytic streptococci dissolve skin grafts while *Pseudomonas pyocyaneus* produces so much pus that the graft floats off its bed. Some of the characteristics of a split-skin graft are given in Box 23.1.

Full-thickness skin grafts (Wolfe grafts; Fig. 23.5)

Full-thickness grafts are often used in facial reconstruction, syndactyly, hypospadias repair and nipple reconstruction.

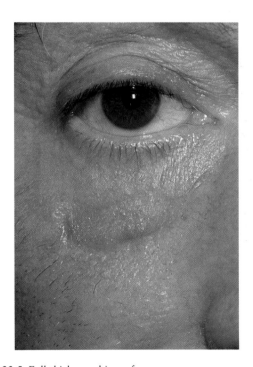

Figure 23.5 Full-thickness skin graft.

The advantages of full-thickness grafts over split-skin grafts are:
• A full-thickness graft is less likely to contract than a split-skin graft and this may be useful in conditions such as syndactyly release, repair of eyelids and correction of scar contracture.

• Because a full-thickness graft may be taken close to the recipient site (for example, from the nasolabial fold for application to the nose) the colour match is likely to be better than a split-skin graft.
• In certain circumstances full-thickness hair-bearing grafts may be used as, for example, in eyebrow reconstruction.

The disadvantages are:
• Because the full thickness of the skin is removed in a Wolfe graft, the donor defect has to be closed primarily (i.e. with sutures or staples). Thus the sites from which Wolfe grafts may be taken (e.g. nasolabial fold, upper eyelid, postauricular, supraclavicular, groin) are rather limited.
• Because a Wolfe graft is thicker than a split-skin graft, it takes longer for the graft to take and a pressure-type dressing is always required.

Skin flaps

The blood supply of the skin

Three types of artery supply blood to the skin:
• Direct cutaneous arteries and veins emerge from deeper vessels and run in a horizontal linear fashion for some distance in the subcutis. Many of these emerge in the axillae and groins (e.g. superficial thoracic artery, superficial inferior epigastric artery), but also at other sites, such as on the anterior chest wall (Fig. 23.6a).
• Musculocutaneous perforating arteries emerge from the surfaces of muscles to supply the integument. Generally these muscles are broad flat ones which largely exist on the trunk (Fig. 23.6b).
• Fasciocutaneous perforating arteries pass along an intermuscular or intercompartmental fascial septum to reach and supply the deep fascia. Generally these vessels are found on the limbs (Fig. 23.6c).

Irrespective of how it gets there, each vessel ascending through the subcutis feeds into the subdermal plexus over a certain area whose boundaries are not absolutely fixed. This area is known as the *territory* of that vessel.

Types of skin flap (Table 23.2)

Random pattern flap This was the only type of flap available until the 1970s. Because the blood supply to these flaps is haphazard, it is not possible to raise them as large flaps. In general the length of the flap should not exceed the width of the base (Fig. 23.7). However, they are still used to cover defects around the head and neck. Random pattern skin flaps may be categorized as advancement, rotation, transposition and island flaps. A z-plasty is an example of a transposition flap (Fig. 23.8).

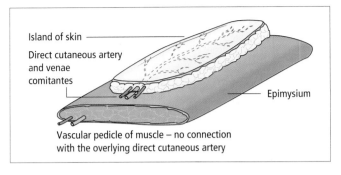

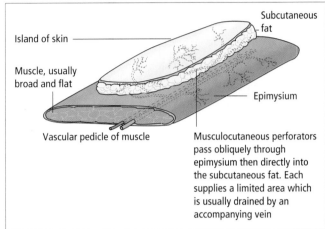

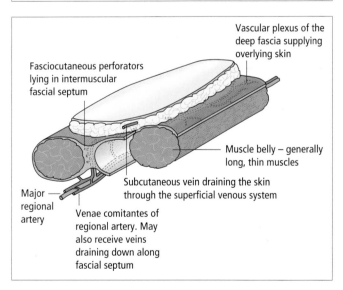

Figure 23.6 (a) Schematic representation of the principles of the blood supply to skin from direct cutaneous arteries. (b) Schematic representation of the principles of the blood supply to skin from musculocutaneous perforators. (c) Schematic representation of the principles of the blood supply to skin from perforators of the fasciocutaneous system.

Table 23.2 Types of flap.

Type of flap	Blood supply	Example
Random pattern flap	Dermal and subdermal plexus	Rotation flap on face
Axial pattern flap	Direct cutaneous vessels	Deltopectoral flap
Musculocutaneous flap	Musculocutaneous perforating vessels	Latissimus dorsi flap
Fasciocutaneous flap	Fasciocutaneous perforating vessels	Radial forearm flap

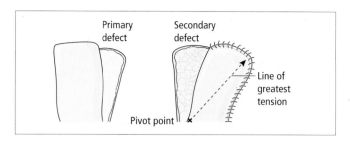

Figure 23.7 Schematic representation of a transposition flap. The secondary defect is often closed with a split-skin graft.

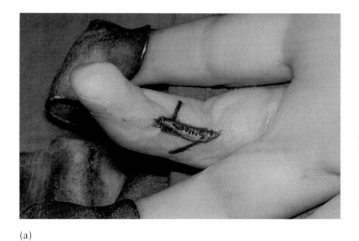

(a)

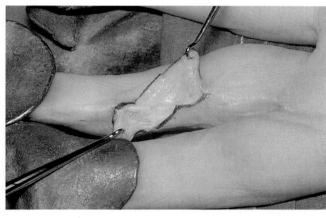

(b)

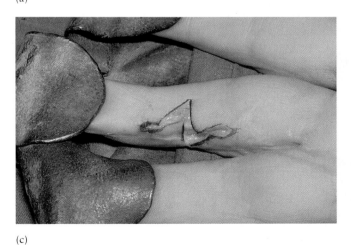

(c)

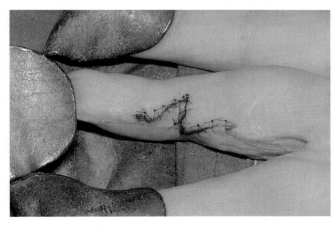

(d)

Figure 23.8 (a) There is scar contracture of the ring finger limiting extension at the interphalangeal joints. The planned z-plasty is drawn on the skin of the finger with the central limb incorporating a slender ellipse to allow excision of the scar. (b) The longitudinal scar has been excised; the z-plasty flaps are shown elevated prior to transposition. (c) After release of the scar, note that the finger will now extend a good deal further. In a well-planned z-plasty the flaps tend to transpose naturally into the final position, as shown here. (d) The flaps have been sutured into position. In effect, scar length in the finger has been increased by bringing in skin from the sides, accounting for the slight wasting of the finger at the level of the z-plasty.

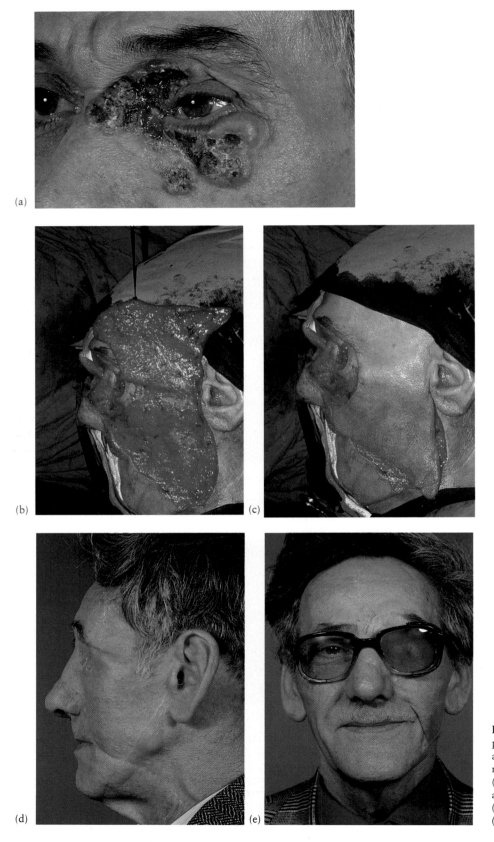

Figure 23.9 (a) A neglected case of periorbital basal cell carcinoma presenting at a late stage. (b) Excision of the tumour necessitated exenteration of the orbit. (c) A cervicofacial flap has been dissected and will be used to reconstruct the defect. (d) Postoperative result, lateral view. (e) Final result with patient wearing glasses.

Axial pattern flap In the early 1970s it was discovered that certain areas of the body already had axially oriented arteries and veins within them. Thus, a large skin flap based on these vessels can be raised, giving an immediate long length-to-breadth ratio (Fig. 23.9). Examples of this type of flap include the groin flap, forehead flap and deltopectoral flap. The axial pattern flaps later led to the concept of free tissue transfer since it was realized that the arteries and veins could be divided and rejoined at a recipient site, thereby transferring the whole flap from one site to another. However, because of the relative difficulty in raising these flaps, they are not often used now for free tissue transfers. They have been superseded by newer flaps such as muscle and fasciocutaneous flaps.

Musculocutaneous flaps These flaps involve the transfer of muscle, subcutaneous tissue and skin. The blood supply is reliable and comes via the muscle. The advent of the muscle and musculocutaneous flap system enabled plastic surgeons greatly to expand their reconstructive capabilities. For example, the gastrocnemius muscle or musculocutaneous flaps could be used to cover compound fractures of the lower limb, thereby saving many limbs that might otherwise have been amputated. These flaps can also be used for breast, head and neck or trunk reconstructions. Skin cover is achieved by split-skin grafts when the muscle alone is used, while compound musculocutaneous flaps are raised with a paddle of skin over them (Fig. 23.10).

Fasciocutaneous flaps Fasciocutaneous flaps consist of skin and subcutaneous fascia supplied by perforating arteries and veins in vascular territories. Because the pedicle of the flap is essentially a small artery, the flaps can be designed with either proximal or distally based pedicles (Figs 23.11 and 23.12).

Free flaps The term *free flap* is applied to any flap (axial, muscle, musculocutaneous or fasciocutaneous) in which the vascular pedicle is divided and transferred to another site where the arteries and veins are anastomosed to appropriate recipient vessels.

Expanded skin flaps Tissue expanders have become popular in plastic surgery to provide 'extra' skin for a local flap. An inflatable balloon is placed under the skin and when the wound is healed the balloon is inflated. Over a period of time a considerable amount of skin can be stretched over the balloon, thus providing more tissue locally to repair a defect (Fig. 23.13).

Surgery for congenital deformities

Congenital head and neck problems

Cleft lip and palate

Cleft lip and palate is one of the commonest congenital abnormalities, occurring in about 1 in 700 live births. The aetiology is unknown but there is a definite family inheritance (about 5% overall) and exposure to certain environmental factors during pregnancy (e.g. rubella, toxoplasmosis, steroids) may also predispose to it. Cleft lip and palate may occur separately or together and may be uni- or bilateral.

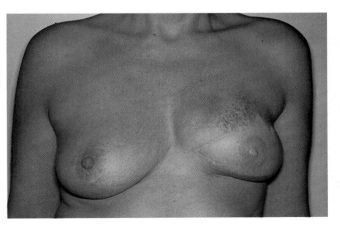

(a)

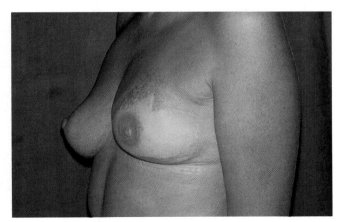

(b)

Figure 23.10 This woman has had a partial mastectomy and radiotherapy for breast cancer. Reconstruction was achieved using a pedicled latissimus dorsi myocutaneous flap. (a) Frontal view; (b) left oblique view.

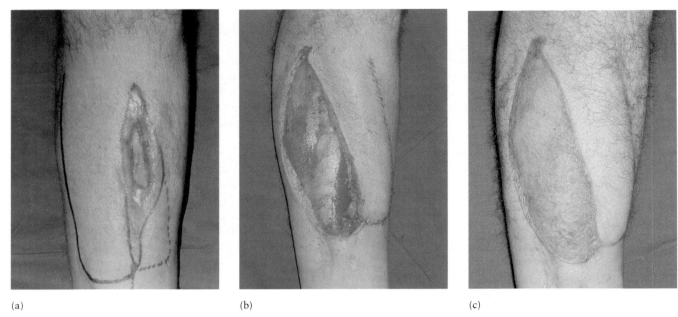

(a)   (b)   (c)

Figure 23.11 (a) Lower limb trauma has resulted in an exposed tibia. A simple proximally based fasciocutaneous flap has been outlined. (b) After wound debridement the flap has been raised, transposed and inset. (c) Final result after the donor area has been covered with a split-skin graft.

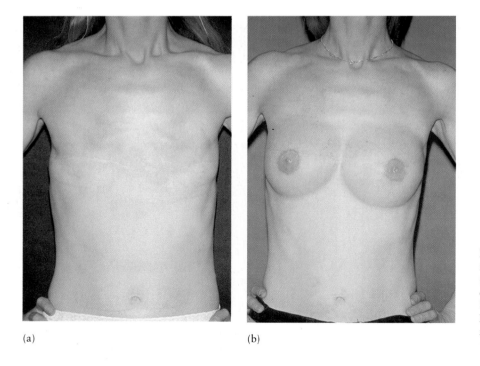

(a)   (b)

Figure 23.13 (a) This woman had bilateral mastectomies for carcinoma.
(b) Reconstruction has involved tissue expansion of the skin envelope followed by bilateral insertion of silicone breast implants. In this patient the nipples have also been reconstructed using full-thickness skin grafts.

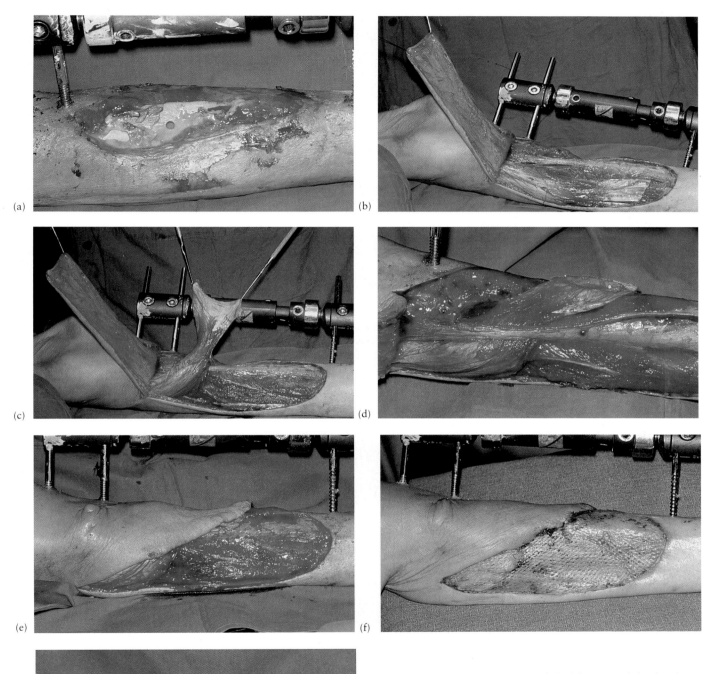

Figure 23.12 (a) Infected compound tibial fracture stabilized with external fixation. There is a large area of tissue loss with exposed bare bone. (b) After debridement of the wound, a fasciocutaneous flap has been raised. (c) In this patient a medial gastrocnemius muscle flap has also been raised to provide muscle cover of the exposed bone. (d) The gastrocnemius flap has been transposed to cover the fracture site. (e) The fasciocutaneous flap has now been transposed and the remaining area will be covered with a meshed split-skin graft (f). (g) Excellent late result. The fracture has united, allowing removal of the external fixator. Note that the split-skin graft has also matured, resulting in an improved aesthetic appearance.

- Cleft lip and palate: 50% (Fig. 23.14a);
- Cleft lip alone: 25% (Fig. 23.14b);
- Cleft palate alone: 25%.

Submucous clefts also occur, in which the mucosa across the soft palate is intact but there is a failure of muscle union. Clefts start at the lip or the uvula and extend towards a point just behind the alveolus. The degree of deformity depends on the extent of the failure of fusion of the mesenchymal processes that make up the nose, lip and palate.

Management

Several problems have to be dealt with when managing a severe cleft lip/palate.

- *Feeding* is difficult and the baby will have difficulty sucking if there is a large defect.

- *Surgical repair* is carried out in stages. Timing varies greatly between surgeons but the trend now is towards early (neonatal) repair of lip and repair of the palate at 6 months.
- Most patients require *orthodontic treatment* throughout the growth period with greater emphasis in the early phase of permanent dentition. Bone grafting to the alveolar defect generally at around the age of 10–12 will allow the teeth to be migrated into normal position in the line of the cleft.
- *Rhinoplasty and submucous resection* to correct the deformity of the nasal bone and septum may be necessary when growth is complete at around the age of 18 years.
- Shortness of the palate, either alone or combined with an inadequate nasopharyngeal sphincter, is evidenced by characteristic cleft palate speech in which there is nasal escape of air. *Speech therapy* is important from the outset and approximately 80% of children can be expected to speak normally.

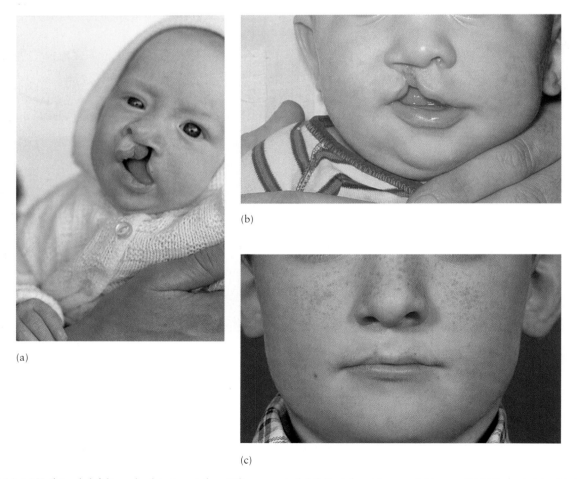

(a)

(b)

(c)

Figure 23.14 (a) Unilateral cleft lip and palate in an infant. Fifty per cent of cleft lip deformities are of this type. (b) Unilateral right-sided incomplete cleft lip. (c) Several operations later, the appearance of the repaired lip is satisfactory.

• *Counselling of parents* is essential in the early stages of treatment so that they are fully appraised of what lies ahead for them and the child and of the generally favourable result that can be achieved with surgical repair (Fig. 23.14c).

Miscellaneous congenital head and neck disorders

• *Prominent (bat) ears*: This is a relatively common problem in which the ear stands away from the side of the head, producing the typical jug-handle appearance (Fig. 23.15). Treat-

ment is by reshaping the cartilaginous framework so that the ear is brought nearer to the side of the head.

• *Accessory auricles* represent ectopic ear tissue which has not become incorporated into the pinna during development (Fig. 23.16). They are treated by excision. It is important to make sure that the cartilaginous element is removed.

• *A dermoid cyst* or *external angular dermoid* occurs most frequently at the outer end of the eyebrow but may also be seen close to the root of the nose (Fig. 23.17). They arise

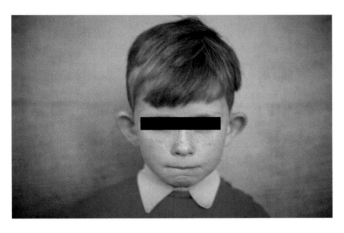

Figure 23.15 A young boy with prominent (bat) ears.

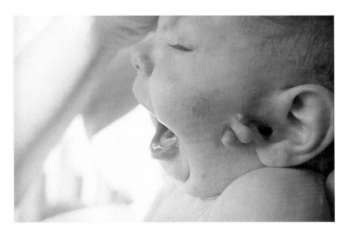

Figure 23.16 An infant with accessory auricles. Note the ectopic ear tissue anterior to the external auditory meatus.

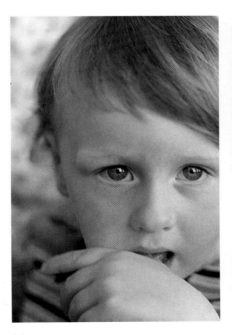

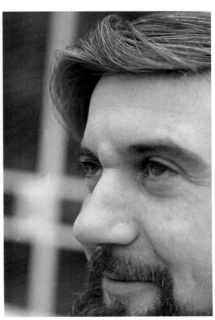

Figure 23.17 (a) External and (b) internal angular dermoids.

(a)

(b)

from developmental epithelial rests. Treatment is by complete excision of the epithelial-lined cyst.

• *Congenital ptosis* results from deficient formation of the levator oculi muscle. There is an obvious droop of the upper lid and children will tilt the head backwards to be able to see. Treatment is by shortening the levator muscle sufficiently to bring the lid margin to the correct level.

• A *branchial cyst* or *fistula* results from persistence of the second branchial cleft, which results in a fistula if the track opens on to the skin and a cyst if it is covered by the skin. Typically a branchial cyst presents as a swelling under the angle of the jaw in front of the sternomastoid muscle. It has a characteristic soft feeling to it and it fluctuates. Although they are congenital lesions, they usually present in adolescence or early adult life. Treatment is by excision.

• *Facial clefts* result from failure of fusion of the mesodermal masses that merge to form the face. These deformities are extremely rare. An example of macrostomia is shown in Fig. 23.18, in which failure of fusion of the lateral facial cleft results in an abnormally large mouth.

Congenital upper limb deformities

Deformities of the upper limb occur approximately once in every 600 live births. Five per cent of these are inherited but the large majority are of undetermined aetiology. Drugs are

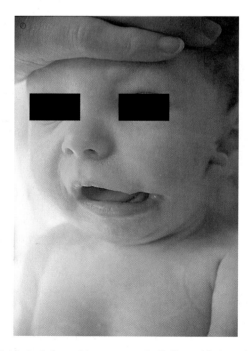

Figure 23.18 An infant with macrostomia. Failure of fusion of the lateral facial cleft on the left side has resulted in a lateral extension of the oral orifice.

a rare cause of congenital malformations but were highlighted by thalidomide which causes phocomelia (absence of all long bones) when taken by expectant mothers in the first trimester of pregnancy. Polydactyly and syndactyly are the commonest upper limb deformities.

Polydactyly

Polydactyly is the presence of an extra digit, which can range from a simple soft-tissue mass that does not attach to the skeleton, to a complete articulating digit. Polydactyly occurs most commonly in association with the small finger. The thumb is the next most frequently affected digit, with central polydactyly being very rare. Simple excision will adequately treat the non-articulating soft-tissue masses. In more complex polydactyly cases, associated hypoplasia leaves a smaller digit despite reconstructive efforts (Henry VIII's second wife, Anne Boleyn, had a rudimentary sixth finger on her left hand — a feature not lost on her enemies who said that it was a sure sign that she was a sorceress.)

Syndactyly

Syndactyly is a failure of the digits to separate during development, leaving a web between them. Males are affected twice as commonly as females, and in some cases inheritance is autosomal dominant with variable penetrance. The third web space (between the long and ring fingers) is most frequently affected, followed in decreasing incidence by the fourth, second and first web spaces. Syndactyly is incomplete when the web does not extend beyond the level of the distal interphalangeal joint (DIPJ) and in these cases only the soft tissues are affected. Complete syndactyly extends beyond the DIPJ and may involve the nail bed. Surgery should be performed early in cases affecting the first web space and also in complex cases where the bony fusions may cause further deformity by abnormal growth.

Treatment of upper limb deformities aims to maximize both function and cosmetic appearance without limiting growth. Predicting the functional deficit at birth can be difficult because children with major deformities can often develop clever alternative methods of manipulating objects. When possible, surgery is performed before the child is 12 months old and should be completed before the child goes to school in order to limit teasing by other children. Orthotic splints are occasionally required prior to surgery to lengthen tendons and improve the alignment of the limb. Prosthetic limbs may also be used alone or in combination with surgery. These range from simple static prostheses for cosmesis to advanced electromechanical devices.

Hand surgery

Introduction

Hand trauma is one of the most frequent reasons for attendance at casualty departments. It is also a major cause of lost working days because the specialized functions of the hand can be severely affected by even quite minor trauma. Despite the use of modern reconstructive techniques, a severe injury may lead to long-term unemployment or require the patient to seek retraining in less skilled work.

When managing hand trauma it is important at each stage to consider the five principal requirements for good function:

- a good blood supply;
- a stable skeleton;
- soft pliable skin cover (which does not restrict mobility);
- innervation (both motor and sensory); and
- motion (provided by smoothly gliding tendons).

Assessment of the injured hand

- The history should establish how the injury occurred, as this will help predict the structures that are likely to have been damaged. It is important to identify the patient's dominant hand, occupation and hobbies, and whether these involve precise hand movements. These factors, in conjunction with the patient's general health and personal circumstances, are important in deciding the appropriate treatment.
- Examination (Box 23.2) of an injured hand must be thorough yet avoid causing unnecessary discomfort to the patient.

The definitive examination is surgical exploration, which is necessary for any wound that is not clearly superficial, especially those involving penetrating glass. This should be performed in theatre where good anaesthesia, lighting and instruments are available.

Hand injuries

Principles of management

Incorrect early management of hand injuries leads to fixed contractures which may permanently limit function (Fig. 23.19). The inflammatory response to injury causes *oedema*, and due to the confined space this swelling may cause pain and splint the hand. A swollen hand will adopt a standard posture of flexion of the interphalangeal joints and extension of the metacarpophalangeal (MCP) joints. This occurs because the lateral skin of the digits is attached

Examination of the injured hand

Integrity of the blood supply
This can be assessed by three methods:
- Colour: Ischaemia will cause the affected area to appear pale and venous obstruction will produce a livid purplish hue. After a prolonged period of insufficiency the skin generally becomes mottled
- Capillary refill time: After a short period of firm compression of the skin or nail bed, the area will initially be pale and then steadily return to a normal colour. A slow return (you can use your own skin for comparison) indicates that the arterial flow is poor and a rapid return indicates that there is venous obstruction
- Pulp compression: Firm compression of the digital pulp for 20 seconds produces an indentation that re-expands over a few seconds. Failure of the pulp to re-expand indicates an inadequate arterial inflow

Skeletal stability
Good quality X-rays, both antero-posterior view and a true lateral are necessary to exclude a fracture or radio opaque foreign body

Skin cover
Actual skin loss will be obvious, but degloving injuries leave skin attached with an inadequate blood supply. This is most easily assessed in theatre when serial debridement is performed until dermal bleeding is seen. Intravenous fluorescein used in conjunction with a blue light is also valuable in identifying which areas are vascularized

Innervation
Denervation leads to immediate loss of sweating in the distribution of the affected nerve. A simple test that has been described is to run a plastic pen across the skin, where there is no sweating there will be reduced skin friction. This test has the benefit that it does not require patient co-operation and is particularly valuable for examination of the unconscious or in children. Sensory testing using light touch and pinprick are less reliable signs as these can be temporarily preserved if the divided nerve ends are in close approximation

Motion (tendon injury)
The digits at rest are normally aligned in an even cascade, from the index finger in least flexion to the small finger in most flexion. Complete division of both flexor tendons to a digit will lead to the classical pointing sign, the affected finger being extended. Any alteration in this cascade and therefore damage to the tendons is made more obvious by the tenodesis test – passive flexion of the wrist causes the digits and the thumb to extend at the MCP and IP joints and the opposite effect is achieved by passive extension of the wrist

Box 23.2

obliquely to the phalanges by Cleland's ligaments; as these tighten, the proximal interphalangeal joint flexes. As a result, the forces of the flexor and extensor tendons are balanced by extension of the MCP joint (tenodesis effect). In this position the collateral ligaments at the MCP joints are slack and will contract.

After an injury it is important to place the hand in *high elevation* and *commence mobilization at the earliest possible time*. When a period of immobilization is necessary, a splint should be used to hold the MCP joints in flexion of 90° and

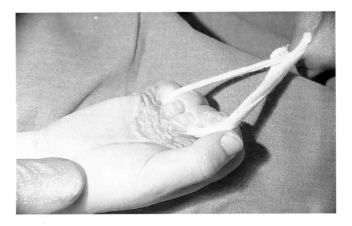

Figure 23.19 Fixed contractures of the fingers following a burn.

the interphalangeal joints in extension. This is commonly referred to as the position of function and should also include placing the thumb in abduction from the palm and extension at the MCP and interphalangeal joints.

Treatment of hand injuries (Fig. 23.20)

Integrity of blood supply

• Anastomosis of small blood vessels can be performed under the operating microscope and these techniques are used to reperfuse the hand. Replantation is technically possible for amputations ranging from distal fingertip amputation to amputation of the entire upper limb. However, each case must be assessed individually as there are many factors to consider in deciding if replantation is appropriate.

• Time delay until surgery must be minimized because prolonged ischaemia causes permanent tissue damage.

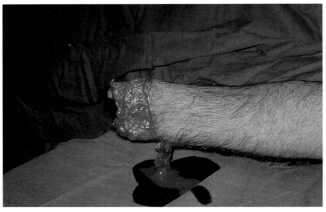

(a)

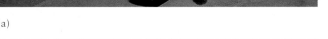

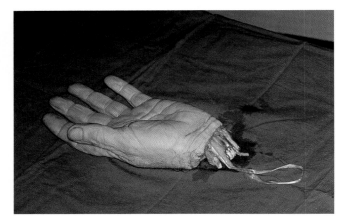

(b)

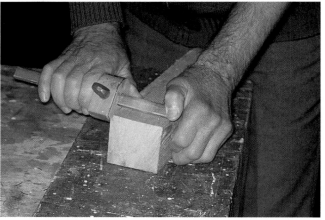

(c)

Figure 23.20 (a) Traumatic amputation of the right hand resulting from an industrial accident. In such cases it is important to ascertain whether there was a significant element of crushing or degloving in the injury, as this will affect the likelihood of successful replantation. (b) Ideally, two teams of surgeons prepare the arm and the severed hand simultaneously to reduce the ischaemia time. Bone fixation is always performed first to provide stability for the rest of the surgery. The tendons are repaired next before proceeding to microsurgical procedures — repair of the veins, arteries and nerves. (c) Twelve months later, after intensive occupational therapy and physiotherapy, there has been a gratifying return of function in the implanted hand.

However, the permissible ischaemia time is longer for parts which do not contain muscle and can be lengthened by cooling the amputated part. This should be done by wrapping the amputated part in a saline-soaked swab and then sealing it in a dry polythene bag. The ideal storage temperature is 4°C, and placing the amputated part *on* melting crushed ice is satisfactory. It should not be placed *in* ice as this will freeze the tissues and cause irreversible damage.

Skeletal stability (fractures)

Fractures can occur at multiple sites in all hand bones. Specific management of each is beyond the scope of this text. Determining the correct treatment requires experience and all hand fractures should be followed up at a hand or fracture clinic. Where possible, the aim is to mobilize the hand early and in stable fractures this may be possible immediately. Most unstable fractures can be treated by immobilizing the hand in the position of function for 3–4 weeks but this runs the risk of stiffness. Fractures or loose small fragments near the articular surfaces may represent avulsion of tendon or ligament insertions and these will often require surgery.

Skin cover (loss)

• Failure to provide adequate skin cover will impair the result of any reconstruction. In the initial period, good-quality skin cover will promote primary healing. This reduces stiffness by limiting the formation of granulation tissue, preventing infection and preserving the viability of exposed deep structures. In the long term, good-quality skin cover in the hand has to be durable, provide the best possible sensation (particularly to key points), allow unrestricted movement and allow late reconstruction of deep tissues, if this is necessary.

• Replacement of skin may need to cover large areas or simply provide additional tissue where linear shortage or scar contracture limits mobility. Split-skin grafts are valuable in the initial management of hand trauma because they are simple and reliable, but long-term they may not be sufficiently durable, can contract and often provide a poor cosmetic result. As it is often necessary to provide supple tissue to areas of the hand for mobility, a large number of specific flaps have been designed, both local and distant.

Innervation (nerve repair)

• Following division of a peripheral nerve, the axon in the distal segment undergoes Wallerian degeneration. In the proximal segment regeneration commences, providing the cell body has not been damaged. Axon sprouts attempt to cross the gap between the segments but fibroblastic proliferation is the most prominent feature in the early stage. Minimal tension will encourage moulding and linear orientation of the collagen, thereby improving the potential for axons to cross the gap. Once the axons have crossed the injury site they advance at approximately 1 mm/day and this can be monitored by the advancing Tinel sign (see below). The quality of recovery depends on the degree of reinnervation of the motor and sensory terminals. These terminals have a decreased ability to recover with increasing time from the injury, so more proximal nerve injuries have poorer results.

The aim of surgery is carefully to approximate the nerve ends in accurate alignment, creating the best possible environment for axon regeneration. If it is likely that the nerve might be under too much tension or direct approximation is not possible, a nerve graft is required. This usually involves sacrifice of a nerve from another site (e.g. sural nerve), although other biological and synthetic tissues are being evaluated as alternatives for small gaps.

Motion (tendon repair)

• The tendons in the hand provide a precisely balanced mechanism for individual fine control of each digit. Following trauma, functional return is maximized by immediate repair. Injuries to flexor tendons are more difficult to repair than extensor tendons because there are two flexor tendons for each digit which glide over each other. The two tendons are in closest approximation between the distal palmar crease and the insertion of the flexor digitorum superficialis where they are enclosed in a narrow sheath surrounded by pulleys.

• Repair of flexor tendons requires a central stitch to take the tension and a peripheral continuous suture to align the ends so that it can continue to glide in the narrow space of the tendon sheath. The pulleys need to be preserved as they prevent bowstringing of the tendons and allow even transmission of forces to the digit. Following repair, the tensile strength at the site of injury will gradually increase but will not return to normal. The repair should not be stressed severely for at least 12 weeks.

• Whilst early excessive use may rupture the repair, inactivity will lead to adhesions, and reduced tendon gliding and mobility. Several postoperative regimes exist: dynamic mobilization, passive mobilization and, most recently, active mobilization. Each has its merits but they all require regular hand therapy and review in outpatients to achieve satisfactory results. If the initial wound is dirty, delayed primary repair can be performed.

• If a repair ruptures it may be possible to resuture it, providing it is identified at an early stage; otherwise later tendon grafting is necessary, and this is to be performed in two stages. If adhesions occur which cannot be corrected by hand therapy they are divided surgically (tenolysis).

Foreign bodies

Removal of foreign bodies from a hand is often difficult if they are not directly visible. This is therefore best performed in theatre under anaesthesia with tourniquet control and an image intensifier (if it is radiopaque) and magnification.

Fingertip injuries

The normal fingertip is stable, padded, durable and has good sensation for performing fine manipulative skills. It is important that these same features are maintained after injury to prevent permanent disability occurring. If there is less than 1 cm diameter defect in the pulp without exposure of bone, conservative treatment will allow the defect to contract and heal, leaving only a small area of altered sensibility. Larger defects and injuries exposing bone will generally require surgical treatment. Injury of the nail bed also requires careful acute repair as late reconstruction is difficult. This includes maintaining the eponychial fold and the lateral nail folds, which is achieved by replacing the nail or using a splint.

High-pressure injection injuries

Accidental injection of material from spray guns often only results in a small entry wound which is easily missed. The fluids involved are usually oil-based and with the high pressure diffuse widely in the tissues. These injuries require extensive exploration to remove all the foreign material and associated necrotic fat. Even with early exploration, this injury may result in significant loss of function.

Follow-up of hand trauma

Hand injuries require regular hand therapy and outpatient review. This allows early detection of cases which are not progressing satisfactorily, so that further treatment can be instituted to ensure the best possible recovery of function.

Assessment of residual problems after hand trauma generally requires a more detailed history and examination. This should be directed at identifying the specific functional impairment. This will include identifying the presence of deformity or contractures of the skin, soft tissues or bone. Further signs that can be elicited are Allen's test and the Tinel sign.

Allen's test

Allen's test assesses the patency of the ulnar and radial arteries. Both the arteries are compressed at the wrist and the residual blood in the hand is pumped out by asking the patient rapidly to open and close the fist. The compression is maintained for at least 10 s to exclude the presence of a median artery. The radial artery is then released whilst maintaining pressure on the ulnar artery. Rapid capillary refill indicates a patent radial artery. The process is then repeated for the ulnar artery. If either of the arteries is occluded, then capillary refill will be sluggish on releasing pressure on that side.

Tinel sign

Tinel sign is used to assess the progress of nerve regeneration. The line of the affected nerve is percussed with the fingertip, commencing distally. Percussion over regenerating axon sprouts induces tingling. Thus, the progress of a nerve repair can be followed using this test.

Posttraumatic (reflex) sympathetic dystrophy (RSD, or Sudek's disease)

This condition can develop after any injury to the hand and is often seen after nerve injuries. It initially causes disproportionate pain and poor progress in regaining hand movement. On examination the hand is swollen, hyperaemic and sweaty. Due to the pain the patient will avoid using the hand and protect it from any contact. If untreated, the pain, oedema and disuse all lead to stiffness and osteoporosis. In the long term and pain may resolve, and the skin becomes dry and vasoconstricted.

The aetiology of this condition is uncertain but it is considered to be a prolonged and exaggerated sympathetic response to injury. It often develops in the early postoperative period, when the diagnosis can be delayed because the clinician believes the patient to have a low pain threshold. Early treatment, however, is more likely to lead to a rapid resolution of the symptoms. This requires regular sympathetic blockade, usually by intravenous regional anaesthesia with guanethidine, in conjunction with intensive physiotherapy.

Hand infection

Inadequate or late treatment of infections in the hand may lead to permanent incapacity with stiffness and reduced grip strength. Many hand infections occur as a result of minor penetrating wounds, particularly when there is retention of organic foreign material. The majority are caused by *Staphylococcus aureus* and the first-choice antibiotic is therefore flucloxacillin. The requirement for tetanus prophylaxis should also be remembered.

Infections can affect several sites in the hand:
- paronychia — an infection of the soft tissue adjacent to the nail;
- pulp space;
- web space;
- palmar spaces; and
- tendon sheath infections.

Tendon sheath infections are rare but serious, requiring early irrigation using fine catheters to limit stiffness and prevent rupture of the tendons. Infections in the palm can be due to local penetrating wounds but can occur from proximal spread of web space and flexor sheath infections. The fascial planes of the palm may lead to 'collar-stud' abscesses and it is therefore important to ensure that there is no deep connection.

If infection is identified at an early stage, when there is no localization of pus, treatment is by systemic intravenous antibiotics and elevation of the hand splinted in the position of function. Daily review is necessary to confirm resolution. Patients who present with throbbing pain in the hand that is causing loss of sleep generally have a collection of pus that requires incision and drainage. Local anaesthesia is often ineffective in the presence of infection, so regional or general anaesthesia should be used. After drainage the wound margins should be held apart with a wick to allow continued drainage but tight packing should be avoided. Once the inflammation is resolving, physiotherapy is necessary to mobilize the hand.

Human and animal bites contain mixed pathogens, including steptococci, anaerobes and unusual Gram-negative bacilli, so the first-choice antibiotic is penicillin. *Erysipeloid* is caused by a Gram-positive bacillus (*Erysipelothrix rhusiopathiae*) present on animals and fish and is therefore common in butchers and fish handlers. It is also sensitive to penicillin. *Orf* is a large poxvirus which causes ulceration around the mouths of sheep. It may enter wounds on the hands of vets, farmers or abattoir workers and form painless granulomas. The condition is self-limiting and does not respond to antibiotics.

Lower limb trauma

Soft-tissue injury

Flap lacerations

Flap lacerations, especially in the pretibial region, are a common problem. They are low-velocity soft-tissue injuries, often affecting the elderly, especially those taking long-term steroids which render the skin thin and fragile.

Management

Often the skin flap is of doubtful viability, requiring debridement and cover with a split-skin graft. In most cases, this procedure can be carried out under local anaesthetic. Skin flaps and undermined or compromised skin edges are trimmed. Loose fat and haematoma are also evacuated and haemostasis secured. A split-skin graft of appropriate size is harvested from the thigh and meshed to a ratio of 1 : 1.5. This allows drainage of exudate and improves graft take. The skin graft is applied to the wound on the leg and dressed using a double layer of paraffin tulle, a foam sponge, and held in place with a crepe and a support bandage.

Postoperatively, these patients have conventionally been treated with 1 week of bedrest. However, early mobilization after 48 h of bedrest does not affect the graft take and at the same time avoids the complications associated with immobilization.

The first change of dressing is carried out at 5 days. A non-adherent protective dressing is then applied for a further 2 weeks. By this time the graft is sufficiently stable to be left exposed.

Soft-tissue injury with fractures

High-energy lower limb trauma causes soft-tissue damage, open fractures and vascular/nerve trauma. Such injury represents a high proportion of non-fatal trauma in both military and civilian practice. A major impetus for the development of modern reconstructive surgery came from the two World Wars and from the post-World War II military conflicts in Korea and Vietnam. Injuries sustained to limbs from explosions and high-velocity missiles resulted in a high rate of amputations. In peace time, similar casualties arise from road traffic accidents involving high-speed vehicles, sport injuries and gunshot wounds. Involvement of soft tissues, bone and vessels in these injuries has necessitated the cooperation of orthopaedic, vascular and plastic surgeons in preoperative planning, timing and application of technical skills to obtain optimal functional salvage of the extremity. Many limbs previously doomed to amputation can now be saved by this combined approach in reconstructive surgery.

Management

The management of the severely traumatized lower extremity involving soft-tissue loss associated with open fractures can be divided into three phases: emergency evaluation, emergency wound management and further wound management.

Emergency evaluation

- History: mechanism of injury; contamination at the scene; tetanus immunization status.
- General examination: assessment of the patient to deal first with any life-threatening injuries to head, chest and abdomen.
- Examination of the limb: site and extent of the soft-tissue injury; neurovascular status; appropriate X-rays to determine the severity of fractures.
- General management: patient should be resuscitated if in shock (Chapter 4); broad-spectrum antibiotics intravenously; tetanus immunoglobulin and toxoid if indicated; culture swabs from the wound.
- Wound management: the wound is then covered with sterile dressings and the limb is splinted before transferring the patient to the operating theatre.

Emergency wound management

The patient is transferred to theatre where further assessment of the injury is made. A high proportion of such extensive injuries are associated with compartment syndrome and therefore require compartment pressure measurements. If the pressure exceeds 30 mmHg, decompression fasciotomies are performed to prevent further damage to muscles and nerves. All gross contamination is removed with saline irrigation or jet lavage. Devitalized skin, muscle and free bone fragments are debrided. The fracture is stabilized, usually with external fixation. If a vascular injury is present it must be repaired as a priority. No attempt should be made to close the wound, which is packed with suitable dressings.

Further wound management

Quite often the zone of injury in these wounds is not demarcated on presentation. Tissues of marginal viability may become non-viable. Therefore re-exploration and further debridement may be necessary 48–72 h later. In the meantime the wound requires bedside dressing changes and adequate leg elevation.

Soft-tissue cover Once the viability of remaining tissue is beyond doubt and the patient has been stabilized from major trauma, an appropriate method of reconstruction is chosen depending upon the site and extent of soft-tissue loss.
- simple split-skin graft;
- local muscle flap;

- local fasciocutaneous flap;
- free tissue transfer using micro and surgical techniques.

Bone reconstruction This is required in fractures with extensive loss of bone and is usually performed 4–6 weeks after providing soft-tissue cover. By this time the soft-tissue cover has healed and stabilized.

In general, bone defects <8 cm are bridged with cancellous bone grafts, whereas defects >8 cm require vascularized bone as a free tissue transfer.

Avulsion injuries

These are usually caused by motor vehicle accidents. Those resulting from being run over by a bus or truck are the most serious. The broad tyres of these vehicles distribute shearing forces over a wide area, which can result in circumferential avulsion of the entire skin and subcutaneous tissues of the leg.

Depending upon the extent of damage, avulsion injuries are of two types:
- *Type 1 avulsion injuries*: Open wound due to degloving of the skin and subcutaneous fat with a narrow zone of undermined tissue around the periphery of the wound. Management consists of debridement of all degloved and undermined soft tissue, skin grafting of the wound and fracture stabilization where appropriate.
- *Type 2 avulsion injuries*: Extensive undermining of soft tissues with a relatively small open wound. The initial assessment of these wounds frequently underestimates the extent of damage as most of the leg appears normal, apart from the presence of tyre marks and patches of ecchymosis. The full extent of soft-tissue loss eventually appears several days later and may give rise to systemic sepsis due to necrosis of large amounts of subcutaneous fat underneath the normal-looking skin. Early intervention and operative assessment are therefore indicated. Fluoroscein injected intravenously circulates only to viable tissue and is a method of identifying all dead tissue (which does not fluoresce), which is excised. Primary or delayed split-skin grafting is performed, sometimes by taking skin graft off the removed devitalized tissue if the degloving injury is extensive. This requires the use of a special graft knife (Gibson–Ross dermatome).

Facial injuries

Introduction

The aesthetic significance of injuries to the face is self-evident. However, proper management from a functional point of view is equally important. Failure to recognize and treat facial fractures can lead to trismus or malocclusion. Untreated orbital floor fractures result in diplopia and nasal fractures lead to airway obstruction. Facial injuries range from simple lacerations and abrasions to major maxillofacial trauma seen as a result of high-velocity road accidents.

Two-thirds of victims of multiple trauma sustain injuries to the head and face. Isolated facial injuries are only rarely the cause of shock and other serious injuries should be sought and excluded in a shocked patient. As with any other form of major trauma, the patient is assessed for ABCD (airways, breathing, circulation, determination of cause; see Chapter 3). After stabilization of life-threatening injuries, a secondary survey of the maxillofacial area is performed. Any associated head injury must also be assessed (see Chapter 21).

Evaluation of maxillofacial injury

Airway control

Airway obstruction may be caused by broken teeth, dentures, bone fragments, haematomata or foreign bodies. In a supine patient with a bilateral *mandibular* fracture the tongue can fall back and obstruct the oropharynx. A towel clip or a suture may be used to pull the tongue anteriorly, or the fractured mandibular fragment may be pulled forwards in order to clear the airway. A posteroinferiorly displaced fractured *maxilla* may cause airway obstruction. The fractured fragment should be disimpacted by pulling it anteriorly, by means of two fingers hooked behind the posterior border of the hard palate. Orotracheal intubation is often necessary, but must be performed without moving the neck unless a cervical spine injury has been ruled out. In extremely urgent cases, where oral or nasal intubation is not possible, a cricothyroidotomy may be performed. Early tracheostomy is advantageous in patients with extensive facial fractures.

Haemorrhage

Direct pressure is usually sufficient to control bleeding from most wounds. A moist pressure dressing will prevent desiccation of the tissues while the patient is being stabilized. Occasionally it may be necessary to clamp or ligate bleeding vessels, though this is usually best left until a formal exploration in theatre is possible. Anterior and posterior nasal packing may be indicated in cases of severe bleeding from the nose and ethmoids.

Examination of maxillofacial injuries

Clinical evaluation

- Bleeding, or leakage of cerebrospinal fluid from the nose or ears suggests a fractured cranial base and the need for antibiotic prophylaxis.
- The eyes should be examined for the presence of foreign bodies, subconjunctival haematomata and visual acuity before periorbital oedema makes this difficult. A retrobulbar haematoma can cause proptosis and decreased vision. Enophthalmos, unequal pupillary levels, restriction of external ocular movements or diplopia suggests a fracture of the orbital floor or wall. Impaired sensation may be noted in the distribution of the infraorbital and inferior alveolar nerves in maxillary and mandibular fractures, respectively. Surgical emphysema suggests fractures of the walls of the paranasal sinuses.
- Rapidly developing oedema in facial injuries often masks the deformity caused by facial fractures and it is important to palpate the bony margins of the orbit, the zygoma and the mandible for any asymmetry, step deformity or localized tenderness.
- Intraoral examination for malocclusion, soft-tissue injury or haematoma is essential. In a conscious patient, the patient's subjective impression of malocclusion may be helpful. The premaxillary teeth should be gripped and rocked back and forth to detect any abnormal mobility of the middle third of the face, which would indicate the presence of a Le Fort fracture.
- Nasal fractures result in nasal deformity, crepitus and airway obstruction.

Radiological examination

Special views, including orthopantomograms for mandibular fractures, need to be obtained to assess facial bones radiologically. One such view (Water's view) is useful in the diagnosis of fractures of the maxilla, maxillary sinuses, orbital floor, zygomatic bone and zygomatic arches. Further specific views as well as computed tomographic scans and preinjury photographs may be used to plan the treatment of severe facial fractures.

Management of maxillofacial injury

Management of soft-tissue injuries

- The face is very vascular and heals well. Therefore, only severely traumatized or contaminated tissue need be debrided. Debridement should be conservative, especially when specialized tissue is involved, e.g. eyebrows, eyelids, nostril margins and lips. However, failure to remove all the dirt from a wound can result in unsightly 'tattooing' of the scar.

(a) Simple facial lacerations may be treated in the A & E department but, where possible, injuries involving specialized structures should be referred to experienced surgeons. In order to prevent cross-hatching of the scars, fine sutures, which are removed on about the fifth postoperative day, are used. Structures like the eyebrows and skin–vermilion junction of the lip should be accurately aligned. Both sides of the face should be exposed to achieve symmetry in the repair. The muscles of facial expression, unlike those elsewhere in the body, are inserted into the skin, and are often involved in soft-tissue lacerations of the face. These injuries should be sutured in two layers, to restore good function of the facial muscles, and to prevent stretched or depressed and tethered scars.

(b) Facial nerve injuries and division of the parotid duct require microsurgical repair which offers the best chance of a successful outcome.

Management of bony injuries

Fractures of the zygomatic arch are elevated and may be wired or plated if they are unstable after reduction. Fractures of the maxilla or mandible are internally fixed with wires or plates. These fractures may also be treated by intermaxillary fixation, which involves fixation of the teeth in occlusion, by means of eyelet wires or arch bars, held together with wires or strong rubber bands. This immobilizes the bone fragments and achieves proper occlusion. External fixators are also used to immobilize fractured facial bones against the cranium.

Decubitus ulcer (pressure sore)

Introduction

Pressure sores (also called bedsores or decubitus ulcers) are lesions caused by prolonged compression of skin and subcutaneous tissues, usually overlying bony prominences. they usually occur in bed-ridden patients, those in a restrictive cast or appliance, or those with large insensate areas. Better management and decreased mortality of paraplegic and quadriplegic patients have also meant an increase in the incidence of pressure sores requiring treatment.

The sites for the development of pressure sores are:
Common
- sacrum (Fig, 23.21a);
- greater trochanter;

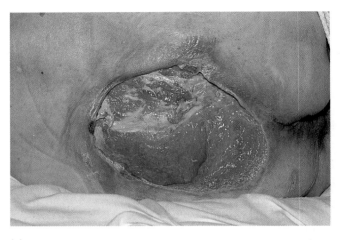

(a)

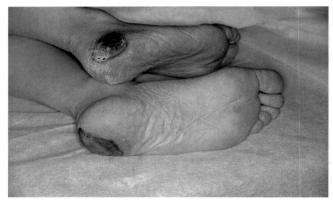

(b)

Figure 23.21 Decubitus ulcers or pressure sores over (a) the sacrum; (b) the heels.

- ischium;
- heel (Fig. 23.21b); and
- malleoli.
Rare
- spinal prominences;
- scapula;
- elbow;
- zygoma and ears; and
- occiput.

The pathophysiological process leading to decubitus ulcer is that prolonged extrinsic pressure leads to ischaemia of the underlying tissues progressing to necrosis and ulceration. Fat and muscle are more vulnerable to ischaemic damage than skin; hence the extent of underlying tissue damage may be much more than is visible on the skin. Unrelieved pressure for even 4–6 h can lead to irreversible ischaemic tissue damage and subsequent development of a pressure sore. Although extrinsic pressure is the single most important aetiological factor, malnutrition, anaemia, sepsis and other systemic illnesses are often significant contributory factors in the development and subsequent poor healing of pressure sores.

Management

Prevention

The cornerstone of the management of pressure sores is prevention in susceptible patients. This is achieved by:
- frequent (i.e. at least every 2 h) position changes in bedridden patients;
- avoidance of tight-fitting casts, braces, splints and other appliances and frequent checking of the underlying skin when they are used;
- use of specialized beds for bed-ridden patients (e.g. flotation bed systems) to distribute pressure evenly.

Treatment

The management of an established pressure sore involves careful assessment of the lesion as well as the patient's general condition:
- bacteriology of the ulcer, preferably by quantitative tissue biopsies. The presence of >100 000 organisms/g of tissue is usually indicative of infection and appropriate antibiotics are used;
- radiographs of the underlying bone to detect osteomyelitis; contrast studies are useful to delineate sinus tracts leading away from the ulcer;
- evaluation of the patient's nutritional status, anaemia, coagulation profile, blood chemistry and urine cultures and institution of appropriate corrective measures are essential before embarking on operative intervention.

The aims of surgical intervention are:
- thorough debridement of the ulcer, all necrotic tissue and the underlying bursa;
- resection of the underlying bone, which is often unhealthy or frankly osteomyelitic;
- coverage of the defect, usually with well-vascularized tissue.

In general, large regional skin or musculocutaneous flaps are used as rotation or advancement flaps to cover the defect. Examples include gluteus maximus flap for sacral or ischial pressure sores and tensor fascia lata flap for trochanteric sores. Occasionally it is possible to provide sensation to the area by the use of innervated flaps, e.g. the tensor fascia lata flap incorporating the lateral femoral cutaneous nerve.

Postoperatively it is important to avoid pressure on the flap for at least 3–4 weeks.

Since recurrence of pressure sores is common and progressively more difficult to treat, prevention is vital in these patients.

Aesthetic surgery

Aesthetic or cosmetic surgery involves the correction of problems which patients perceive as making them look different or abnormal. Various procedures are utilized in trying to approach a 'normal' or 'ideal' appearance. The term 'cosmetic' derives from the cosmeticians who were employed to paint public statues in the Roman era. In a sense most, if not all, plastic surgery includes the consideration of aesthetics, and indeed there are large areas where reconstructive and aesthetic surgery overlap, as when facelift procedures are performed for facial nerve palsy, or neurofibromatosis affecting the face.

People have always been concerned by appearance, both in terms of outer adornments such as clothing and make-up, and by temporary or permanent alterations to the body with tattooing, scarification, filing of teeth, etc. More recent examples include seeking changes in body form by various dietary regimes, and body-building. Several studies have shown that external appearance is important not only in relation to self-image, but also in relation to how people perceive and react towards you. The patient presenting for aesthetic surgery is often very self-conscious of the perceived deformity, and this can lead to a vicious circle: being self-conscious gives rise to loss of confidence and awkwardness in social interaction; withdrawal from interaction with other people then further increases self-consciousness, confirming the lack of self-image. Aesthetic surgery can dramatically change the quality of life in suitable cases. However, patient selection is crucial and in some instances the desire for aesthetic surgery is masking an underlying but quite different problem. The various procedures are briefly outlined below.
- *Facelift (rhytidectomy)*: This procedure involves tightening of sagging skin in the face and neck.
- *Blepharoplasty*: Baggy lower eyelids and drooping upper ones can be corrected by excision of excess skin, with or without muscle, and associated fatty pads.
- *Aesthetic rhinoplasty*: Nasal surgery to improve appearance is usually performed via incisions inside the nose, and can include removal of a prominent hump, refining the nasal tip and making the root of the nose slimmer. Reconstructive procedures to correct posttraumatic deformities and airway problems are also frequently done, hence septo-

plasty or submucous resection of the septum may be combined with the rhinoplasty.

• *Chin or cheek augmentation*: Augmenting the chin or cheeks with either prosthetic or autogenous material can be performed alone, or sometimes with aesthetic rhinoplasty when a prominent nose is associated with a receding chin (correction of one deformity alone will not achieve a balanced profile in this situation).

• *Breast reduction*: There are now a large number of techniques for correction of the hypertrophic breast. The particular technique chosen will depend on age, degree of hypertrophy, and whether the patient has completed her family or intends to have further children and breast-feed.

• *Mastopexy*: Mastopexy is performed when the breasts are ptotic, to improve the contour and resite the nipple to a higher position on the breast.

• *Breast augmentation*: Hypoplastic breast development can be corrected by the use of prosthetic implants (Fig. 23.22).

• *Abdominoplasty*: This procedure can be performed to improve the appearance of the lower abdominal outline and to tighten a weak abdomen stretched from extreme weight or pregnancy.

• *Liposuction*: Using special cannulae, suction removal of fat is possible in most parts of the body. The technique allows relative sparing of damage to blood vessels and nerves, as the blunt cannulae should slip around these structures. The technique works best where there are specific confined areas of excessive fat, and where there is sufficient elasticity of The skin to allow contraction over the new reduced volume of subcutaneous tissue.

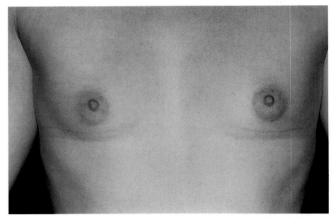

(a)

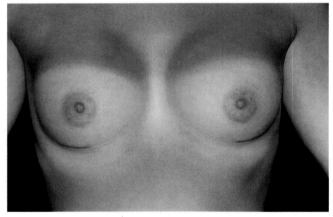

(b)

Figure 23.22 Preoperative (a) and postoperative (b) breast augmentation using silicone implants.

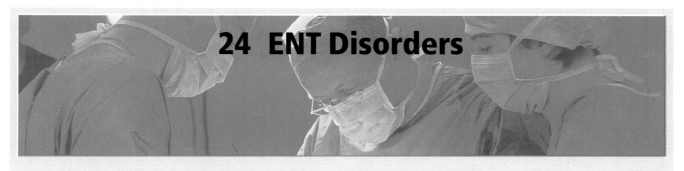

24 ENT Disorders

Laugh and the world laughs with you, snore and you snore alone. (Mark Twain 1835–1910)

Introduction

Many are put off ENT by the intricacy of otolaryngological anatomy, but the vast majority of ENT problems presenting to the non-specialist can be managed without reference to anatomical refinements. Excellent colour atlases, thanks to the advent of fibreoptic illumination, are now able to illustrate in colour the depths of previously inaccessible orifices. Two general points in the history require to be highlighted. The first is the patient's smoking habit which, due to the commendable reduction in smoking among the medical profession, is all too often overlooked. The level of urgency associated with the referral of a patient with hoarseness is directly related to the smoking history. Second, occupation is important not only in relation to industrial deafness but also to dust or allergen exposure.

This chapter discusses the principal causes of the major ENT symptoms. This requires some simplification as no disease ever gives rise only to one symptom but it is intended to give a framework with which to approach ENT patients.

The ear

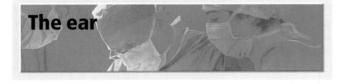

Evaluation of the patient

Clinical assessment

Symptoms

The common symptoms of ear disease are given in Table 24.1
• *Deafness*, which may vary greatly in degree, is the most common symptom of ear disease and may conveniently be divided into two large groups:

(a) *Conductive deafness*, which occurs because of a problem with the conducting mechanism of the ear (e.g. otosclerosis), is characterized by reduced but not distorted sound levels. This type of deafness responds well to amplification.

(b) *Sensorineural deafness*, which is caused by lesions in the cochlea or auditory nerve, presents with reduced and distorted sound levels. Usually the higher frequencies are lost, making speech comprehension difficult for the

Table 24.1 Common symptoms of ear disease.

Deafness
Ear discharge
Pain
Itching
Tinnitus
Vertigo

patient. This type of deafness does not respond to amplification.

• *Discharge* from the ear has many causes. Discharge from the external auditory canal is serous or purulent while that from the inner ear may be mucopurulent or consist of pus. Bleeding from the ear may be due to granulation tissue from chronic otitis media or occasionally malignant disease. Cerebrospinal fluid may leak from the ear after head injury or occasionally after ear surgery.

• *Pain*: Several pathological processes involving the auricle, the external auditory canal, the middle ear and the mastoid may result in ear pain and having the patient point to the exact site of pain may give a clue as to the cause. Pain around the tragus indicates external auditory canal pathology while pain deep in the ear may result from a lesion in the middle ear or mastoid. Ear pain may also be referred from another site, e.g. a diseased tooth may present with earache.

• *Itching* is a symptom of otitis externa.
• *Tinnitus* is a subjective sensation of sound caused by irritation of the upper auditory pathways or the cochlea. There are many causes of this common condition (see below).
• *Vertigo* is a very distressing symptom and indicates a lesion in the vestibular system. Usually the patient complains of a sensation of rotation but a history of staggering to one side may also indicate vertigo.

Physical examination and investigations of the ear (Table 24.2)

External examination

Inspect the shape and set of the pinna (outer ear). Look for skin disease, mastoid swelling or general inflammation and for anterior (endaural) or postaural scars.

Otoscopy

The external auditory canal slopes downwards and forwards in the adult. The pinna should, therefore, be pulled upwards and backwards with the left hand while the right hand holds the auriscope to look in the right ear. Reverse the hand positions for the left ear. The speculum is inserted under direct vision to avoid tympanic membrane trauma; this is a particular hazard in children where the drum lies superficially as the tympanic ring and mastoid process are

Table 24.2 Investigations for assessment of the ear.

Investigation	Comment
Visual	
Otoscopy	Using an auriscope the external auditory canal and the tympanic membrane can be inspected
	Ear discharge and the colour, position and integrity of the drum should be noted
Auditory function	
Tuning-fork tests	
Rinne's test	Compares air conduction with bone conduction. Air conduction is better in the normal ear
Weber test	Lateralizes unilateral deafness. In conductive deafness the sound is best heard in the affected ear. In sensorineural deafness sound is heard best in the non-affected ear
Audiometry	Air and bone conduction are tested at frequencies ranging from 125 to 8000 Hz
Tympanometry	A small probe plays a tone into the ear. The amount of sound absorbed by the middle ear is assessed. Provides useful information about the state of the middle ear
Electrophysiological tests	Assess auditory pathway
Vestibular function	
Caloric tests	Cold (30°C) and hot (44°C) water irrigated into the ear induces nystagmus by stimulating endolymph flow in the semicircular canals. Nystagmus will not be induced if there is a vestibular lesion causing canal paresis
Electronystagmography (ENG)	Electrodes placed on the eye exploit the corneoretinal electric potential (300–1300 μV) to provide sophisticated

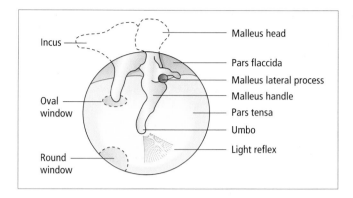

Figure 24.1 The right tympanic membrane and associated structures.

not developed. The vascularity, colour, integrity and position of the tympanic membrane should be noted (Fig. 24.1). If the drum is not intact, an estimate should be made of the size (as a percentage of the drum area) and state (dry, moist, wet) of any perforation. Some commercially available hand-held aurisopes have a pneumatic attachment. The principle of pneumatic otoscopy is that, if there is a hole in the tympanic membrane, it will not move when a puff of air is gently directed towards it, as the air goes down the hole and escapes via the eustachian tube which connects the middle ear cleft to the postnasal space. If there is no hole, the light reflex of the drum moves. A common mistake is the misinterpretation of tympanosclerosis — white (chalk) patches in the drum, usually a sign of burnt-out infection or previous surgery.

Much the best way to learn how to use an auriscope is to look at as many normal drums as possible, starting with your colleagues. In the same way, you will never be able to detect pathological splitting of the second heart sound until you have listened to a great many normal precordia. Examination of the ear is not complete until the neck has been carefully palpated for the presence of nodes, and the nose and postnasal space inspected.

Auditory function

The assessment of auditory function starts with the tuning-fork tests. A 256 or 512 Hz fork is preferable, struck on a padded surface such as a chairback or your elbow to generate a pure tone. Many people get confused about hearing tests.

• In *Rinne's test* air conduction is compared to bone conduction. The vibrating tuning fork is held near the ear and then while it is still vibrating is applied with its base to the mastoid process. The patient is asked which is heard louder. In a normal person air conduction should be better than bone conduction, i.e. the test is positive. Rinne-positive is perfectly normal. It is normal to hear through the air — the telephone receiver is applied to the ear canal, not plastered on to the mastoid process and thus normal air conduction is louder than bone conduction. Air-conducted sounds are naturally amplified by, first, the lever system of the three ossicles — malleus moulded to the drum, stapes sitting in the oval window and incus in between; second, the relative size of the drum and oval window; and third, the separation of sound between the oval and round windows. If these mechanisms for sound amplification are interfered with (conductive hearing loss), then the bone conduction becomes better than the air conduction (Rinne-negative).

• In the *Weber test*, the tuning fork is placed centrally on the head. You would expect this sound to be heard better in the better ear. And so it is — provided any deficit is of a sensorineural type. If the air sounds are not conducted properly, then the fork is heard in the worse ear. You can test this by placing the fork centrally on your own forehead and putting a finger in one ear. The fork is heard in the occluded ear. Why? The answer is not altogether clear. Because natural (ambient) noises are not being conducted into the ear, there is less interference with the vibrating tone of the fork in the affected ear. But this is probably not the whole story. The Weber is a very sensitive test and is lateralized to the side of a unilateral conductive deafness of as little as 10–15 dB.

• *Audiometry*: Hearing is tested by pure-tone audiometry at octave steps from 125 to 8000 Hz in patients of 4 years of age and older (Fig. 24.2). Air conduction and bone conduction are both measured in one ear while the other ear is masked. In distraction audiometry the child (aged between 6 and 12 months) is tested by inducing a head-turning response. At 2 years children can be conditioned to make a movement (building a tower of bricks) in response to an audiometric tone.

• *Tympanometry*: Conductive deafness can be further defined by tympanometry (Fig. 24.3). A small probe plays a tone which is partly absorbed by the ear. Maximum absorption occurs when the ear pressure in the external auditory canal equals middle-ear pressure. The amount of sound reflected out is measured by a microphone within the probe. The more compliant the middle ear, the greater the sound absorption. Reduced pressure in the middle ear, e.g. in eustachian tube dysfunction, gives a point of maximum compliance when the canal pressure is also subatmospheric (type C tympanogram). Fluid in the middle ear is incompressible and generates a flat tympanogram (type B).

• *Electrophysiological tests* of hearing such as brainstem evoked response audiometry can be used to locate a lesion on the auditory pathway or to establish thresholds in children, particularly those with multiple handicaps, or in cases

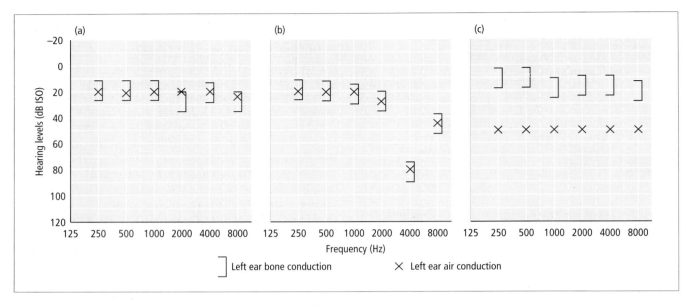

Figure 24.2 Pure-tone audiogram. (a) Normal; (b) noise-induced hearing loss; (c) conductive hearing loss.

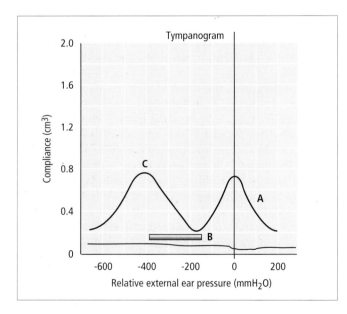

Figure 24.3 Tympanometry. — Type A = normal; type B = secretory otitis media; type C = reduced middle ear pressure.

of possible non-organic hearing loss. Electrical impulses occuring in the region of the brainstem in response to a click stimulus are detected by surface electrodes placed over the mastoid, forehead and vertex by means of computer averaging. The N1 and N5 waves are usually most prominent.

Vestibular function

- *Nystagmus*: The physical sign of a vestibular disorder is nystagmus, which is defined as an involuntary deviation of the eyes away from the direction of gaze followed by a return of the eyes to their original position. Nystagmus may have vestibular, ocular or central causes. Vestibular function may be assessed by caloric tests and electronystagmography (ENG).
- *Caloric test*: In these tests the lateral semicircular canals are subjected to caloric stimulation by irrigation of the ear canals with water at 30 and 44°C. Nystagmus is normally induced by these manoeuvres. Where there is depression of vestibular function on one side the response to cold and hot irrigation is reduced. This response is called canal paresis and is suggestive of a lesion in the vestibular apparatus on that side. The test is not a diagnostic test for dizziness and rarely gives a conclusive answer when used in isolation.
- *Electronystagmography* is a sophisticated method for assessing vestibular function. ENG is performed by placing electrodes on either side of the eyes and picking up electrical signals from oscillations of the corneoretinal potential. This investigation will detect spontaneous nystagmus with the eyes open or closed, differentiate between central and peripheral nystagmus and indicate which side is affected if it is peripheral.

Disorders of the ear

Sensorineural deafness

Sudden sensorineural deafness is a medical emergency and should be referred to an ENT department for investigation and treatment at once — not several days later, as some cases are reversible by the use of vasodilators and steroids. Presbyacusis is the auditory equivalent of presbyopia — hearing loss due to ageing. The sensory (cochlear) components of sensorineural deafness give a high tone loss while the neural component affects discrimination. Thus the patient experiences difficulty in unravelling complex speech sounds, especially in the presence of background noise, even when the volume of sound is increased. This is because the number of nerve fibres available to carry the sound-induced impulses centrally is reduced.

- *Non-organic hearing loss*: The astute audiometrician may detect a discrepancy between the patient's response to questions posed with the headphones on and the level of acuity on the audiogram. Evoked response audiometry, or special testing with two audiometers, can also be used to pick up cases of psychogenic deafness or malingering.
- *Noise-induced deafness* may be occupational (boiler-making, riveting or weaving) or recreational (motor cycles, guns or music). The initial temporary threshold shift later becomes permanent and is maximum at 4 kHz (Fig. 24.2b). Ultimately, all frequencies are affected and all parts of the cochlea — hair cells, membrane and nerve fibres — show signs of damage. At present there is an industrial safety limit on noise exposure of 90 dB for 8 h/day for a 5-day week. Because of the logarithmic nature of the decibel scale, 93 dB is a safe level for only 4 h daily. Some people with sensitive ears can be damaged by less noise exposure. The most effective form of ear protectors are ear muffs but these provide attenuation only of 30 dB at the lower frequencies. Acute noise trauma can occur during blast injuries.
- *Congenital sensorineural deafness* is significant and bilateral in 1 per 1000 live births. Deaf children should be identified under 1 year, preferably under 9 months, as most language is acquired within the first 2 years. Sadly, many deaf children are not identified until after the second birthday. Aids can be fitted as early as 3 months. Many rare sex-linked or recessive syndromes are associated with deafness. Dominant syndromes include:
    (a) Waardenburg's syndrome: deafness, a white forelock and bushy eyebrows;
    (b) Alport's syndrome: deafness with progressive glomerulonephritis; and

(c) Treacher Collins syndrome: deafness, hypoplasia of the first branchial arch, an underdeveloped mandible and low-set ears.

Non-hereditary prenatal deafness arises from maternal infections, not only rubella but also cytomegalovirus and infectious mononucleosis when contracted in the first trimester. Perinatal risk factors include prematurity, low birth weight, hypoxia and hyperbilirubinaemia.

Neonatal deafness screening programmes usually attempt to screen all special care unit babies. Postnatal deafness is specifically associated with meningitis, mumps and measles. Mumps tend to cause a unilateral deafness. When deafness in a child is suspected, it is worth remembering that, by the age of 1 year, most children have two or three words and by 18 months, 18 words. By 2 years words are beginning to be strung together into phrases and short sentences. A child diagnosed as having a profound hearing impairment is nowadays usually managed in a special paediatric hearing assessment unit with input from ENT, paediatrics, visiting teachers of the deaf, an educational psychologist and a speech therapist. There is no doubt that some children do very poorly educationally unless they are allowed to use signing for the deaf. Fortunately this group is now a very small minority and the integration of hearing-impaired children into the normal educational system supported by visiting teachers of the hearing-impaired has been made possible by radio aids with direct input from the teacher or parent.

- *Traumatic deafness*: Temporal bone fracture can be missed on X-ray but may produce Battle's sign — bruising over the mastoid process. The common type runs along the long axis of the temporal bone (longitudinal fracture) and usually spares the inner ear, which is protected by the hard bone of the otic capsule. Conductive deafness results from involvement of the canal, tympanic membrane and middle ear. If there is cerebrospinal fluid otorrhoea, systemic antibiotics which cross the uninflamed blood–brain barrier, e.g. a cephalosporin, should be used. An occipital blow can cause a transverse fracture from the foramen magnum to the foramen lacerum, involving the inner ear and facial nerve.

Inner ear trauma also results from labyrinthine window rupture, either explosive (coughing, sneezing or straining) or implosive (blast, closed-head injury or barotrauma). There is fluctuating hearing loss, tinnitus and vertigo. The symptoms can be reproduced by carrying out pneumatic otoscopy. It may be possible to repair the leak of perilymph with a small piece of fat.

- *Ototoxic drugs*: The most notorious ototoxic drugs are the aminoglycoside antibiotics, including streptomycin, gentamicin and neomycin. Their nephrotoxicity can enhance the risk of ototoxicity. Neomycin principally affects the cochlea but streptomycin and gentamicin are vestibulotoxic. The ototoxic diuretics are frusemide and ethacrynic acid. Salicylates can cause a sensorineural hearing loss which is almost always reversible. Many drugs are only occasionally ototoxic and almost any medication may be responsible for a hearing defect.

• *Acoustic neuroma*: A great deal of ENT energy is expended on excluding this rare benign neurilemmoma of the eighth nerve in subjects with unilateral deafness, but 5% of the population have a slight asymmetry in hearing. Acoustic neuromas are very slow-growing but, as the tumour expands out of the internal auditory meatus (IAM), it compresses the brainstem and trigeminal nerve (causing loss of the corneal reflex). Despite its origin from the vestibular division, vertigo is rare because the very slow expansion is accompanied by central compensation of balance. Brainstem evoked response audiometry shows a characteristic delay in the N5 wave and computed tomographic (CT) scanning can display tumours greater than 1 cm within the cerebellopontine angle. Tumours entirely confined to the IAM are detectable by magnetic resonance imaging with gadolinium.

Conductive deafness

The common causes of conductive deafness are secretory otitis media, congenital conductive deafness and otosclerosis. Conductive deafness responds to amplification and it is the patient with certain types of conductive deafness that benefits most from hearing aids.

• *Secretory otitis media*: This is the commonest cause of conductive deafness in children, although adults can develop a secretion of fluid within the middle ear after a cold. Contributing factors are said to be adenoid hypertrophy, allergy, anatomy of the child's eustachian tube (short and fat) and antibiotic therapy in a subtherapeutic dose for acute otitis media. It should be remembered that otoscopy is far from 100% reliable in diagnosis and audiometry and/or tympanometry should be carried out in cases of doubt. Because middle ear effusion is very common and can resolve spontaneously, it has been difficult to obtain adequately controlled data on the best treatment.

Some advocate adenoidectomy as the cornerstone of treatment but more recently it has been suggested that in the absence of adenoid symptoms, insertion of ventilation tubes through the drums (grommets) may produce the optimum hearing results. Children who persistently reaccumulate middle ear effusions and require repeated grommet insertion may suffer from scarring of the drum. This group may ultimately benefit more from the fitting of a hearing aid until the problem is outgrown. Occasionally such children have a reservoir of serous fluid in the mastoid cells which requires to be drained. It should be noted that children with cleft palate have disordered eustachian tube function and rely on their adenoid pad to close off the nose during swallowing. Adenoidectomy is thus strictly contraindicated, even in children with only a bifid uvula, who may also have a submucous palatal cleft, and may develop gross hypernasal speech postoperatively.

• *Congenital conductive deafness*: Meatal atresia may be unilateral or bilateral, complete or incomplete. If both ears are involved, surgery should be considered between the ages of 18 months and 2 years. If the cochlea is normal and a middle ear space with ossicular chain has been demonstrated by tomography, surgery is indicated, accepting the potential hazard to the facial nerve which may run an abnormal course in this congenitally abnormal ear.

• *Otosclerosis*: Beethoven's famed deafness began in 1798 and was due to otosclerosis, the commonest non-infective cause of conductive deafness in adults. Although it occurs congenitally in association with brittle bone disease, the onset is usually between the ages of 18 and 30 years. The formation of spongy new bone around the stapes footplate leads to fixation of the footplate and to a conductive or mixed deafness. There is a female preponderance and a positive family history in 50% of cases. Sometimes patients hear better in a noisy background (paracusis of Willis) as the speaker's voice volume is increased in a noisy environment. In 10% of cases, otoscopy shows a flamingo-pink blush due to the vascular bone but most have normal tympanic membranes.

Conservative treatment is with a hearing aid. For patients under 60 years of age, surgical treatment by (partial) stapedectomy is offered. The drum is reflected forward (tympanotomy) and the superstructure of the stapes is removed. A small hole is made in the footplate and a Teflon piston is attached to the incus and protrudes through this hole to conduct sound into the perilymph of the inner ear. The patient must appreciate the small risk of sudden and complete postoperative deafness.

Hearing aids

Hearing aids comprise a microphone to pick up sound, a small amplifier and a receiver. The National Health Service behind-ear (BE series) hearing aids have varying strengths and microphone positions. The body-worn (BW series) aids are preferable for more severe deafness or those with arthritis who cannot manipulate the BE aid controls. Some aids have an automatic volume control to avoid amplification of very loud sounds. The range of amplification is 250–4000 Hz (the speech frequencies). A poorly fitting or inadequately inserted mould produces feedback (squealing). Most hearing aids have a T (Telecoil) position in addition to the M (microphone) position. Users in public places with an electromagnetic induction loop, e.g. theatres and cinemas, can switch to the T position. An improved quality of sound is then transmitted by electromagnetic induction of the aid coil rather than via the microphone. Ancillary aids include loud telephone bells, flashing door bells and fittings for television sets. Cochlear implants use sound waves to produce electrical stimulation of the cochlear nerve. At present, the number of different impulses which can be delivered is limited, so that cochlear implants benefit only the most profoundly deaf and not those whose hearing can be successfully amplified with a hearing aid.

Tinnitus

Tinnitus is a sensation of sound which is entirely subjective, i.e. not caused by a noise in the environment. It is important to realize that the annoyance of the noise is out of proportion to its measured volume. When a patient is asked to match noise intensity with tinnitus, the volume is only about 10–20 dB, much quieter than a conversational voice. But because it is a noise over which the patient has no control, it is *extremely annoying*. This is analogous to the annoyance caused by the distant sound of a neighbour's machine while no such annoyance is caused by the much louder sounds emanating from one's own appliances. Minor degrees of non-intrusive tinnitus are extremely common and often idiopathic. Up to 1% of the adult population has what can be defined as annoying tinnitus. Pseudotinnitus is a noise caused by a true environmental sound, e.g. the hum of electricity pylons, or of a refrigerator.

Causes of tinnitus

Sometimes tinnitus is caused by inner ear disease or by wax impinging on the eardrum or debris from otitis externa. Pulsatile tinnitus may be of vascular origin and it is always worth checking the patient's blood pressure and listening to the neck for a cervical bruit. More rarely, pulsatile tinnitus is caused by a vascular tumour (chemodectoma) such as a glomus tympanicum or glomus jugulare. General precipitating factors of non-pulsatile tinnitus include excessive coffee, aspirin or cigarette consumption, which should be eliminated.

Management of tinnitus

No drug treatment is effective but a hearing aid, by bringing in an increased volume of ambient noise, will act as a masker, i.e. drown out the noise and distract the patient's attention. The hours before sleeping are often the worst as there is little ambient noise, and a radio played quietly may help the patient get to sleep. A more sophisticated device is a tinnitus masker which looks like a hearing aid but which generates a sound which can be matched to the patient's tinnitus. Because this is a sound over which the patient has complete control, it is much less annoying. As an added bonus, occasionally patients get residual inhibition, i.e. for a very short period of time after use, the tinnitus is abolished. Patients may also be referred to the British Tinnitus Association, affiliated to the Royal National Institute for the Deaf.

Discharge from the ear

• *Otitis externa*: This localized dermatitis is the commonest cause of ear discharge in adult patients. The ear canal is the only blind-ending skin-lined tract in the body and normally is self-cleansing with a complex system of wax formation and skin migration. This may be interrupted by the ingress of water, chemicals, cotton buds or an allergenic hearing aid mould. Bacteriology swabs usually have a mixed growth, including *Pseudomonas*. The cornerstone of treatment is keeping the ears dry. Hair should not be washed in a shower or bath. The ears should be plugged with cotton wool, generously covered in petroleum jelly, or with well-fitting ear plugs or with commercial malleable wax plugs. Swimming is contraindicated in the active stages of the disease. For chronic sufferers who wish to swim, plugs can be worn with a cap and without diving or submersing the head. The debris is best cleared by cotton wool on a wire carrier but in chronic cases, where the eardrum is known to be intact, there may be a place for gentle syringing with warm saline. In this situation obviously the eardrum then has to be dried carefully. Pope's otowicks are small deliquescent wicks which expand when drops are applied to the surface. Useful preparations are Locorten-Vioform drops and Vioform-Hydrocortisone ointment which is an antiseptic-steroid combination. As they contain no antibiotic, they rarely induce contact sensitivity.

• *Acute suppurative otitis media*: This is commonest in children, often following a cold, but it can also follow the entry of water via a pre-existing membrane perforation. In infants, the peak incidence is 16–24 months and discharge or pyrexia of unknown origin are often the first symptoms. Acute ear infection should always be suspected in a child who is generally unwell or who pulls at his or her ears. Eustachian tube obstruction and pain are followed by pyrexia as the middle ear begins to develop an exudate. When the pus builds up, the eardrum bulges and ultimately perforates. The pain subsides, the ear discharges and, in most cases, heals spontaneously.

The disease can be arrested by the early use of antibiotics and decongestion by topical pseudoephedrine or Otrlvine nose drops, together with steam and possibly systemic decongestant such as Sudafed (paediatric elixir or, in adults, 60 mg t.i.d.). Decongestant therapy is helpful for those who wish to fly with a blocked eustachian tube and prevents the severe pain on descent of the aeroplane where the tube fails to open and equalize the low pressure in the middle ear with the atmospheric pressure on the ground. The antibiotic should be active against *Haemophilus influenzae* (amoxycillin, Augmentin). The rare complication of acute mastoiditis, which was once very common, gives a velvety feel to the periosteum over the mastoid bone, sometimes a subperiosteal abscess and the ear tends to protrude on the affected side. There may be swelling of the posterosuperior canal wall. If there is no response to systemic antibiotic therapy within 48 h the mastoid is explored and a cortical mastoidectomy carried out by drilling all the air sinuses into continuity.

• *Chronic suppurative otitis media*: This disease is conveniently subdivided into cases with and without cholesteatoma.

(a) *With cholesteatoma*: Cholesteatoma is a sac of keratinizing squamous epithelium rather like an aggressive sebaceous cyst surrounded by granulation tissue and enzymes which erode bone, particularly when infected. The sac can be congenital and grows slowly by expansion within the middle ear or petrous bone. Often it is difficult to diagnose cholesteatoma because the opening at the drum, usually in the attic or posterosuperior segment, may be quite small and there is only a scanty, offensive discharge. The patient may have a hearing loss disproportionate to the apparent disease. Untreated cholesteatoma can lead to petrositis, suppurative labyrinthitis, facial nerve palsy and intracranial complications, including extradural abscess, sigmoid sinus thrombosis, meningitis, subdural and cerebral abscess. Some of these conditions still carry a 50% mortality and so the standard treatment is to carry out a radical mastoidectomy which involves removing the drum and ossicles, except the stapes footplate, and drilling down the posterior canal wall so that it is thrown into one large cavity with the drilled-out mastoid air cells. Nowadays, a modified radical mastoidectomy is more usual and non-diseased portions of the drum, malleus and stapes may be left, although the incus is generally removed. The meatus of the ear is enlarged — meatoplasty — giving the appearance of a very large earhole. The complications of mastoid surgery include facial nerve palsy, conductive or sensorineural deafness and dizziness.

(b) *Without cholesteatoma*: Chronic suppurative otitis media without cholesteatoma is a much more benign disease. There is usually a central perforation with a copious mucoid discharge. The treatment may be conservative with drops and advice to keep the ear dry in patients who wish to accept an occasionally discharging perforation. Alternatively, attempts may be made to dry the ear and to repair the perforation with a graft of temporalis fascia inserted beneath the tympanic membrane — myringoplasty. In a discharging ear, a (cortical) mastoidectomy may also be required. Reconstitution of the ossicular chain may also be performed — ossiculoplasty. Middle ear carcinoma is a rare late complication of chronic suppurative otitis media with gradually worsening symptoms so that the discharge may become bloody with a facial nerve palsy, intractable pain and increasing deafness or dizziness. The treatment is a combination of radiotherapy and radical surgery with a low success rate. Anyone with a chronic ear discharge who develops new symptoms should, therefore, be sent for specialist assessment and biopsy.

Otalgia

The causes of earache are legion. This is because the ear is densely innervated and many structures give rise to referred pain. Dental disease and sinusitis are among the commonest causes of referred otalgia but a careful search should be made at more distant sites. This may require specialist referral to exclude, for example, a laryngeal carcinoma.

• *Furunculosis*: Boils in the ear canal are extremely painful. The redness, swelling and extreme tenderness are usually fairly obvious but can be confused with acute mastoiditis. Where possible, a meatal dressing or a Pope's otowick should be inserted and an oral 5-day course of flucloxacillin given.

• *Viral disorders*: Viral infection of the outer ear by herpes zoster may involve the geniculate ganglion with a facial palsy — *Ramsay Hunt syndrome*. Myringitis bullosa haemorrhagica is an uncommon complication of viral infection with very painful characteristic serosanguineous vesicles on the tympanic membrane. Treatment is to give simple analgesia and keep the ear dry.

• *Temporomandibular joint dysfunction* is a very common cause of ear pain, particularly in women who have had posterior teeth extracted or who have an overclosure of the bite. Specific treatment includes dental splintage, amitriptyline therapy and transcutaneous electrical nerve stimulation.

• *Laryngopharyngeal causes* of otalgia induce referred pain via the glossopharyngeal and vagus nerves. Probably the commonest are tonsillitis and tonsillectomy but in older patients, particularly those with a history of heavy smoking and drinking, head and neck tumours should always be borne in mind. Cervical spondylitis can also cause otalgia by involvement of the second and third cervical nerves.

Vertigo

Non-specific dizziness can be caused by a multitude of diseases from agoraphobia to uncontrolled diabetes. True *vertigo* is a sensation of movement of the patient relative to the surroundings. Vestibular disorders are often accompanied by nystagmus (see above).

Causes of vertigo

• *Viral labyrinthitis* is the commonest cause in young adults. There is a short history of rotatory dizziness, usually following an upper respiratory infection. Initially the patient may be confined to bed but, as central compensation and recovery of the affected labyrinth occur, balance gradually improves. In middle-aged subjects, there may be a recurrent form of vestibular neuronitis.

• *Vertebrobasilar ischaemia*: In older subjects especially smokers, this is probably the commonest cause of rotatory dizziness. Classically there are associated symptoms such as drop attacks and dysphagia but in practice many patients appear to have isolated dizziness which may have a component of cervical spondylosis.

• *Benign paroxysmal positional nystagmus*: The name is self-explanatory. Short bursts of rotatory vertigo are provoked by a head position. In benign positional nystagmus, there is fatigue and adaptation of the nystagmus on repeat positional testing in the clinic. Rehabilitation can involve avoidance of the provoking position. The many other causes of dizziness include trauma, ototoxicity, middle ear surgery and Ménière's disease.

• *Ménière's disease* is said to have affected Julius Caesar and Van Gogh. It has not been given a prominent place in the present summary because Ménière's disease is rare and overdiagnosed. Probably much of the Ménière's triad of dizziness, tinnitus and deafness is due to vertebrobasilar ischaemia. Ménière's disease is caused by a build-up of excessive endolymph within the inner ear. The eventual rupture of the membranous labyrinth casues an acute attack of vertigo which can last anything from about half an hour up to several hours. The patient is usually prostrate and may notice an exacerbation of deafness and tinnitus during the attack but is often so dizzy that these are peripheral concerns. The strict diagnostic criteria for Ménière's disease — a fluctuating hearing loss, usually maximum in the low tones and specific ENG features — preclude diagnosis by a non-specialist. Medical treatment is inner ear vasodilation, e.g. by naftidrofuryl oxalate (Praxilene) 100 mg t.i.d or diuretics. During the acute phase of any labyrnthine vertigo, the sedative prochlorperazine (Stemetil) gives symptomatic relief but does nothing to prevent long-term hearing loss. In refractory cases, surgi-cal decompression of the endolymphatic sac is of great benefit.

Facial nerve palsy

Central causes of facial nerve palsy, e.g. a stroke, may spare the forehead muscles because their bilateral cortical representation allows retention of function in supranuclear lesions. Peripheral causes of lower motor neuron facial nerve palsy, such as parotid gland tumours or facial trauma, may be obvious on clinical examination. The extent of paralysis can be assessed by electroneuronography. The nerve is stimulated at the stylomastoid foramen and recordings made from the facial muscles in response to a supramaximal stimulus. If less than 5% of the nerve fibres on the paralysed side are functioning compared with the good side and if there is a lesion such as a bone spicule from a fractured temporal bone, then surgical decompression of the nerve may be justified.

Bell's palsy

Bell's palsy is the commonest intratemporal facial nerve palsy but the aetiology remains unknown. It was once known as 'cabbie's face' as it occurred frequently among cab drivers in London. Various causes such as spasm of the small artery supplying the facial nerve or viral inflammation have been proposed. Well over 90% of patients have a full recovery. In older subjects, if there is total paralysis and severe pain, only 20% will have a good recovery. There is no specific treatment. Steroids have been tried by some but are of no proven benefit and are hazardous in the elderly. For the non-specialist perhaps the most important thing is to think about referring the patient if there is any doubt about the diagnosis, remembering that acoustic neuromas, congenital cholesteatomas, middle ear carcinoma or suppuration and other lesions such as sarcoidosis, diabetic cranial nerve palsy and arachnoid cysts or meningiomas of the cerebellopontine angle may all cause a facial nerve palsy.

Ear wax

Finally, we must consider ear wax because many patients regard the mere presence of wax as a symptom. Most health centres will carry out hundreds of ear syringings per annum but it is important to ascertain that the patient has a true complaint before undertaking the procedure. There are several potential hazards to ear syringing, including otitis externa, tympanic membrane perforation or vertigo, particularly in the presence of a pre-existing perforation. Syringing is the commonest source of iatrogenic ear disease in general practice. Where it is indicated, for example, to inspect the tympanic membrane, or if there is pain or tinnitus associated with the wax, then the wax should be softened with oil or sodium bicarbonate ear drops. It is quite safe to insert oil into a mastoid cavity. It is quite safe to use proprietary ear drops in the stated dose where there is a perforation. It is quite safe to fly with perforations or a grommet *in situ* — indeed these patients are at an advantage because they do not have any problems in equilibrating middle ear pressure. It is *not* safe, however, to syringe cavities, perforation or grommets. When in doubt, refer to a specialist.

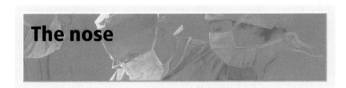

The nose

Evaluation of the patient

Clinical assessment

Symptoms

The main symptoms of nasal disorders are nasal blockage, sneezing, rhinorrhoea, postnasal drip, epistaxis, snoring, facial pain, halitosis, deformity of the nose and disorders of smell (Table 24.3). The time of onset of symptoms, exacerbating or relieving factors and variability with time of day of year should be sought. A history of allergies and smoking and an assessment of the patient's environment is also important.

Physical examination and investigation of the nose

First look at the shape of the nose. Is there any deviation and, if so, is it worse high up in the nasal bones or lower

Table 24.3 Symptoms of nasal disorders.

Nasal blockage
Sneezing
Rhinorrhoea
Postnasal drip
Epistaxis
Snoring
Facial pain
Halitosis
Deformity of the nose
Disorders of smell

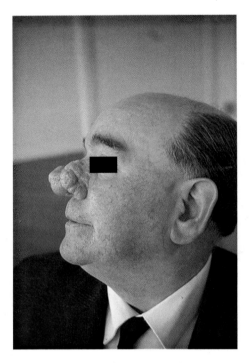

Figure 24.4 Patient with extensive rhinophyma.

down in the cartilage? Sometimes skin discoloration will signal systemic disease, e.g. lupus vulgaris (cutaneous tuberculosis), sarcoid or systemic lupus erythematosus. There may be evidence of tumour or of the much commoner rhinophyma — a bulbous nasal tip due to excessive seborrhoeic tissue (Fig. 24.4).

Now get the patient to tilt up the chin and look at the nostrils. They may be asymmetrical due to trauma, surgery or congenital abnormality, perhaps with an associated cleft lip or palate. Examination of the interior of the nose or anterior rhinoscopy is preceded by assessment of nasal airway. In a child, hold a mirror or metal tongue under the nostrils and inspect the two steam marks. Complete absence of one may indicate choanal atresia — failure of perforation *in utero* of the membrane at the back of the nose. Bilateral choanal atresia is a neonatal emergency — the baby is an obligate nose breather. Periodic oral gulps of air are drawn in as cyanosis develops. Treatment is insertion of an oral airway. In the adult, each nostril should be gently occluded by applying the pad of the (gloved) thumb, taking care not to push the septum into the test nostril, and asking the patient to sniff.

The tip of the nose should then be pushed gently up by the thumb and the interior illuminated by either a torch of an auriscope. A wide aural speculum gives a good view with a greater depth of field. The septum is examined for deviation and bleeding points and the cavity for discharge, polyps, tumour and, in children, foreign bodies. The side walls carry the three lateral swellings (conchae) which, in clinical practice, are known as the superior, middle and inferior turbinates. The superior turbinate is hidden, the middle turbinate may be swollen and, if in contact with the septum high up, may be a source of pain. The inferior is much the largest turbinate. It is important to realize that turbinates are normally salmon pink but that inflammatory nasal polyps are shiny grey.

Examination is completed by examination of the postnasal space and neck. Only the latter is possible without special instruments but occasionally large postnasal lesions — polyps, adenoids or tumours — hang down into the mouth. CT scanning is the most useful imaging technique for assessment of the nasal sinuses (Fig. 24.5).

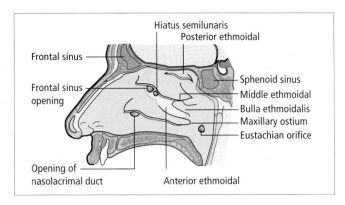

Figure 24.6 The lateral wall of the right nasal cavity: the turbinates have been partially removed.

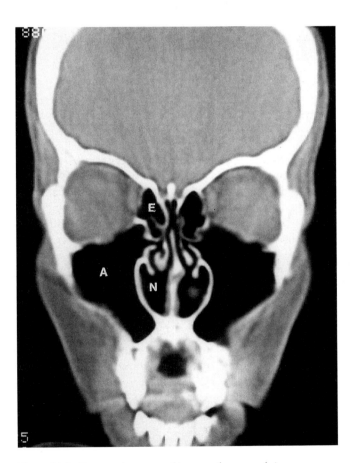

Figure 24.5 Computed tomographic scan of paranasal sinuses. E, ethmoid cells; A, maxillary antrum; N, nasal cavity.

Disorders of the nose

Nasal obstruction and rhinorrhoea

• *Adenoids* (Fig. 24.6) may give rise to nasal symptoms through enlargement or through acute or chronic infection. The child may be reported to snore, mouth-breathe and have hyponasal speech, chronic cough and vestibulitis. Adenoid tissue is very scanty under the age of 2 years and usually regresses in later childhood. It is probably more common nowadays for adenoidectomy to be carried out as part of the treatment for secretory otitis media.

• *Juvenile nasopharyngeal angiofibroma* is a much less common condition affecting largely prepubescent or pubertal males and may have a hormonal basis. Surgery requires careful planning with preoperative CT scanning, angiography and either a lateral rhinotomy or transpalatal approach. Always remember that nasal polyps are extremely rare in childhood and a polypoid lesion in a child should, therefore, be considered a tumour, or meningocele until proven otherwise, unless the child has cystic fibrosis.

• *Simple inflammatory nasal polyps* are related to intrinsic asthma and aspirin sensitivity but not to classical type 1 allergy. Conservative treatment is now favoured by some with, for example, Betnesol drops instilled into the nose in the kneeling, head-down (Mecca) position. Simple nasal polypectomy with wire snares may not be effective in the long term. Patients requiring many polypectomies may opt to have a more definitive procedure. This entails clearing out the ethmoid cells — polyps are simple hypertrophied, prolapsing ethmoid sinus lining.

• *Allergic rhinitis* affects 10% of the western population. The commonly inhaled allergens are dust, house dust mite protein, pollen, spores and animal dander. There may be associated sneezing and a history of eczema or extrinsic asthma in the subject or family. It is diagnosed on the basis of positive skin tests and, as desensitization is now banned on safety grounds, the mainstay of treatment is topical nasal steroid preparations such as Beconase and Rhinocort, or a selective H_1-antihistamine; this is much less sedative than the original antihistamines which have anticholinergic side-effects.

• *Vasomotor rhinitis* is a disorder of the autonomic control mechanisms which act to adjust the inspired air with changing conditions of temperature and humidity. (It is a normal experience on a cold winter morning when leaving a warm environment to have an engorged and dripping nose.) Some patients have an allergic component and respond to topical steroids. Others require surgical decongestion with submucosal diathermy or removal of the inferior turbinates.

• A *deviated nasal septum* may also cause nasal obstruction. This may be present from birth or be caused later by trauma or by a growth deformity. The nasal septum is the only midline-growing structure in the face and all of us have some degree of fascial asymmetry. The treatment is submucous resection of the nasal septum. Repositioning the septum — septoplasty — is used if there is an associated external deviation, in children or if the procedure is performed in conjunction with straightening of the nasal bones — rhinoplasty.

• *Nasal tumours* are very rare. One of the best known is the *inverted papilloma* which is essentially a benign growth but with a marked propensity for local recurrence and about an 8% malignant transformation rate. *Wegener's granuloma* is a systemic condition which also affects the lungs and kidneys and *Stewart's granuloma* is a type of localized lymphoma. In many parts of the world, *nasopharyngeal carcinoma* is a major disease, particularly in South-East Asia where it can account for 18% of all malignant tumours. Any person of Chinese extraction with cranial nerve palsies, epistaxis or unusual nasal symptoms should be suspected of having this disease and undergo specialist examination. Aetiology is complex but there appears to be an association with Epstein–Barr Virus. Cancer of the nose and sinuses is rare (1 per 300 000 population). The majority are squamous cell carcinomas which may cause nasal obstruction, polyps, bleeding, dental pain, loosening of teeth or dentures or a non-healing socket after tooth extraction. Extension may cause eye symptoms or cheek swelling. Patients tend to present late and the survival rate overall for sinus tumours is only 25%.

• *Cerebrospinal fluid*: Fracture of the cribriform plate following nasal or head trauma may lead to cerebrospinal fluid rhinorrhoea. Lesser leaks may close spontaneously but sometimes a craniotomy and formal repair of the dura are required to stop the leak.

Mucopurulent nasal discharge

• *Bacterial superinfection* following the common cold is the commonest cause of this symptom. The nasal lining may be damaged by addiction to topical pseudoephedrine preparation — rhinitis medicamentosa, best treated by topical nasal steroids. Discharge may also follow the presence of a foreign body or rhinolith, or primary ciliary dyskinesia with bronchiectasis and sometimes situs inversus (Kartagener's syndrome).

• *Sinusitis* affects the maxillary, ethmoid, frontal and sphenoid sinuses in that order of frequency. It follows mechanical or inflammatory obstruction of the natural ostium of the sinus (adenoids, polyps, deviated nasal septum, rhinitis). The discharge may be scanty and is accompanied by pain over the sinus or vertex, increased by bending, and peaking in the afternoon. Treatment of the acute phase is by decongestants and antibiotic therapy. Surgery is minimal to limit spread of infection.

There are few physical signs of chronic sinusitis. Beware the mucosal increase observed on plain sinus X-rays which accompanies any inflammation of the nose. There is a fitted carpet lining the whole of the nose and sinuses and patients with allergic rhinitis will also have mucosal swelling in the sinuses. Only CT scanning and nasoendoscopy can assess the ethmoid sinuses, the middle meatus and maxillary ostia. Classical operations include intranasal antrostomy to ventilate the antrum, or a Caldwell–Luc procedure where irreversibly diseased mucosa is removed through an anterior window. The rare frontal sinusitis is usually treated by an external frontoethmoidectomy or by an osteoplastic flap, where the front of the sinus is uncapped, like taking the top off an egg. With the emergence of endoscopic sinus surgery, which is more conservative, some of these radical procedures may become obsolete. The complications of sinusitis include orbital cellulitis, osteomyelitis with subperiosteal abscesses over the frontal bone (Pott's puffy tumour), cavernous sinus thrombosis and intracranial abscess. Any patient with suspected meningitis secondary to sinus disease should have a CT scan carried out to exclude an intracranial collection.

Epistaxis

Causes

• *Trauma*: Sometimes nasal bleeding follows obvious trauma. A fracture of the nasal bones, often associated with a fracture-dislocation of the septal cartilage, can be corrected with nasal manipulation under the briefest of general anaesthetics within the first 2 weeks following injury. If the procedure fails, then a formal rhinoplasty will be required at a later date. Major facial fractures, including the Le Fort maxillary fractures, may also cause epistaxis. Always check for a malar fracture, which may require zygomatic elevation in a patient with nasal injury. If there is a step on the infraorbital ridge, or infraorbital nerve paraesthesiae, there may be sufficient orbital blow-out to require open reduction via a Caldwell–Luc approach.

• Much commoner is epistaxis due to *microtrauma of Little's area* on the anteroinferior aspect of the septum. Insert your right index finger into the right vestibule — the pad of the distal phalanx rests on Little's area. Bleeding may be due to drying, particularly in the presence of the deviated nasal septum, and exacerbated by manual interference by the patient.

• It is hard to assess the role of *hypertension* in epistaxis. Attendance at hospital tends to elevate the blood pressure, while blood loss tends to reduce it. Coagulation defects, anticoagulation therapy and the extremes of age and climate are all predisposing factors.

Management of epistaxis

The simplest treatment is to press hard on the anterior, soft tip of the nose over Little's area. The patient leans forward and spits out any oral blood and sucks ice cubes. If this fails after 10 min of constant pressure then intervention is necessary. Good vasoconstriction and local anaesthesia are achieved by a pack of 2 ml of 4% cocaine on a 1 cm ribbon gauze dressing. If cocaine is not available then lignocaine and topical adrenaline solution may be used. After 15 to 20 min this will have arrested bleeding and anaesthetized the nasal cavity. Cautery of anterior bleeding points may be with silver nitrate, chromium trioxide, trichloracetic acid or electrocautery. Failing this, a nasal pack, traditionally soaked in bismuth iodoform paraffin paste (BIPP), is inserted. A postnasal pack or postnasal balloon may be required to control bleeding. The last resort is to carry out ethmoid, maxillary or even external carotid arterial ligation.

Snoring

The debate continues about whether or not snoring is an independent risk factor for cardiovascular disease. Nasal snoring results from a deviated nasal septum. In pharyngeal snoring vibration of the soft palate, sometimes in the presence of obesity narrowing the pharyngeal airway, or increased depths of sleep induced by alcohol, culminates in a low-grade form of obstructive sleep apnoea. The obstructive sleep apnoea can really be diagnosed only by formal study in a sleep lab where a low Po_2 and disturbed sleep pattern may be documented. In children, enormous hypertrophy of the tonsils and adenoids can lead to cor pulmonale. The treatment for severe snoring is uvulo-palatopharyngoplasty, an extended tonsillectomy involving removal of the uvula and soft palate. The principal postoperative complications are hypernasality and pharyngeal scarring.

Facial pain

• Much the commonest cause of facial pain is *dental disease* involving the pulp space or periodontal membrane.

• *Trigeminal neuralgia* is the commonest primary neuralgia, although the glossopharyngeal nerve can give rise to similar stabbing sharp pains, often triggered by chewing or other stimuli.

• *Postherpetic neuralgia* follows severe shingles (herpes zoster).

• Any *central lesion* of the brainstem causes ill-defined facial pain, as do base-of-skull tumours, including deep lobe parotid tumours. Lesions involving the trigeminal or glossopharyngeal nerves directly, for example sinus neoplasms or an elongated styloid process, are painful.

• *Sluder's neuralgia* results from pressure of the middle turbinate on the septum which gives pain around the bridge of the nose and inner canthus.

• *Periodic migrainous neuralgia* wakes the patient, typically a stressed or obsessional middle-aged man, in the early hours of the morning with unilateral pain associated with flushing, lacrimation, nasal blockage and rhinorrhoea.

• *Giant cell arteritis* affects older people and is diagnosed by an index of suspicion and a high erythrocyte sedimentation rate (ESR). Once confirmed by temporal artery biopsy, steroid therapy in instituted as a matter of urgency to prevent the complicating blindness which may occur.

• *Atypical facial pain* typically affects middle-aged women and has a psychological origin but exclusion of an organic cause for facial pain is no easy matter.

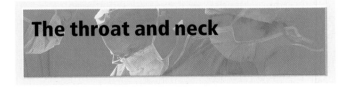

The throat and neck

Evaluation of the patient

Clinical assessment

Symptoms

The common symptoms of throat disorders are pain (tonsillitis), dysphagia (carcinoma of the hypopharynx or oesophagus), regurgitation (pharyngeal pouch), hoarseness, nasal and ear symptoms and a lump in the neck (nasopharyngeal tumours).

Physical examination and investigations

Mouth and throat

Having removed any dentures a close examination should be made of the lips, teeth, gums, buccal surfaces, parotid duct orifices and tongue, whose base is palpated, as it is a notorious area for silent head and neck cancers. Palpate the floor of the mouth bimanually in patients with suspected calculi or tumour. If the lower alveolar teeth are not within the upper alveolar ring there is bite over-closure. The oropharynx begins at the level of the anterior pillars of the fauces, behind which sit the palatine tonsils (Fig. 24.7). Medial displacement of the tonsil may be due to a deep parotid tumour or another mass deep in the neck in the parapharyngeal space. The rest of Waldeyer's ring of lymphoid tissue (lingual tonsils and adenoids) is usually not visible, although you may see patches of lymphoid tissue or lateral pharyngeal bands behind the posterior pillar of the fauces on the posterior pharyngeal wall. Check your own pharynx for these next time you have a cold. Check palatal movement and the gag reflex. Ask the patient to count to five and observe the voice quality. Vocal cord palsy is associated with gross air escape. Learning to perform indirect (mirror) examination of the larynx (Fig. 24.8) using a bull's-eye lamp focused by a head mirror takes several weeks and you should take every available opportunity to examine all visible landmarks at direct laryngoscopy in the anaesthetic room.

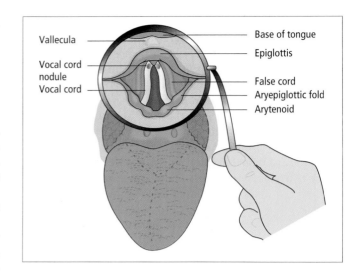

Figure 24.8 Mirror examination of the larynx in a patient with vocal nodules.

Neck

After inspection for obvious swellings, systematic bilateral palpation of the neck from behind should be performed. Palpate down along the trapezius muscles, up over the posterior triangles to the mastoid processes and down again anterior to the sternomastoids. Come up the central structures — thyroid, larynx, hyoid, — to the submental triangle and finally the submandibular area. Do not press on the salivary glands until you have looked at the duct orifices for the expression of pus.

Investigations

Laboratory investigation A full blood count and ESR should be performed in all patients. These are particularly useful in patients with suspected infection. The monospot test is performed in patients with suspected infectious mononucleosis. Patients with dysphagia should have serum proteins estimated, as albumin levels are usually reduced in these people. Serum iron and iron-binding capacity should be checked in those with suspected Plummer–Vinson syndrome (dysphagia, hypochromic microcytic anaemia, angular stomatitis, glossitis and koilonychia).

Imaging Plain film lateral radiographs are useful to give an indication of the size of a mass in the nasopharynx or hypopharynx. Barium swallow will detect oesophageal web, pharyngeal pouch or hypopharyngeal or oesophageal tumour. CT scanning is essential in defining naso-, oro- and

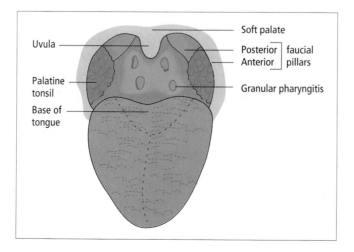

Figure 24.7 Examination of the oropharynx.

hypopharyngeal lesions and occasionally arteriography is indicated.

Disorders of the throat

Oral ulceration

Benign ulceration

Aphthous ulcers are essentially of unknown aetiology, although they appear to be increased by stress and are less common in cigarette smokers. Some are *herpetic* or *traumatic*, for example from ill-fitting dentures. In recurrent oral ulceration, B_{12} or *folate deficiency* may contribute. There is an increased incidence of a flat coeliac-type jejunum and an autoimmune component, particularly in *Behçets disease*, which is associated with human leucocyte antigen (HLA)-DR5.

Oral tumours

• Oral tumours may be preceded by *leukoplakia*, which has a 15% incidence of malignant transformation, or by *erythroplakia*, which has a very high malignant potential. *Squamous carcinoma* comprises 95% of all oral tumours, with a male to female ratio of 2 : 1 and a peak age in the seventh decade (Fig. 24.9). Patients may present with painful dysphagia and submandibular or upper deep cervical chain lymphadenopathy. Radiotherapy gives a 60% cure. The occurrence of *minor salivary gland tumours* within the oral cavity means that small oral lesions should not be subjected to an incisional biopsy because of the risk of implantation of a pleomorphic adenoma. *Malignant melanoma* at this site shares the uniformly gloomy prognosis of mucosal head and neck melanomas.

Vincent's angina

• Vincent's angina, a synergistic infection of a fusiform bacillus and a spirochaete, was formerly known as trench mouth but is now usually seen as a secondary infection of a malignant lesion, causing a horrible foetor. It can be treated successfully with antibiotics (e.g. penicillin or erythromycin and metronidazole). Because of its infectious nature patients should be barrier-nursed. Other rarer causes of oral ulceration include leukaemia, acquired immune deficiency syndrome (AIDS) and syphilis (e.g. primary chancre of the lip or tonsil; secondary syphilic lesions occur anywhere in the oral cavity and are highly contagious).

Sore throat

Infections

• In *viral sore throat* in children, look for Koplik's spots — a prodromal sign of measles.

• *Granular pharyngitis* is common in the British climate (Fig. 24.7). Other aetiological factors are chronic obstructive airways disease, gastro-oesophageal reflux and postnasal drip.

• *Tonsillitis* is now considered to justify tonsillectomy if it occurs in six mild or three to four severe attacks per annum. The patient has a high temperature, white spots on the tonsil and painful dysphagia. The principal hazards of tonsillectomy are haemorrhage and having to re-anaesthetize a patient whose pharynx is full of blood. Untreated tonsillitis can progress in young adults to a *peritonsillar abscess* or *quinsy*. This gives muffled speech or palatal swelling and displacement of the uvula of the contralateral side. It is treated either by aspiration or incision and drainage under topical anaesthesia. The differential diagnosis includes infectious mononucleosis and, in developing countries, diphtheria. Secondary infection may occur in the retropharyngeal, parapharyngeal or submandibular spaces. Infection of the submandibular space (Ludwig's angina) produces a strangulated voice and can be rapidly fatal because of airway obstruction.

Malignancy

• *Cancer of the oropharynx* is squamous cell-type in 75% of cases. The rest are lymphomas. In 20% of tonsil carcinomas, the only symptom will be of a lymph node in the neck.

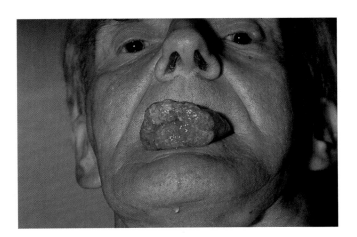

Figure 24.9 Carcinoma of the tongue.

Twenty per cent of oropharyngeal cancers are incurable because of advanced local disease (Horner's sign or trismus) or spread to bilateral nodes or distant sites. Where nodes are present, surgery is the treatment of choice — the commando operation (combined oral mandibular operation) with reconstruction by a pectoralis major myocutaneous flap. A radical neck dissection is also required. It should be appreciated that head and neck cancer is essentially a local disease. Aggressive local surgery is much more appropriate than in, for example, breast cancer where there are early distant metastases. In a radical neck dissection, an attempt is made to remove all the major lymph nodes in the neck, together with the internal jugular vein, sternomastoid muscle tail of parotid, submandibular gland and accessory nerve. Paralysis of the accessory gland often results in some painful drooping of the shoulder.

• Extensive lymphatic drainage gives *cancer of the base of tongue* a worse prognosis than soft palatal and posterior pharyngeal wall tumours, which are also more easily observed following radiotherapy.

Hoarseness

It is a useful rule that if hoarseness persists for more than 6 weeks, the patient should be referred to a specialist because of the risk of tumour being present.

• The commonest cause of hoarseness is, of course, *acute laryngitis* which accompanies an upper respiratory tract infection. A professional singer with acute laryngitis must cancel performances or risk a bleed into the vocal cords which may cause irreparable damage and nodule formation.

• *Voice strain* is common in teachers or amateur singers, particularly those singing at too high a pitch with tense laryngeal muscles and air escape. Fibreoptic video laryngoscopy is useful to the speech therapist to demonstrate the abnormality to the patient and also to follow the progress of therapy. Untreated voice strain can lead to vocal nodules (Fig. 24.8), otherwise known as screamer's nodes. These also occur in children. They occur at the point of maximum vibration of the vocal cord. Because the posterior one-third of the vocal cord is cartilaginous, the point of maximum vibration is situated at the junction of the anterior one-third and the posterior two-thirds of the vocal cords.

• *Spasmodic dysphonia* gives a somewhat strangled voice, often precipitated by trauma and exacerbated by stress. It was thought for many years to be of psychosomatic origin but there is a current fashion to use botulinum toxin injections to the vocal cord in treatment.

• *Chronic laryngitis* is caused by smoking, vocal abuse and, when occurring in the posterior third, probably also by gastro-oesophageal reflux. Unlike carcinoma, the changes are symmetrical. A fluid collection in the subepithelial space of the cords is known as Reinke's oedema, which tends to occur in middle-aged women who smoke.

• *Tuberculosis* is now a rare cause of laryngeal inflammation.

• In a *laryngocele* an air-filled sac develops in the laryngeal ventricle. It may present as a swelling in the neck and is clearly visible on an X-ray of the neck during a Valsalva manoeuvre. Treatment is by excision.

• *Benign tumours* of the larynx include *viral papillomas* which occur predominantly in childhood or adolescence. *Intubation granuloma* is now a rare sequel of intensive care unit therapy due to the use of high-volume, low-pressure cuffed endotracheal tubes with minimal movement. It can, however, follow a long operation on a too lightly anaesthetized patient and occasionally it leads to subglottic stenosis in premature babies managed in special care baby units for prolonged periods of time.

• *Cancer of the larynx* as elsewhere in the head and neck, is usually squamous carcinoma. Fortunately, the glottis is the commonest site as this tends to present early because of the hoarseness due to incomplete closure of the vocal cords. Those in the subglottis tend to present with inspiratory and expiratory (tracheal) stridor while those in the supraglottis can present late with a mass in the neck or dysphagia. Glottic carcinoma can be preceded by dysplasia, whose malignant potential depends on the severity of the epithelial abnormality. In general, T1 and T2 tumours, i.e. those involving one of two regions of the larynx but with mobile vocal cords, are adequately treated by radiotherapy, provided the patient stops smoking. T1 tumours of the glottis have a greater than 95% cure rate. T3 tumours (fixed vocal cords) or T4 tumours (spread outside the larynx) are more likely to require primary surgery, which in this country is almost always total laryngectomy. Social support is available from the National Association of Laryngectomy Clubs and voice rehabilitation is possible with oesophageal speech, neoglottis valve or a cervical or oral vibrator.

• *Vocal cord paralysis* is commoner on the left because of the longer course of the left recurrent laryngeal nerve. Recurrent nerve palsy is caused by carcinoma of the bronchus (at the left hilium or right lung apex), thyroid surgery or cancer, oesophageal cancer, pharyngeal pouch surgery, cricopharyngeal myotomy and left atrial hypertrophy, or may be idiopathic or viral. The vagal trunk is affected by base-of-skull disease or by bulbar palsy due to vascular or motor neuron disease. If one vocal cord is abducted it can be medialized by an injection of Teflon or collagen, or insertion of a Silastic strut — thyroplasty. One adducted cord is not a major problem but if both cords are adducted, giving stridor, one may require to be lateralized, or a tracheostomy fashioned.

Cervical dysphagia

- Any *lower oesophageal cause* of dysphagia can be perceived by the patient to be cervical in origin.
- True cervical dysphagia can be caused by any of the *painful oropharyngeal conditions* already alluded to.
- Acute dysphagia following *foreign body impaction* is particularly common in the edentulous. A gas shadow may be seen on lateral soft-tissue neck X-ray above the obstruction. Remember that fish bones and false teeth are frequently radiolucent. A fish bone felt to be above the hyoid is often seen in the tonsil. Patients with suspected bolus obstruction should be referred to hospital. Left untreated, oesophageal perforation can ensue. *Upper oesophageal webs* are seen as fine anterior radiographic indentations at the pharyngo-oesophageal junction, mostly in women and probably increased by iron deficiency. Treatment is by oesophageal dilatation and iron supplementation. *Pharyngeal pouch* (Fig. 24.10) is a midline posterior pulsion diverticulum through Killian's dehiscence, between the thyropharyngeus and cricopharyngeus portions of the inferior constrictor, commonest in the seventh decade. It may be

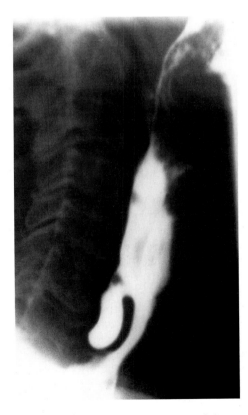

Figure 24.10 Lateral barium swallow radiograph of pharyngeal pouch.

due to muscle dysfunction, although this does not explain the six-fold male preponderance. Treatment of small pouches is by dilatation, perhaps with the addition of cricopharyngeal myotomy. Larger pouches require, in addition to the myotomy, to be excised or inverted (diverticulopexy).

- *Hypopharyngeal carcinoma* arises between the floor of the vallecula and the inferior margin of the cricoid cartilage (pharyngo-oesophageal junction). Three subdivisions of the hypopharynx are recognized. The *posterior hypopharyngeal wall* runs from the level of the hyoid to the inferior margin of the cricoid and 10% of hypopharyngeal tumours arise here. The *postcricoid region* itself is the short area on the back of the cricoid lamina, the only head and neck site with a female preponderance of squamous carcinoma which may be associated with a web. The third region of the hypopharynx comprises the *piriform fossae*, a pair of pouches posterolateral to the larynx on each side of the oesophageal inlet. Imagine looking down on the larynx and pushing a finger down each side of the laryngeal inlet. The tips will lodge in the piriform fossae which lie immediately deep to the thyrohyoid membrane. About 60% of hypopharyngeal tumours occur in this area, whose rich lymphatic drainage results in early nodal metastasis. CT scanning may be useful to define the extent of the disease and to plan treatment. In general, large tumours with large nodes are best managed with primary surgery and early disease by radical radiotherapy. After resection there may be primary closure of the pharynx, partial replacement with a pectoralis major flap or a total laryngectomy and replacement of the pharynx by a free jejunal graft with microvascular anastomosis to cervical vessels. If there is involvement of the cervical oesophagus then a laryngopharyngo-oesophagectomy is required, usually with replacement by a stomach pull-up or colon interposition.

Globus sensation

The symptom of a feeling of something in the throat is known as globus hystericus (Latin *globus* = ball; Greek *hysteros* = womb) — the ancients thought it was due to a migrant uterus. The condition is around three times commoner in women and, while organic theories such as gastro-oesophageal reflux and cricopharyngeal spasm were popular in the 1970s it now seems that at least a significant minority of patients with globus sensation are psychologically distressed. The commonest associations are somatization disorders, threatening life events and anxiety. Patients with long-standing globus should be referred for specialist reassurance which can itself have a therapeutic effect for the patient and allows detection of any associated structural lesion. Any patient who has atypical features such as pain, true dysphagia or weight loss should be referred as a matter of urgency.

Stridor

Stridor is a noise caused by obstruction to the upper respiratory tract. By convention, stridor refers to the inspiratory noise caused by obstruction above the level of the larynx or to the inspiratory and expiratory noise caused by obstruction in the trachea. Obstruction of the lower airways which causes noise on expiration is known as wheeze. The distinction might appear to be clearcut but many expert clinicians have been embarrassed by failing to diagnose stridor and treating the patient for asthma (see also Chapter 19).

• *Congenital stridor* can be caused by a laryngeal web, a cyst, vocal cord paralysis, vascular abnormalities, micrognathia, laryngeal cleft, and a variety of benign tumours. The commonest cause of stridor in infancy, however, is laryngomalacia, in which floppy laryngeal cartilages collapse on exertional respiration.

Beyond infancy, stridor is either infective or inflammatory or structural in origin.

• *Inflammatory causes* of stridor include *acute epiglottitis* which is often caused by *Haemophilus influenzae* and is commoner in children, although it can occur in adults. George Washington died within 24 h with fever, severe pain in the throat and respiratory distress, almost certainly due to epiglottitis. In the stridulous child, minor stress such as attempted examination or X-ray can precipitate respiratory arrest and both activities are strictly contraindicated. Treatment is by chloramphenicol and steroids, with upper airway protection (see below).

• Another childhood inflammation is *acute laryngotracheobronchitis* or croup. This is a viral infection which may often be adequately managed by placing the child in the moist air of a croupette.

• *Infectious mononucleosis* can cause fatal upper airway obstruction in adults if the tonsillar and pharyngeal swelling becomes sufficiently marked.

• *Inhaled foreign bodies* in children are a well-known source of upper respiratory obstruction. A large sweet, for example, can be aspirated or a coin swallowed and lodged, usually at the level of the vocal cords. Sometimes this obstruction can be relieved by the Heimlich manoeuvre or by tilting the child and giving a sharp slap between the shoulder blades. Failing this, laryngotomy may be necessary or the child may die before being hospitalized.

• *Laryngeal trauma*, either mechanical or due to thermal injury, may also cause stridor.

• Frequently in adults, however, the cause is *transglottic laryngeal carcinoma* or other upper aerodigestive tract neoplasm. This may cause stridor either by mechanical obstruction or by involvement of the recurrent laryngeal nerves.

• The commonest cause of bilateral recurrent laryngeal nerve palsy, however, is as a result of *thyroid surgery*.

Management of upper airway obstruction

In children with acute upper airway obstruction, endotracheal intubation by a paediatric anaesthetist may be possible with an otolaryngologist standing by to intervene if necessary. In adults with acute respiratory obstruction, surgery is usually the treatment of choice. For the nonspecialist, the relief of acute upper airway obstruction at the bedside, or indeed on the top of a bus, is best effected by inserting a penknife through the cricothyroid membrane — laryngotomy — a frequent procedure in the days of endemic diphtheria.

Laryngotomy

Extend your neck and feel the ridge of the cricoid. The cricothyroid membrane is just above this. Keep strictly in the midline. There are no intervening vessels. The vocal cords are very much higher, behind the midpoint of the thyroid cartilage. The scalpel, penknife blade or biro tubing may be used to hold the membrane open. An alternative is to insert one or two large-bore intravenous cannulae through this avascular superficial structure (see Fig. 3.3).

Tracheostomy

In contrast, incisions on the front of the trachea encounter not only the thyroid isthmus but also the anterior jugular veins and strap muscles. Only an expert can readily perform an emergency tracheotomy, although this is the only way to relieve airway obstruction at the level of the cricoid cartilage or below. The old aphorism that 'the time to do a tracheotomy is the time that it is first considered' remains true. Unlike respiratory failure due to lower airway obstruction, there is no gradual change in blood gases which signals the right time to perform the operation. Because of compensatory hyperventilation, the patient will not become hypoxic or hypercarbic until respiratory arrest is imminent. It is unwise to let any patient go to sleep with impending airway obstruction because respiratory failure may supervene overnight and pass unnoticed.

Cervical swelling

The causes of cervical swelling are legion (Fig. 24.11). Their differential diagnosis has been greatly simplified by

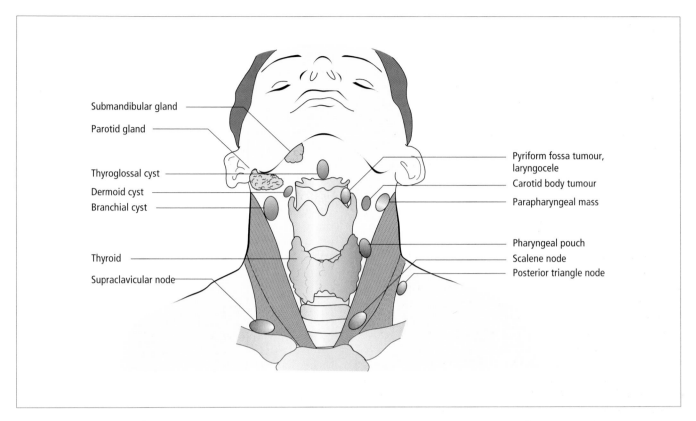

Figure 24.11 Cervical swellings.

the advent of fine-needle aspiration cytology, which has a high level of accuracy (over 90%) in the head and neck. Also, because of the wide variety of anatomical structures and pathologies which can occur in the head and neck area, the early use of fine-needle aspiration allows subsequent investigations to be directed. Thus, if a lesion is found at an early stage to be lymphoma, the subsequent investigation is quite different than if it were of thyroid origin or a metastatic adenocarcinoma metastatic from some distant site.

25 Ophthalmic Disorders

It so happens that if there is one thing I am good at, it is taking things out of eyes; cinders, flies, gnats on picnics or whatever it may be.   (P.G. Wodehouse 1881–1975)

Introduction

The medical student traditionally worries about ocular disease. Sight is such an important faculty and the eye seems to be small and difficult to examine. It is not surprising then that students are apprehensive about ocular signs. In fact, things are relatively uncomplicated, for the symptoms are usually confined to pain or blurring of vision — just occasionally double vision. A basic understanding of the anatomy of the eye and visual pathways is mandatory and can be found in any student's anatomy textbook. The following chapter attempts to give a résumé of the important ocular conditions that will allow a sufficient ophthalmic knowledge to carry students through their exams and then hopefully on the wards as a house officer in casualty departments or in general practice.

Evaluation of the patient

Clinical assessment

Symptoms

Most ophthalmic problems can be diagnosed with a good history and careful clinical examination. As many systemic diseases affect the eye, a good general history needs to be obtained first. General points to consider are:

- Medical history: hypertension, diabetes mellitus, sarcoidosis, inflammatory bowel disease.
- Family history: squint and some types of glaucoma may be familial.
- Drug history: some drugs affect the eye, e.g. chloroquine, ethambutol, systemic steroids.
  The specific points to consider in eye disease include:
- Ocular history: short- or long-sightedness; history of trauma, previous eye surgery.
- Eye pain: mode of onset, severity, gritty feeling, associated discharge/redness, photophobia.
- Visual symptoms: monocular or binocular blurring or loss of vision, related to posture, rate of onset, flashing lights, field loss, double vision, amaurosis fugax (see Chapter 18).

Physical examination

For the purpose of physical examination, the eye includes the following elements: eyelids, the conjunctiva, the cornea, sclera, the orbits and the eye ball. An assessment of eye function is made by examining visual acuity, the visual fields, the pupillary reflexes and the eye movements. The fundi may be examined with the ophthalmoscope.

The elements

- Eyelids: look for ptosis, xanthelasma, exophthalmos (lid lag), ectropion, basal cell carcinoma, stye (chalazion).

- Conjunctiva: pallor, injection, chemosis.
- Cornea: ulcer, arcus senilis.
- Anterior chamber: check for blood (hyphaema) or pus.
- Sclera: yellow in jaundice, blue in osteogenesis imperfecta.
- Orbit: palpate for tenderness: anaesthesia or hypo-aesthesia of the cheek indicates inferior orbital nerve damage.
- Eyeball: palpate to get an impression of intraorbital pressure.

Eye function

- Visual acuity: this is usually checked using a standard Snellen chart at 6 m with glasses if worn or pinhole.
- Visual fields: the patient sits facing the examiner and both examiner and patient cover their respective eyes not being tested, e.g. the patient covers the right eye and the examiner covers the left eye. The patient looks at the examiner's face while the examiner moves a red-headed pin into the visual field from the periphery. The patient indicates when he or she first sees red.
- Pupillary reflexes: The direct and consensual light reflex and the accommodation reflex are a simple way of checking the integrity of the anterior visual pathways.
- Swinging light reflex: The symmetry of pupil responses should be checked by the swinging light test which will detect a relative defect in the afferent input in one eye compared with the other — as with an optic nerve lesion on one side. As the light moves from the normal to the defective eye, the pupil response is to dilate, rather than to constrict. This difference is made more obvious if the light is moved repeatedly from one eye to the other.
- Eye movements: The eyes should be assessed for movement in all directions to check the function of third, fourth and sixth cranial nerves. Fatigability of eye muscles should be tested by continuous upward gaze. In myasthenia gravis the muscles tire and ptosis occurs. In Horner's syndrome the pupil is small but reactive (miosis); there is also ptosis and lack of sweating (anhydrosis). In third-nerve palsy, the pupil may be large, with ptosis and sometimes abnormal eye movement.
- Corneal reflex: The patient blinks when the cornea is stimulated. This checks the integrity of cranial nerve V.

Investigations

The general investigations depend on the clinical evaluation and the need to identify an underlying cause for the eye signs, e.g. a CT scan would be indicated in someone with bitemporal hemianopia to confirm the presence of a pituitary lesion; a carotid duplex scan would be indicated in a patient with a history of amaurosis fugax. However, simple specific eye investigations include fluorescein testing and ophthalmoscopy.

- *Ophthalmoscopy*: The 'red reflex' should be elicited first. The ophthalmoscope is set at the 0 lens and the eye is viewed from about 60 cm away. The reflection from the fundus is seen as red; this is the red reflex. (It is also seen in photographs of people taken with a flash.) Any opacity between the cornea and the fundus will disrupt the reflex: the commonest cause is a cataract. The ophthalmoscope is then brought close to the patient's eye and the lens setting is altered until a clear view of the retina can be obtained (Fig. 25.1). The optic disc is sought, The edges of the disc are examined (a blurred edge may indicate a cerebral tumour) and the retina should be scanned for exudates, haemorrhage or new vessel formation. Finally the macula should be examined (macular exudates may be seen in diabetes; see Fig. 25.6).
- *Fluorescein testing*: A few drops of fluorescein are instilled on to the cornea and the cornea is examined with a blue light. Any abrasion or ulceration of the cornea will easily be seen as a green lesion on the corea.
- *Dilating the pupil*: Most optic discs are visible through a normal pupil but dilating drops should be used if the pupils are too small, if there is a cataract, or if the retina in general (particularly the fovea) needs to be inspected. Tropicamide 1%, available as a single-dose 'minim', dilates the pupil within 20 min and wanes after about 2 hours. Do not dilate if acute neurological observation is needed. Using this agent the risk of precipitating acute glaucoma is extremely low.

More sophisticated investigation requires referral to an ophthalmologist.

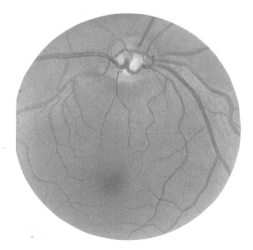

Figure 25.1 Normal fundus showing optic nerve head (disc) and macula, which surrounds the central fovea.

Table 25.1 Causes of an acute red eye.

Conjunctivitis
    Bacterial
    Viral
    Chlamydial
    Allergic
    Foreign body
Acute anterior uveitis (iritis, iridocyclitis)
Acute glaucoma
Episcleritis and scleritis

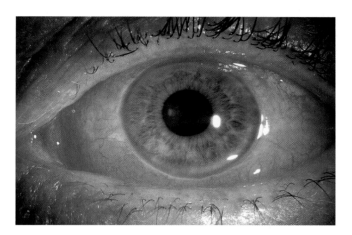

Figure 25.2 Red eye due to adenovirus conjunctivitis. Note the swelling of conjunctiva and scanty discharge.

The acute red eye

For the medical student the acute red eye is the principal ocular emergency. The categories that need to be considered are given in Table 25.1.

Acute conjunctivitis

Bacterial

The common bacterial invasions are usually from *Staphylococcus aureus*, although *Haemophilus influenzae* may occur in epidemics. Pneumococcal conjunctivitis may be unpleasant, particularly in children, and *pseudomonas* may invade the conjunctiva in debilitated patients, especially those in intensive care units. The eyes generally are very red with a sticky discharge. Patients usually describe a gritty sensation rather than pain in the eyes. The lids may be stuck together on waking in the morning. Unless the cornea is involved, photophobia is rare and generally the vision is good and unimpaired by the condition beyond minor blurring. The pupil reaction is always normal. The treatment of bacterial conjunctivitis is generally intensive topical antibiotics, with chloramphenicol being the most common used. It is important to instill the drops on a 2-hourly basis for at least 24 h before tailing off the treatment, otherwise insufficient application will produce relatively little improvement.

Viral

Viral conjunctivitis is more common and may accompany a flu-like illness, particularly that due to the adenovirus. Type 8 adenovirus may be responsible for epidemics of keratoconjunctivitis. If the cornea is involved there may be quite acute photophobia and pain. Viral conjunctivitis tends to settle spontaneously, but topical antibiotics will do no harm (Fig. 25.2).

Chlamydial

An increasingly common form of conjunctivitis is due to *Chlamydia trachomatis*, which is often found in young people and may be sexually transmitted, such that there is chlamydial infection in the genitourinary tract as well as the eye (see Chapter 20). Chlamydial conjunctivitis is best treated with tetracycline or erythromycin orally unless there is some contraindication, such as pregnancy. If the disease is found in a young child or pregnant adult, he or she should not be given tetracycline as it causes staining in developing teeth. Tetracycline ointment used five times daily is also necessary.

Ophthalmia neonatorum is contracted at birth from an infected cervix or vagina and used to be due to the gonococcus (Box 25.1). Now it is far more commonly due to

---

Elizabeth Blackwell

Elizabeth Blackwell (1821–1910) graduated from Geneva Medical College NY in 1849, the first woman to become a medical doctor. She wanted to be a gynaecological surgeon but being a woman in a male dominated profession she could only obtain training as a midwife in La Maternite Hospital in Paris. One night she was syringing the eyes of a baby with ophthalmia neonatorum when the water splashed up into her own eyes. She rapidly developed a purulent conjunctivitis which left her completely blind in one eye and partially blind in the other. Undaunted she abandoned her surgical ambitions, applied herself to medicine and eventually established a medical practice in New York. She also opened a hospital and founded a medical school for training women doctors in the USA and eventually returned to her native England where she became professor of gynaecology at the London School of Medicine for Women.

Box 25.1

Chlamydia. It is a notifiable disease. Any eye discharge within 3 weeks of birth is considered notifiable. Treatment is as described for chlamydial conjunctivitis after swabs have been taken. Generally speaking, this has to be combined with topical antibiotics and small babies need to be admitted, for the treatment is really very difficult to administer without expertise from trained nursing staff.

Allergic

Atopic patients are often susceptible to outbreaks of allergic disease of the conjunctiva, particularly during the pollen season, when the eye may become acutely congested and extremely itchy. Sticky discharge is generally described as white, in contrast to the yellow pus associated with infective conjunctivitis, and is stringy in texture.

Allergy may be seen with a form of contact sensitivity in the eye due to the application of make-up or the use of astringent drops purchased without prescription from a pharmacist when the skin takes on a typical look of contact dermatitis.

The treatment for acute allergic conjunctivitis in the atopic patient is topical steroid combined with Opticrom drops. The steroid is tailed off rapidly once the inflammation has come under control. The use of Opticrom should prevent further attacks and patients tend to manage the condition themselves once they have been educated. The pros and cons of using topical steroid will be discussed below.

Foreign body

A conjunctival or corneal foreign body may induce a painful red eye and this is a commonly seen problem in casualty departments. Usually there is a history of trauma, but sometimes patients have no recollection of injury. It is important to recognize and remove foreign bodies as soon as possible. Local anaesthetic eye drops will be required to examine the eye properly. The upper lid should be everted to exclude or remove a subtarsal foreign body. A superficial foreign body may be washed out of the eye or removed with a cotton-wool bud, but foreign bodies that are embedded in the cornea may have to be removed with a needle tip or special drill under local anaesthetic. Following removal, chloramphenicol ointment and a pad should be applied to the eye for 24–48 h. More serious eye injuries require expert management by eye surgeons.

Acute anterior uveitis, iritis, iridocyclitis

The uveal tract is made up of the iris, ciliary body and choroid; if the inflammation is mainly anterior it is termed anterior uveitis, iritis or iridocyclitis.

Anterior uveitis/iritis is a serious cause of the acute red eye. Classically the eye redness is most marked adjacent to the corneal margin. This is unlike conjunctivitis where the whole eye tends to be red. A small pupil is common with spasm of the iris sphincter from inflammation. There will be cells in the anterior chamber, but this is often only seen on examination with a slit lamp. In severe cases the inflammation may build up as a hypopyon if the outflow from the eye is obstructed and the intraocular pressure rises. Adhesions between the iris and the lens are known as posterior synechiae and cause distortion of the pupil which is most obvious when the pupil is dilated. If the posterior synechiae are confluent all the way round the pupil margin, aqueous cannot drain through the pupil; this causes an iris bombe with severe secondary glaucoma.

Anterior uveitis/iritis is painful and, unlike conjunctivitis, this pain is aching rather than 'gritty'. Closing the eyes or bathing does not relieve any of the symptoms. The eye is often excessively light-sensitive — so-called photophobia. Acute iritis often takes 2 or 3 days to develop into a painful red eye. Patients who have previous attacks sense that things are building up again and they confusingly present themselves at casualty departments with a white eye and relatively little to find. The experienced practitioner however will ensure that careful slit-lamp examination is carried out.

In practical terms most anterior uveitis/iritis is of unknown aetiology and is treated using topical steroids and pupillary dilators to prevent synechiae forming between the lens and the posterior iris. Moreover, dilatation paralyses the muscles of the iris and ciliary body and relieves painful spasm. It is therefore particularly important when treating a patient with a red eye to distinguish between anterior uveitis/iritis, sometimes with a small pupil that requires pupillary dilatation, and acute glaucoma with a large oval pupil which requires pupillary constriction.

Acute glaucoma

Acute glaucoma is a rare condition. To understand it a basic knowledge of the anatomy of aqueous production and drainage within the eye is required (Fig. 25.3). Aqueous is normally produced in the ciliary body by a process of ultrafiltration and active secretion. The aqueous passes into the posterior chamber, circulates through the pupil into the anterior chamber and is able to escape from the eye through the trabecular meshwork. This links up with the canal of Schlemm and then into the episcleral veins and main circulation. The angle between the iris and the trabecular meshwork is called the drainage angle.

Most drainage angles are wide open, with easy access from the anterior chamber to the trabecular meshwork.

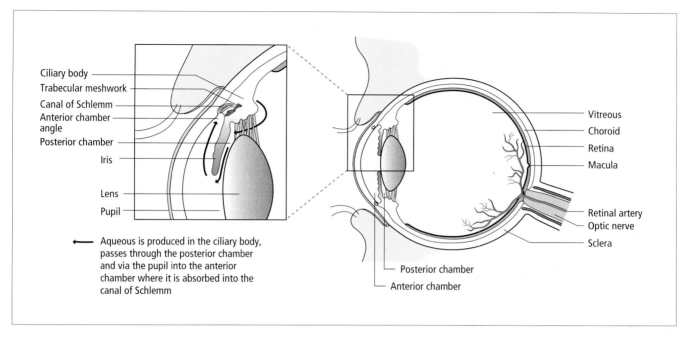

Figure 25.3 The anatomy of the eye and (inset) the aqueous circulation.

Some eyes, however, have very narrow drainage channels. These are usually small eyes and patients with small eyes tend to be long-sighted, for the optical power of the eye cannot overcome the short axial length. If for some reason the drainage channel between the iris and cornea narrows in patients with already narrow drainage angles, complete closure of the angle may take place, leading to acute obstruction to the circulation of aqueous. This process is called *acute-angle closure glaucoma*. This can be provoked by the pupillary-dilating effects of topical mydriatics or the anticholinergic effect of many medications, e.g. tricyclic antidepressants, antiemetics and antispasmodics. Similarly, the drainage angle may narrow with age or an increase in lens size due to a cataract will result in the lens pushing forwards to obliterate the angle.

The sudden rise in intraocular pressure provoked by acute angle closure may cause corneal oedema due to interference with normal corneal endothelial cell function. This produces the visual symptoms of haloes with a rainbow pattern around white lights. This is very striking and may cause the patient some consternation. It is different from the haloes produced by cataracts, which tend not to be coloured. The patient may have intermittent symptoms of glaucoma with spontaneous resolution for months prior to an acute attack.

Once the pressure has risen and the cornea becomes oedematous, the eye rapidly becomes ischaemic. The iris becomes enlarged and oval. The pain is intense; it is described as an aching pain and is often severe enough to provoke vomiting. Sight is lost due to the high pressure affecting the ocular circulation and it is only a matter of hours before irreversible blindness occurs. Patients with acute glaucoma are often misdiagnosed in casualty departments. The most common fault is to assume that the vomiting is due to some sort of acute abdominal problem and they are shipped off to the surgical ward.

The difference between acute glaucoma and other causes of a red eye is the degree of visual deterioration and the irregular, oval, slightly dilated pupil. The pain tends to be far worse than that produced by other forms of acute red eye, except perhaps intense scleritis, in which there is also a mixture of ischaemia and inflammation.

As far as treatment is concerned, the most important medication to administer is intravenous acetazolamide (Diamox) 500 mg. This will reduce aqueous production in the eye. Pilocarpine drops are then instilled; this may constrict the pupil and pull the iris away from the closed angle. There is no point in giving pilocarpine if the pressure is very high, for the iris is too ischaemic to respond to pilocarpine stimulation. Topical steroids and β-blocking agents such as timolol may also need to be used to bring the pressure down. Sometimes these measures are ineffective and intravenous mannitol is required. Surgery as a means of treating acute glaucoma is hazardous unless the pressure is brought down medically first. Laser iridotomy may be necessary.

The use of potent agents such as intravenous acetazolamide or mannitol must be measured against the patient's general health. They can be detrimental in diabetics (where intense dehydration or acidosis may be produced) or in patients with chronic renal failure. However, unless these medications are given the sight will be lost.

In suspected cases of acute glaucoma it is generally best to commence therapy with acetazolamide tablets immediately if there may be a delay in referring the patient to an ophthalmologist, by which time severe damage may have occurred in the eye. It is always possible to diagnose angle-closure glaucoma in retrospect, so there is no need to fear that the medication will interfere with later assessment.

Corneal ulcers

Corneal ulceration is most commonly viral, bacterial or traumatic. An ulcer characteristically causes pain, watering and photophobia. Ulcers are highlighted with fluorescein, especially if viewed with a blue light. Herpes simplex often produces a dendritic or branching pattern in the acute stage; herpes zoster may cause a similar appearance. Traumatic ulcers may become secondarily infected with bacteria, especially with contact lens wear. Hypersensitivity to chronic staphylococcal infection of the eyelids (blepharitis) may cause marginal ulcers at the edge of the cornea, which tend to be recurrent. Each type of ulcer needs specific treatment, so patients should be referred without delay to an ophthalmic specialist, otherwise a corneal scar may result.

Episcleritis and scleritis

The inflammatory causes of a red eye include episcleritis and scleritis. These may or may not be associated with systemic diseases, particularly rheumatoid arthritis, polyarteritis nodosa and Wegener's granulomatosis.

Episcleritis presents classically as an uncomfortable red eye or sometimes the eye may simply be red with no other features at all. The pupil is not involved and vision is unimpaired.

Scleritis can be very severe. It is a potentially blinding disease. There is a distinction between scleritis which simply forms inflammatory painful nodules and a form where a vasculitis leads to painful ischaemia. These conditions are termed either nodular scleritis, which is relatively benign, or severe necrotizing scleritis.

Treatment of episcleritis is confined to the use of topical steroid or non-steroidal anti-inflammatory ointments, such as a variation of phenylbutazone. Scleritis which threatens

sight requires an oral agent such as flurbiprofen (Froben) or high doses of systemic steroids and is a matter for expert assessment as an inpatient.

Topical steroids and the red eye

If the herpes simplex virus was responsible for the initial redness, corneal ulceration will probably worsen and blindness may follow. Allergic eye disease will improve dramatically with steroids, but the problem is weaning patients off the medication. If used for a prolonged period, topical steroids provoke a rise in intraocular pressure with irreversible damage to the optic nerve. Topical steroids may be used in patients with iritis if the diagnosis is established, but supervision by an ophthalmologist is necessary. Generally, the red eye should not be treated with topical steroids unless the diagnosis is certain and the treatment appropriate.

Conclusion

In conclusion, the acute red eye is one of the most important topics for the medical student. A detailed history and a careful but simple examination should differentiate between the various causes and the patient can be directed towards the appropriate management or expert.

Sudden loss of vision (Table 25.2)

Bilateral visual loss

Bilateral visual loss of sudden onset is extremely rare and is usually caused by disease of the visual pathways or visual cortex.

Table 25.2 Causes of sudden loss of vision.

Bilateral visual loss
Cerebrovascular accident
Toxic substances, e.g. methyl alcohol
Bilateral ocular disease
Unilateral visual loss
Arterial occlusion
Retinal artery occlusion
Ciliary artery occlusion (giant cell arteritis)
Venous occlusion
Inflammatory conditions
Optic neuritis
Leber's optic neuropathy
Optic nerve compression
Vitreous haemorrhage

The acute red eye at a glance

DEFINITION

The *acute red eye* is a physical sign characterized by redness of all or part of the conjunctiva or sclera ± discomfort in the eye

CAUSES OF AN ACUTE RED EYE

- Conjunctivitis
- Foreign body
- Anterior uveitis, iritis, iridocyclitis
- Corneal ulcer
- Acute glaucoma
- Episcleritis and scleritis
- Subconjunctival haemorrhage

CONJUNCTIVITIS

Clinical features

- Inflammation of the conjunctiva
- Red eye with sticky discharge, especially after sleep
- Pupil is normal and vision is not impaired

Causes
- *Staphylococcus aureus, Haemophilus influenzae, Pseudomonas*
- Virus
- *Chlamydia trachomatis*
- Herpes simplex
- Allergic reaction

Treatment
- Topical antibiotics 2-hourly

- Settles spontaneously
- Tetracycline–systemic or topical
- Idoxuridine, acyclovir
- Topical steroids, but only under expert supervision

FOREIGN BODY

- A conjunctival or corneal foreign body (FB) is a common cause of red eye. May or may not be history of trauma

Clinical features

- Painful, 'gritty' eye
- Pupil normal and vision not impaired

Treatment
- Topical anaesthesia to examine eye properly
- Evert upper lid to exclude subtarsal FB
- Irrigate out superficial FB or remove with cotton wool
- FB embedded in cornea has to be removed with needle tip or drill
- Topical antibiotics and eye pad for 24–48 h following removal

UVEITIS, IRITIS, IRIDOCYCLITIS

- Inflammation of all or part of the uveal tract

Clinical features

- Red eye with circumcorneal injection
- Constant 'aching' pain in eye and photophobia
- The pupil is *small* and fixed and the anterior chamber may be turgid
- Intraocular pressure is normal

Causes
- Ankylosing spondylitis
- Psoriasis
- Sarcoidosis

Treatment
- Treat underlying cause
- Topical steroids
- Pupillary dilators

- Crohn's disease
- Ulcerative colitis
- Syphilis, tuberculosis

CORNEAL ULCER

- Ulcer of the cornea caused by viruses, bacteria or trauma

Clinical features

- Pain, watering and photophobia
- Highlighted with fluorescein in blue light

Treatment
- Identify and treat cause
- Neglected ulcers lead to corneal scarring

ACUTE GLAUCOMA

- Precipitated by narrowing of the drainage angle between iris and cornea. This is a medical emergency, as blindness will ensue if not treated promptly

Clinical features

- Red eye with injected conjunctiva and iris
- Severe 'aching' pain
- Patient sees haloes with rainbow pattern around white light
- Pupil is dilated, fixed and oval
- Intraocular pressure is very high

Treatment
- Acetazolamide 500 mg IV to reduce aqueous production
- Pilocarpine drops to constrict the pupil and widen the drainage angle
- Topical steroids and ß-blockers to reduce intraocular pressure
- Occasionally IV mannitol is required

EPISCLERITIS AND SCLERITIS

- Localized inflammation of the sclera
- Small oval, slightly raised red area on the sclera
- May be 'aching' pain or not

Causes
- Allergic
- Rheumatoid arthritis
- Polyarteritis nodosa
- Wegener's granulomatosis

Treatment
- Treat underlying cause, if any is identified
- Topical steroids

CONJUNCTIVAL AND SUBCONJUNCTIVAL HAEMORRHAGE

- A conjunctival haemorrhage is in the conjunctiva and is usually due to trauma
- A subconjunctival haemorrhage is a painless collection of blood under the conjunctiva. It is associated with anterior cranial fossa fracture and the posterior limit of the haematoma cannot be defined
- Neither requires specific treatment

- The most common cause of sudden bilateral visual loss is cerebrovascular accident affecting the visual cortex. Here, although the eyes see perfectly well, there is nowhere to send the visual message. In these circumstances the pupil reactions remain normal, for they do not require an intact visual cortex, merely depending on the pupillary pathway which passes through the upper mid-brain.
- Occasionally visual loss occurs due to ingestion of toxic substance, for example methyl alcohol or drugs such as quinine in large doses.
- Rarely, causes of unilateral visual loss affect both eyes simultaneously, as for example with acute bilateral optic neuritis, but this is excessively unusual.

Unilateral visual loss

Generally sudden loss of vision occurs in one eye and is due either to arterial or venous vascular occlusion or to an inflammatory disease of the optic nerve.

Arterial occlusions

Arterial occlusions may affect either the circulation in the retina or the optic nerve.

Retinal arterial occlusion

Occlusion of the retinal artery may be preceded by premonitory symptoms of episodes of visual loss lasting for 10–15 min at a time. The vision is usually more or less completely obscured and then comes back slowly. The patient may be otherwise perfectly well and the signs are unilateral (Fig. 25.4). Emboli from the heart or the carotid arteries may lodge in the retina. Management is directed towards locating the source of emboli and then the appropriate medical or surgical treatment. Simply listening to the carotid arteries or heart may reveal a murmur or bruit and further investigations include echocardiography, 24-h electrocardiogram (Holter) monitoring and duplex scanning of the carotid arteries. Patients found not to have significant cardiac or carotid disease may obtain symptomatic relief from low-dose aspirin therapy.

Ciliary artery occlusion

The optic nerve may be damaged by occlusion of the ciliary circulation. This is separate to the retinal circulation and is usually involved as part of an ischaemic optic neuropathy. Occlusion of the posterior ciliary arteries may lead to infarction of the head of the optic nerve. The patient simply wakes up or suddenly experiences visual loss of all or part of the visual field. Classically inferior field is lost.

Giant cell arteritis

In elderly patients the most important underlying disease to consider is giant cell (temporal or cranial) arteritis. In this case the visual disturbance may be preceded by headache, particularly in the temporal area, and symptoms of polymyalgia rheumatica with stiffness around the shoulder girdle and pelvis. Whenever optic neuropathy is suspected, a full blood count and erythrocyte sedimentation rate (ESR) must carried out. If the ESR is >50 mm/h then it should be repeated and C-reactive protein also estimated. A temporal arterial biopsy must be carried out to exclude giant cell arteritis. It is rare to see temporal arteritis in patients under 60 years old. The immediate treatment of giant cell arteritis consists of high-dose systemic steroids, i.e. methylprednisolone 500 mg intravenously initially followed by oral prednisolone 60 mg daily. Justification for this sort of dose of steroid in elderly patients really does require a temporal artery biopsy to confirm the diagnosis of giant cell arteritis. The morbidity of temporal arteritis is essentially confined to the eye, although involvement of the vertebral arteries may cause a stroke and sometimes the coronary arteries are involved. It is a very important condition to recognize and treat properly.

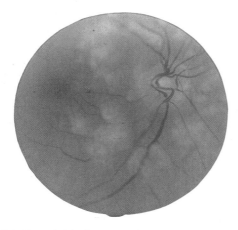

Figure 25.4 Central retinal artery occlusion responsible for acute loss of vision. There is pallor of the retina and narrowed branch arteries without haemorrhage.

Retinal venous occlusion

Retinal venous occlusion is generally not as devastating as arterial occlusion. Visual loss is mostly confined to blurring of vision, but if the central retinal vein is involved symptoms may be more severe. Predisposing factors for retinal venous occlusion are smoking, diabetes mellitus, myeloma,

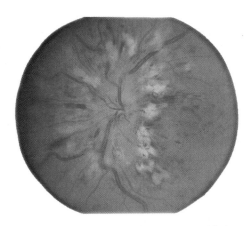

Figure 25.5 Central retinal vein occlusion responsible for acute loss of vision. There are retinal haemorrhages, a swollen disc, dilated veins and pale cotton-wool spots.

hyperlipidaemia and glaucoma. The patients are usually hypertensive and as a consequence the thickened retinal arteries impinge on the retinal veins at arteriovenous crossings, impairing venous flow. Flame haemorrhages and cotton-wool spots may be seen on ophthalmoscopy, the latter indicating an ischaemic retina and a bad prognosis (Fig. 25.5). Retinal ischaemia induces neovascularization, which may lead to glaucoma. Fluorescein angiography further delineates the diseased retina, which can be ablated by panretinal photocoagulation to prevent neovascularization and bleeding.

Inflammatory conditions

Inflammatory conditions which provoke sudden visual loss are less common.

Optic neuritis

Optic neuritis as part of demyelination is the commonest inflammatory cause of unilateral visual loss. The patients are usually young and may have other symptoms suggesting demyelinating disease. The visual loss is very variable and tends at least in the first attack to recover subjectively, although there are objective signs that the optic nerve has been damaged. These signs include failure of the afferent pupil defect to resolve and a colour vision deficit. A careful visual field test generally shows central loss. There is no good treatment for optic neuritis, although high doses of systemic steroids relieve the pain and possibly accelerate recovery. The condition may be mimicked by sarcoidosis or indeed any other inflammatory cause of optic nerve disease. Syphilis must never be forgotten and just occasionally there

can be metastatic malignant infiltration of the nerve which may mimic optic neuritis.

Compression of the optic nerve

Compression of the optic nerve is rare. Haemorrhage in to a pituitary tumour may compress the optic chiasm acutely leading to bilateral visual loss. This 'pituitary apoplexy' is a rare condition where there are symptoms and signs of hypopituitarism accompanied by bilateral visual loss. Very high doses of systemic steroid and urgent neurosurgical consultation are required.

Vitreous haemorrhage

Vitreous haemorrhage may occur from spontaneous or traumatic rupture of vessels or bleeding from new vessels. Rarely, generalized bleeding diathesis may be associated with vitreous haemorrhage. The commonest cause of vitreous haemorrhage is the sudden movement of the vitreous jelly within the eye, tearing the peripheral capillaries and sometimes the retina as well. The ageing process allows vitreous jelly to move into the centre of the eye, but if the peripheral attachments are firm then structures may be pulled along with the vitreous. Premonitory symptoms of flashing lights accompanied by floaters may herald this.

This main problem with vitreous haemorrhage is identifying the cause. About 75% is idiopathic and the cause is never strictly determined, though diabetes should be sought. There may of course be a tear in the retina and an underlying retinal detachment which cannot be treated until the haemorrhage has been removed. In general terms the management of vitreous haemorrhage includes bedrest (with patients being allowed up only for ablutions) for 48 h. If the haemorrhage has not cleared, ultrasound investigation is necessary to determine whether there is or is not a detachment. Management of retinal detachment is highly specialized.

From the student's point of view, patients with flashing lights and floaters must be assumed to have vitreoretinal pathology until proved otherwise and an urgent consultation is sought, requiring dilatation of the pupil and examination of the peripheral retina. Ophthalmological referral is therefore mandatory.

Diabetes mellitus

Blindness is a feared complication for many diabetics. It remains the most common cause of blindness in the UK for patients between the ages of 30 and 64 years. Screening of diabetic patients to identify early sight-threatening retinopathy is of paramount importance. A hospital clinician or general practitioner has the responsibility to include a careful retinal examination in the assessment of a diabetic patient. Serious retinopathy may be present without the patient having any untoward symptoms in the early stages. Laser treatment is effective in controlling the two main categories of sight-threatening retinopathy — diabetic maculopathy and proliferative retinopathy. Good diabetic control unfortunately does not protect an individual from developing serious retinopathy. Indeed, there is not a close relationship between control and the development of diabetic retinopathy. However, early treatment yields better results than late treatment.

Classification of retinopathy

• *Background retinopathy*: This is characterized by the presence of microaneurysms and haemorrhages scattered over the posterior fundus, i.e. within the arcades of major vessels. There may also be scattered exudates but to fit within this classification they must not involve the macular area. Background retinopathy may progress to maculopathy or proliferative retinopathy or a combination of both.

• *Diabetic maculopathy*: This is the commonest cause of visual loss in diabetes. It is due to the accumulation of oedema fluid or lipoprotein which has leaked from abnormal capilliaries. The underlying problem is abnormal permeability of the retinal capillaries. The lipoprotein collects as exudates often in a circinate (or circular) pattern. These are easily seen with the ophthalmoscope as yellow/white collections (Fig. 25.6). Macular oedema may also occur due to leakage of fluid, producing blurring or distortion of vision.

• *Proliferative retinopathy*: Proliferation refers to the development of abnormal blood vessels on the surface of the retina or on the optic disc. This proliferation of new vessels may lead to the serious complication of vitreous haemorrhage. Neovascularization occurs in response to retinal ischaemia. The new blood vessels grow forwards from the retinal surface into the vitreous gel. These vessels are friable and bleed easily, often resulting in profound and sudden loss of vision when the vitreous gel fills with blood. Repeated bleeding produces a fibrotic process which may result in retinal detachment by bands, and blindness.

• *Preproliferative retinopathy*: Before the development of true neovascularization, changes in the retina can be identified, indicating significant ischaemia. The changes to be noted are multiple cotton-wool spots, retinal venous dilatation, large dark haemorrhages and intraretinal vascular abnormalities. These patients require regular assessment as they are very likely to develop proliferative retinopathy. In patients who smoke these changes may improve if they discontinue cigarette smoking. All diabetic patients should be strongly encouraged not to smoke.

• *Cataract*: Opacification of the intraocular lens occurs earlier in diabetic patients; indeed a patient presenting with cataract in mid-life must be tested to exclude diabetes mellitus. The cataract may develop quite suddenly in young patients — so-called 'snow-storm' cataract (Fig. 25.7).

Treatment

• *Photocoagulation*: The main treatment for diabetic retinopathy is photocoagulation with the argon laser. Treatment is delivered via a contact lens with local anaesthesia. Maculopathy is treated by directing the laser at the areas of leakage, allowing the exudate to absorb. Prolifera-

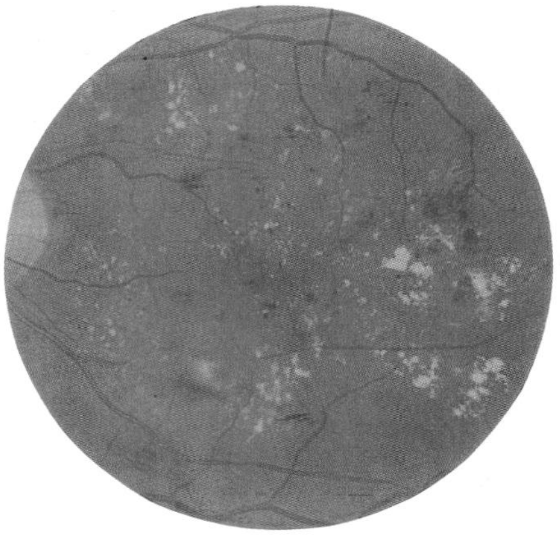

Figure 25.6 Diabetic macular changes showing pale hard exudates and blot haemorrhages.

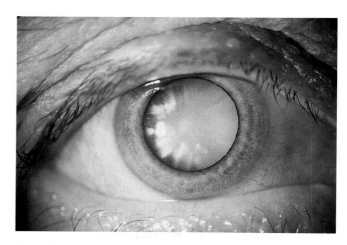

Figure 25.7 Cataract (lens opacity) causes whitening of the pupil.

tive retinopathy is treated with panretinal photocoagulation. With this treatment the more peripheral retina is covered with laser burns, leaving only untreated the central retina consisting of the macula and the neuroretina extending from the macula to the optic disc. This treatment alters the perfusion of the retina and should result in resolution of neovascularization. Retinal photocoagulation is considered to work by reducing the stimulus of retinal ischaemia which induces the abnormal vascularization, by destroying the stimulation retinal areas.

• *Vitrectomy*: Vitrectomy is necessary in advanced cases of proliferative retinopathy when there has been recurrent vitreous haemorrhage and/or a detachment of the retina. The vitreous is removed by microsurgery using a vitreous cutting instrument passed into the eye immediately behind the lens.

• *Education*: As with all aspects of diabetes, the patient must be educated as to the seriousness of the complications which may develop and attend for regular assessment, reporting any visual disturbance early.

The macula

The macula is the central and critical area of retina which serves detailed acuity and colour vision. The macular receptors are exclusively cones. The paramacular area consists of a combination of cones and rods. The remaining retina is made of rod photoreceptors. Sensitivity of the macula is increased at the fovea as the transmission layers of the retina are shelved, forming a central pit. A normal macula may be identified with the ophthalmoscope by the light reflex (the foveal reflex) in which the viewing light is reflected out from the foveal pit. The macular area is free of retinal capillaries and receives its principal blood supply from the underlying choroidal vessels. Symptoms of macular disease are early reduction of central vision which may be associated with distortion.

Macular degeneration

Degeneration of the macula with loss of central vision is common in the elderly and is the principal cause of registerable blindness in the over-64-year-old age group. The degenerative process results in disruption of the normal retinal architecture with loss of support for the photoreceptors. The process is principally an age-related degenerative process. Exposure to excessive ultraviolet light may be a risk factor in patients with presenile macular degeneration.

• *Atrophic degeneration*: In this condition vision gradually deteriorates over a number of years. Clumps of pigment with areas of depigmentation at the macula are seen on the retina. Visual acuity is generally in the range 6/36. Affected individuals therefore remain independent with preservation of peripheral vision.

• *Haemorrhagic macular disease*: This is a serious condition characterized by disruption of the retinal layer, including a break in the membrane separating the choroidal layer from the pigment epithelial layer. Blood vessels then grow through the break in this membrane and may bleed under the retinal surface, causing acute disruption and eventual destruction of cones due to scarring. The loss of vision is more abrupt, usually associated with distortion, and is generally more profound than that which occurs in atrophic macular disease. Retinal examination in an established case reveals an irregular grey area of scarring covering the macula. In the acute phase there is an elevated central area with surrounding retinal haemorrhage.

• *Drusen (colloid bodies)*: Drusen appear as collections of yellow/white round bodies in the retina. They are collections of material at the level of Bruch's membrane of the retina and are associated with macular degeneration. They are commonly seen in the macular and paramacular area of elderly patients. They may be difficult to distinguish from collections of exudate for the inexperienced ophthalmoscopist. Exudates, however, usually collect in a focal, sometimes circinate pattern in the retina. Drusen are spread more randomly and do not collect in circles (Fig. 25.8).

• *Hereditary macular disease*: There are a number of rare macular degenerative conditions which result in visual deterioration in childhood or early adult life.

• *Drug-induced macular problems*: Certain drugs specifically affect the retina, chloroquine being the principal example. This drug binds to the retinal pigment epithelium, resulting in disturbance of macular function.

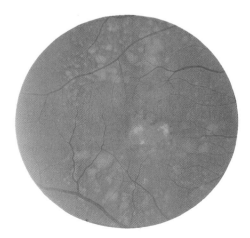

Figure 25.8 Age-related macular change with scattered pale retinal drusen.

Treatment

No effective treatment is known for atrophic macular degeneration. In a small number of cases of haemorrhagic macular degeneration, laser photocoagulation directed at the abnormal collections of blood vessels may be effective in preventing progression of the condition. Magnifying and telescopic low-vision aids are very valuable for maximizing the limited vision for patients with macular degeneration. Good lighting conditions are important when using these aids.

Squint (strabismus)

Squint or strabismus is the term applied to misalignment of the visual axis of the eyes. The visual system is arranged to achieve binocular single vision. Both eyes, therefore, must be aligned to allow an object of view to project on to the fovea of both eyes simultaneously. The convergence reflex provides the mechanism for continued binocular vision when the object of view becomes progressively closer to the eye. The visual cortex has cells which receive an input from each eye (binocular cells). During infancy and early childhood the visual system continues to develop and the normal adult state of binocular single vision is achieved only if the eyes are aligned and if each eye is projecting a focused image to the cortex. Amblyopia or lazy eye develops when this system fails. The child's visual system is 'plastic' up to the age of approximately 8 years, and therefore lazy eye may be reversible up to this age. The results of treatment are, however, much better the earlier the defect is corrected.

- *Concomitant squint*: The angle of misalignment does not alter in different positions of gaze. This is the classical squint of childhood. An infant may be born with squint or develop it within a few months of life. The cause is not known but there is often a family history of a similar condition in siblings or the parents. When examining the infant, full abduction of the squinting eye must be demonstrated to exclude a lateral rectus palsy.

  The infant's visual system has the capacity to suppress the image from the squinting eye to prevent double vision. Treatment of the condition is initially to induce free alternation of the squint by patching the non-squinting eye. This will prevent the squinting eye from becoming amblyopic (lazy). Uncorrected, the child will have permanently reduced vision in the affected eye. Corrective surgery is generally performed at the age of 18 months.
- *Paralytic or inconcomitant squint*: The deviation alters in different gaze positions, for example, sixth nerve palsy, as there is weakness of particular eye muscles.

Accommodation and convergent squint

Children who have a high degree of hypermetropia (longsightedness) may develop convergent squint due to the increased accommodative effort required to see clearly. There is an accommodation convergence reflex which normally results in convergence when viewing close objects. A child with a high degree of hypermetropia has to employ a significant amount of accommodation even to see in the near distance.

Correction of the hypermetropia with spectacles will in many cases correct the squint. Surgery for many of these children is therefore unnecessary. This type of squint generally develops at the age of 3 or 4 years.

Divergent squint

Divergent squint may be present at birth but this is uncommon. Divergence is usually intermittent and occurs in childhood. It tends to become gradually less intermittent and more permanent. Corrective surgery is then necessary.

Retinal disease causing squint

Poor central vision in a child will result in a squint. It is therefore very important to exclude a retinal condition as the cause. Retinoblastoma, a rare tumour of childhood, is an example in which the child may present initially with a squint and possibly whitening of the pupil. All children who are squinting or suspected of squinting should be referred for assessment by an ophthalmologist.

Pseudosquint

Many infants have a broad bridge to the nose with a large epicanthus. This results in the appearance of a convergent squint. The corneal reflections are seen to be symmetrical on the cornea of each eye excluding a true squint. With normal growth of the face the appearance of pseudosquint due to epicanthus gradually disappears.

Diseases of the eyelid

Blepharitis

Eyelid inflammation is a common condition. The underlying problem is abnormal secretion from the meibomian glands of the lid. This results in secondary bacterial infection with commensal staphylococci (*Staphylococcus epidermidis*). There may be an associated skin condition of rosacea. Blepharitis results in conjunctivitis with ocular irritation and redness. Treatment consists of regular cleansing of the lid margins and the use of appropriate topical or oral antibiotics.

Stye

This is a common condition and is simply an infection of the lash follicles. A stye generally resolves without specific antibiotic treatment. However, recurrent styes in childhood may require topical or oral antibiotics.

Meibomian cyst (chalazion)

This is a retention cyst of a meibomian gland due to obstruction of the outlet duct in the lid margin. The cyst may rupture into the lid tissue, causing an acute reaction and the development of a foreign-body granuloma. Meibomian cysts are removed by incision through the conjunctiva, but only if they persist.

Ectropion and entropion

Ectropion is an outturning of the eyelid, generally of the lower lid. This usually occurs in the elderly due to the loss of normal muscle tone of the lid. It results in watering of the eye and discomfort due to drying of the exposed conjunctiva. Ectropion may also result from scarring of the eyelid skin following trauma.

Entropion is an inturning of the lid, again generally of the lower eyelid. This also occurs as a senile change due to loss of muscle tone. Irritation occurs due to the eye lashes turning in and abrading the cornea (trichiasis). Senile entropion and ectropion are corrected surgically, generally with local anaesthesia.

Eyelid malignancy

Basal cell carcinoma (rodent ulcer) is the most common malignant eyelid tumour. It is more common in fair-skinned individuals who have had excessive exposure to sunlight. The typical appearances are of a pearl-like appearance with rolled edges. Treatment is by wide excision or by radiotherapy. *Squamous cell carcinoma* is rare but a serious condition as it may metastasize.

Ptosis

The position of the eyelid is controlled principally by the levator muscle. This is made up mainly of striated muscles supplied by the third nerve but also has a smooth-muscle portion (Müller's) supplied by the sympathetic nerve supply. The eyelid position is also influenced by the action of the frontalis muscles.

- *Third-nerve palsy* results in ptosis but there may also be interruption of the supply to the extraocular muscles, resulting in outward and downward deviation of the eye, sometimes with dilated pupil.
- *Horner's syndrome* occurs when there is disruption of the sympathetic nerve supply. This results in a small degree of ptosis, generally 2 mm and also pupillary miosis. Miosis is due to unopposed action of the parasympathetic supply to the sphincter pupillae muscle. Horner's syndrome is caused by damage to the sympathetic pathway. Surgical injury and malignant injury from lymph nodes or an apical lung tumour are common causes.

Thyroid eye disease

Upper eyelid retraction occurs due to abnormal stimulation of the smooth-muscle part of the levator due to circulating sympathomimetic agents (see also Chapter 15).

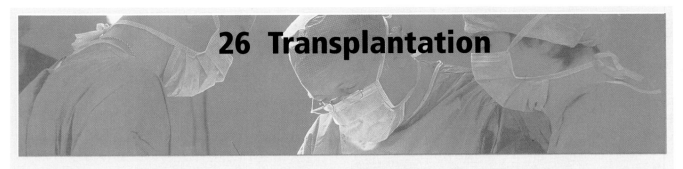

26 Transplantation

A new kind of surgeon–scientist was called into being by the growth of therapeutic organ transplantation — a procedure which makes special demands on the technical skills, knowledge and physiological understanding of the surgeon.

(Peter Medawar)

Introduction

Saints Cosmos and Damian, travelling Christian physicians who lived in the third century AD, are reported to have successfully transplanted a leg from a recently deceased Moor to a Caucasian cancer victim whose leg they had amputated. Unfortunately, attempts by others since then to transplant tissues from one person to another have not been as successful due to the uncompromising (one might say ungrateful!) way the recipient rejects the donated tissue. It is only in the last 50 years that this phenomenon has begun to be understood and it has been the successful management of rejection which has permitted the startling advances in transplantation that have occurred over the last two decades. The definitions of common terms used in transplantation are given in Box 26.1.

Histocompatibility

The major difficulty with transplanting tissues from one individual to another is the recipient's immune response against the donor's antigens leading to rejection. The fate of the graft is determined by the genetic relationship between the donor and the recipient. The greater the genetic similarity between donor and recipient, the more likely is graft acceptance.

Major and minor histocompatibility complex

The histocompatibility antigens are the most important for organ transplantation. Two types of histocompatibility

Glossary of transplantation terms

Transplantation
• The transfer of a graft (i.e. living cells, tissues or organs) from one individual to another

Donor
• The individual from whom the graft is taken

Recipient (Host)
• The individual into whom the graft is transplanted

Allogeneic graft
• Transplantation of a graft from one individual to another of the same species, e.g. blood transfusion and all organ transplants

Xenogeneic graft
• Transplantation of a graft from one individual to another of a different species, e.g. baboon liver to human

Orthotopic graft
• The transplanted graft is placed in the normal anatomic site for that tissue in the recipient, e.g. heart transplant

Heterotopic graft
• The transplanted graft is placed in a location other than the normal anatomic site for that tissue in the recipient, e.g. kidney transplant, pancreas transplant

Antigen
• Complex macromolecules (e.g. proteins) that interact with T- or B-cell receptors usually leading to an immune response. Antigens are usually foreign (alloantigens, xenoantigens), but non-foreign antigens (autoantigens) also exist

Allograft reaction
• An immunological reaction occurring in response to the presence of the graft
• Host versus graft reaction (rejection) occurs when the recipients cells attack and destroy the graft
• Graft versus host reaction occurs when immunologically competent donor cells in the graft attack the host

Box 26.1

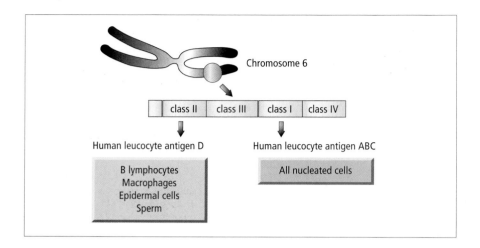

Figure 26.1 Components of the major histocompatibility complex.

antigens exist — major and minor. In humans the major group of antigens are encoded by genes located on the short arm of chromosome 6, known as the *major histocompatibility complex (MHC)*. The genes of the MHC comprise class I genes that encode for human leukocyte antigens (HLA) A, B and C, which are present on all nucleated cells and class II genes that encode for HLA-D antigens, which are found only on B lymphocytes, macrophages, epidermal cells and sperm (Fig. 26.1). A difference in the MHC antigens between donor and recipient results in rapid graft rejection. The genes of the *minor histocompatibility complex (MIH)* are scattered across the genome. The only feature that these genes have in common is that they code for proteins that are capable of initiating an allograft reaction. A difference in one MIH gene usually leads to slow rejection.

Human leukocyte antigen (HLA)

All human cells express molecules that are recognized by other individuals as foreign antigens. The *ABO blood group antigens* on erythrocytes are important for blood transfusion while the *HLAs* are important for organ transplantation. HLAs are found on the surface of all nucleated cells and their expression is controlled by the MHC (see above). In the various subgroups (HLA-A–D), there are over 147 possible HLAs that may be expressed on the cell surface. The function of HLAs is to act as receptors for foreign antigens and present them to the recipient's CD4 (helper/inducer) or CD8 (killer) T cells, thus provoking an immune response. (The initials CD stand for cluster differentiation; the number, which may be from 1 to 60, refers to the surface features of the T cell which differentiate one functional type from another.)

Identical twins are of course HLA-identical, but it is also not uncommon for two siblings to be HLA-identical. The MHC locus on chromosome 6 tends to be inherited intact, so that each individual will have inherited a paternal and a maternal haplotype. There is a one in four chance that two siblings will inherit the same paternal and maternal haplotypes, thus making them HLA-identical.

HLA matching

HLA matching is a technique used in transplantation for selecting the best recipient for a given donor. It is used in renal transplantation and is very important in bone marrow transplants but it is impracticable for most other organ transplants due to the lack of artificial organs. HLA typing is performed by reacting lymphocytes from the individual being typed (who could either be a donor or a recipient) with commercially available HLA antisera. The lymphocytes are plated on to microtitre plates which contain, in wells, different specific HLA antisera. Complement is added to each well, the reaction proceeds and if cytotoxicity occurs, a dye is taken up by the dead cells. From the pattern of the dye uptake the HLA type of the individual can be determined. The HLA types of potential recipients for renal transplantation are held by national and international agencies. When a cadaver kidney becomes available, it is typed and then offered to the recipient with the closest HLA match and compatible for ABO. The national centre for the UK is in Bristol.

Organ procurement

Most organ transplantation is performed using grafts obtained from cadavers. Exceptions are living related renal transplantation and liver or lung lobe transplantation, usually from a parent to a child. Before an organ may be removed for cadaveric transplantation brain death has to be established in the donor. The guidelines for declaring a person brain-dead are given in Chapter 21. The body from which the organ is removed should be free from infection (bacterial, fungal, viral) and malignancy. The majority of donors are young patients with severe head injury or sub-arachnoid haemorrhage.

The donor's circulation is supported until the organs have been removed. Once the organ has been removed, its vascular bed is flushed through with cold preservation solution and the organ is stored in a sterile cold container at 0–4°C. Hypothermia is effective because it slows metabolism and prolongs the period of ischaemia required to cause irreversible tissue destruction. However, to reduce cell swelling which occurs with ischaemia, preservation solutions have been developed which contain large molecules (impermeants) that retard water absorption by the cell. These solutions also contain adenosine to stimulate adenosine triphosphate production on reperfusion and free radical scavengers to reduce the level of reperfusion injury. The most widely used preservation solution today is University of Wisconsin solution which was developed in 1987 (Table 26.1).

Table 26.1 Composition of University of Wisconsin (UW) solution.

Potassium phosphate	25 mmol/l
Magnesium sulphate	5 mmol/l
Lactobionate	100 mmol/l
Adenosine	5 mmol/l
Allopurinol	1 mmol/l
Raffinose	30 mmol/l
Glutathione	3 mmol/l
Starch	50 g/l

Using organ preservation, the kidney may be kept satisfactorily for 36 h, the liver and pancreas for 20 h and the heart and lungs for 5–6 h. With living related transplantation, two surgical teams operate simultaneously and the donated organ is immediately transplanted into the recipient.

Allograft reaction

An allograft reaction is an immunological reaction occurring in response to the presence of the transplanted cells. Two types of reaction are recognized:

- *Host-versus-graft reaction (HvGR; rejection)* occurs when the host's immune system attacks and destroys and the graft.
- *Graft-versus-host reaction (GvHR)* occurs when immunologically competent transplanted cells (e.g. bone marrow transplant) attack the host environment.

Host-versus-graft reaction (HvGR; rejection)

Types of rejection

A spectrum of graft rejection has been identified and has been divided into four types on a temporal basis (Table 26.2).

Table 26.2 Timing of reactions which may occur following transplantation.

	Time to reaction	Mechanism
Host-versus-graft reaction		
Hyperacute rejection	Minutes or hours	Humoral
Accelerated rejection	First 4 days	Humoral/cellular
Acute rejection	First month	Cellular
Chronic rejection	Several months	Humoral/cellular
Graft-versus-host reaction		
Acute	2–10 weeks	Unknown
Chronic	3–18 months	Unknown

- *Hyperacute rejection* occurs within minutes of transplantation. It is caused by the interaction between preformed cytotoxic antibodies circulating in the host and graft antigen expressed on the graft endothelium. The result is complement activation, kinin release, coagulation, microvascular thrombosis and graft infarction. Hyperacute rejection occurs when there is ABO incompatibility between donor kidney and recipient. Anti-A or anti-B antibodies interact with the corresponding antigen in the kidney, triggering an inflammatory response. Similarly, patients who have had a previous failed transplant are at risk.
- *Accelerated rejection* occurs in the first 4 days after transplantation. It includes both cellular and humoral components and occurs in individuals previously sensitized against donor antigens.
- *Acute rejection* is a cell (T-lymphocyte)-mediated response that occurs during the first month after transplantation (see below).

• *Chronic rejection* is probably a humoral response and is characterized by fibrosis of the graft and decreasing function over a period of months or years.

Mechanism of rejection

Graft rejection can be divided into afferent and efferent phases.
• The afferent phase (sensitization) is the mechanism by which the transplanted tissue induces change and proliferation in the host immune system. The antigens on several different cells in the graft may be involved in provoking the immune response in the host. These include epidermal cells, vascular endothelium, donor 'passenger' leukocytes and dendritic cells, so-called because, like nerve cells, they send out branches.
• The efferent phase is the method of host immune attack on the graft (graft destruction). Both cellular and humoral factors are needed to initiate the efferent immune response.

(a) *Cellular response:* CD4 and CD8 T cells are activated in response to the presence of donor antigens. CD8 T cells are directly cytotoxic to graft cells, while CD4 cells release lymphokines which attract monocytes to the graft where they become activated macrophages and attack the graft.
(b) *Humoral response:* Antibodies also play an important role in graft destruction. In response to soluble antigen, B lymphocytes develop into plasma cells, which secrete antibodies specific to the graft antigen.

Graft-versus-host reaction

If immunocompetent cells are transplanted they will respond to and mount an immune response against the host's antigens. This phenomenon is termed graft-versus-host disease (GvHD) and is seen following bone marrow transplantation. The mechanism of injury of GvHD is unknown. Almost half of the patients with acute GvHD will die, usually from uncontrollable infection. Chronic GvHD has a better prognosis.

Prevention of allograft reaction

Manipulation of either the afferent or efferent arms of the immune response should block a rejection response. If the host cannot recognize the graft as non-self, a response will not be mounted (tolerance) and blocking the effectors of the response should protect the graft (immunosuppression).

Tolerance

Immunotolerance is a state of immunological inactivity in the presence of antigens which would normally elicit an immune response. The immune system has developed mechanisms which make it unresponsive to self antigens. Exposure to antigens *in utero* results in clonal deletion of the B and T cells which recognize those antigens, from bone marrow and thymus, respectively. Exposure to a foreign antigen *in utero* will also produce tolerance to that antigen. There are also a number of privileged sites in the body where antigens are confined and are not exposed to lymphocytes. The anterior chamber of the eye, the brain and the testicle are examples of privileged sites. Transplantation into these areas will not result in an immune response.

Immunosuppression

Suppression of the efferent arm of the immune response has been the principal method of manipulating the immune

Table 26.3 Immunosuppressive agents.

Name	Mode of action	Side-effects
Azathioprine	Blocks DNA synthesis in CD4 and CD8 cells	Leukopenia, hepatotoxicity, GIT disturbances
Corticosteroids	Anti-inflammatory actions Stabilize cell membranes Reduce antigen presentation Decrease numbers of circulating lymphocytes	Infection, poor wound healing and skin striae, diabetes, Cushing's syndrome, gastric ulceration, hypertension and psychoses
Cyclosporin	T-cell suppression Blocks the release of IL-2	Nephrotoxicity, Epstein–Barr virus-induced lymphoma
FK506	T-cell suppression Blocks the release of IL-2	Nephrotoxicity
RS-61443	Inhibits purine synthesis in lymphocytes	Very low toxicity

GIT, Gastrointestinal tract; IL-2, interleukin-2.

response after transplantation. Ionizing radiation effectively blocks the immune system but the host is then susceptible to overwhelming viral, bacterial or fungal infection. Pharmacological immunosuppression is now used to suppress effector cells following transplantation. The drugs most frequently used today are given in Table 26.3.

Antibodies against human lymphocytes have been used to induce immune suppression. Antilymphocytic globulin (ALG) is a *non-specific* immunosuppressant which is active against all lymphocytes and removes mature T lymphocytes from the circulation. It is raised by injecting human lymphocytes into animals, from whom the antibody-containing globulin is obtained and administered to the patient. Unfortunately, the patient will make antibodies against ALG, necessitating larger doses or switching to another species to obtain ALG. Severe leukopenia is also a serious complication of ALG therapy.

Using monoclonal antibodies (MAB), *specific* immunosuppression against human lymphocytes is also now available. The MAB that has been used most frequently is an antibody to the CD3 complex on human lymphocytes called Orthoclone OKT3; it prevents the activation and generation of CD8 killer T lymphocytes. Side-effects include pulmonary oedema, fever and headaches.

Treatment of GvHD

The best treatment is prevention by limiting bone marrow transplantation to HLA-identical siblings. However, even in this group minor histocompatibility incompatibility can induce GvHD. Two strategies are currently used to prevent GvHD:
- *Donor T-cell depletion:* Depleting the donor marrow of T lymphocytes is achieved by exposing T cells to specific monoclonal antibodies and complement which will lyse mature T cells. This therapy reduces the incidence of GvHD but is associated with a higher rate of engraftment failure and relapse of leukaemia.
- *Chemotherapy* is also effective in preventing GvHD. Cyclosporin with or without methotrexate is administered to the recipient for several days before transplantation and continued for months thereafter. If GvHD occurs, pulse doses of prednisolone are administered and immunosuppressive therapy is increased. However, the prognosis from established GvHD is poor.

Specific organ transplantation

Renal transplantation

Renal or kidney transplantation is the longest established and most successful of the major organ transplantations.

The first renal transplant was performed in Boston in 1954. The indication for renal transplantation is end-stage chronic renal failure and kidney transplant is probably the treatment of choice for this group of patients who would otherwise require long-term dialysis. Two types of donor are used: cadaver and living related donors. It is essential that the donor has good renal function, no infection (especially human immunodeficiency virus or cytomegalovirus) and no malignancy. Matching donor and recipient is performed by ABO blood typing and HLA tissue typing.

The kidney is transplanted into an extraperitoneal site in the pelvis; the recipient's own non-functioning kidney is usually left *in situ*. The renal artery and vein are anastomosed to the iliac artery and vein and the ureter is implanted into the bladder (Fig. 26.2). Complications include acute tubular necrosis, infection and rejection. Immuno-

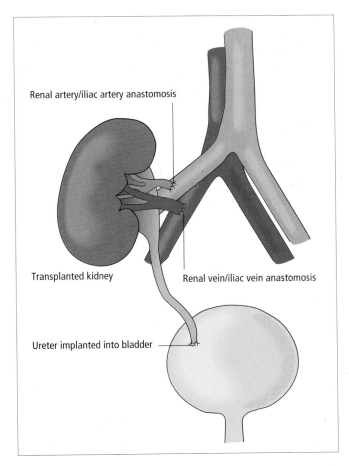

Renal artery/iliac artery anastomosis

Transplanted kidney

Renal vein/iliac vein anastomosis

Ureter implanted into bladder

Figure 26.2 Renal transplantation. The donor kidney is transplanted into an extraperitoneal site in the pelvis. The patient's own kidney is left *in situ*. The donor renal vessels are anastomosed to the recipient's iliac vessels and the ureter is implanted into the bladder.

suppression with cyclosporin A, azathioprine and steroids is started immediately following transplantation and renal function is assessed regularly. Rejection is confirmed by a transcutaneous needle biopsy of the engrafted kidney. Results of renal transplantation are good, with graft survival rates of approximately 80% at 1 year and 60% at 5 years.

Liver transplantation

Liver transplantation is now a very successful technique for the management of terminal liver disease. The first liver transplant was undertaken by Starzl in Denver in 1963. The indications for hepatic transplantation include liver failure and end-stage non-malignant liver disease (chronic active hepatitis, posthepatic or biliary cirrhosis, alcoholic liver disease) in adults and biliary atresia in children. Alcoholics, in general, are not good candidates for liver transplantation as they soon begin to expose the new liver to the same abuse which led them to transplantation in the first place. Transplantation for primary liver malignancy is considered by some centres but the prognosis is less favourable than in patients with benign disease. As with renal transplantation, cadaveric and live related donors (who undergo a partial hepatectomy) are used. HLA matching is often impracticable (as there is no hepatic equivalent to renal dialysis, recipients cannot wait for a suitable donor to become available) and it is not clear that matching is beneficial in liver transplantation.

The surgery of liver transplantation is formidable (Fig. 26.3). During the transplantation operation blood loss may be considerable because of clotting abnormalities sec-ondary to liver failure, difficult vascular anastomoses and portal hypertension. Biliary tract complications may occur; the bile duct anastomosis is prone to ischaemic dehiscence and occasionally a form of rejection specifically targeted against the biliary epithelium (the vanishing bile duct syndrome) occurs. The survival rate at 1 year for liver transplantation is 80% and almost 60% survive 5 years.

Heart and lung transplantation

Heart transplantation is now well-established, having been first performed in a blaze of publicity by Barnard in South Africa in 1966. It is indicated in young patients with end-stage ischaemic heart disease and cardiomyopathies. HLA matching is not practical as it is virtually impossible to support the recipient until a suitable donor becomes available. However, HLA-DR-matched transplants appear to have better graft survival rates than unmatched transplants.

The surgical procedure consists of suturing the ventricles of the donor heart to the atria of the recipient heart (Fig. 26.4). The advent of cyclosporin-A greatly facilitated heart transplantation. Rejection, if it occurs, is a major problem and regular biopsies are required to detect early signs of rejection so that maximum immunosuppressive therapy can be administered. Irreversible rejection will require retransplantation. Accelerated atherosclerosis in the graft coronary arteries is also a problem. The 1 year survival rate following heart transplantation is now approximately 80%.

Single- and double-lung as well as combined heart and lung transplantations have been performed and although many difficulties remain to be overcome, the technique is

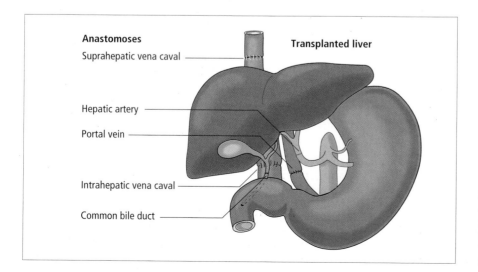

Figure 26.3 Liver transplantation. The recipient's liver is removed. The donor liver is implanted using the following sequence of anastomoses: superior vena cava, inferior vena cava, portal vein, hepatic artery and bile duct.

Anastomoses

Suprahepatic vena caval

Transplanted liver

Hepatic artery

Portal vein

Intrahepatic vena caval

Common bile duct

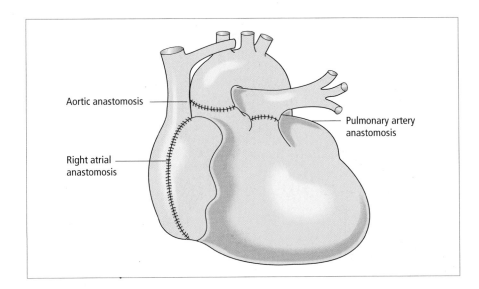

Figure 26.4 Heart transplantation. The recipient's atria are left *in situ*. The donor heart is anastomosed to the atria, the pulmonary artery and the aorta.

promising. The indications for lung transplantation are idiopathic pulmonary fibrosis, cystic fibrosis, emphysema and pulmonary hypertension. Opportunistic infections and obliterative bronchiolitis are two long-term problems following lung transplantation. Survival following heart and lung transplantation is 60% at 1 year and 40% at 5 years.

Pancreas transplantation

Pancreas transplantation, first performed in Minneapolis in 1966, has been attempted as a cure for diabetes. Pancreatic islet transplantation, performed following separation of the islets of Langerhans from the exocrine pancreatic tissue, has not been very successful. Currently, whole-organ pancreatic transplantation is indicated for patients undergoing renal transplantation for end-stage renal disease secondary to diabetes mellitus. The splenic and superior mesenteric artery blood supply to the pancreas is preserved and the pancreatic duct is implanted with a cuff of duodenum into the bladder (Fig. 26.5). Pancreatic function can be monitored by measuring urinary amylase and early rejection detected. The graft survival rate at 1 year is approximately 70%.

Small-bowel transplantation

A number of attempts have been made to transplant small bowel either alone or as part of a multivisceral or cluster transplant (liver ± pancreas and duodenum, small intestine). The indication is usually short-bowel syndrome. Living related and cadaveric grafts have been used. The best results appear to be with single intestinal transplantation but further studies are needed before small-bowel transplantation becomes a routine procedure.

Bone marrow transplantation

Bone marrow transplantation is now well-established as a treatment for marrow disease. It is indicated in patients with severe aplastic anaemia, some leukaemias and in a number of inherited deficiency states, e.g. thalassaemia. Because of GvHD, transplantation is confined to HLA-identical siblings. To ensure that HvGD (rejection) does not occur, suppression of the recipient's immune system (*conditioning*) is undertaken immediately prior to grafting. This is achieved by high-dose chemotherapy combined with whole-body irradiation. The transplantation process is simple. Marrow is aspirated from the donor's iliac crest and infused intravenously into the recipient. The complications of bone marrow transplantation are failure of engraftment, infection (usually herpes simplex, cytomegalovirus and varicella-zoster) and GvHD. The results depend on the indication for grafting. Long-term survival following transplantation for aplastic anaemia is about 50%, and 60–70% for leukaemias.

Conclusion

Transplantation is an expanding area of surgical science. There have been tremendous advances over the last 10–15 years with the scope and indications for transplantation constantly expanding. Better methods of organ preserva-

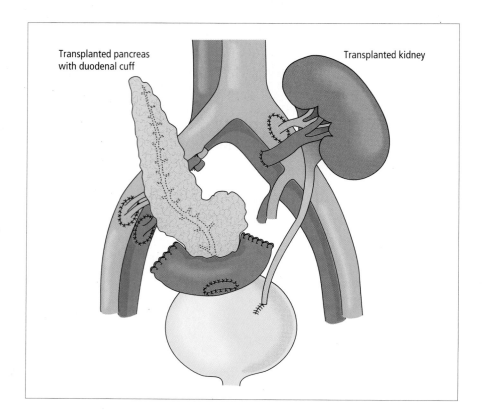

Transplanted pancreas
with duodenal cuff

Transplanted kidney

Figure 26.5 Combined kidney and pancreas transplantation.

tion and newer drugs for immunosuppression have improved results. Unfortunately, there are far more patients awaiting transplant operations than there are organs and organ donation remains a problem. The use of xenografts (from one species to another) have not proved successful but the development of transgenic animals (e.g. pigs that have had human genes inserted into their genome) may provide a ready supply of suitable organs for transplantation. However, the use of such donors raises a number of ethical problems which society must address.

PART 4 Perioperative Care

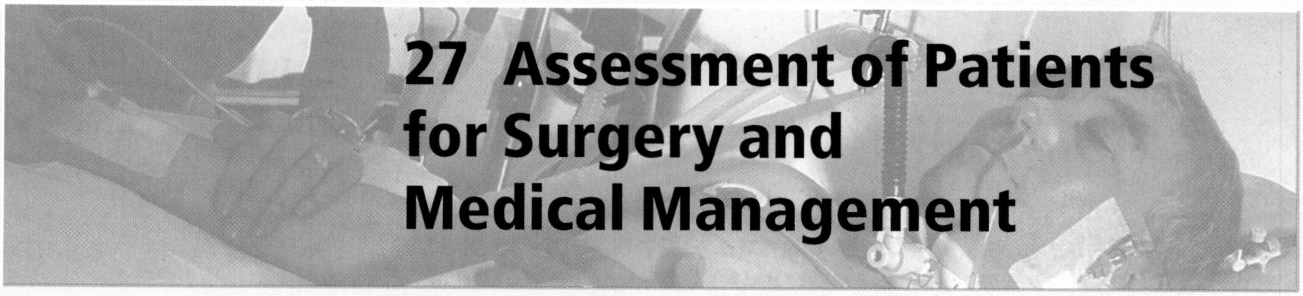

27 Assessment of Patients for Surgery and Medical Management

Dr Snow gave that blessed chloroform and the effect was soothing, quieting and delightful beyond measure.
(Queen Victoria 1819–1901)

Patient selection

Good surgical treatment demands careful patient selection whereby the benefit from the proposed surgical operation is balanced against the risk of the procedure to the patient. Patient selection is therefore a two-stage process (Fig. 27.1):
- the determination that a specific operation provides the best treatment for the disease;
- the risk to the patient's life imposed by the operation and general anaesthesia should be minimal.

Thus, a particular operation, though effective in curing the patient's illness, may be contraindicated if the patient is unfit for the procedure. In the emergency treatment of patients with life-threatening disorders or trauma the decision to operate may be straightforward. However, in the elective situation the decision to operate can be difficult, especially in elderly or high-risk patients with intercurrent cardiorespiratory disease.

Another aspect of patient selection relates to the early recognition of the failure of conservative management. The lowest overall operative mortality after surgery is observed when operations are undertaken electively. Thus, for example, the mortality following colectomy for ulcerative colitis is highest when this is performed as an emergency because of colonic perforation, intermediate when undertaken for toxic dilatation and lowest when the procedure is carried out electively because of failed medical therapy.

Fitness for surgery and general anaesthesia

Introduction

Death on the operating table is rare and is usually the result of an unexpected catastrophic event, e.g. sudden massive uncontrollable haemorrhage or myocardial infarction. The assessment of fitness for surgery relates to the chances of survival of the patient beyond the postoperative period (i.e. within 30 days of the operation or before discharge from hospital). Postoperative death, which is usually due to a combination of intercurrent disease, surgical complications and the adverse cardiopulmonary effects of general anaesthesia, is as much an operative death as is demise on the operating table. Assuming that there will be no surgical complications, the physiological state of the patient before surgery is the most important consideration influencing the fitness of operation. This is categorized by the Physical Status Scale proposed by the American Society of Anesthesiologists (ASA) and is shown in Table 27.1.

Routine preoperative evaluation

The preoperative evaluation of patients before surgical treatment is based on history and physical examination, supplemented by investigations when indicated (Table 27.2).

Special investigations are needed in specific groups, such as blood-clotting studies in jaundiced patients, detailed spirometry in patients with significant chronic pulmonary disease and those undergoing pulmonary surgery and screening for sickle cells in the appropriate ethnic groups.

Does a specific operation provide the best treatment for the disease?	Vs	What is the risk to the patient from the operation and the anaesthetic?

Figure 27.1 Balancing the benefits and risks of an operation.

Table 27.1 Physical status scale: American Society of Anesthesiologists (ASA).

ASA class	Physical status
1	A normally healthy individual: no organic, physiological, biochemical or psychiatric disturbance
2	A patient with mild to moderate systemic disturbance: this may or may not be related to the disorder requiring surgical treatment, e.g. diabetes mellitus, hypertension
3	A patient with severe systemic disease which is not incapacitating, e.g. heart disease with limited exercise tolerance, uncontrolled hypertension or diabetes
4	A patient with incapacitating systemic disease that is a constant threat to life with or without surgery, e.g. congestive cardiac failure, severe angina
5	A moribund patient who is not expected to live and where surgery is performed as a last resort, e.g. ruptured aortic aneurysm
E	A patient who requires an emergency operation

Table 27.2 Routine preoperative evaluation.

History
Respiratory disease, smoking
Cardiovascular disease, including DVT
Other medical disorders, e.g. bleeding diathesis, hypertension, diabetes
Previous general anaesthesia
Drugs and alcohol intake

Physical examination
Nutrition
Mental state
Dentures
Abnormalities of jaw and neck
Respiratory system
Cardiovascular system

Investigations
Hb, blood group and antibody screen
Ward urinalysis
Chest X-ray (in patients with cardiovascular and respiratory disease, elderly and smokers)
ECG (in patients >50 years, cardiac disease and hypertension)
Blood urea and electrolytes (in patients undergoing major surgery, patients on diuretics, those with suspected renal impairment and patients on IV fluids)

DVT, Deep vein thrombosis; Hb, haemoglobin; ECG, electrocardiogram.

High-risk groups

An increased risk is encountered in certain patient groups (Table 27.3) and these require special therapeutic and sup-

Table 27.3 High-risk groups.

Elderly patients
Patients with respiratory disease and smokers
Patients with cardiovascular disease
Obese patients
Patients with diabetes mellitus
Jaundiced patients
Patients on chronic drug medication
Females on oral contraceptives
Patients with bleeding disorders

portive measures including, in some instances, elective transfer to a high-dependence or intensive care unit after surgery.

Elderly patients

Elderly patients incur an enhanced risk which is the result of limited mobility, frequent presence of intercurrent disease and diminished reserve of cardiac, respiratory and renal function. They require more time in hospital after a given operation and, largely for this reason, have higher in-hospital postoperative wound infection rates than patients under the age of 50 years.

A postoperative stroke occurs in 1% of patients over 65 years of age. There does not appear to be an increased incidence of postoperative stroke in patients with a history of old cerebrovascular accident and in those with an asymptomatic carotid bruit, although a recent stroke (within 2–3 months of the operation) is thought to enhance the risk of a recurrent episode. As the autoregulation of the cerebral circulation becomes impaired with age, extremes of hypotension and hypertension must be avoided throughout the perioperative period. Old people are more prone to postoperative delirium, deep venous thrombosis, circulatory overload and cardiac decompensation.

Respiratory disease and smoking

Obstructive airways disease (chronic bronchitis and asthma) is followed by a higher incidence of postoperative pulmonary complications than restrictive airways disease. Patients with significant chronic pulmonary disease require careful preoperative evaluation by blood gas analysis, spirometry and exercise tolerance testing. Active breathing exercises and physiotherapy are started before the operation and a sputum culture is obtained. In the postoperative period oxygen administration, active physiotherapy and incentive spirometry are used to prevent hypoxaemia, pulmonary collapse and infection, and some patients will require assisted ventilation in the intensive care unit. Patients with asthma can be managed effectively in the postoperative period with selective β_2-adrenoceptor stimulants (e.g. salbutamol or terbutaline) administered via a nebulizer. Secretional airway obstruction is commonly managed by bronchoscopic lavage and minitracheostomy.

Smoking increases the risk of surgery and anaesthesia because of its adverse effects on the cardiovascular and respiratory system. Carbon monoxide and nicotine are responsible for the immediate cardiovascular effects of smoking:

• *Carbon monoxide*: Smoking leads to the formation of carboxyhaemoglobin which reduces the amount of haemoglobin available for combination with oxygen. In addition, it alters the oxygen dissociation curve such that the affinity for oxygen is increased (less oxygen is released for tissue oxygenation).

• *Nicotine* enhances the demand for the myocardium by increasing the heart rate and blood pressure. Elimination of both carbon monoxide and nicotine with improvement in the cardiovascular reserve is complete after a 24-h abstinence from smoking.

Smoking results in a sixfold increase in postoperative respiratory morbidity. In both smokers and in patients with chronic bronchitis, the underlying pathophysiological response after general surgery and anaesthesia is secretional airway obstruction leading to pulmonary collapse and infection. This response is due to:

• the production of an excessive amount of viscid mucus (bronchorrhoea);

• impaired tracheobronchial clearance of the mucus from impaired ciliary activity;

• decreased and unproductive cough response because of pain.

Smoking also impairs the immune function. A period of 6–8 weeks' abstinence from smoking is required to improve pulmonary function and reduce the postoperative pulmonary morbidity in smokers. However, even cessation of smoking for 24 h before an operation will result in improved cardiovascular function and is especially important in patients with ischaemic heart disease.

Cardiovascular disease

Although the mortality of patients with cardiovascular disease undergoing both cardiac and non-cardiac surgery has declined considerably during the last 10 years, none the less these patients are at an increased risk of both life-threatening complications and cardiac death in the perioperative period. The important cardiac risk factors which have been identified by Goldman and his colleagues in patients undergoing non-cardiac surgery are shown in Table 27.4.

• Patients with *congestive cardiac failure* require aggressive medical treatment prior to surgery because of the high

Table 27.4 Goldman cardiac risk factors in non-cardiac surgical operations listed in descending order of weighting risk.

Factor	Score
Signs of congestive heart failure	11
Myocardial infarction in the past 6 months	10
Premature ventricular beats (>5/min)	7
Arrhythmias	7
70 or more years old	5
Emergency surgery	4
Vascular, intrathoracic, upper abdominal surgery	3
Aortic stenosis	3
Poor general condition	3

risk of severe pulmonary oedema which often develops within 1 h of reversal of general anaesthesia.

• The risk of postoperative *myocardial infarction* is low in patients who have no prior history but is extremely high in those with a recent infarction (30% within 3 months) and continues to be elevated until 6 months have elapsed, when it stabilizes at 5%. Thus, elective surgery should not be performed on any patient within 6 months of a myocardial infarction.

• Operation is also postponed in patients with *uncontrolled hypertension*. The aim in these patients is to achieve a stable diastolic pressure of <110 mmHg, at which stage surgery can be undertaken with low risk. In patients with controlled hypertension, the antihypertensives are continued over the perioperative period.

• Although patients with *stable angina* exhibit an increased risk, operative intervention to revascularize the myocardium before their general surgical operation is not indicated as the combined risk of the two procedures exceeds or equals that following the general surgical intervention alone. However, prior cardiac surgery to revascularize the myocardium is needed in patients with *unstable angina* as 15% of these patients would otherwise develop a myocardial infarction during or immediately after the general surgical operation.

• Specific antibiotic prophylaxis against *bacterial endocarditis* is needed in patients with prosthetic valves, valvular heart disease, hypertrophic obstructive cardiomyopathy, mitral valve prolapse and insufficiency, and prior history of bacterial endocarditis.

Obese patients

Obese patients have an increased risk of respiratory complications, deep vein thrombosis, wound infection and dehiscence. Their mobility is restricted and the frequent presence of hypertension further increases the overall risk of surgery.

In addition, the operation is more difficult to perform, as a result of which the risk of iatrogenic injury to adjacent organs during the procedure is increased. Weight reduction should be actively encouraged before elective surgery. Morbidly obese patients undergoing surgical intervention designed to achieve weight reduction (bariatric surgery) require assisted ventilation and intensive care management in the postoperative period.

Diabetes mellitus

The management of diabetic patients undergoing surgical treatment depends on the magnitude of the operation and the type and severity of the diabetes.

Type of operation

- No special preoperative treatment is needed for operations performed under local anaesthesia.
- Patients having an operation under regional or general anaesthesia should be managed as follows:

Type II (maturity-onset) diabetes

- Patients controlled on diet alone: These patients require no special perioperative measures but their glucose levels should be monitored perioperatively.
- Patients controlled with diet and oral hypoglycaemic agents: The use of long-acting oral hypoglycaemics (chlorpropamide and metformin) should be avoided in patients who are to have surgery. Short-acting sulphonylureas (tolbutamide) should be used instead. On the day of surgery starve the patient and omit the morning dose of oral hypoglycaemic agent. The blood glucose should be monitored regularly during the perioperative period and if the level rises above 13 mmol/l, small doses of soluble insulin may be given subcutaneously. Oral hypoglycaemics should be reintroduced when the patient starts eating again. If major surgery is anticipated then glucose and insulin infusions should be used.

Type I (insulin-dependent) diabetes

The management of patients with insulin-dependent diabetes entails close cooperation between surgeon, anaesthetist and physician:
- establish good diabetic control preoperatively;
- put the patient first on the operating list;
- omit the morning dose of insulin;
- check blood glucose and electrolytes on the morning of the operation;
- set up a 5% dextrose intravenous infusion (100–125 ml/h) before surgery;

Table 27.5 Management of insulin-dependent diabetic patients having surgery.

Surgery should be performed in the morning
Omit morning insulin on day of surgery
Commence dextrose 5% (125 ml/h) at 6.00 am
Commence insulin infusion at 6.00 am
Test blood sugar hourly
Titrate insulin infusion according to sliding scale:

Blood glucose (mmol/l)	Units of insulin per hour
<4.0	0
4.1–7.0	1
7.1–10.0	2
10.1–14.0	4
>14.0	6

Recommence subcutaneous insulin when patient is eating normally

- set up an insulin infusion pump and titrate the rate of insulin infusion against hourly blood glucose estimations using the sliding scale given in Table 27.5. The aim should be to maintain the blood sugar at 8 mmol/l;
- blood glucose is estimated at hourly intervals throughout the immediate perioperative period and 2–4-hourly after that;
- check electrolytes postoperatively;
- postoperatively, intravenous 5% dextrose or dextrose saline with potassium (20 mmol/l) is administered at 125 ml/h until oral feeding is commenced; and
- when the patient is taking a full diet, recommence patient's preoperative insulin regime.

Jaundiced patients

Patients who are heavily jaundiced and who require surgical treatment for bile duct obstruction (impacted ductal calculi, carcinoma) are at risk of developing a number of serious complications during the perioperative period. The most important are:
- bleeding due to malabsorption of vitamin K (prolonged prothrombin time);
- increased risk of infection including cholangitis due to depression of the reticuloendothelial system;
- renal failure consequent on circulating endotoxinaemia (hepatorenal syndrome) secondary to absorption of endotoxin from the gut, which occurs even in the absence of infection in these patients.

Prophylactic support measures include:
- parenteral administration of synthetic vitamin K analogue to reverse the bleeding tendency;

• adequate hydration (set up an intravenous infusion the night before surgery) and natriuresis by the administration of an osmotic (mannitol) or loop diuretic (frusemide) at the time of induction of anaesthesia;

• systemic antibiotics (usually a cephalosporin with or without metronidazole).

If the hepatocyte function is not grossly impaired, the administration of intramuscular vitamin K analogue should correct the prolonged bleeding time within 48 h. As these patients require constant monitoring of the urine output on an hourly basis throughout the perioperative period, the urinary bladder is catheterized. A further dose of diuretic is administered if, in the presence of good hydration, the urine output falls below 30 ml/h in the postoperative period. Despite these measures, some of these patients still develop acute renal failure and require haemodialysis or haemofiltration at some stage after their operation.

Patients on chronic drug medication

Details of drug medication in patients undergoing surgery must be obtained in every patient. Some drugs have to be continued throughout the perioperative period and parenteral substitutes administered during the period when the patient is unable to take oral medication. Examples include *antihypertensive drugs, cardiac inotropes and steroids*. The suppression of the adrenal cortex in patients on steroid therapy is covered by the use of parenteral hydrocortisone until such time as the patient is able to resume oral intake.

Some drugs must be discontinued for a few weeks before surgery and anaesthesia because of adverse effects and drug interactions with anaesthetic agents and neuromuscular blocking drugs. These include monoamine oxidase inhibitors, tricyclic antidepressants, fenfluramine, lithium and phenothiazines.

Oral contraceptives

Females taking the combined oestrogen and progesterone contraceptive pill exhibit an enhanced risk of postoperative deep vein thrombosis. This is related to a reduction in the activity of antithrombin III induced by the additive effect of the combined pill and general anaesthesia. This enhanced risk is not seen with the progesterone-only pill or with hormone replacement therapy (HRT), which need not be stopped prior to surgery.

Although some advocate cessation of the oestrogen-containing contraceptives for at least 4 weeks prior to surgery to reduce the risk of deep vein thrombosis, others argue that this policy will incur added risk from unwanted pregnancies. When the intended operation is likely to result in early ambulation, the majority view is that cessation of

the combined pill before surgery is not needed. If the operation is major, alternative contraceptive measures (e.g. Depo-Provera) are used for several weeks before surgery. Patients on the combined pill requiring emergency surgery should receive chemoprophylaxis with low-dose subcutaneous heparin.

Bleeding disorders

Bleeding disorders may be inherited or acquired. Although rare, inherited bleeding disorders cause recurrent spontaneous bleeding episodes. Acquired bleeding disorders are much more commonly encountered and are secondary to disease or drug therapy.

Hereditary bleeding disorders

Introduction

Hereditary bleeding disorders may affect all the components of the haemostatic process: vascular, coagulation, platelet function and the fibrinolytic system (Table 27.6). All are rare and the important group is that comprised by the genetically determined defects of coagulation.

Haemophilia A and Christmas disease (haemophilia B)

Both of these disorders have similar clinical features. Haemophilia A results from a deficiency of the procoagulant portion of factor VIII (FVIII Act), whereas Christmas disease is due to a lack of factor IX (see Chapter 18). Both proteins are crucial to the intrinsic system of blood coagulation and the genes which control them are located on the X chromosome. This explains the recessive sex-linked pattern of inheritance whereby males are affected and females act as the carriers. Although this is largely true in the sense that clinical problems are predominantly confined to males, some female carriers may have a bleeding tendency which becomes obvious only when major surgery is undertaken.

Aside from the family and genetic history, both conditions are diagnosed by documentation of prolonged activated partial thromboplastin time (APTT), a normal prothrombin time (PT) and assay of factors VIII and IX. In both disorders the deficiency varies from mild (5–20% of normal level of the respective clotting factor) to moderate (1–5% of normal activity) and severe (<1% of normal activity).

The clinical picture is dominated by recurrent bleeds, most commonly in the muscles and joints (haemarthroses), especially in toddlers and children, although neonatal

Table 27.6 Hereditary bleeding disorders.

Name	Defect
Genetically determined defects of coagulation	
Haemophilia A	Factor VIII deficiency
Christmas disease	Factor IX deficiency
von Willebrand's disease	von Willebrand factor deficiency
Vascular and connective tissue disorders	
Osler – Weber – Rendu syndrome	Hereditary haemorrhagic telangiectasia
Ehlers – Danlos syndrome	Hereditary disorder of collagen
Marfan's syndrome	Defective collagen cross-linking
Osteogenesis imperfecta	Abnormal type I procollagen
*Disorders of platelet function**	
Glanzmann's thrombasthenia	Absence of specific surface glycoproteins
Grey platelet syndrome	Defects in secretory granules
Wiscott – Aldrich disease	

*Affected individuals exhibit a prolonged bleeding time but have a normal coagulation screen. These patients are liable to spontaneous bleeding and require platelet transfusion.

bleeding is not uncommon. Haematuria is fairly frequent and intracranial bleeding (intracerebral subarachnoid and subdural) may be fatal. Gastrointestinal haemorrhage is usually secondary to disease such as peptic ulceration and may be precipitated by non-steroidal anti-inflammatory agents which are contraindicated in these patients. The most common chronic disability is severe arthropathy from recurrent intra-articular bleeds and this often requires orthopaedic treatment.

Replacement therapy with clotting factors is required for the management of active bleeding episodes and to cover surgical treatment or dental extraction. Such treatment consists of the intravenous infusion of *plasma-derived factor VIII concentrates* for haemophilia A and *factor IX concentrates* for Christmas disease. Factor VIII concentrates are heat-treated to inactivate human immunodeficiency virus (HIV) and are available as lyophilized powder in vials containing 250 IU. Factor IX concentrates also contain prothrombin and factor X. They are heat-treated against HIV and packaged in vials containing 300 IU. *Cryoprecipitate*, which is rich in factor VIII (100 IU/pack), fibrinogen and fibronectin, can be used as an alternative to factor VIII concentrates in haemophilia A. As cryoprecipitate does not contain factor IX, it is ineffective in Christmas disease. The dose of the respective concentrate needed in the individual patient depends on the severity of the defect, the nature of the intended operation and the presence of acquired coagulation inhibitors (antibodies which develop in some patients). As the half-life of factor VIII is only 8–12 h, twice-daily administration is necessary to maintain thera-

peutic levels in haemophilia A. By contrast, in Christmas disease single daily dosing is usually sufficient as the half-life of factor IX is 18–24 h.

Elective surgery in haemophilia A and Christmas disease patients must be planned several weeks beforehand and requires that adequate notice be given to the blood transfusion or haemophilia centre. The preoperative work-up must include a coagulation-inhibition screen test. The first dose of concentrate or cryoprecipitate is administered 1 h before surgery and is followed by an assay of the factor level in a sample of the patient's blood taken 30 min later. Postoperative factor assays are also performed and replacement therapy continued to maintain a level >40% for the first 10 postoperative days. Patients with haemophilia A and Christmas disease must never receive intramuscular injections of any sort.

The complications of clotting factor therapy include:
- urticarial reactions (common);
- severe anaphylactoid reactions (rare);
- viral hepatitis (usually due to hepatitis C virus);
- HIV infection;
- development of antibodies to factor VIII.

In the early 1980s contaminated clotting factor concentrates resulted tragically in widespread seroconversion, especially in patients receiving factor VIII concentrates. Currently some 40% of UK haemophiliacs are HIV-positive, although the number is declining as many of the patients have died from acquired immune deficiency syndrome (AIDS).

Isoantibodies to factor VIII concentrate develop in some 6–12% of patients with haemophilia A. Their presence poses great difficulty in replacement therapy and these patients must be managed in specialist centres.

von Willebrand's disease

This familial bleeding disorder was first described by von Willebrand in the inhabitants of the Alland Islands in the Baltic sea. The disease is inherited as an autosomal dominant trait and therefore appears in consecutive generations affecting both males and females equally. It is caused by a deficiency of von Willebrand factor (vWF) normally produced by the endothelial cells and the megakaryocytes and is present in both plasma and platelets as high-molecular-weight molecules of varying sizes. vWF is essential for platelet adhesion to subendothelial tissues following vascular injury and as a carrier molecule for factor VIII which it stabilizes (factor VIII/vWF complex). Several variants of the disorder are recognized but the classical disease is characterized by:
* prolongation of the skin bleeding time;
* prolongation of the APTT;
* normal PT;
* reduced FVIII Act;
* reduced vWF antigen; and
* reduced vWFRCo (*in vitro* cofactor activity for platelet aggregation).

Clinically, von Willebrand's disease presents with bleeding, mainly from skin and mucous membranes and often after surgical intervention (particularly ear, nose and throat operations) or dental extraction. In women, menorrhagia is a common feature. In contrast to haemophilia A and Christmas disease, haemarthroses are rare.

Fresh frozen plasma (FFP), cryoprecipitate and some intermediate-purity factor VIII concentrate will restore the bleeding time and the coagulation defect to normal. Preparation of patients for surgery is similar to that previously described for haemophilia A and Christmas disease. In some cases (type I disease) intravenous infusion of deamino-D-arginine vasopressin (DDAVP, desmopressin) will increase the plasma FVIII Act and vWF levels and is therefore used as an alternative to replacement therapy in these patients to cover dental extractions or minor surgical operations. As desmopressin also stimulates the release of plasminogen activator, it is administered in conjunction with an antifibrinolytic agent such as tranexamic acid.

Acquired bleeding disorders

Acquired bleeding disorders are common and often involve more than one function of the haemostatic response. The most common abnormality encountered in clinical practice is bleeding caused by *oral anticoagulation* therapy. In some patients with malignant tumours impaired platelet function may lead to purpuric bruising but major disturbances of coagulation are rare, although some neoplasms may release products and cytokines which activate the coagulation cascade and lead to disseminated intravascular coagulation.

The major acquired bleeding problems usually arise on a background of acute or *chronic liver disease*. The bleeding diathesis in this situation reflects a complex picture due to defective synthesis of clotting factors (II, VII, X and the vitamin K-dependent factors), with the exception of factor VIII which is elevated, abnormal (hypo- or acarboxylated) clotting factors, abnormal fibrinogen (excess sialic acid which impairs polymerization), increased fibrinolysis and thrombocytopenia. In jaundiced patients due to large bile duct obstruction, the defective synthesis of the vitamin K-dependent factors is rapidly reversed by parenteral vitamin K analogue. Lack of response with persistence of the prolonged PT despite vitamin K therapy indicates severe hepatocyte malfunction.

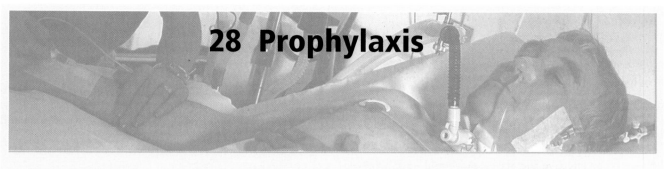

28 Prophylaxis

My father invented a cure for which there was no disease and unfortunately my mother caught it and died of it.
(Victor Borge 1909–)

Introduction

Prevention is always better than cure and so a careful assessment of relative risks is the first rule of management planning. Once the diagnosis has been established and the indications for surgery assessed, the potential benefits of the procedure must be offset against the risks of the procedure for the individual. In situations of very high risk a decision not to proceed may be reasonable (see also Chapter 27). However, most risks are relative and many per- and postoperative problems can be avoided by careful planning, anticipation and the institution of prophylactic measures designed to minimize or ideally eliminate potential complications. Of course, prophylactic treatment itself must carry minimum risk and certainly the benefits of prophylaxis must outweigh any risk many thousands of times.

Clinicians should also give consideration to their own and their colleagues' protection. It is important to appreciate that diseases can be transmitted from patient to doctor and vice versa. In past times many clinicians contracted tuberculosis which, although serious, is treatable. Many modern diseases, including hepatitis and acquired immune deficiency syndrome (AIDS), are not curable and may result in loss of ability to practise medicine and, in the case of AIDS, in premature death.

Principles of prophylaxis

• To be effective, prophylaxis must commence before the operation or procedure and be continued until the risk period has passed. Thus, for example, prophylactic heparin is started preoperatively and continued until the patient is ambulant postoperatively.

• The prophylactic measure must be effective and carry very little risk of itself.

There are two principal indications of prophylaxis:
• where the particular risk is relatively common and the prophylactic measure is safe, e.g. prophylactic antibiotics to prevent infection after bowel surgery, where the peritoneal cavity may become contaminated by lower bowel luminal organisms; and
• where the risk is rare but its consequences are very serious — such as death — and the prophylactic measure is relatively safe, e.g. administration of subcutaneous heparin to prevent deep vein thrombosis and antibiotics to avoid joint infection following arthroplasty.

Specific prophylaxis

Prophylaxis against infection

Following surgery there is nothing more frustrating than to see an excellent operation destroyed by infection. Over the last 100 years or so several measures have been introduced to try and reduce postoperative infection by minimizing the numbers of organisms which get into the wound (see also Chapter 30). No surgical wound is sterile but provided bacterial counts are kept low the body's normal immune defence system will cope. The following measures all help in this respect:
• short operations;
• skin cleansing with antibacterial chemicals and detergents;
• filtering of the air;
• channelling of filtered air by pumping;
• occlusive surgical masks and clothing; and
• prophylactic antibiotics.

Prophylactic antibiotics

Some operations carry a higher risk of being complicated by infection than others and wounds have been classified according to this risk (Table 28.1).

The indications for prophylactic antibiotics are given below. To be effective the antibiotic should have achieved *high tissue levels* at the time of contamination and *bactericidal* antibiotics should be used. Usually one preoperative dose of antibiotic given intravenously 1 h before the operation is sufficient.

Potentially contaminated wounds

The risk of postoperative wound infection is greatly increased if the surgical procedure includes opening the alimentary, the urinary, the biliary or respiratory tract. The risk is also increased if the patient already has an infection, particularly in or close to the operative field, e.g. an appendicular abscess. In such circumstances antibiotics should be given before and during surgery. If it has been possible to determine the microbiology of the infection and the sensitivity of the organisms in advance, the appropriate antibiotic should be given. If not, broad-spectrum antibiotic should be used in prophylaxis.

Joint replacement surgery

Prophylactic antibiotic cover should also be provided in procedures such as joint replacement when organisms which are not normally pathogenic multiply more readily in the presence of foreign material. The consequences of infection in an artificial joint replacement are serious. Loosening and mechanical failure are almost inevitable if infection ensues. It is important to appreciate that such infections are often caused by normal skin commensals not normally regarded as pathogens, e.g. *Staphylococcus albus*. Protection against these and more clearly recognized pathogens, e.g.

S. aureus, requires the administration of a broad-spectrum antibiotic perioperatively and immediately postoperatively. Antibiotics are commenced at induction of anaesthesia and continued for 16–24 h.

Following trauma

All *open wounds* are contaminated with microorganisms and with debris such as bits of clothing, grit, etc. The addition of soft-tissue injury, including ischaemic muscle, produces low tissue oxygen tension, thus creating an ideal milieu for anaerobic infection. Of particular concern are spore-bearing Gram-positive organisms, including clostridia, which may cause gas gangrene (*Clostridium welchii*) or tetanus (*C. tetani*). Other organisms may be present in particular situations, such as mouth organisms after a bite; human bites produce particularly nasty infections. Most patients have received active tetanus immunity in childhood, although few sustain booster injections into adult life. If active immunization has not been administered in the last 5 years a booster dose should be given. In any case, where the wound is very dirty passive immunity with human antitetanus globulin (Humotet) should be offered. This is now a very safe substance with few side-effects and a low incidence of anaphylactoid reaction.

First-line treatment of all open wounds includes surgical exploration and removal of dead tissue (*debridement*). Wounds should be left open, at least initially, and regularly inspected. If possible, wounds should be allowed to heal naturally, although some may be closed by delayed suturing if clean.

The role of antibiotics in open wounds is controversial. Fresh and relatively clean wounds may not demand prophylaxis. If there is any delay or wounds are dirty or they communicate with a fracture, a course of broad-spectrum antibiotics effective against Gram-positive organisms should be administered intravenously.

Table 28.1 Incidence of infection in relation to wound classification.

Type of wound	Definition	Examples	Incidence of wound infection (%)
Clean	No contamination from GI, GU or respiratory tracts	Thyroidectomy, hernia repair	1–5
Clean-contaminated	Minimal contamination from GI, GU or respiratory tracts	Cholecystectomy, TURP, pneumonectomy	7–10
Contaminated	Significant contamination from GI, GU or respiratory tracts	Elective colonic surgery	15–20
Dirty	Operations in the presence of infection	Bowel perforation Pelvic abscess	30–40

GI, Gastrointestinal; GU, genitourinary; TURP, transurethral resection of the prostate.

• Prophylaxis should also be employed in *closed-limb injury* because of the extensive soft-tissue damage which may occur. In such injuries prophylactic policy mirrors that of elective joint replacement. After trauma there is also the added risk associated with increased soft-tissue ischaemia through small blood vessel damage which causes bruising. This combination of damaged tissues and poor blood supply is a particular risk.

Surgery in the presence of valvular heart disease

Patients with damaged heart valves (e.g. post rheumatic fever) or with prosthetic heart valves are at risk of developing infective endocarditis during procedures which cause a transient bacteraemia; dental extraction is the classical example. The incidence of endocarditis is low following such procedures but the consequences are devastating and therefore the use of prophylactic antibiotics is mandatory. While Gram-positive cocci (*Streptococcus viridans*) are the commonest causative organisms, coliforms or even fungi may also be responsible.

Postsplenectomy

Following splenectomy there is a considerable risk of overwhelming postsplenectomy infection by encapsulated organisms, particularly *Streptococcus pneumoniae*. In this respect, splenic preservation is particularly indicated in children who are more at risk of this complication than adults. All young patients undergoing splenectomy should be vaccinated with the polyvalent pneumococcal vaccine (Pneumovax). Furthermore, any fever should be treated aggressively with antibiotics and small children should probably receive prophylactic penicillin (see Chapter 8).

Prophylaxis against thrombosis (see also Chapter 18)

Deep vein thrombosis is not uncommon, depending on the type of patient and the kind of operative procedure being performed. Not all, but many, patients with deep vein thrombosis will go on to have pulmonary embolism and many of these will be fatal. Thrombosis in the pelvic veins is particularly associated with pulmonary embolism. Overweight, immobility, smoking, oestrogens and pelvic surgery are all associated with increased risk of venous thromboembolism.

Simple prophylactic measures include cessation of smoking, weight loss, maintenance of mobility and avoidance of oestrogen for 6 weeks prior to surgery. Women taking low oestrogen pills or hormone replacement therapy (HRT) do not need to discontinue their drugs. If it is deemed necessary to stop contraceptive agents then the patient must be counselled about alternative methods of birth control.

In the operating theatre physical methods have been shown to aid prophylaxis against deep vein thrombosis. These include:
• ensuring the calves are not restricted by resting on the operative table;
• actively pumping blood around the calves either by pneumatic compression or with a system designed to stimulate the foot muscles; and
• certain drugs are of proven effectiveness although most have the problem of increased risk of postoperative bleeding. Common agents include heparin given subcutaneously, low-molecular-weight dextran, the coumarins and indanediones. These substances are discussed in detail in Chapter 18.

Postoperatively early mobilization will reduce risk and any chemoprophylactic measure should be continued until regular mobility has been established.

Prevention of pressure sores

Patients lying in bed for long periods are at risk of developing pressure sores (also called bedsores or decubitus ulcers) (see Fig. 23.21). These are skin ulcers which result from excessive pressure leading to reduced tissue perfusion and ischaemic necrosis. Shearing of soft tissues over bony points adds to the risks of tissue damage and ischaemia. Common sites are the heels, the buttocks and over the greater trochanters of the femurs. Shearing, particularly over the buttocks, is potentiated by awkward sitting. All patients who are *immobile* for long periods are at risk; however, some groups are in particular danger. These include the *old*, those who are *confused*, those without cutaneous sensation, including some *diabetics*, those with *vascular disease*, *rheumatoid arthritis*, those with *spinal cord injury* and those taking *steroids*.

Most pressure sores are preventable by ensuring that the patient is not left in the same position for long periods of time. Thus, regular turning of those unable to turn themselves and the avoidance of sharp or projecting objects coming into contact with the patient are essential. Most important, however, is regular inspection of areas at risk and this should be the responsibility of the whole clinical team.

Prevention of chest and urinary problems

Chest problems

Prolonged immobility may lead to bronchopneumonia through poor ventilation. The passage of air in and out of the chest is restricted by recumbency. Ideally patients should stop smoking for several weeks before operations. Deep breathing exercises under the direction of a physiotherapist and incentive spirometry for some days before operation are also useful. Regular postoperative breathing exercises, incentive spirometry and coughing, particularly after abdominal surgery, will also minimize risk. In selected patients with bronchospasm, bronchodilators (usually administered by aerosol inhalation) may be very valuable.

Urinary problems

Recumbency also makes emptying the bladder less than efficient. This, plus the difficulties of maintaining good personal cleanliness while confined to bed, makes the risk of bladder infection greater. This may be avoided by permitting the patient to stand or sit to void where possible. Women are particularly at risk from urinary tract infection because of the short female urethra.

Prolonged recumbency also puts patients at risk from urinary calculus formation. This is brought on by a combination of low fluid intake and mobilization of bone calcium induced by inactivity. Prevention is largely dealt with by early mobilization and maintenance of an adequate oral fluid intake.

Prevention of stress ulceration (see also Chapter 13)

Stress ulceration is most likely to occur in patients who have had severe trauma (especially burns) or after major surgery (including neurosurgery). Many have associated severe infection. The ulceration may be a single ulcer in the duodenum or multiple erosions involving the gastric antrum and body of the stomach. Prevention involves the use of antacids to maintain a pH of 6, the administration of parenteral H_2-receptor antagonists (e.g. cimetidine or ranitidine) or mucosal protectants (e.g. sucralfate). All patients undergoing major surgery should receive some form of prophylaxis against stress ulceration. Operative intervention is rarely required but, if serious bleeding cannot be controlled, truncal vagotomy and antrectomy is probably the operation of choice.

Protection against AIDS and hepatitis

Health care workers are at risk of coming into contact with patients' tissues (open wounds), secretions (sputum, naso-gastric aspirate, faeces) and body fluids (blood and urine). Overall the risks of contracting a disease from a patient are very small but if one is unfortunate enough to contract a disease the consequences may be dire. Many health care workers have died of hepatitis and a growing number have contracted the AIDS virus (human immunodeficiency virus; HIV).

In general, everyday contact with infected patients does not increase the risk of contamination unless one is handling their tissues or body wastes. No health worker has contracted AIDS from routine nursing duties. Most cases have been associated with either massive transfusion of infected blood or sharp injury with contaminated needles or during surgery. There is a greater risk of acquiring hepatitis than becoming HIV-positive on exposure to the blood of patients with these respective conditions. Furthermore, the risk of contracting AIDS is increased if the patient has AIDS rather than is simply HIV-positive. In other words, the more viral particles in the blood stream or the greater the volume of contaminated blood one comes in contact with, the higher the risk.

All health care workers, including medical students, should be actively immunized against hepatitis. This is a safe and efficient vaccine provided immunity is confirmed by serology. There is no vaccine for HIV and so care against needlestick injury is paramount. Precautions when handling sharp instruments should become second nature both in the wards and in the operating theatres and sharps should always be placed in designated containers to protect ancillary workers.

Medical workers who become hepatitis antigen-positive or who contract HIV infection cannot continue to come in contact with patients. In the latter situation such infected workers will die of AIDS. The risk of infecting patients is high and so there is an ethical obligation to give up practice, with all the personal consequences that entails. Care and good practice must prevail!

29 Transfusion of Blood and Blood Products

Will all great Neptune's ocean wash this blood
Clean from my hand? No, this my hand will rather
The multitudinous seas incarnadine,
Making the green one red.   (Macbeth ii. 61)

Introduction

Modern blood transfusion is based on the philosophy that only those components of blood which are deficient in a particular patient should be infused, rather than whole blood. This practice ensures the safe, economic use of blood products and increases the therapeutic scope. Thus, a single blood donation may be used for treating a variety of disorders. The blood products available in the majority of hospitals are shown in Table 29.1.

Transfusion of blood and blood products

In elective surgery, the predicted transfusion needs are best calculated by the adoption of a *blood tariff policy* whereby the requirements for a specific operation are calculated on the basis of average usage. For some operations no blood is required and patients are simply blood-grouped and a sample of their serum saved. It should be noted that there is no medical or surgical condition which justifies the transfusion of less than 2 units of blood.

Stored whole blood

Whole blood is only indicated for the treatment of acute haemorrhage; hypovolaemia is accompanied by an acute reduction in red cell mass, resulting in impaired oxygen-carrying capacity at a time when tissue perfusion is compromised. Even in this situation, its use must be reserved for

Table 29.1 Blood products available for therapy.

*Red cell preparations**
Whole blood
Red cell concentrate
Leukocyte-poor red cell concentrates
Frozen red cells (not available generally)
Autologous blood

*Platelets**
Random donor pooled
Single-donor apheresis
HLA-matched
Cross-matched

Plasma components
Plasma protein fraction (5% albumin in buffered saline)
Salt-poor human albumin (25%)
Fresh frozen plasma (plasma + all clotting factors)*
Cryoprecipitate (factor VIII, vWF, fibrinogen)*
Factor VIII concentrate
Factor VIIa
Factors II, IX, X
Factor VII
vWF
Antithrombin III
Intravenous immunoglobulin G (IgG)
   Human normal IgG
   Specific hyperimmune IgG (Rh anti-D, tetanus, etc.)

Fibrin sealant (glue)

* ABO compatibility essential.
HLA, Human leukocyte antigen; vWF, von Willebrand factor.

those patients with substantial blood loss and a haematocrit of 30% or less after volume replacement with crystalloids and plasma expanders.

Stored blood has a number of unwanted features. These include:

- citrate anticoagulant;
- an acid pH (6.6–6.8);
- high levels of K+ (from the stored red blood cells);
- ammonia (from erythrocyte adenosine);
- reduced red-cell 2,3-diphosphoglycerate (2,3 DPG; which leads to impaired release of oxygen from oxyhaemoglobin).

The use of stored whole blood is rapidly decreasing because of increasing demand for individual blood products and for economic reasons.

Red cell concentrates

Packed red cells have the same oxygen-carrying capacity of blood but a lower volume. They are thus ideal for the treatment of *anaemic patients* who invariably have a normal blood volume and are at risk from circulatory overload. Even so, unless the anaemia is severe and symptomatic, transfusion is no substitute for haematinic (promotion of blood production) therapy and is only indicated in patients who:

- do not respond to haematinic treatment (refractory anaemia);
- are unable to adapt to the reduced oxygen-carrying capacity of the blood and exhibit signs of incipient cardiovascular failure;
- require urgent surgery.

Up to 10% of patients develop alloimmunization to leukocyte antigens, usually after repeated red cell infusions. The antibodies cause severe febrile reactions which can only be prevented by the use of leukocyte-poor red cell concentrates.

Autologous blood

The use of autologous blood, donated by the patient for his or her later use, is becoming more common. This is obviously applicable to elective surgery and autologous blood donation can be enhanced by treatment with recombinant human erythropoietin. Very close collaboration between the haematology and surgery departments is required for such a service to run smoothly and as yet facilities for autologous transfusion are not universally available. The patient's own blood may also be collected during surgery and returned to the circulation via a cell saver. This technique is used in operations where blood loss is likely to be considerable, e.g. liver transplantation, but is contraindicated if there is contamination by bowel content. Blood is

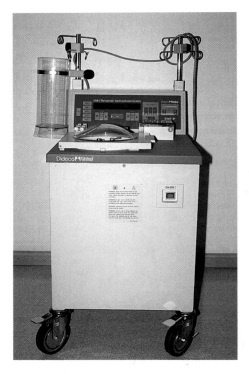

Figure 29.1 Cell saver.

collected by suction from the operation site and the cells are washed and resuspended in physiological solution before transfusion. Considerable amounts of red cells can be recycled in this way (Fig. 29.1).

Frozen red cells

With the use of cryoprotective agents (glycerol, hydroxyethyl starch), satisfactory storage of red cells at –80°C to 196°C (mechanical freezing or liquid nitrogen storage) for long periods (up to 10 years) can be achieved. This method of storage removes leukocytes, platelets and any viral particles, thereby reducing the incidence of both transmission of viral disease and alloimmunization to leukocyte and platelet antigens. Red cells recovered from a frozen bank are of particular value to patients on renal dialysis programmes, those with refractory anaemias and patients with rare cell types and complex antibody mixtures. However, frozen red cells are very expensive and impractical for most patients.

Platelet concentrates

Platelet concentrates can be obtained by centrifugation of blood from several donors or by plateletpheresis from a single donation. Because of the variable but significant con-

Table 29.2 Indications for platelet transfusion.

Surgical
Bleeding and thrombocytopenia
Limited cover for operative interventions:
  Platelet count below 40×10^9/l (40 000/mm³)
  Platelet dysfunction
Acute disseminated intravascular coagulation (with fresh frozen plasma)
Massive blood transfusion (washout thrombocytopenia)
Postcardiac bypass platelet loss and/or dysfunction

Medical
Marrow-suppressed patients (intensive chemotherapy)
Aplastic anaemia

tamination with red cells, platelet concentrates have to be obtained from ABO/Rh-compatible donors. Some human leukocyte antigens (HLAs) are expressed on platelets and determine the survival of platelets after transfusion. They lead to alloimmunization in patients requiring repeated platelet transfusions. The antibodies generated cause rapid destruction of the transfused platelets and account for the progressive inefficacy of repeated transfusions. For these patients, HLA-matched platelet concentrates are needed. The indications for platelet transfusions are shown in Table 29.2. In surgical practice platelet transfusions are most commonly used to stop bleeding in thrombocytopenic patients, to cover surgery if the platelet count is below 40×10^9/l and in patients with platelet dysfunction.

Clotting factors

The most common fraction used in surgical practice is *fresh frozen plasma*, for which ABO compatibility is essential. It is indicated in bleeding states associated with multifactorial deficiencies, such as disseminated intravascular coagulation (DIC), massive transfusion of stored blood, overdose with oral anticoagulants (warfarin) and acute fulminant or chronic liver disease. *Cryoprecipitate* (factor VIII, von Willebrand factor, fibrinogen) is used in haemophilia, von Willebrand's disease and in fibrinogen deficiency. However, because of the risk of transmitted infection, cryoprecipitate is now used much less for haemophilia. *Factor VIII concentrate* is preferred as it is safer and gives a more certain dose. *Factor IX concentrate* is indicated to arrest acute bleeding and cover operative interventions in patients with Christmas disease. Factor VIII and IX therapy requires expert guidance.

Other plasma components

The availability of synthetic gelatin and starch plasma expanders has made redundant the use of *plasma protein* *fraction* for volume replacement. Human *salt-poor albumin* solution (25%) is administered selectively in patients with severe hypoalbuminaemia, particularly when this is accompanied by reduced glomerular filtration, usually in patients with chronic liver disease. Immunoglobulin (IgG) is administered in patients with hypogammaglobulinaemia and as a prophylaxis against viral disease in non-immunized patients. *Hyperimmune IgG* is partially effective in the prophylaxis and disease attenuation of tetanus and herpes zoster infections.

Adverse effects of transfusion of blood and blood products

The mechanisms of transfusion reactions are varied, depending on the cause. Hence, the complications of transfusion are usually classified according to aetiology; they may also be either acute or delayed (Table 29.3).

Table 29.3 Complications of transfusion of blood and blood products.

Acute
Non-haemolytic reactions
  Pyrogenic (febrile) reactions
  Hypersensitivity reactions
Haemolytic reactions
Metabolic, respiratory and haemostatic complications
Circulatory overload
Septic shock (bacterially infected units)

Delayed
Delayed haemolytic
Infective

Bacterial	Brucellosis, syphilis
Helminthic	Filariasis
Protozoal	Babesiosis, Chagas disease, kala-azar, malaria, trypanosomiasis, toxoplasmosis
Rickettsial	Relapsing fever, Rocky Mountain spotted fever
Viral	B19, cytomegalovirus, Epstein–Barr virus, HIV 1 and 2, HTLV 1 and 2, hepatitis and yellow fever

Sensitization/alloimmunization
  Haemolytic disease of the newborn
  Immune suppression (increased infective risk and increased tumour recurrence rate)
  Posttransfusion purpura
  Platelet refractoriness
Transfusion iron overload (haemosiderosis)

HIV, Human immunodeficiency virus; HTLV, human T-lymphotrophic virus.

Acute reactions

Acute non-haemolytic reactions

The routine establishment of quality control in the manufacture of both intravenous fluids and disposable giving sets has virtually eliminated pyrogenic reactions. Pyrexia following blood transfusion is nowadays the result of alloimmunization to leukocyte and platelet antigens in patients requiring repeated blood transfusions. This is the commonest cause of severe febrile reactions. Although the reaction is usually self-limiting and benign, the transfusion must be stopped to exclude the possibility of a more serious haemolytic reaction. Febrile reactions in alloimmunized patients can be prevented by using red cell concentrates, from which most of the other formed elements have been removed (leukocytes, platelets, soluble histocompatibility antigens).

The other non-haemolytic reactions include severe immediate hypersensitivity reactions and mild allergic or anaphylactoid reactions. The causes of these reactions are rarely established. The reaction results in the release of vasoactive peptides and activation of complement. The severe anaphylactic reaction is accompanied by profound hypotension, laryngeal and/or bronchospasm and cutaneous flushing. It is fortunately rare (1 in 20 000 transfusions) and responds to *stopping the transfusion*, adrenalin, intravenous antihistamines and hydrocortisone. *Adrenaline* (0.5–1.0 mg) is given immediately either by the subcutaneous or intramuscular route and the dose repeated, if necessary, every 10 min, depending on the improvement of the blood pressure and pulse. *Antihistamines* are administered by slow intravenous injection after the adrenaline treatment and should be continued for 24–48 h. Because of its delayed action, *hydrocortisone* is of secondary value in this severe complication but its use prevents further deterioration. Antihistamines are also employed in the prophylaxis and active treatment of urticarial reactions.

Acute haemolytic reactions

Acute haemolytic reactions are usually the result of *ABO incompatibility* caused by human error at the bedside (blood given to the wrong patient) or in the laboratory (faulty cross-matching). Incompatible blood transfusion is a serious complication and carries an average mortality of 3%, which is higher if more than 200 ml of incompatible blood is administered. The clinical features include pain at the infusion site and along the vein, chest and back pain, fever and rigors. The patient becomes flushed, hypotensive and develops oozing from vascular access sites and wounds (DIC). The extensive intravascular haemolysis results in haemoglobinaemia and haemoglobinuria. Oliguria rapidly supervenes and progresses to acute renal failure.

Management entails immediate recognition with *cessation of the transfusion* and replacement of the giving set. Adequate hydration is maintained by *intravenous infusion of crystalloids* (isotonic saline or Hartmann's solution) and an attempt is made at forced diuresis with intravenous large-dose *frusemide* (150 mg). If this fails, a 20% solution of *mannitol* (100 ml) is administered. If diuresis is obtained, a high urine output is maintained (100 ml/h) by large-volume crystalloid infusions. Often, however, these patients progress to acute renal failure, necessitating *haemodialysis*.

The other problem which requires immediate support is the development of DIC and bleeding. After the initial resuscitation is completed, the investigation of such an incident is essential and is outlined in Table 29.4.

Table 29.4 Investigation of an acute haemolytic transfusion episode.

Report incident to the blood transfusion department
Establish that the unit of blood had been issued to the patient who received it
Obtain fresh samples of patient's blood (clotted and in EDTA) for repeat cross-matching and serological testing
Send the unit of blood to the blood transfusion department for culture and further investigation
Obtain further blood samples from patient for clinical chemistry (electrolytes, urea, free haemoglobin) and coagulation screen
Discuss any further transfusion requirements with the blood transfusion officer
EDTA, Ethylenediaminetetraacetic acid.

Acute haemolytic reactions giving a similar picture may arise from acute haemolysis caused by preformed antibodies in the patient's blood as a result of alloimmunization to minor blood group antigens in the donated unit. This may be encountered in patients requiring repeated blood transfusions.

Metabolic, haemostatic and respiratory complications

These complications are confined to patients who, because of severe haemorrhage, receive a massive blood transfusion of stored blood. *Massive blood transfusion is defined as that which is equivalent to or exceeds the patient's own blood volume within 12 h.* Apart from being cold (4°C), stored blood has an acid pH, contains citrate anticoagulant, has elevated plasma potassium and ammonia and a reduced 2,3 DPG. The metabolic consequences therefore include:

- *Hypothermia*: This may lead to cardiac arrhythmias, including ventricular fibrillation and asystole. For this reason, blood warming is necessary if the transfusion rate exceeds 50 ml/min. Unfortunately, the heating coils increase the resistance of the giving circuit but none the less their use is essential in these patients.
- *Acidosis*.
- *Increased affinity of oxyhaemoglobin for oxygen*, which is thus not readily released to the tissue, thereby contributing to defective tissue oxygen uptake. However, increased oxygen affinity reverses after transfusion.
- *Citrate intoxication* is due to the chelation of ionized calcium which may result in prolongation of the QT interval, but this does not usually materially affect cardiac function and the ionized calcium levels rapidly return to normal after the transfusion as the excess citrate is metabolized and excreted. Thus, the use of supplemental calcium is not justified, particularly as it may itself give rise to arrhythmias.
- *Hyperkalaemia* is seldom a problem as the excess plasma K+ enters the red blood cells, with warming to body temperature. It is, however, a consideration in patients with acidosis and renal failure when calcium is administered as the physiological antidote.
- Stored blood is *deficient in platelets and labile clotting factors* (V and VIII). For this reason, massive transfusion of stored blood induces a dilution of the labile clotting factors in addition to a moderate thrombocytopenia. The deficiency of the labile clotting factors can be circumvented by the administration of two units of fresh frozen plasma for every 8 units of blood. The transfusion-related thrombocytopenia is seldom significant and can usually be ignored.

Pulmonary oedema is common after massive blood transfusion, although adult respiratory distress syndrome (ARDS) is rare nowadays. The oedema is often due to an element of left ventricular failure. There is controversy with regard to the aetiology of ARDS (see Chapter 19). Undoubtedly, microaggregates of platelets, leukocytes and fibrin (50–200 μm) are present in stored blood but the extent of pulmonary microvascular occlusion which these may cause is unknown. None the less, the use of microaggregate filters when more than 5 units of blood are administered is a sensible practice. They do, however, reduce blood flow — a practical problem with massive transfusion.

Circulatory overload

Circulatory overload is encountered in the transfusion of anaemic patients, particularly those with severe and long-standing anaemia. These patients must be transfused very slowly and only with packed cells (with or without concomitant diuretic therapy). In some patients, an exchange transfusion has to be carried out to avoid severe congestive failure.

Delayed reactions

Transmission of infectious disease

A wide spectrum of infectious disease can be transmitted by the transfusion of blood and blood products. However, with screening of blood donors and heat treatment of blood protein products, the risk is now small. The most commonly transmitted viral disease is hepatitis C (non-A non-B hepatitis), but this occurs in less than 0.1% of transfusions (see Table 29.3).

Immune suppression

There is no doubt about the immunosuppressive effect of blood transfusion. Indeed, blood transfusion has been employed specifically for this purpose in patients prior to renal transplantation to improve graft survival. In the context of general surgery, perioperative blood transfusion, by virtue of this immunosuppressive effect, which is additive to that inherent to the operative trauma, has undoubted undesirable consequences. The important ones are an enhanced risk of infective complications and a poorer prognosis following cancer surgery, manifested by an increased recurrence rate and reduced disease-free survival.

Transfusion haemosiderosis

Iron overload of the monocyte–macrophage system is caused by repeated red-cell transfusions over many years. This becomes significant after 100 units have been administered, when the liver, pancreas, myocardium and the endocrine glands become damaged. It is especially a problem in childhood anaemias (e.g. thalassaemia) and in patients with chronic refractory anaemia. Iron overload is reduced in these patients by iron chelation therapy with desferrioxamine.

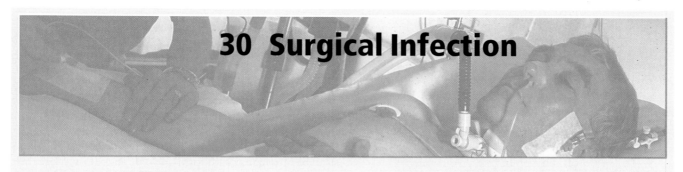

30 Surgical Infection

Humanity has three great enemies:
Fever, famine and war,
Of these by far the greatest,
By far the most terrible is fever.   (William Osler 1849–1919)

Introduction

Surgical infections are as old as surgery itself and surgeons encounter infection in two ways:
- patients present with an infection that requires surgical treatment, e.g. drainage of an abscess; or
- infection complicates a surgical procedure, e.g. wound infection. This problem was almost universal prior to the development of aseptic surgery in the last century but, in spite of our more sophisticated understanding of the nature of infection and an arsenal of antimicrobial agents, infection still remains a major surgical problem today. An infection acquired in hospital is called a *nosocomial* infection.

Most surgical infection is due to bacterial and, more rarely, fungal infection. Viruses, such as human immunodeficiency virus (HIV) and the hepatitis B and C viruses, are important to surgeons because they may contract these diseases from their patients and due care has to be taken when managing such patients. Spirochaetal diseases rarely come to the attention of surgeons now, although *noma* and *tropical phagedenic ulcer*, from which *Borelia vincentii* and various bacteria are isolated, are common in some parts of the world. Most of this chapter will be devoted to the problem of bacterial infection.

Pathophysiology of infection

Like the rich and the poor, microorganisms are always with (and *within*!) us, but for most of the time we coexist happily with them. Infection occurs when microorganisms in sufficient numbers and virulence (i.e. with an innate capacity to cause disease either by invasion or toxin production) breach the body's defensive barriers and initiate an inflammatory response.

Establishing an infection

Generally, various combinations of three elements are important for bacterial infection:
- *An inoculum of bacteria.* The number of bacteria required to establish an infection depends on the virulence of that bacterium. Relatively small numbers of a very virulent organism (e.g. *β-haemolytic streptococcus*) or large numbers of organisms with low virulence (e.g. *Staphylococcus epidermidis*) may cause an infection. However, in most established surgical infections there are 100 000 organisms per millilitre of exudate, gram of tissue or square millimetre of infected surface area. A single organism or mixtures of organisms can establish an infection and synergistic infections can be particularly severe (e.g. Vincent's angina, which is caused by Gram-negative anaerobic *Fusobacterium* species and a spirochaete *B. vincenti*). The elements of aseptic surgery (i.e. sterilization of instruments and drapes, skin preparation with antiseptics, e.g. povidone-iodine, wearing of special clothing in theatre) were introduced to reduce the size of any potential inoculum which might enter the body via the wounds made during surgery. It is almost impossible to create a germ-*free* surgical environment.
- A '*bacteria-friendly*' *environment.* We know from bacteriology that bacteria grow best in culture media that

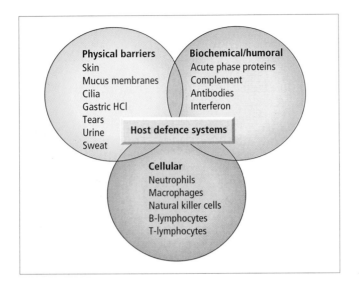

Figure 30.1 The elements of the immune system which counter bacterial infection.

contain water, electrolytes, carbohydrate, protein digests and blood; some also like air (aerobes), some do not (anaerobes). Any *in vivo* situation which provides these elements will facilitate bacterial growth and infection. Thus, patients with diabetes mellitus, whose tissues contain excess amounts of glucose, are more prone to infection than non-diabetics. Accumulations of blood or serum, e.g. in surgical wounds or after trauma, and ischaemic or necrotic tissues are all likely to promote bacterial growth.
• *Diminished host resistance.* The very complicated systems which protect us from a hostile environment are summarized in Fig. 30.1. Anything which reduces the host's resistance will allow an infection to become established even with a relatively small inoculum. During an operation the physical barriers are breached but the risk of infection is greatly increased if the host is also immunocompromised (e.g. if the patients has acquired immune deficiency syndrome; AIDS). Patients who are malnourished, have malignancy or are taking steroids or other immunosuppressive agents are all more susceptible to bacterial infections.

Bacterial secretions

Bacteria cause some of their ill effects by releasing various compounds. These are:
• *Enzymes* (e.g. haemolysins, streptokinase, hyaluronidase) which help the organism become established.
• *Exotoxins* are proteins which are released from the intact bacterial cell wall of (mostly) Gram-positive bacteria. They spread by the blood stream or in some cases (e.g. tetanus)

via nerves. Exotoxins produce ill effects both at the site of infection and remote sites. In tetanus (see below) the bacteria stay in the wound but the clinical features of the disease are caused by the action of the exotoxin. (Diphtheria produces its ill effects in a similar manner.) Exotoxins can be attenuated with formaldehyde so that they lose their toxicity but retain their antigenicity. The attenuated toxin is called *toxoid* and is used as a vaccine.
• *Endotoxins* are composed of lipopolysaccharides (LPS) in the bacterial cell wall of Gram-negative bacteria. They are liberated only on the death of the bacterium. LPS stimulate macrophages and endothelial cells to release cytokines which mediate the inflammatory response and play an important role in the pathogenesis of septic shock (see Chapter 7).

Natural history of infection

Prior to the introduction of antibiotics, little could be done to halt the progress of an infection and a patient's survival depended on the ability of his or her immune system to deal with the invading organism (Box 30.1). It is the body's reaction to an invading microorganism which produces the classical inflammatory response resulting in the clinical features of infection:

The tragedy of Ignaz Semmelweis (1818–1865) and puerperal sepsis

Throughout history young mothers frequently died from infection (puerperal fever) following childbirth. Ignaz Semmelweis, a Hungarian doctor working in Vienna in the 1840s, noticed that the maternal death rate in one of the two maternity wards of the Allgemeines Krankenhaus was 10% compared to only 3% in the other. He observed that the first ward was run by doctors and that frequently medical students would come to this ward straight from the autopsy room and perform vaginal examinations on the women in labour. The second ward was run by midwives who paid a lot of attention to personal cleanliness. Medical students did not come to this ward.

Semmelweis conducted some animal experiments in which he transmitted fatal puerperal sepsis to rabbits by introducing into the rabbit's vagina pus he had obtained from women dying from puerperal fever. The use of chlorinated lime prevented the sepsis. On the maternity ward he introduced a programme of compulsory hand washing with chlorinated lime and immediately reduced the mortality rate to 3%. Thus, he performed an important and very good piece of research; he identified a problem, he tested his hypothesis in the laboratory and applied his solution to patients resulting in considerable reduction in mortality.

Was Semmelweis hailed as a hero and given a medal? He was dismissed from his post and forgotten. He returned to Budapest where he published a little-read monograph on puerperal fever and its prophylaxis. In 1865 he was committed to a mental institution and died shortly thereafter.

Box 30.1

- rubor (redness);
- tumor (swelling);
- dolor (pain);
- calor (heat).

In acute infection these clinical features may be accompanied by a swinging pyrexia, leukocytosis, raised C-reactive protein and, if the infection spreads, bacteraemia (see Chapter 7). Following an acute inflammatory response a number of outcomes are possible:

- *Resolution*: If tissue damage is minimal, the inflammatory response settles completely and the tissue returns to normal.
- *Spreading infection*: An infection may spread from its initial site:
  (a) by direct spread into adjacent tissues;
  (b) along tissue planes, e.g. tendon sheaths;
  (c) via the lymphatic channels, producing the characteristic red lines of lymphangitis and enlarged tender lymph nodes (acute lymphadenitis); or
  (d) via the blood stream causing bacteraemia (the presence of bacteria in the blood stream) or septicaemia (the presence of propagating organisms in the blood stream).
- *Abscess formation*: An abscess is defined as a localized collection of pus. Pus is composed of neutrophils, exudate and bacteria. The common pus-producing organisms (pyogenic) are *Staphylococcus aureus*, *Streptococcus pyogenes*, *Escherichia coli* and *Bacteroides*. An abscess which is not drained surgically may discharge spontaneously, e.g. through the skin, and resolve, or it may lead to septicaemia and death (Fig. 30.2).
- *Organization*: Following acute inflammation with tissue damage or drainage of an abscess, repair of the tissues is achieved by organization, laying down of granulation tissue and fibrosis.
- *Chronic inflammation*: If the injuring agent persists in the tissues (e.g. a foreign body), a chronic inflammatory response is established. Such responses are characterized histologically by macrophages and giant cells and often the presence of granulomas. Certain microorganisms cause most of their damage by chronic inflammation, e.g. *Mycobacterium tuberculosis*.

Management of surgical infections

Prevention of infection

Several prophylactic measures are now available to prevent infection. These are discussed fully in Chapter 28.

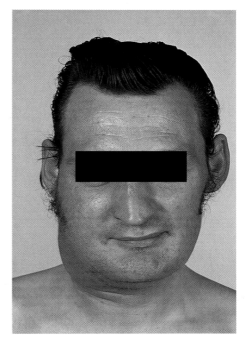

Figure 30.2 Abscess on the right side of the neck.

Management of established infection

- *Diagnosis*: The presence of an infection will be suspected from the clinical picture. Wherever possible, infected material should be obtained for culture before commencing antibiotics. Swabs should be obtained from infected skin lesions and discharging wounds. Material from deep-seated infections, e.g. a subphrenic abscess, may be obtained by needle aspiration, possibly with computed tomographic (CT) or ultrasound imaging to guide the needle. The tips of infected intravenous lines should be cultured and blood cultures obtained in anyone with an unknown pyrexia. Urine and sputum should be cultured as appropriate.
- *Antibiotics*: The use of antibiotics has revolutionized the management of surgical infection and where possible antibiotics should be administered on the basis of the culture results. However, until the culture result becomes available, treatment should be given on the basis of the most likely organisms present. A Gram stain of the material sent for culture will usually give a clue as to what is present, e.g. Gram-positive cocci, Gram-negative bacilli, and an appropriate antibiotic may be chosen.
- *Drainage*: Drainage is essential once an abscess has become established and antibiotics play only a secondary role in the management of abscesses. Traditionally all abscesses were drained surgically but more recently many abscesses have been drained successfully by interventional

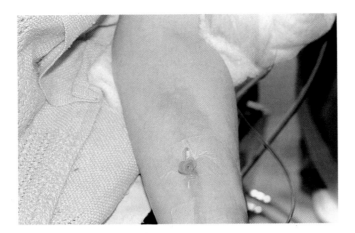

Figure 30.3 Cellulitis from an infected intravenous line.

radiology techniques. Whichever method is employed the principle is the same — the pus should be removed and a track should be established for free drainage.

Specific surgical infections

Cellulitis

Cellulitis is defined as an infection of the subcutaneous tissues. Two distinct types are recognized.

• The common type is *acute pyogenic cellulitis*, which is caused by *Streptococcus pyogenes* and presents as a spreading infection (facilitated by streptokinase and hyaluronidase) of the skin and subcutaneous tissues (Fig. 30.3). It is characterized by a dark-red skin discoloration, heat and oedema and it is often associated with lymphangitis and lymphadenopathy (see above). The most virulent form of this streptococcal infection is called *erysipelas*, which most frequently affects the face, producing a characteristic butterfly erythema. Erysipelas is a rarely seen condition today.

Treatment consists of immobilization, elevation of the affected part and intravenous antibiotics (penicillin or erythromycin).

• *Anaerobic cellulitis*. The second type of cellulitis is much more sinister and fortunately rare. This is the so-called 'flesh-eating' infection (also Meleney's gangrene) and is caused, not by a single organism, but by a combination of aerobes (*Streptococcus pyogenes, Staphylococcus aureus, Escherichia coli, Proteus, Klebsiella, Pseudomonas aeruginosa*) and anaerobes (*Bacteroides, anaerobic cocci, Clostridium*). These act synergistically to cause extensive tissue destruction and death. Two clinical syndromes are recognized from this type of infection:

(a) *Progressive bacterial synergistic gangrene* in which the skin becomes dark red and purple with areas of necrosis. This infection classically arose around infected closed wounds, e.g. abdominal wound, or a stoma but can complicate a simple abrasion. It spreads very rapidly and a whole limb can be involved in a few hours. When it affects the penoscrotal region it is called Fournier's gangrene (see Chapter 20).

(b) *Necrotizing fasciitis* is a deep cellulitis affecting the fascial planes. Initially the overlying skin is relatively normal while the necrotic process proceeds underneath. The patient becomes extremely toxic and later the skin becomes painful, red and necrotic as it is deprived of its blood supply.

Treatment of anaerobic cellulitis includes surgery to remove the necrotic tissue, appropriate antibiotics depending on sensitivity (e.g. combinations of flucloxacillin, benzylpenicillin, cephalosporins, erythromycin or gentamicin for the aerobes and metronidazole for the anaerobes) and systemic support in an intensive care unit (see Chapter 18). The mortality from anaerobic cellulitis is high.

Staphylococcal infections

Staphylococci are Gram-positive organisms which cause a spectrum of skin infections (boils, styes, carbuncles, abscesses and sycosis barbae) as well as osteomyelitis and deeper abscesses (e.g. breast abscess). The pathogenic species is *Staphylococcus aureus*. Staphylococci are normal skin commensals; *Staph. epidermidis* is found on all skin and rarely causes disease. Some 10–30% of the population carry *Staph. aureus* in the nares or perineum.

A *boil (furuncle)* is a skin abscess which involves a hair follicle and its associated gland. They are found commonly on the face, neck and axilla. Treatment is by incision and drainage and better hygiene. Systemic antibiotics are not indicated.

A *stye* is a self-limited staphylococcal infection of the eyelash follicles.

A *carbuncle* is a serious infection characterized by an area of subcutaneous necrosis with a honeycomb of small abscesses. It is particularly common in diabetics and can cause considerable disability. Treatment is with antibiotics and, rarely, surgery (Fig. 30.4).

Sycosis barbae is a staphylococcal infection of the shaving area caused by minor trauma made by a razor. This is one of the few conditions which should be treated with topical antibiotics.

Most strains of staphylococci are now resistant to penicillin due to their ability to produce an enzyme (β-lactamase) which breaks the β-lactam ring of the

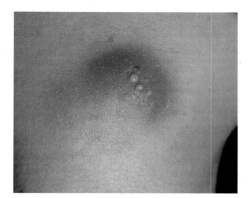

Figure 30.4 Carbuncle.

penicillin molecule. However, penicillinase-resistant antibiotics (e.g. flucloxacillin) remain effective against most species and are the first line of treatment for staphylococcal infections. In recent years a species of staphylococcus has been identified (usually in hospitals) which is resistant to most antibiotics. This is called *methicillin-resistant Staphylococcus aureus (MRSA)* and radical measures (e.g. patient isolation, barrier nursing, ward closure and disinfection) have to be taken when it is isolated to prevent its spread throughout a unit.

Hidradenitis

Hidradenitis suppurativa is an infection of the apocrine glands in the skin. It is common in the axilla and the groin. Irritation by deodorants and excessive sweating have been implicated as precipitating factors. The patient presents with multiple tender swellings under the arm or in the groin; these enlarge and discharge pus. Unless the area is kept very clean, recurrence is common and often surgery is required to excise the involved skin (Fig. 30.5).

Tetanus

Tetanus is a clostridial infection caused by the organism *Clostridium tetani*. This is now a rare infection in the western world due to universal vaccination but it is an important cause of death in the Third World. The infection is established when a penetrating wound, often of a minor nature, is contaminated by soil or animal manure containing *C. tetani* spores. In anaerobic conditions the spores germinate to produce bacilli which form an exotoxin. The bacteria are confined to the wound but produce their ill effects by the exotoxin which is absorbed at the motor nerve endings and travels via the nerves to the anterior horn cells.

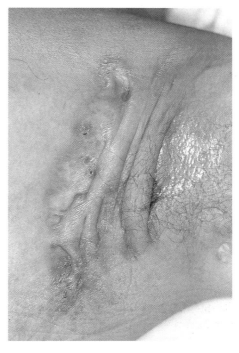

Figure 30.5 Hidradenitis suppurativa affecting the axilla.

The exotoxin is composed of two elements:
- *a neurotoxin* which acts on neuromuscular end-organs, producing spastic contractions and trismus (lockjaw), spasm of the facial muscles (risus sardonicus), rigidity and generalized convulsions so severe that only the patient's heels and head touch the bed (opisthotonos). Death, when it occurs, is due to asphyxia from spasm of the respiratory muscles and cardiovascular complications;
- a *haemolytic toxin* which lyses red blood cells.

Management

Tetanus prophylaxis

- Prevention is the ideal and in the UK active immunization with tetanus toxoid is administered to all children as part of the triple vaccine during the first year of life, with a booster dose at 5 years and at the end of schooling.
- If a patient presents to a casualty department with a potentially contaminated wound and has previously been fully immunized, then a booster dose of tetanus toxoid is administered.
- If a patient *has not* been vaccinated or is unsure of status, passive immunization with human antitetanus immunoglobulin is given and a full course of active immunization with toxoid is commenced.

Treatment

Antibiotics (penicillins) are administered to eliminate the contaminating organisms in a potentially infected wound. In an established case artificial ventilation with muscle relaxation is required and antitetanus immunoglobulin is administered in large doses. Antibiotics should be given to destroy the bacteria and prevent further toxin production.

Gas gangrene

Gas gangrene, the scourge of all wounded soldiers since men began to assault each other, is rare in civilian practice. Occasionally gas gangrene follows operations such as amputation for lower limb ischaemia. It is a spreading gangrene of the muscles accompanied by oedema, blackening of the tissues, crepitus (from gas production), profound toxaemia and shock. It is caused by contamination of extensive, necrotic wounds with soil or animal manure containing clostridial species (*C. perfringens* 65% of cases; *C. novyi* 30%: *C. septicum* 15%) that secrete powerful toxins. The toxins produce further tissue destruction and anaerobic conditions which enhance the spread of the infection. There is usually a foul-smelling discharge.

Treatment consists of wide excision or amputation of all necrotic and ischaemic tissue with free drainage and high-dose antibiotic therapy, including penicillin and metronidazole. Hyperbaric oxygen may be helpful in some cases and should be administered if available. Antitoxin has been used in military practice but with little benefit. The outlook for patients with this condition is still grim.

Postoperative infection

Postoperative infections are most frequently seen in surgical wounds, the abdominal cavity, chest, urinary tract and catheter sites. Clinically infection may present as cellulitis or abscess formation. Local symptoms and signs are pain, tenderness, swelling and heat. Systemic signs are fever, rigors and malaise. Uncontrolled infection may spread to the blood stream, producing septicaemia and septic shock.

Wound infections

The incidence of wound infection depends on whether the wound was initially clean, clean-contaminated, contaminated or dirty (see Table 28.1). A mild infection may present as no more than a cellulitis with pain, tenderness, swelling and redness and may subside with rest and antibiotics. Most wound infections, however, progress to abscess formation and require incision and drainage. The wound should be left open and secondary suture employed when the infection has subsided.

Intra-abdominal infections

Postoperative intra-abdominal infections present in one of two ways:
• *Generalized peritonitis* is usually a preoperative event but generalized peritonitis may also occur postoperatively (e.g. due to suture line dehiscence in gastrointestinal surgery). Postoperative peritonitis is a polymicrobial infection commonly caused by *E. coli*, *Klebsiella*, *Proteus*, *Strep. faecalis* and *Bacteroides*. The rapid spread of infection throughout the peritoneal cavity is a consequence of the virulence of the organisms, diminished host resistance and the failure to wall off the infection and confine it locally with omentum, loops of intestine and fibrinous deposits.

Clinical features include pain, rigidity and absence of bowel sounds. Fever and leukocytosis are present and septic shock rapidly supervenes. Treatment consists of intravenous fluids for resuscitation, elimination of the source of infection (e.g. closure of perforated viscus), removal of necrotic material and appropriate therapy.
• *Intra-abdominal abscess* occurs in association with severe inflammation of abdominal organs such as the appendix, pancreas, colon, etc. They are well-defined collections of pus which have been walled off from the rest of the peritoneal cavity by omentum, intestinal loops and fibrin. Abscesses represent victory for the peritoneal host defence mechanisms; the infection is contained and prevented from reaching the blood stream. An intra-abdominal abscess causes local pain and tenderness and sometimes a palpable mass. Fluctuating fever and rigors are characteristic. Common sites for intra-abdominal abscess are right or left iliac fossae due to appendicitis or diverticulitis respectively, subphrenic abscess following cholecystitis, pancreatitis or leaking suture lines from upper gastrointestinal surgery, and pelvic abscess, often associated with appendicitis or inflammation of pelvic organs.

General support of the patient, adequate drainage of the abscess and antibiotic cover are the mainstays of treatment. Drainage may be achieved by percutaneous drainage techniques or by surgery. Over 85% of abscesses can now be drained percutaneously with the aid of ultrasonography or CT scanning. Surgical drainage is associated with a higher morbidity and mortality than percutaneous drainage. However, in many cases a surgical approach is necessary in order to deal with the underlying pathology (e.g. perforated viscus) or to divert the faecal stream (i.e. create a stoma).

Respiratory infection

Pulmonary infection is common after surgery. Factors which predispose to postoperative respiratory infection are:
- *pre-existing pulmonary disease*, e.g. chronic obstructive airways disease;
- *smoking*, which causes mucus production and ciliary dysfunction;
- *starvation and fluid restriction* prior to surgery, which leads to dehydration;
- *anaesthesia*, which paralyses the respiratory epithelial ciliary activity; and
- *postoperative pain*, which makes deep breathing and coughing difficult and predisposes to atelectasis.

Preventive measures include vigorous preoperative physiotherapy with incentive spirometry, cessation of smoking and postponement of surgery in the presence of acute infection.

Physiotherapy and antibiotics are the mainstay of treatment for an established infection with bronchoscopy and bronchial aspiration for atelectasis. Minitracheostomy may be helpful when regular bronchial toilet is needed (see also Chapter 19).

Urinary tract infection

Postoperative urinary tract infection is commonly related to the presence of urinary catheters. Catheterization of the urinary bladder should be employed only when necessary and should be discontinued as soon as possible. A strict sterile technique should be observed during catheterization and a closed system should be used for drainage. Culture of the urine and appropriate antibiotic therapy should be employed when infection occurs (see Chapter 20).

Intravenous central line infection

Avoidance of intravenous central-line sepsis is achieved by strict aseptic technique during the insertion of the catheter and careful maintenance of the line, with removal after a limited time. It is important to avoid using central lines for administration of drugs. Similarly, all of a patient's parenteral nutrition requirements should be provided in a single bag which is infused over a 24-h period. Once the bag has been made up in the pharmacy, nothing should be added to it. Sepsis is manifested by pyrexia and sometimes rigors. The catheter should be removed, the tip cultured and antibiotics should be given.

Pseudomembranous enterocolitis

Pseudomembranous enterocolitis is an infection caused by *Clostridium difficile*. It is seen in postoperative patients who have received antibiotics (cephalosporins, ampicillin) and is characterized by diarrhoea, abdominal discomfort, leukocytosis and the presence of a typical (pseudomembranous) membrane in the colon. The infection develops because antibiotics alter the normal flora, allowing the overgrowth of *C. difficile*, a normal bowel organism in 5% of people. *C. difficile* produces an enterotoxin which is responsible for most of the gut symptoms. Treatment consists of withdrawing current antibiotics and giving oral vancomycin, to which *C. difficile* is sensitive.

Viral diseases of surgical importance

Hepatitis B and C

Hepatitis B is a viral infection which causes hepatitis. It is spread by infected blood products (e.g. among intravenous drug abusers) or secretions (sexual contact). Health care workers, especially those who handle blood products, are at high risk of contracting hepatitis B. The symptoms of hepatitis are fever, malaise, anorexia, nausea, vomiting and upper abdominal discomfort. The patient becomes jaundiced with a hepatitic picture (cholestasis with elevated enzymes; see Chapter 13).

There are three hepatitis B antigens:
- a surface antigen (HepBsAg) which appears in the blood at 6 weeks;
- an internal antigen (HepBeAg) which is also present from 6 weeks to 3 months and indicates high infectivity;
- a core antigen (HepBcAg) which is usually found only in the liver.

The majority of patients require supportive treatment only. Spontaneous recovery is usual but a majority of patients (5%) become carriers with persistent HepBsAg in the blood and may progress to chronic hepatitis and hepatocellular carcinoma.

High-risk groups should be vaccinated against hepatitis B. This is achieved with three injections of recombinant HepBsAg.

Hepatitis C is also transmitted parenterally from contaminated blood products and is clinically similar to hepatitis B.

Acquired immune deficiency syndrome

AIDS is caused by HIV. First recognized in 1981, the virus is transmitted by sexual contact or by direct injection from contaminated syringes or blood products. Although the majority of cases have been reported in homosexual men, intravenous drug abusers and haemophiliacs, the groups recently noted to be increasing in incidence at the greatest rate are heterosexual women and men. Symptoms of HIV infection are absent in early cases; however, those infected commonly go on to develop weight loss, night sweats and pyrexia. Generalized lymphadenopathy, oral candidiasis and Kaposi's sarcoma are also seen. The disease causes a decrease in T-helper lymphocytes and an abnormal decrease in the ratio of T-helper to T-suppressor cells, making patients more susceptible to opportunistic infections, including Pneumocystis pneumonia, toxoplasmosis and cryptococcal meningitis. Testing of HIV infection utilizes the enzyme-linked immunosorbent assay (ELISA) test and the Western blot test which together have greater than 99% sensitivity and specificity. Treatment has recently been shown to benefit some patients with HIV infection using azidothymidine (AZT). Although no cure or vaccine is presently available, AZT will help slow the progression of the disease in some patients.

All members of the health care profession must be aware of the rapidly growing incidence of this disease and practise universal precautions when dealing with all patients to eliminate direct contact with blood and secretions. This is the most appropriate strategy for prevention of transmission of the virus.

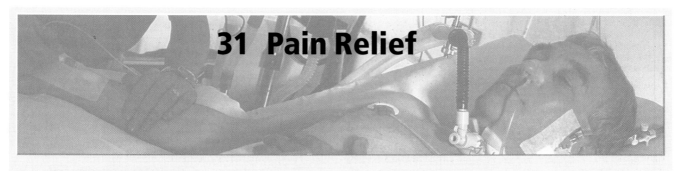

31 Pain Relief

There was a faith healer of Deal
Who said 'Although pain isn't real
If I sit on a pin
And it punctures the skin
I dislike what I fancy I feel'.   (Anonymous)

Introduction

Satisfactory relief of pain is an essential component of good postoperative care. It enables good respiratory exchange and effective coughing to take place and ensures sleep and early mobilization. Although the response to surgery is not abolished by good analgesia, its severity is reduced by adequate pain control. In truth, postoperative pain is poorly managed and it has been estimated that 40% of patients are in severe pain following elective abdominal operations. The various methods of pain relief used in surgical practice are shown in Table 31.1 and some of the commonly used agents are given in Table 31.2.

Table 31.1 Methods of postoperative analgesia.

Oral analgesia
Intramuscular injection of opioids
Intravenous infusions
Subcutaneous infusions
Patient-controlled analgesia
Spinal opioids
Rectal opioids
Transdermal opioids
Local anaesthesia
   Infiltration
   Nerve block
   Epidural
Cryoanalgesia

Methods of postoperative analgesia

Oral analgesia

This is the simplest method of achieving pain relief and oral agents in appropriate doses may provide effective analgesia. Oral analgesia is indicated after outpatient surgery (e.g. day-case varicose vein surgery) and can frequently replace parenteral drugs 12–24 h after surgery or as soon as oral intake is possible. Patients may also regulate their own analgesia if provided with a supply of drugs. This is the simplest method of patient-controlled analgesia (PCA; see below).

Intermittent intramuscular opioid injections (prn regimen)

Intramuscular opioid injection is used after operations when the duration of the painful period is limited to a few hours after surgery, e.g. laparoscopic cholecystectomy. After major surgical intervention, this intermittent injection technique is inadequate, as a significant number of patients experience an unacceptable degree of pain when this regimen is used. Aside from humane considerations, painful postoperative periods have adverse psychological effects on patients. Studies have shown that patients who have had good postoperative pain relief in the past react positively to the prospect of further surgical intervention, as opposed to those who experienced poor relief. Thus the conventional method of intramuscular opioid analgesia, prn regimen, is

Table 31.2 Commonly used postoperative analgesic agents.

Name	Pain level	Route	Dose	Side-effects
Simple analgesics				
Paracetamol	Mild to moderate	PO	500–1000 mg/4-hourly	Liver damage with overdose
Aspirin	Mild to moderate	PO	300–900 mg/4-hourly	GI irritation/hypersensitivity reactions
Codeine	Mild to moderate	PO/IM	30–60 mg/4-hourly	Constipation/dependence
Compound analgesics				
Co-proxamol	Moderate	PO	2 tablets/6-hourly	Liver damage and heart failure
(Paracetamol 325 mg + propoxyphene 32.5 mg)				with overdose
Co-dydramol	Moderate	PO	2 tablets/6-hourly	Liver damage with overdose
(Paracetamol 500 mg + dihydrocodeine 10 mg)				
NSAIDs				
Ibuprofen	Moderate	PO	200–300 mg/4-hourly	GI irritation/nausea/diarrhoea bleeding/
Indomethacin	Moderate	PO/PR	50 mg/6-hourly	hypersensitivity reactions/headache/dizziness
Opioid analgesics				
Pethidine	Moderate to severe	IM/SC/PO	50 mg/4-hourly	Constipation/respiratory depression/urinary
Morphine	Moderate to severe	IM/SC/PO	10 mg/4-hourly	retention/nausea/tolerance
Diamorphine	Severe	IM/SC	5 mg/4-hourly	
Buprenorphine	Moderate to severe	SL*/IM	200 μg/8-hourly	Drowsiness/nausea/vomiting
				dizziness/sweating

* SL, sublingual; GI, Gastrointestinal.

unsatisfactory and should be abandoned as the routine analgesic policy in patients undergoing major surgery.

Intravenous pump infusion

Intravenous infusions (pump-driven) result in better control of pain. The underlying principle entails the production and maintenance of a steady-state concentration of the drug that is sufficient to achieve good pain control without serious side-effects. There are however some disadvantages to this approach. Thus it may take several hours to achieve the right plasma steady-state concentration of the opioid and, indeed, the concentration of the drug may suddenly overshoot to reach levels which cause respiratory depression and hypoxia. For this reason careful respiratory monitoring (or pulse oximetry) is required in patients receiving opioid intravenous infusions.

Continuous subcutaneous infusion

The continuous subcutaneous infusion of more soluble opioids, such as diamorphine, subcutaneously through a butterfly needle achieves the same results with less risk of respiratory depression and is preferred in some hospitals.

Patient-controlled analgesia

With PCA systems, the opioid is contained in a delivery system which will administer a preset bolus dose when a button is pressed by the patient, i.e. within the permissible total dosage, the delivery rate is controlled by the patient (Fig. 31.1). The system incorporates certain intrinsic safety features designed to prevent overdosing: bolus dose, lockout interval, background infusion and maximum dose. All these are preset for a given patient before the system is used. The bolus dose is the dose which the machine will deliver when the patient presses the button. The lock-out time is the period after a given dose during which any further demands by the patient are ignored by the system. The background infusion relates to a continuous infusion of opioid by the machine which is delivered throughout the period in addition to the bolus injections activated by the patient's commands. The maximum dose is the total dose (boluses and continuous infusion) which the system will deliver during a given 24-h period. PCA undoubtedly produces excellent analgesia which is comparable to that of epidural analgesia. The system is, however, not in widespread use for a variety of reasons. It is costly, familiarity with its use by the nursing staff is essential, instrument failure may occur on rare occasions, as can respiratory

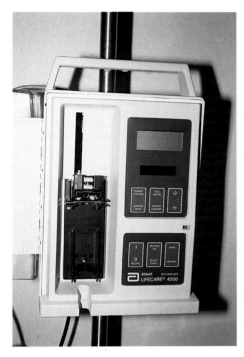

Figure 31.1 Patient-controlled analgesia (PCA) pump used for pain control.

depression. Thus continuous nursing care or pulse oximetry is essential.

Spinal opioid analgesia

This refers to the instillation of opioids through special catheters introduced in the epidural space or in the cerebrospinal fluid. Although effective, this method has a number of disadvantages (technically difficult, time-consuming) and adverse reactions (nausea and vomiting, urinary retention and respiratory depression). The most important and potentially fatal complication is respiratory depression (especially with morphine) since this may be delayed several hours after the spinal injection.

Rectal suppositories

Rectal formulations of opioid preparations are available which result in reasonable blood concentration levels following administration as suppositories. The technique has not been sufficiently evaluated but holds promise particularly for children.

Transdermal techniques

The transdermal opioid technique employs the use of a patch containing fat-soluble synthetic opioid fentanyl. Early clinical trials have indicated that this simple technique is as effective as continuous intravenous infusions.

Local infiltration anaesthesia

Local anaesthetic techniques, which include local infiltration, nerve block and epidural analgesia, give excellent pain control. Infiltration may entail simple injection around the wound of a long-acting local anaesthetic or, preferably, the insertion of special fine J-catheters which permit repeated top-ups.

Epidural analgesia

Excellent pain relief is achieved by epidural injection of local anaesthetic agents but this is a specialized procedure which must always be carried out by experts and in the presence of continuous monitoring and facilities for advanced resuscitation techniques, i.e. in the intensive care or high-dependence units. The dangers of epidural block are twofold: hypotension because several nerves are involved, and inadvertent injection of the local anaesthetic agent into the cerebrospinal fluid. This results in severe hypotension and profound generalized paralysis which may require immediate ventilation and mechanical ventilation.

Cryoanalgesia

This technique, which is rarely used, involves the freezing of sensory nerves, such as the intercostal nerves during thoracotomy, by a liquid nitrogen probe. Although it reduces the amount of opioid administration needed in the postoperative period, its effects are variable and the recovery of nerve function (numbness) takes several weeks to months.

32 Rehabilitation

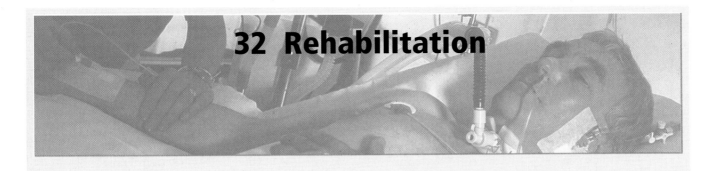

Introduction

Rehabilitation is the process whereby a patient is actively helped to return to a maximum potential lifestyle — physical, mental and social — after a major illness or accident. This work is carried out by a team and initially starts in hospital but rapidly progresses to include rehabilitation in the community. Ultimately, rehabilitation takes place exclusively in an environment most suited to the patient — preferably at home. Rehabilitation may be carried out by individual medical or surgical specialties. However, specialists in rehabilitation medicine provide a professional and cost-effective approach and may save time and effort through their expertise.

Principles of rehabilitation

Rehabilitation should begin as soon as possible and potential disabilities should be anticipated. Disability may be either:
• *primary* (i.e. directly due to the disease or injury), e.g. direct trauma, amputation, stroke; or
• *secondary* (i.e. as a complication of the disease or injury), e.g. muscle atrophy, joint contractures, decubitus ulcers, depression.
  Rehabilitation is a team effort and demands the services and enthusiasm of several people to be effective. These include doctors, nurses, physiotherapists, occupational therapists, social workers, prosthetists, speech therapists, psychologists, the patient and the patient's family. The aim of the team must be to prepare a plan of action culminating not in the patient's discharge from hospital, but in the restoration to as normal a pre-injury lifestyle as is

practical. However, rehabilitation should not be overly ambitious and limitations set by disability must be appreciated. The setting of unrealistic and overoptimistic goals is as counterproductive as setting no goals at all.

Physiotherapy

Physiotherapists use a variety of techniques to prevent patients developing complications, to relieve pain and to enhance physical activity. These techniques include the following.
• Chest physiotherapy: deep breathing exercises, incentive spirometry, coughing, chest percussion.
• Muscle exercise and re-education: active and passive exercises, stretching, joint movements. Electrotherapy may be used to stimulate denervated muscles.
• Walking: teaching patients to stand and walk, initially with support (physiotherapists, parallel bars, walker frames, crutches, stick) and then without support, progressing to walking up stairs.
• Pain relief: both heat (superficial and deep) and cold are used to relieve pain. Transcutaneous electrical nerve stimulation (TENS) is also commonly used in the management of chronic pain. Massage may be combined with heat to reduce oedema and relax muscle tension.
• Ultraviolet therapy: some decubitus ulcers (pressure sores) respond favourably to ultraviolet light.
• Hydrotherapy: helps to relieve pain, reduce muscle spasm and induce relaxation.

Occupational therapy

The aims of occupational therapy are:
• to assist in increasing the physical rehabilitation of the patient;

581

• to assess and maximize the patient's ability to perform daily activities, including self-care, mobility and communication. These are known as *activities of daily living* (ADL);
• to provide splints and other prostheses to facilitate independent daily living;
• to give emotional and motivational support to patients during rehabilitation.

Social services

The social services should be contacted as early as possible so that the particular services required for a given patient will be available when the patient is ready for discharge from hospital. The social worker will:
• inform the patient what services are available;
• evaluate which services will be appropriate for a patient, e.g. whether the patient should go home and be provided with meals on wheels, home help and district nursing or offered supervised accommodation, etc.;
• coordinate the provision of services for the patient; and
• maximize financial benefits for their patients.

Rehabilitation in surgery

Rehabilitation in musculoskeletal disorders

Rehabilitation of the musculoskeletal system may be viewed as the recovery from trauma caused by chance accident or surgery. In both cases the needs of the whole patient and family must be catered for and must, if possible, span the whole of the subject's lifestyle, including pastimes and work.

Rehabilitation after trauma

Mostly following *simple injuries*, patients may be taught simple exercises which they can carry out at home with supervision at outpatient follow-up. Whilst in hospital an attitude of progress towards recovery must be engendered from the first day as otherwise a state of regression to a dependent state rapidly becomes established. The role of physical rehabilitation after simple injuries is often taken for granted, although in times of scant resources it would be better if its use were confined to those accurately assessed as gaining useful benefit. For example, therapy following even quite minor hand injury may be essential to ensure early return to work, but commonly provided mass rehabilitation classes such as back or knee groups have not been proved to be a valuable use of resources.

After *multiple injuries*, often associated with head injury, rehabilitation needs to be instituted as soon as medical and surgical management permits. In these cases commitment of large resources may be required to ensure optimal recovery. For example, following a head injury which may have involved many months in bed, vigorous physiotherapy will be required to re-establish motor function; speech therapy may be required to re-establish the patient's ability to speak and occupational therapy to help the patient back to independent living. Careful psychological examination will also be essential as the presence of psychological disturbance is often underestimated unless a full assessment is performed. The long-term effects of head injury can be one of the most difficult areas in rehabilitation as the behaviour and personality changes may make reintegration into the community very difficult indeed.

Rehabilitation after amputation

Patients following amputation have very specific problems to cope with and this group of patients presents an ideal model to illustrate all aspects of rehabilitation.

The trauma of the surgery has profound psychological effects on the individual concerned.

For the *traumatic amputee* there has been no warning or preparation prior to limb loss. The majority of these patients are young and following the accident there may be considerable anguish, disbelief and despair at the amputation and the perceived problems that may follow. The initial postoperative period requires considerable care and understanding and should be handled by experienced staff. Full explanations must include realistic consideration of likely outcome and description of the rehabilitation process that is to follow.

In contrast, the elderly *vascular amputee* has usually had a period of pain and suffering prior to surgery. The patient will have often chosen amputation as a means of relieving the severe pain of an ischaemic limb. Counselling patients preoperatively is extremely valuable and should wherever possible be undertaken by experienced staff. In addition, relatives need to be included in these discussions as their understanding and reassurance can help the patient overcome the natural fear of the future.

The rehabilitation of the amputee and consequent independence depend on several factors (Fig. 32.1).
• In the first instance the *level of lower limb amputation* can profoundly affect the ability of the patient to walk with a prosthesis and gain the fullest mobility possible. The higher the amputations, the greater the psychological effect on the patient, and the greater the effort required to walk.
• The expertise of the *rehabilitation team* and the facilities at their disposal can similarly affect the ultimate success of

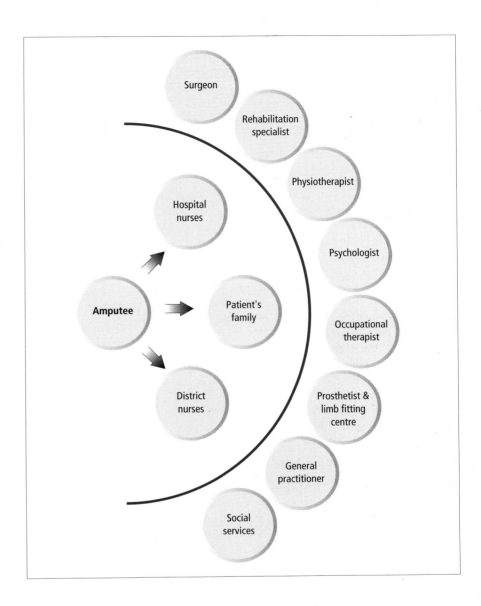

Figure 32.1 A summary of the various people involved in the rehabilitation of a patient following amputation.

the rehabilitation process. The rehabilitation team which cares for the amputee of whatever age must be a closely integrated group of professionals who work together. This ensures the amputee is given total care in a constructive coordinated environment, which should be cheerful and encouraging. The medical team should include the operating surgeon and the rehabilitation specialist. In some areas the medical team will vary but in all cases there must be a specialist responsible for prosthesis prescription. The responsibility for the overall medical care rests with the medical staff.

• The *nursing staff* provide day-to-day care of the patient with particular attention to pressure areas and to the care of the stump.

• *Physiotherapy* provides assessment of early mobilization of the patient. The patient should be mobilized 24 h after surgery if possible. Chest physiotherapy is used to avoid chest infections and early mobility to avoid deep venous thrombosis. The use of early walking aids has greatly enhanced the ability of the patient to mobilize. Once the stump is healed, mobility with a prosthesis is undertaken under the supervision of a physiotherapist and the prosthetist.

• the *prosthetist*, the specialist responsible for the manufacture, fitting and maintenance of artificial limbs, works closely with the therapists. A wide range of prostheses are available for the amputee.

• The *occupational therapist* is specially trained to teach aids to daily living skills and assess home circumstances.

The latter assessment involves domiciliary visits at home with patients. The advice provided ensures that services are altered to the needs of the individual once discharged. The training in ADL is undertaken in the hospital and concentrates on self-hygiene, personal independence and domestic skills in a kitchen.

- Close liaison with *social services* is essential. All team members may need to discuss patient care with them; in particular, the occupational therapist and nursing staff may need to liaise with the social worker. The social workers are often attached to hospitals and wherever possible should be part of the rehabilitation team. The social worker can arrange domiciliary services, e.g. home help, meals-on-wheels, and may help with financial matters.

- In addition to the social worker, the *general practitioner*, who will provide the care once discharge has occurred, should be informed as to the progress and likely prognosis of the patient.

- *District nurses* are essential to ensure nursing skills are available in a home situation.

The whole team should meet regularly to discuss the patient's progress and decide on realistic goals which the patient can achieve. Patients should be involved in the discussion so that they are aware of what is to be achieved. Family members also need to be kept aware of progress and of the problems as they arise. The goals may need to be modified as the rehabilitation process proceeds in the light of progress.

In the case of a young amputee the *return to work* can be an important issue. The social worker and occupational therapist can give initial guidelines and discussion with the employers which can be helpful. In a situation where a return to the former work is not possible the patient is referred to the *Disablement Employment Adviser*, who has a statutory responsibility to advise on retraining programmes and potential employers. Local charitable organizations may also offer employment advice and these services are often worth considering.

Social reintegration is important. The amputee may initially feel isolated and handicapped by surgery. Family and friends play a vital role in encouraging the patient to get back into society. The rehabilitation team should be aware of this isolation and encourage the patient to get out. The use of clubs and societies (e.g. National Association for Limbless Disabled) can be extremely valuable. To encourage this reintegration, rapid discharge home is important but this should be undertaken once prosthetic fitting has been completed and the occupational therapist has assessed the patient's home. If discharged too early, demoralization of both patients and relatives can reduce the ability to achieve full potential.

The patient will need to remain in contact with a *limb-fitting centre* for the rest of his or her life for the maintenance

and provision of prosthesis. Regular reviews are initially necessary as the stump matures and the patient adapts to the new situation. The review clinics act as both a stump and prosthetic review but also as an opportunity for open discussion on how the patient has managed at home. In this way, shortfalls in service provision and the identification of areas in which help can be provided are assessed.

Amputees can be seen to be a very specific group of patients with whom a rehabilitation team can work closely. All patients may require varying degrees of rehabilitation, but the most important factor in achieving the optimum recovery is the close cooperation between all members of the team, with full and frank discussion of the patient's needs.

Rehabilitation of patients with specific problems

Patients with neurological problems

Patients following head injury or those with paraplegia require intensive rehabilitation to get them to achieve their maximum potential. They may require chest care (to avoid infection), protection of pressure areas, assistance with bladder and bowel function, feeding, mobilization and speech therapy. The patients and their relatives also need constant support and encouragement. The detailed management of patients with neurological problems is given in Chapter 19.

Stoma care

Patients in whom stomas have been created have specific concerns and needs and require expert advice concerning the management of the stoma. The various stomas which can be created have been described in the relevant chapters but colostomy and ileostomy (including ileal conduit) are the types most frequently encountered. The patients are mostly concerned about leakage, odour and, in the case of colostomies, noisy expulsion of gas. Ileostomies may also be associated with skin irritation and preventive measures need to be taken to avoid dermatitis.

If the stoma is created electively then the skin can be marked preoperatively and the stoma created in the most optimal site for the patient. Postoperatively the patient should be encouraged to take charge of stoma care as soon as is practicable. Most hospitals now have a stoma nurse or therapist dedicated to dealing with patients who have stomas. A wide variety of appliances are now available which attach securely to the abdominal wall, do not leak and do not allow any malodorous gas escape. The stoma therapist will help the patient choose the most suitable appliance and give dietary advice. A number of 'ostomy' support groups also exist which provide assistance to patients with stomas. Most patients learn to manage their stoma very efficiently and live relatively normal lives.

Laryngectomy

Total laryngectomy leaves the patient with a tracheostomy and complete loss of speech. The patient has to be instructed in the management of the tracheostomy and speech training, under the supervision of a speech therapist, should commence as soon as possible after surgery. Voice rehabilitation is possible with either oesophageal speech (successful in 75% of patients), or a cervical or oral vibrator. In some patients good restoration of speech can be achieved with a neoglottis valve. Social support is available from the National Association of Laryngectomy Clubs.

Conclusion

Rehabilitation is an extremely important part of the care of patients and is the responsibility of every physician who cares for potentially disabled patients. Disability is a substantial problem in the community, with approximately 2% of the population having some form of locomotor disability. The main features of a rehabilitation programme can be summarized as follows:
- assessment of patients' abilities and disabilities in terms of physical, mental and social factors;
- establishing a comprehensive treatment programme with well-defined, realistic goals;
- coordination of the various professionals and agencies involved with rehabilitation.

With such programmes patients can be helped to achieve their potential and to have a good quality of life.

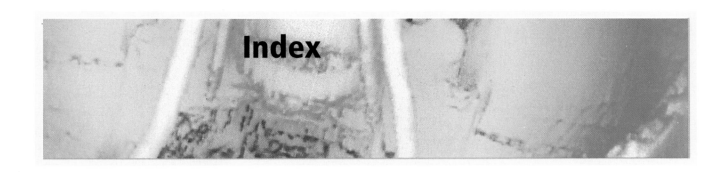

Index

Page references to figures appear in *italic* type and those for tables appear in **bold** type